Supportive care
in heart failure

Supportive Care Series

Volumes in the series:

Supportive care in heart failure

Edited by

James Beattie

Consultant Cardiologist,
Heart of England NHS Foundation Trust,
and National Clinical Lead, NHS
Heart Improvement Programme, UK

and

Sarah J. Goodlin

President, Patient-Centered
Education and Research,
Salt Lake City, Utah, USA

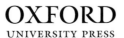

OXFORD
UNIVERSITY PRESS

OXFORD
UNIVERSITY PRESS

Great Clarendon Street, Oxford OX2 6DP

Oxford University Press is a department of the University of Oxford.
It furthers the University's objective of excellence in research, scholarship,
and education by publishing worldwide in

Oxford New York

Auckland Cape Town Dar es Salaam Hong Kong Karachi
Kuala Lumpur Madrid Melbourne Mexico City Nairobi
New Delhi Shanghai Taipei Toronto

With offices in

Argentina Austria Brazil Chile Czech Republic France Greece
Guatemala Hungary Italy Japan Poland Portugal Singapore
South Korea Switzerland Thailand Turkey Ukraine Vietnam

Oxford is a registered trade mark of Oxford University Press
in the UK and in certain other countries

Published in the United States
by Oxford University Press Inc., New York

A catalogue record for this title is available from the British Library

Data available

Library of Congress Cataloging in Publication Data

Typeset by Cepha Imaging Private Ltd., Bangalore, India
Printed in Great Britain
on acid-free paper by
Biddles Ltd., King's Lynn, Norfolk, UK

ISBN 978-0-19-857028-8

10 9 8 7 6 5 4 3 2 1

Preface to the Supportive Care Series

Supportive care is the multidisciplinary holistic care of patients with chronic and life-limiting illnesses and their families – from the time around diagnosis, through treatments aimed at cure or prolonging life, and into the phase currently acknowledged as palliative care: It involves recognizing and caring for the side-effects of active therapies as well as patients' symptoms, co-morbidities, psychological, social, and spiritual concerns. It also values the role of family carers and helps them in supporting the patient, as well as attending to their own special needs. Supportive care is a domain of health and social care that utilizes a network of professionals and voluntary carers in a 'virtual team'. It is increasingly recognized by health-care providers and governments as a modern response to complex disease management, but so far it can lay claim to little dedicated literature.

This is therefore one volume in a unique new series of textbooks on supportive care, published by Oxford University Press which has already established itself as a leading publisher for palliative care. Unlike 'traditional' palliative care, which grew from terminal care of cancer patients, supportive care is not restricted to dying patients nor to cancer. Thus this series covers the support of patients with a variety of long-term conditions, who are currently largely managed by specialist and general teams in hospitals and by primary-care teams in community settings. It will therefore provide a practical guide to supportive care of the patient at all stages of the illness, providing up-to-date knowledge of the scientific basis of palliation and also practical guidance on delivering high-quality multidisciplinary care across health-care sectors. The volumes, edited by acknowledged leaders in the specific field of each volume, will bring together research, health-care management, economics, and ethics through contributions from an international panel of experts of all disciplines. The underlying theme of all the books is the application of the latest evidence-based knowledge, in a humane way, for patients with advancing disease.

As Series Editors, we bring between us over four decades of research and clinical experience of acute medicine and palliative care. Our work has spanned St Christopher's Hospice and the Leicestershire Hospice in England – both of which have been inspirational leaders in traditional palliative care; the Academic Unit of Supportive Care at the University of Sheffield, England and the Harry Horvitz Center for Palliative Medicine in The Cleveland Clinic Foundation, USA. We have independently and jointly advocated the supportive care approach to cancer and other chronic disease management and are delighted to be collaborating on this series. We are both committed to delivering high-quality of end-of-life care when it is necessary but we are constantly seeking to influence our colleagues in all relevant health-care disciplines to adopt the principles of modern supportive care to benefit a wider range of patients at earlier stages of illness. We aim

through this series to inform and inspire other doctors, nurses, allied health professionals, pharmacists, social and spiritual care providers, and students, to improve the quality
of living for all patients and families in their care

Sam Hjelmeland Ahmedzai
Professor of Palliative Medicine
Academic Unit of Supportive Care
The University of Sheffield
Royal Hallamshire Hospital
Sheffield, UK

Declan Walsh
Professor and Director
Harry Horvitz Center for Palliative Medicine
The Cleveland Clinic Foundation
Cleveland, Ohio, USA

Foreword

Heart failure (HF) occurs in almost epidemic proportions, affecting many millions of people worldwide. This condition confers a major burden on affected individuals and their families and demands a significant proportion of health-care resources. As demographic studies suggest a relative ageing of the population in industrial countries in response to better medical care and social conditions, we can only anticipate an increasing prevalence. Planning for the complex social and health-care needs of this increasingly dependant cohort with all their attendant co-morbidities will be a challenge for cardiovascular medicine, public health professionals, and society as a whole.

In recent years we have made enormous strides in our understanding of the pathophysiology of the complex clinical syndromes that comprise clinical HF and there has been a widespread adoption of evidence-based treatment for the various stages of this condition. With the many advances in pharmacological, device, and surgical therapies, the previously inexorable progression of HF may no longer be inevitable, but the gain in increased life expectancy is often conditional on accepting a more prolonged phase of symptomatic ill health prior to death. Despite our best efforts, HF remains a generally progressive condition with significant symptoms, a poor quality of life, and a high mortality.

The recognition of the similarity between the symptomatic burden and mortality risk for HF and cancer has led to a realisation that incorporation of the principles and practice of palliative medicine might improve the care of those with advanced HF. Many of the skills of palliative care that have been honed in the treatment of those with cancer are transferable to other life-limiting diseases. An increasing proportion of patients with non-malignant conditions are now offered the many facets of supportive care that enables patients and their families to live as well as possible through the course of their illness, as well as end-of-life care when death is anticipated. The very complexity of modern HF care demands this approach. Treatment dilemmas are common and there is a constant need to examine patient and clinician perspectives and reappraise earlier decisions on therapy to maintain optimal goals of care. Cardiologists primarily concerned with the investigation and treatment of HF may not appreciate that patients' concerns may lie more in refractory non-cardiac symptoms or the psychosocial and spiritual aspects of their condition, issues that are intrinsic to palliative care.

Cardiology and palliative care professionals have only recently started to work together to optimize HF care, and challenges remain in prognostication, in the need to balance continuing active and symptomatic care, and to ensure provision of this integrated approach in all care settings. A successful outcome demands close collaboration between these disciplines and liaison with a range of allied health professionals and other agencies. This book is timely in providing an academic basis for this new alliance and Dr Beattie and Dr Goodlin have persuaded an international group of leaders in cardiology and palliative care to contribute authoritative reviews relevant to the comprehensive care of those with advanced HF. This publication offers a synthesis of their collective expertise and I commend it to you.

Kim Fox, MD FESC
President of the European Society of Cardiology

Preface

The care for patients with heart failure (HF) has evolved significantly over the past several decades as our knowledge and understanding of the pathophysiology of HF has developed. The significant growth in the incidence and prevalence of HF now means that the syndrome presents major impacts on the financial and clinical resources of health-care systems. HF also has a significant impact upon the quality of life of individual patients and their families.

The complexity of HF care argues for a team approach. At fortunate centers, a team of professionals (physicians, social workers, nurses, pharmacists) is organized to provide HF care; however, most clinicians will need to create virtual teams. The virtual team will incorporate clinicians at a variety of sites of care within the community and create an integrated multidisciplinary approach to HF care. Teams may also span the spectrum of acute hospital care, outpatient management, nursing homes, home care, and end-of-life or hospice care.

This book on *Supportive Care in Heart Failure* strives to meet the needs of the varied members of both formal and virtual HF care teams. Clinicians well versed in palliative care will benefit from the discussions of pathophysiology, epidemiology, and evidence-based HF care, while those who are expert in clinical HF care will gain insight into their work from the chapters addressing management of common symptoms, problems, communication, and support.

As editors we have been privileged to invite internationally recognized experts to contribute to this book. The book begins with an introduction to the concept of support-ive care. Part One of the book addresses the state of knowledge in the epidemiology, pathophysiology, and evidence-based management of HF with medications, surgery, and devices. Part Two addresses the burden of HF on quality of life, symptoms, and specific clinical problems and aspects of HF care throughout its course. Part Three focuses on prognostication, communication and decision-making. Specific chapters address ethical aspects, transcultural issues, and conclude with an exploration of the physician coping with patient death, a topic heretofore not well addressed in HF care.

Supportive Care in Heart Failure is a unique book that brings together authorities from a broad range of clinical and research expertise. We anticipate that clinicians and researchers from a similarly broad experience will find value in many parts of this book.

As editors we would like to express our gratitude to the many individuals who made this book possible. We are enormously grateful to the authors who contributed to the book. The donation of their expertise, time, and effort truly were essential, and we thank them. The book also would not have been possible without the dedicated assistance of the commissioning team at Oxford University Press—initially Catherine Barnes, and then Georgia Pinteau and Clare Caruana. The support and encouragement of Sam Ahmedzai as Series Editor was also essential.

Sarah J. Goodlin, MD and James Beattie, FRCP, FESC

Contents

Contributors

Julia M. Addington-Hall
Professor in End of Life Care, Department
of Nursing and Midwifery, University of
Southampton, UK

Stefan D. Anker
Professor for Applied Cachexia Research
Division of Applied Cachexia Research,
Department of Cardiology,
Campus Virchow Clinic, Charité –
Universitätsmedizin Berlin,
Germany; Department of Cardiac
Medicine, National Heart & Lung
Institute, London, UK

Peter C. Austin
Institute for Clinical Evaluative Sciences,
Toronto, Canada; Departments of
Public Health Sciences and Health Policy,
Management and Evaluation,
University of Toronto, Canada

James Beattie
Consultant Cardiologist,
Heart of England Foundation Trust,
Birmingham, UK;
National Clinical Lead, NHS
Heart Improvement Programme

David Bekelman
Assistant Professor of Medicine,
Division of General Internal Medicine,
University of Colorado Denver School of
Medicine; Director, Suppportive Care
Program, Univerisity of Colorado
Hospital Heart Center, Denver,
Colorado, USA

Roberto Bernabei
Department of Gerontology, Catholic
University, Rome, Italy

Gabriele B. Bertoni
II Division of Cardiovascular Surgery
Cardiovascular centre "E. Malan"
Policlinico San Donato
University of Milan
Milan Italy

Rebecca Boxer
Heart and Vascular Institute,
University Hospital,
Case Medical Center,
Cleveland, Ohio, USA

Katrina A. Bramstedt
Department of Bioethics and Transplant
Centre, Cleveland Clinic, Cleveland,
Ohio, USA

Eric J. Cassell
Professor of Public Health Emeritus,
Weill Cornell Medical College;
Adjunct Professor of Medicine, faculty of
Medicine, McGill University, USA

John G. F. Cleland
Department of Cardiology,
University of Hull, UK

Diane Snyder Cowan
Director, Elisabeth Severance, Prentiss
Bereavement Center,
Hospice of the Western Reserve,
Cleveland, OH, USA

Patricia M. Davidson
Professor of Cardiovascular
and Chronic Care, Centre for
Cardiovascular and Chronic Care,
Curtin University of Technology,
Sydney, Australia

John E. Ellershaw
Professor of Palliative Medicine,
University of Liverpool; Director,
Marie Curie Palliative Care Institute
Liverpool, UK

Mark W. Elliott
Department of Respiratory Medicine,
St James' University Hospital, Leeds, UK

Neil D. Gillespie
Senior Lecturer in Medicine (Ageing and
Health); Honorary Consultant Physician,
Ninewells Hospital and Medical School,
Dundee, UK

Ronald Gillilan
Medical Director of Preventive Cardiology
St Agnes Hospital,
Baltimore, MD, USA

Cynthia R. Goh
Head, Department of Palliative Medicine,
National Cancer Centre, Singapore;
Program Director, Lien Centre for
Palliative Care, Duke-National University
of Singapore Graduate Medical School

Sarah J. Goodlin
President, Patient-centered Education and
Research, Salt Lake City, Utah, USA

Karen Hatfield
Team Leader, Counseling Services,
Hospice of the Western Reserve,
Cleveland, Ohio, USA

Yasuhiro Ikeda
Department of Molecular Cardiovascular
Biology, Yamaguchi University School of
Medicine, Ube, Japan

Tiny Jaarsma
Associate Professor of Cardiology
and Heart Failure,
Department of Cardiology
University Medical Centre Groningen
The Netherlands

Miriam Johnson
Senior Lecturer in Palliative Medicine,
Hull-York Medical School; Honorary
Consultant Palliative Physician to
St Catherine's Hospice, Scarborough, UK

Corrine Jurgens
Clinical Associate Professor, School of
Nursing, Stony Brook University;
John A. Hartford Postdoctoral Fellow,
School of Nursing, University of
Pennsylvania, USA

Thomas Köhnlein
Department of Respiratory Medicine,
Hannover Medical School, Hannover,
Germany

Mitja Lainscak
Assistant Professor of Internal Medicine
Division of Applied Cachexia Research,
Department of Cardiology, Campus
Virchow Clinic, Charité –
Universitätsmedizin Berlin, Germany;
Department of Internal Medicine,
General Hospital Murska Sobota,
Murska Sobota, Slovenia

Alice Laudisio
Department of Gerontology, Catholic
University, Rome, Italy

Douglas S. Lee
The Heart & Stroke/Richard Lewar Centre
for Excellence, University of Toronto;
Division of Cardiology, Toronto General
Hospital; Institute for Clinical Evaluative
Sciences, Toronto, Canada

Peter S. Macdonald
Co-Director, Heart Failure and
Transplant Unit,
St Vincents Hospital,
University of NSW,
Sydney, Australia

John J. V. McMurray
Professor of Medical Cardiology,
Department of Cardiology, Western
Infirmary, Glasgow, Scotland, UK

Masunori Matsuzaki
Department of Molecular Cardiovascular
Biology and Department of Medicine and
Clinical Science, Yamaguchi University
School of Medicine, Ube, Japan

Mandeep R. Mehra
Herbert Berger Professor and Head of
Cardiology, University of Maryland
School of Medicine,
Baltimore, MD, USA

Phillip J. Newton
Project Director, Centre for
Cardiovascular and Chronic Care,
Curtin University of Technology,
Sydney, Australia

Maral Ouzounian
The Heart & Stroke/Richard Lewar Centre
for Excellence, University of Toronto;
Division of Cardiology, Toronto General
Hospital, University Health Network,
Toronto; Department of Surgery,
Dalhousie University, Halifax, Canada

Ileana Piña
Professor of Medicine, Case Western
Reserve University, Heart Failure
Transplant, Cleveland, USA

Christina M. Puchalski
Executive Director
The George Washington Institute for
Spirituality and Health; Associate
Professor of Medicine, Healthcare
Sciences The George Washington
University School of Medicine Associate
Professor of Health Management and
Leadership, The George Washington
University School of Public Health

Timothy E. Quill
Professor of Medicine, Psychiatry and
Medical Humanities; Director, Center for
Ethics, Humanities and Palliative Care,
University of Rochester
School of Medicine, USA

Barbara Riegel
Associate Professor, School of Nursing,
University of Pennsylvania, USA

J. Paul Rocchiccioli
Clinical Research Fellow in Cardiology,
Department of Cardiology, Western
Infirmary, Glasgow, Scotland, UK

Angie E. Rogers
Senior Research Fellow – End of Life Care,
Department of Nursing and Midwifery,
University of Southampton, UK

Anja Sandek
Division of Applied Cachexia Research
Department of Cardiology, Campus
Virchow Clinic, Charité –
Universitätsmedizin Berlin, Germany

Mark D. Sullivan
Professor of Psychiatry and Behavioral
Sciences; Adjunct Professor of Medical
History and Ethics, University of
Washington, Seattle, Washington, USA

Jom Suwanno
Assistant Professor, Walailak University,
School of Nursing, Thailand

Lip-Bun Tan
Consultant Cardiologist,
Leeds General Infirmary, Leeds, UK

Jeffrey Teuteberg
Cardiovascular Institute, Section of Heart
failure/Cardiac Transplantation,
University of Pittsburgh, Pittsburgh, PA,
USA

Winifred G. Teuteberg
Section of Palliative Care and Medical
Ethics, Department of Medicine
University of Pittsburgh, Pittsburgh,
PA, USA

Jack V. Tu
Institute for Clinical Evaluative Sciences,
Toronto, Canada; The Heart &
Stroke/Richard Lewar Centre for
Excellence, University of Toronto;
Division of Cardiology,
Schulich Heart Program, Sunnybrook
Health Sciences Centre, University of
Toronto, Toronto, Canada

Christoper Ward
Honorary Consultant Cardiologist,
Ninewells Hospital and Medical School,
Dundee, UK

Stephen Westaby
Consultant Cardiac Surgeon,
John Radcliffe Hospital, Oxford, UK

Mary S. Wheeler
Clinical Educator, Capital Hospice, Falls
Church, Virginia, USA

Sue Wingate
Cardiology Nurse Practitioner, Kaiser
Permanente Mid-Atlantic States, Silver
Spring, Maryland, USA

Takeshi Yamamoto
Department of Medicine and Clinical
Science, Yamaguchi University Graduate
School of Medicine, Ube, Japan

Clyde W. Yancy
Medical Director, Baylor Heart and
Vascular Institute; Chief, Cardiothoracic
Transplantation, Baylor University
Medical Center, Dallas, Texas, USA

Masafumi Yano
Department of Medicine and Clinical
Science, Yamaguchi University Graduate
School of Medicine, Ube, Japan

Giuseppe Zuccalà
Department of Gerontology, Catholic
University, Rome, Italy

Chapter 1

An overview of supportive care in heart failure

Sarah J. Goodlin and James Beattie

Heart failure (HF) is a clinical syndrome characterized by abnormal systolic and/or diastolic function, fluid and sodium overload, cytokine activation, alterations of neuro-hormones, and dysfunction in many organ systems. HF carries a significant sympto-matic, social, and functional burden for patients and their families. It is the only cardiovascular condition that is increasing in prevalence. Worldwide, a rising prevalence and improved survivorship in predisposing cardiovascular conditions such as coronary artery disease and hypertension as well as diabetes mellitus ultimately lead to an increas-ing frequency of HF. Coupled with increasing longevity of the population, growing numbers of people live with HF and this, in turn, presents a real burden to health-care systems.[1] Several decades ago the diagnosis of HF was associated with a 43% mortality within 1 year in men and 36% in women. Only a quarter of men survived for 5 years from their HF diagnosis.[2] Recent epidemiologic analysis demonstrates increasing incidence and improved survival of people with HF,[3] yet death rates remain high.[4]

With a common age at presentation of between 70 and 80 years, HF is often encoun-tered in the growing aging population, with all their attendant co-morbidities.[5] In elderly patients an admission with HF may result in progressive functional decline and increas-ing dependency.[6] Conditions that complicate HF include respiratory disorders, renal dysfunction, anemia, arthritis, cognitive impairment, and depression.[7] While the complex mechanisms underlying symptoms of breathlessness, fluid retention, and fatigue have been studied, their origins and management are incompletely defined, and the background of other aspects of the malaise associated with HF is even less well understood. The quality of life for both the HF patient and his or her family is significantly impaired.

A consensus conference in 2002 to address palliative and supportive care in HF set an agenda for research and approaches to care that are only beginning to be addressed.[8] In 2004, the NHS Heart Improvement Programme in England published a framework document 'Supportive and palliative care for advanced heart failure'.[9] The need to address symptoms, the burden of the illness on the patient and family, communication, psychological and spiritual support, and end-of-life care were emphasized in both these initiatives. This agenda builds on a model of multidisciplinary supportive care proposed for cancer care as illustrated in the 'Sheffield model' (Fig. 1.1).[10] As well as HF, this is also

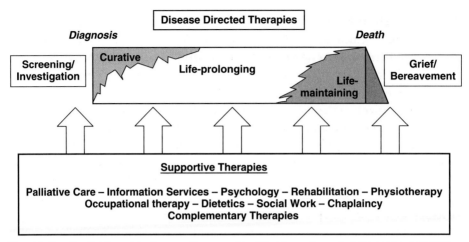

Fig. 1.1 The Sheffield model of supportive care. Modified from Ahmedzai SH, Walsh D (2000). *Semin. Oncol.* **27**: 1–6. Reproduced with permission.

applicable to other chronic progressive illnesses including pulmonary disease, degenerative neurological diseases, and advanced renal disease.

Concepts of supportive and palliative care

'Supportive care' is a concept that originated in cancer care as a response to the need to provide relief from symptoms and other distress throughout the illness, even when the focus was to cure the disease or prolong life. Supportive care is the multidisciplinary holistic care of patients and their families from the time of diagnosis, during treatment aimed at prolonging life, and into the end of life when palliative care is provided. Supportive care involves recognizing and caring for patients' co-morbidities, the psychological, social, and spiritual impacts of the illness, as well as addressing family needs. Supportive care in HF is not restricted to dying patients, rather it should be provided along with evidence-based medical, device, and surgical management.

'Palliative care' developed as an approach to the management of symptoms and other distress and support for the patient and family when it was clear that cure was not possible and life was limited. The definition of palliative care has evolved over the past several decades. While 'palliative', from the Latin 'to hide or cloak' (referring to the cloak worn in ancient Greece), originally denoted care for those recognized to have no curative or life-extending therapies available,[11] the definition by the World Health Organization (WHO) was broadened in 2002 to apply to care throughout the course of a life-limiting illness.[12] The most recent WHO definition also emphasizes the inclusion of diagnostic studies and the use of therapies that may be viewed as life-prolonging. The National Consensus Project in the United States further defined palliative care as both a philosophy of care and an organized system of care delivery that aims to address physical symptoms and other sources of distress for patients and families facing debilitating and life-threatening illness.[13] Thus, the terms 'supportive care' and 'palliative care' are now used by some virtually interchangeably; however, others reserve palliative care for end-of-life care. Differing reimbursement models for health care worldwide impact upon the delivery of specialist palliative care for HF patients. Some delivery systems align palliative care primarily with care for patients with neoplastic disease. Others limit palliative care to end-of-life or hospice care.

In HF, few patients are 'cured', and even cardiac transplantation carries burdens and prolongs life for only an average of 15 years. Care and reimbursement systems that separate or layer supportive and palliative care on life-prolonging care create a false dichotomy.[14] In HF care, therapies such as medications known to prolong life and improve HF status, some electrical devices, as well as left-ventricular assist devices both palliate symptoms and prolong life. Unfortunately documentation of patient-reported symptoms and quality of life responses have been incorporated inconsistently within clinical studies of HF therapy; it is often possible only to presume symptomatic benefit from some treatments.

Delivery of supportive care

The Sheffield model distinguishes the provision of disease-directed therapies and supportive therapies requiring different sets of providers. In settings with specialist HF care, this model would imply collaboration with a second team of health care professionals to provide the multidisciplinary elements inherent in supportive care. The vast majority of HF care is delivered by primary care physicians who offer evidence-based HF care less frequently than HF specialists or cardiologists.[15,16] Thus in their care for HF patients, primary care clinicians must develop expertise both in evidence-based medical and interventional care for HF and provide or facilitate access to supportive care.

Because HF carries a significant symptom burden and impacts upon the patient and family throughout the illness, it is critical that clinicians providing care to HF patients integrate supportive care throughout the course of care. The inter-relation of evidence-based HF care and supportive care requires increased knowledge and skills from all team members about HF and the supportive aspects of care. An understanding of the epidemiology and pathophysiology of HF is no less relevant to appropriate medication and device management of advanced HF by hospice providers at the end of life than to HF clinicians responsible for symptom relief earlier in the course of the illness. Communication skills and the ability to facilitate participatory decision-making are important to all clinicians, at all phases of HF care.

Framework for supportive care in HF

Integrating supportive care into HF care permits clinicians to avoid defining an arbitrary cut point when care should 'shift' to palliation. Figure 1.2 is a schematic diagram of concurrent supportive care and evidence-based HF care (medical, surgical, and device therapies), merged as 'comprehensive HF care'. Supportive care and palliative care address the social, psychological, and physical distress from symptoms and other aspects of the illness in the patient and in the family. The patient and the family are treated as a unit, as it is clear that the well-being of one impacts upon the well-being of the other.[17]

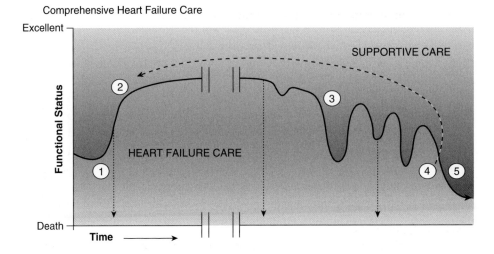

Fig. 1.2 Comprehensive HF care. (1) Initial symptoms of HF develop and HF treatment is initiated. (2) Plateaus of variable length may be reached with initial medical management, or following mechanical support or heart transplant. (3) Functional status declines with variable slope, with intermittent exacerbations of HF that respond to rescue efforts. (4) Stage D HF, with refractory symptoms and limited function. (5) End of life. Sudden death may occur at any point along the course of the illness. Supportive care and HF care are concurrent; amounts of each aspect of care vary with the patient's status. S. Goodlin & D. Renlund, used with permission.

Comprehensive HF care combines evidence-based HF care and supportive care

The evidence-based pharmacological, interventional and surgical treatments specifically related to cardiovascular physiology have been best defined in early and mid-phases of the disease course, and are least clear at the end of life, although increasingly, studies are including people with advanced HF in research. The majority of clinical studies in HF care have evaluated the impact of interventions on mortality or hospitalization; however, many believe that effective HF care also improves symptoms and the quality of life.

At each phase of comprehensive care, the communication and education needs of patients and families vary along with appropriate treatments. Supportive care needs are most intense at the time of diagnosis and initiation of treatment, when there are recurrent exacerbations, and in advanced disease, evaluating and initiating transplantation or device therapy or allowing the end of life. Supportive care remains important during the plateau of improved function usually achieved with HF care; most persons require ongoing supportive interventions to cope with their chronic HF. End-of-life care for HF patients includes intensive supportive and palliative care and evidence-based HF management. Successful supportive care requires an understanding of appropriate evidence-based HF care and ensuring its delivery. Similarly, effective HF care relies on supportive care. These care domains are mutually dependent. Decisions depend on education, communication, and support of the patient and family and rest on knowledge of the available treatments for HF and their likely outcomes.

Future work in supportive care

This book reviews current understanding of HF care and the many aspects of supportive care. Further study is needed to identify how best to enhance quality of life and reduce the symptoms and burdens associated with HF. It appears that some therapies will benefit patients throughout the course of their HF, while others are perhaps appropriately limited to certain phases of the illness. Increasingly, clinical studies must collect data about the impact of interventions on quality of life, physical and cognitive function, and symptom burden. Other important issues such as spirituality and bereavement in patients and families will demand specific focus to improve our ability to provide these aspects of supportive care.

Communication and decision-making are not well studied in HF care. Better information about patient and family needs, and how best to facilitate decision-making, are central to education of clinicians about HF care. While concepts about communication can be translated to HF care from studies in other diseases, we do not know how differently patients and their families understand the course and potential adverse events (including death) from HF. Work to address these issues will be necessary to improve this essential part of care.

Few studies have specifically evaluated palliative therapies and their outcomes for HF patients. Building an evidence base for interventions to manage symptoms is critical to the development of supportive and palliative care in HF. Research is also needed to elucidate the impact of the pathophysiological alterations in HF on specific symptoms and conditions. For example, levels of norepinephrine are elevated in HF and particularly in the presence of sleep apnea in HF patients. Studying how these high norepinephrine levels contribute to symptoms of depression and anxiety may ultimately improve the management of these symptoms. The implications of activation of inflammatory markers in HF are only partially understood. Investigations to understand cachexia and other problems in advanced HF may further our understanding of HF pathophysiology and allow intervention. We need to foster translational research to explore the links between these basic mechanisms fundamental to the HF state, the resultant symptoms, and the potential for their control.

Conclusions

While challenges presented by delivery and reimbursement systems may require organized schemes to achieve comprehensive HF care, framing supportive care as integral to comprehensive HF care allows clinicians to better meet the needs of the patient and family now recognized as essential to 'patient-centered care'.[18] Similarly, embedding supportive care in HF care will invite researchers to understand the clinical correlates of the effects of treatment on symptoms and other sources of distress, as well as their pathophysiological underpinnings. Viewed as a whole, HF is a fascinating, complex syndrome that challenges our scientific models and our clinical expertise, collaboration, and compassion.

References

1. Stewart S, MacIntyre K, Capewell S,McMurray JJ (2003). Heart failure and the aging population: an increasing burden in the 21st century? *Heart* **89**:49–53.
2. Ho KK, Anderson KM, Kannel WB *et al.* (1993). Survival after the onset of congestive heart failure in Framingham Heart Study subjects. *Circulation* **88**:107–15
3. Barker WH, Mullooly JP, Getchell W (2006). Changing incidence and survival for heart failure in a well-defined older population, 1970–1974 and 1990–1994. *Circulation* **113**: 799–805.
4. Cowie MR, Wood DA, Coats AJ *et al.* (2000). Survival of patients with a new diagnosis of heart failure: a population based study. *Heart* **83**: 505–10.
5. Wenger NK (2007). The greying of cardiology: implications for management. *Heart* **93**: 411–12.
6. Formiga F, Chivite D, Sole A *et al.* (2006). Functional outcomes of elderly patients after the first hospital admission for decompensated heart failure. A prospective study. *Arch Gerontol Geriatr* **43**: 175–85.
7. Lang CC, Mancini DM (2007). Non-cardiac comorbidities in chronic heart failure. *Heart* **93**: 665–71.
8. Goodlin SJ, Hauptman PJ, Arnold R *et al.* (2004). Consensus Statement: Palliative and Supportive Care in Advanced Heart Failure. *J Card Fail* **10**: 200–9.
9. NHS Modernisation Agency Coronary Heart Disease Collaborative (2004). *Supportive and Palliative Care for Advanced Heart Failure.* London: NHS Modernisation Agency (http://www.heart.nhs.uk/Heart/Portals/0/docs_2004/Palliative%20Care%20Framework.pdf,accessed 9 November 2007).
10. Ahmedzai SH (2005). The nature of palliation and its contribution to supportive care. In: *Supportive Care in Respiratory Disease* (ed. SH Ahmedzai, MF Muers). Oxford: Oxford University Press.
11. Goodlin SJ (1997). What is palliative care?. *Hosp Pract* **32**: 13.
12. World Health Organization. *WHO Definition of Palliative Care.* Geneva: World Health Organization (http://www.who.int/cancer/palliative/definition/en/, accessed 7 November 2007).
13. National Consensus Project for Quality Palliative Care. *Clinical Practice Guidelines for Quality Palliative Care* (http://www.nationalconsensusproject.org/).
14. Gillick MR (2005). Rethinking the central dogma of palliative care. *J Palliat Med* **8**: 909–13.
15. Baker DW, Hayes RP, Massie BM, Craig CA (1999). Variations in family physicians' and cardiologists' care for patients with heart failure. *Am Heart J* **138**: 826–34.
16. Hobbs FD, Jones MI, Allan TF *et al.* (2000). European survey of primary care physician perceptions on heart failure diagnosis and management (Euro-HF). *Eur Heart J* **21**: 1877–87.
17. Dracup K (2002). Beyond the patient: caring for families. *Commun Nurs Res* **35**: 53–61.
18. Institute of Medicine (2001). *Crossing the Quality Chasm: a New Health System for the 21st Century,* Vol. 6. Washington, DC: National Academy Press.

Part 1

Heart failure

Chapter 2

The epidemiology of heart failure

John G. F. Cleland

Introduction

There is general agreement that heart failure (HF) is a common and deadly problem and yet, because it is a rather heterogeneous and ill-defined entity, the epidemiology remains poorly understood. The burden of HF from the viewpoint of society and health-care services is poorly described by study of its prevalence because few patients remain stable for long periods. Progression of the disease, response to therapy, and high mortality create a dynamic picture that is best described in terms of incidence and duration in various health states. Unfortunately, relevant data are limited.[1–3]

Definition, diagnosis and cause of HF

In order to understand the epidemiology of HF, it is first necessary to consider its definition and causes (Tables 2.1 and 2.2).

HF is defined in terms of pathophysiological principles as the inability to maintain an adequate cardiac output while maintaining normal filling (atrial) pressures (see also Chapter 3 on the pathophysiology of HF). From a clinical perspective, there are numerous problems with this definition, including the limited ability to measure cardiac output and atrial pressure and to define what cardiac output is adequate for the metabolic needs of the body. A clinical definition of HF is: symptoms and signs consistent with HF, mainly breathlessness and ankle swelling, associated with evidence of important cardiac dysfunction. Symptoms are generally thought to be due to fluid accumulation

Table 2.1 Definitions of HF

Pathophysiological	Inability to maintain a cardiac output for the needs of the body while maintaining normal atrial pressure
Clinical	Symptoms (predominantly breathlessness) associated with signs such as peripheral oedema and jugular venous distension due to a cardiac abnormality (usually identified by echocardiography). Symptoms and signs should improve with diuretics
Robust	As for clinical but using an elevated BNP as alternative or additional evidence of cardiac dysfunction[a]

[a] Note that BNP (brain natriuretic peptide) can be increased due to renal dysfunction and this needs to be taken into account.

and therefore relief of symptoms and signs by the use of diuretics adds further weight. However, breathlessness, fatigue and ankle swelling have many causes; ankle swelling regardless of cause may respond to diuretics and the ability of echocardiography to usefully assess diastolic dysfunction remains controversial.[4]

Probably the best measure of cardiac dysfunction is natriuretic peptides, with brain (BNP) or N-terminal pro-brain (NT-proBNP) natriuretic peptides being the most widely studied. Experience suggests that when natriuretic peptides and echocardiography give discordant results that it is very often the echocardiogram that has been evaluated wrongly. Natriuretic peptides are certainly the best prognostic marker available for HF, regardless of its cause,[5] and are consistently better than echocardiography. However, atrial fibrillation and renal dysfunction can cause increases in natriuretic peptides that are disproportionate to the severity of structural heart disease, so BNP testing alone is not perfect either.[6] Ideally, natriuretic peptides should be measured first, followed by assessment of renal function, heart rhythm and echocardiography, whenever it is elevated, to identify the probable cause. Unfortunately, the epidemiology of HF based on these principles has not been adequately described.

HF is the final common pathway of many cardiac problems.[1,7] Most patients have several reasons for developing HF, although there is usually one principal cause with several contributory factors (Table 2.2). The most common pathophysiological causes are left-ventricular systolic dysfunction (LVSD), valve disease, and a less well defined and probably heterogeneous entity called HF with a normal left ejection fraction (HFNEF). HFNEF probably comprises several conditions such as long-axis systolic dysfunction and diastolic dysfunction. Other less common causes of HF are pulmonary hypertension and constrictive pericarditis. Valve disease in affluent countries is predominantly due to degenerative disease, with aortic stenosis and mitral regurgitation being the dominant lesions. Atrial fibrillation[6] and cardiac dyssynchrony[8] lead to uncoordinated and inefficient cardiac contraction that may induce or exacerbate HF. Both are common.

Until recently, epidemiological studies of HF paid little attention to its cause, although many imply that HF secondary to valve disease, other perhaps than mitral regurgitation

Table 2.2 Causes of HF

Lay term	Conventional terminology	Predominant aetiologies
Weak heart	LV systolic dysfunction	Ischaemic heart disease. Dilated cardiomyopathy
Stiff heart	HFNEF (see text) or LV diastolic dysfunction	Hypertension
Overloaded heart	Pressure or volume overload	Hypertension. Aortic stenosis. Anaemia
Leaking heart	Valve regurgitation	Mitral regurgitation
Confused heart	Atrial fibrillation. Cardiac dyssynchrony	Ischaemic heart disease. Dilated cardiomyopathy

which is commonly a consequence of left-ventricular dilatation, was excluded. Accordingly, the epidemiology of HF needs to be described in at least three groups of patients; clinical HF regardless of cause, LVSD, and HFNEF.

One further neglected cohort of patients deserves mention. The diagnosis of HF is refuted in somewhere between 30–90% of referrals. These patients have a variety of medical problems and their prognosis may often also be poor. Their importance in the context of HF is that they represent the diagnostic burden of HF. If the ratio of referral to diagnosis is 3:1 and the incidence of HF is 300 per 100,000 population, then provision might be required for 900 patients to be evaluated each year. This does not appear to be consistent with current clinical activity, and two explanations seem likely. Many patients may not be referred from primary care and many patients are diagnosed as a result of an acute severe episode in hospital. Indeed, epidemiological studies suggest that two-thirds or more of new cases of HF are diagnosed subsequent to a hospital admission.[9,10]

Problems with the interpretation of epidemiological studies

Studies of the epidemiology of HF usually exclude younger patients (e.g. aged less than 25 years) but often also have an upper age limit.[3,11–13] These studies quote incidence and prevalence figures for the population group studied and yet these data are often extrapolated to the general population without correction for demographics. Thus, a prevalence of LVSD of 1% in a population aged 25–75 years cannot be simply applied to the general population, since the prevalence will be much lower in those aged less than 25, who constitute perhaps 30% of the population, and might be higher in those aged over 75.

A second problem is the means used to ascertain which patients have HF. Studies that depend on admission to hospital or referral for specialist advice may reflect a group with advanced HF. Diagnosis by non-specialists without objective confirmatory tests will include many patients with the wrong diagnosis. Accordingly, studies that routinely assess representative population samples are required. However, given that the prevalence of HF may be only about 1%, 1000 patients or more may need to be assessed to identify 10 patients with HF. As 25% or more of patients invited to participate in such surveys decline, considerable uncertainty remains about the epidemiology of HF.

The prevalence of HF must reflect its incidence, persistence, and longevity. Since HF, at least until recently, has been considered incurable, incidence should equal mortality, whilst prevalence will be determined by incidence and longevity. However, only a minority of patients with HF who die are reported to die of HF. The cause of HF is often given as the cause of death. Also, the mortality of HF appears to be biphasic, with 30–40% of patients dying in the first 6 months with a relatively constant hazard of about 5–15% per year thereafter depending on the severity and cause of HF (Fig. 2.1).[14,15]

Finally, epidemiologists often quote age-related incidence or prevalence. This is useful for looking at disease trends from an epidemiological perspective. However, clinicians need to know how many people in the community are in each age band to make practical sense of these data. For instance, graphs show that the age-related incidence of HF increases with age and peaks in people aged over 80 years. However, since there are

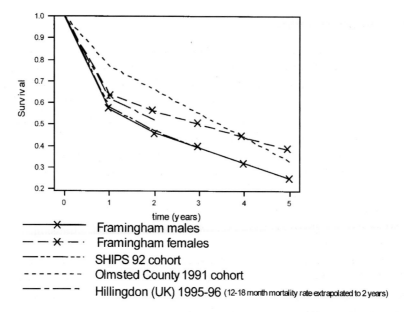

Fig. 2.1 Mortality in HF in epidemiological studies showing higher mortality in the first year after diagnosis. (Reproduced from Khand A, Gemmel I, Clark A, Cleland JGF. Is the prognosis of heart failure improving? *J Am Coll Cardiol* **36**: 2284–6. Copyright ©2000, with permission from Elsevier.)

currently many more people aged 60–80 years than aged over 80 years, most people with HF will be aged less than 80 years (Fig. 2.2).[13] Likewise, an epidemiologist may report an age-related decline in a problem, but if the population has aged, or the intervention has delayed the event to a greater age, the problem may be increasing at an alarming rate. Whenever possible the clinician should look at the number of people with problems rather than the proportions of subgroups of varying size within the population.

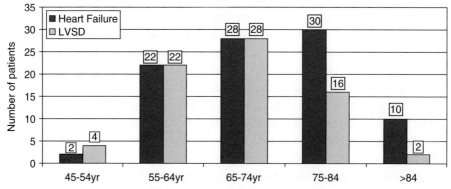

Fig. 2.2 Number of people identified with left-ventricular systolic dysfunction (LVSD) and heart failure (HF) in a UK community epidemiological programme of 3960 subjects.

Epidemiology of clinical HF

The largest body of data on the incidence of HF comes from the Framingham study. This suggested that, regardless of starting age, the life-time risk of developing HF is about one in five.[16] Men and women are equally affected but men are more likely to develop HF at a younger age and due to ischaemic heart disease (IHD). Taking into account the caveats above about the application of data from certain age groups to the general population, the incidence of HF in the overall population is about 300 per 100,000 per year. The data are fairly consistent in suggesting that more than 30% of patients will die in the first 6 months, presumably reflecting a rapid decline in cardiac dysfunction, a high risk of cardiac arrhythmias and sudden death and serious co-morbidities. The mortality is subsequently about 7% per annum or, if rebased to those still alive at 6 months, 10–15% per annum. Thus of 300 incident cases, about 100 will die in the first year, perhaps 20% of survivors in the next year, 15% of survivors in the year after that and about 10% of the survivors each year after that. This leads to a calculated median survival of incident HF of 2–3 years, and of those who survive the first year about 5 years with a few patients surviving for more 10 years. This is consistent with epidemiological data (Fig. 2.1).[14,15]

Using approximate knowledge about incidence and survival, prevalence at a notional steady state can be calculated; this is about 1.5% and is in line with expectations for HF due to LVSD and HFNEF combined. If it is assumed that new treatments can reduce mortality by 20% and/or that the incidence of HF increases by 20% due to changing demographics in the population, then the prevalence of HF is likely to increase substantially. Tables 2.3–2.5 provide approximate models based on existing epidemiology and some projected changes.

The average age of patients with prevalent HF in affluent countries is between 75 and 80 years of age and therefore the age of onset may be expected to be roughly 5 years younger, since most patients in a prevalent population will have had the problem for 3–5 years. The proportion of the population aged over 70 is set to increase, and accordingly an increase in the overall incidence of HF is likely, even if age-related incidence rates fall. However, patients with LVSD tend to be younger, most patients being aged 60–75 years, while patients with HFNEF are on average older than 75. This probably reflects the greater contribution of hypertension, vascular stiffness, and atrial fibrillation to the development of HF at this age and also the very poor prognosis of older patients with LVSD, who will show up in incidence studies but be under-represented in the long-term prevalent population.

Overall, HF affects men and women equally. However, men more often have LVSD and women HFNEF. In other words, a younger man with HF is likely to have LVSD, whilst an older women is very likely to have HFNEF.

The EuroHeart Failure survey of hospital deaths and discharges suggests that of about 6000 patients with a death or discharge diagnosis of HF, about 31% will have LVSD alone, 14% valve disease alone, 23% LVSD with valve disease (predominantly mitral regurgitation), and 32% will have HFNEF, although in a substantial proportion of the

Table 2.3 Population model showing expected prevalence of HF per 100,000 population, given an annual incidence of 300 patients, with approximately 30% mortality in the first year, 20% mortality amongst survivors in the second year, 15% mortality amongst survivors in the third year, and approximately 10% mortality per year thereafter. This gives an expected prevalence at steady state of about 1.6% which is in line with epidemiological expectations for HF due to LVSD and HFNEF combined

Annual cohort →	1	2	3	4	5	6	7	8	9	10	11	12	13	14	15	16	17	18	19	20	21	22	Cumulative number
Duration of follow-up ↓	300																						300
1	200	300																					500
2	160	200	300																				660
3	135	160	200	300																			795
4	115	135	160	200	300																		910
5	100	115	135	160	200	300																	1010
6	90	100	115	135	160	200	300																1100
7	80	90	100	115	135	160	200	300															1180
8	70	80	90	100	115	135	160	200	300														1250
9	60	70	80	90	100	115	135	160	200	300													1310
10	50	60	70	80	90	100	115	135	160	200	300												1360
11	45	50	60	70	80	90	100	115	135	160	200	300											1405
12	40	45	50	60	70	80	90	100	115	135	160	200	300										1445
13	35	40	45	50	60	70	80	90	100	115	135	160	200	300									1480
14	30	35	40	45	50	60	70	80	90	100	115	135	160	200	300								1510
15	25	30	35	40	45	50	60	70	80	90	100	115	135	160	200	300							1535
16	20	25	30	35	40	45	50	60	70	80	90	100	115	135	160	200	300						1555
17	15	20	25	30	35	40	45	50	60	70	80	90	100	115	135	160	200	300					1570
18	10	15	20	25	30	35	40	45	50	60	70	80	90	100	115	135	160	200	300				1580
19	5	10	15	20	25	30	35	40	45	50	60	70	80	90	100	115	135	160	200	300			1585
20	0	5	10	15	20	25	30	35	40	45	50	60	70	80	90	100	115	135	160	200	300		1585
21	0	0	5	10	15	20	25	30	35	40	45	50	60	70	80	90	100	115	135	160	200	300	1585

Table 2.4 Impact of reducing mortality in the first 2 years by 20% and then assuming a 10% annual mortality thereafter (late mortality is assumed not to be lower despite treatment because additional patients surviving in the initial years will presumably have a higher intrinsic risk). Note that prevalence will rise substantially

Annual cohort →	1	2	3	4	5	6	7	8	9	10	11	12	13	14	15	16	17	18	19	20	21	22	Cumulative number
Duration of follow-up ↓	300																						300
1	220	300																					520
2	185	220	300																				705
3	170	185	220	300																			875
4	155	170	185	220	300																		1030
5	140	155	170	185	220	300																	1170
6	125	140	155	170	185	220	300																1295
7	115	125	140	155	170	185	220	300															1410
8	105	115	125	140	155	170	185	220	300														1515
9	95	105	115	125	140	155	170	185	220	300													1610
10	85	95	105	115	125	140	155	170	185	220	300												1695
11	75	85	95	105	115	125	140	155	170	185	220	300											1770
12	65	75	85	95	105	115	125	140	155	170	185	220	300										1835
13	55	65	75	85	95	105	115	125	140	155	170	185	220	300									1890
14	45	55	65	75	85	95	105	115	125	140	155	170	185	220	300								1935
15	40	45	55	65	75	85	95	105	115	125	140	155	170	185	220	300							1975
16	35	40	45	55	65	75	85	95	105	115	125	140	155	170	185	220	300						2010
17	30	35	40	45	55	65	75	85	95	105	115	125	140	155	170	185	220	300					2040
18	25	30	35	40	45	55	65	75	85	95	105	115	125	140	155	170	185	220	300				2065
19	20	25	30	35	40	45	55	65	75	85	95	105	115	125	140	155	170	185	220	300			2085
20	15	20	25	30	35	40	45	55	65	75	85	95	105	115	125	140	155	170	185	220	300		2100
21	10	15	20	25	30	35	40	45	55	65	75	85	95	105	115	125	140	155	170	185	220	300	2110

Table 2.5 Effect of increasing the incidence of HF and applying assumptions as in Table 2.4. Note the further increase in prevalence. Note the longer time required to reach steady state and that the prevalence of HF will increase to about 2.6%

Annual cohort →	1	2	3	4	5	6	7	8	9	10	11	12	13	14	15	16	17	18	19	20	21	22	23	24	25	26	Cumulative number
Duration of follow-up ↓	360																										360
1	270	360																									630
2	230	270	360																								860
3	210	230	270	360																							1070
4	190	210	230	270	360																						1260
5	170	190	210	230	270	360																					1430
6	150	170	190	210	230	270	360																				1580
7	135	150	170	190	210	230	270	360																			1715
8	120	135	150	170	190	210	230	270	360																		1835
9	110	120	135	150	170	190	210	230	270	360																	1945
10	100	110	120	135	150	170	190	210	230	270	360																2045
11	90	100	110	120	135	150	170	190	210	230	270	360															2135
12	80	90	100	110	120	135	150	170	190	210	230	270	360														2215
13	70	80	90	100	110	120	135	150	170	190	210	230	270	360													2285
14	60	70	80	90	100	110	120	135	150	170	190	210	230	270	360												2345
15	50	60	70	80	90	100	110	120	135	150	170	190	210	230	270	360											2395
16	45	50	60	70	80	90	100	110	120	135	150	170	190	210	230	270	360										2440
17	40	45	50	60	70	80	90	100	110	120	135	150	170	190	210	230	270	360									2480
18	35	40	45	50	60	70	80	90	100	110	120	135	150	170	190	210	230	270	360								2515
19	30	35	40	45	50	60	70	80	90	100	110	120	135	150	170	190	210	230	270	360							2545
20	25	30	35	40	45	50	60	70	80	90	100	110	120	135	150	170	190	210	230	270	360						2570
21	20	25	30	35	40	45	50	60	70	80	90	100	110	120	135	150	170	190	210	230	270	360					2590
22	15	20	25	30	35	40	45	50	60	70	80	90	100	110	120	135	150	170	190	210	230	270	360				2605
23	10	15	20	25	30	35	40	45	50	60	70	80	90	100	110	120	135	150	170	190	210	230	270	360			2615
24	5	10	15	20	25	30	35	40	45	50	60	70	80	90	100	110	120	135	150	170	190	210	230	270	360		2620
25	0	5	10	15	20	25	30	35	40	45	50	60	70	80	90	100	110	120	135	150	170	190	210	230	270	360	2620

latter group the diagnosis might be wrong.[17] Surveys of patients in primary care come to similar conclusions (Fig. 2.3).[2]

The epidemiology of LVSD

About half of patients with important LVSD will be symptomatic.[18] Asymptomatic patients have a better prognosis than symptomatic ones.[19–21] The commonest presentation of asymptomatic LVSD is sudden death but a substantial proportion goes on to develop symptoms of HF.[22] Men are more likely to be asymptomatic than women.[18]

LVSD is usually due to IHD. Most patients will have had a myocardial infarction but perhaps one-third will have extensive coronary disease but no classical evidence of myocardial infarction.[1,2,23] Detailed examination using gadolinium delayed-enhancement cardiac magnetic resonance (deCMR) imaging shows that a substantial proportion of those without a history of myocardial infarction have myocardial scarring, suggesting they have had an infarct but also that some patients with classical evidence of an infarct have no scar. As the amount of scar on deCMR appears to be an important determinant of recovery of LV function with beta-blockers or revascularization, it is unlikely that these scars, or lack thereof, are artefacts. Clearly, IHD causes HF in complex ways and IHD acts as the predominant driver that links men, younger age at onset, and LVSD.[1,2]

Less than 10% of LVSD is probably due to dilated cardiomyopathy (DCM), but it causes a relatively high proportion of LVSD in people aged under 50 years. Despite the production of some vague, unhelpful, and contradictory guidelines by the World Health Organization on the definition of cardiomyopathy,[24] most clinicians still regard demonstration of the absence of important coronary disease as a prerequisite for the diagnosis of DCM.

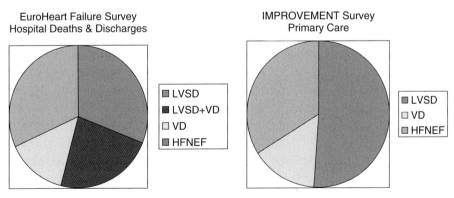

EuroHeart Failure Survey
Hospital Deaths & Discharges

IMPROVEMENT Survey
Primary Care

- LVSD
- LVSD+VD
- VD
- HFNEF

- LVSD
- VD
- HFNEF

LVSD = left ventricular systolic dysfunction
VD = valve disease
HFNEF = heart failure with a normal ejection fraction

Fig. 2.3 Causes of HF in surveys.

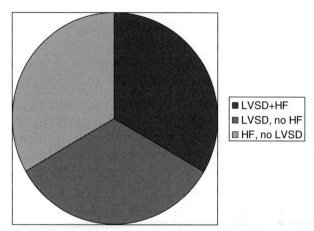

Fig. 2.4 Approximate proportions of patients with heart failure (HF) or left-ventricular systolic dysfunction (LVSD) or both.

Given that about 50% of patients with HF have LVSD and that 50% of LVSD is asymptomatic, then there should be a similar number of patients with LVSD and with clinical HF, that is about 1.5% or 1500 in a population of 100,000. Accordingly, about 0.75% will have both HF *and* LVSD and about 2.25% patients with HF *or* LVSD (Fig. 2.4).

The great majority of hospitalizations and deaths in patients with LVSD are cardiovascular. Sudden death occurs with a fairly monotonous regularity of about 3% per year and most are probably due to arrhythmias, although some will be due to acute vascular events or other causes. It is not clear that patients with a substantially greater risk of sudden death can be identified. The proportion of patients with LVSD that die suddenly will depend greatly on their risk of dying of other things. Thus, if death occurs in an asymptomatic patient it will usually be sudden, and over a 10-year period the risk may be about 30%. On the other hand, a very symptomatic patient may have a somewhat higher risk of sudden death, let's say 6% per year, but if they are destined to die of HF or some other problems within 2 years, the surviving life-time risk of sudden death may be low (6–12%) and even if sudden death is prevented, they may die soon after of another problem (Figs 2.5 and 2.6; see also Chapter 18).[25,26]

The epidemiology of HFNEF

HFNEF is even more complex. It is the most likely diagnosis in older women.[1,2] It appears that echocardiography is unable to distinguish reliably between those with and without HF amongst patients who present with clinical features suggesting HF but a normal ejection fraction. The utility of Doppler criteria is controversial at best. The only echocardiographic feature to provide some diagnostic and prognostic assistance in this setting is size of the left atrium.[27] On the other hand, NT-proBNP does appear useful in identifying patients who are at increased risk of cardiovascular events and death and who respond to treatment.[4] However, rather little is known about the epidemiology of diagnosis guided in this way.

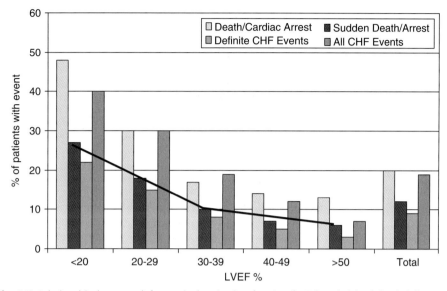

Fig. 2.5 Relationship between left-ventricular ejection fraction (LVEF) and risk of death (all-cause and sudden) and worsening HF events.

Many patients who appear to have HFNEF have symptoms that can be attributed to obesity, arthritis, or respiratory disease, in other words the diagnosis is wrong.[28] However, for some patients the symptoms appear to be cardiac in origin. Many have LV hypertrophy as a legacy of hypertension, atrial fibrillation, and dilated left atria. The problem with these patients is excessively high filling pressures despite adequate contractile LV function (see Chapter 3).

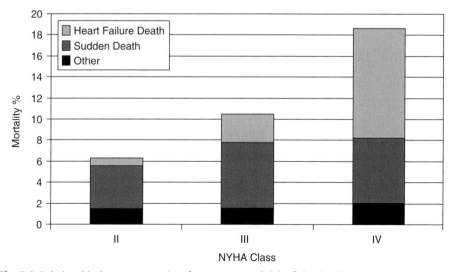

Fig. 2.6 Relationship between severity of symptoms and risk of death, all-cause and sudden.

Epidemiological studies, mainly of hospital discharge populations, suggest that the prognosis of HFNEF is similar to or only slightly better than that of HF due to LVSD.[29,30] However, clinical trials suggest dramatically lower rates of hospitalization with HF and death compared with patients with LVSD.[4,31] This may reflect the effects of non-cardiac co-morbidity. In both epidemiological studies and trials, non-cardiac morbidity and mortality constitute a far higher proportion of events than for patients with LVSD. As patients with serious non-cardiac co-morbidity are usually excluded from clinical trials, this would account for the disparity in prognosis compared with the epidemiology. It also suggests that many of the deaths observed in the epidemiological studies would not be prevented by cardiological interventions.

Amongst patients with HFNEF in the Perindupril in Elderly People with Chronic Heart Failure (PEP-CHF) trial, patients with a near-normal NT-proBNP had a risk of cardiovascular events or death that is similar to that of a normal elderly population.[4] On the other hand, patients with elevated NT-proBNP have event rates not dissimilar to patients with LVSD and obtained similar benefits from ACE inhibitors during the first year of treatment.

Contributory factors

HF is usually the result of a number of different insults conspiring to overwhelm cardio-vascular compensatory mechanisms. By the time the patient has any symptoms of HF the heart has already been severely compromised.

The cause of HF is usually considered to be due to myocardial disease. However, many contributory factors conspire to exacerbate the underlying disease and some

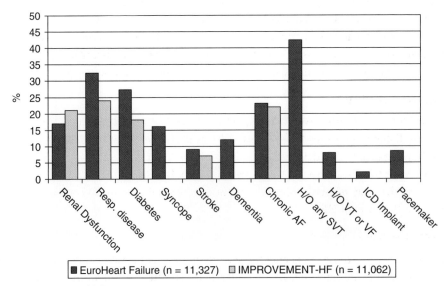

Fig. 2.7 HF co-morbidity.

contributory factors may be a more important cause of HF than the underlying disease (Fig. 2.7).

Arrhythmias

The most common arrhythmia in HF is atrial fibrillation (AF). Fast, persistent AF may cause the heart to dilate and fail (tachy-cardiomyopathy). This is entirely reversible with good heart rate control and warfarin prophylaxis to prevent strokes.[32] Many patients with HFNEF have long-standing hypertension and LV hypertrophy but only develop HF at the onset of AF. Cardioversion can cure their symptoms but the risk of relapse is high and rate control and anti-coagulation are usually preferred. Ventricular arrhythmias can present as worsening HF or syncope, but most often as sudden death. Use of implantable defibrillators (ICDs) can reduce the rate of sudden death by about 2% per year.[8] This is valuable in patients with a good quality of life. On the other hand, for sicker patients, ICDs may prevent sudden death and increase the duration of time spent in terminal HF. Such patients constitute an increasing focus of attention for palliative care, made all the more complex by the need to decide whether to turn the device off (see also Chapters 5 and 24).

Anaemia

About one-quarter of patients with HF are anaemic and about a quarter of these cases will be due to iron deficiency, possibly related to aspirin use.[33] Anaemia will exacerbate symptoms and is associated with a worse prognosis. The safety and efficacy of haematinics and stimulating the bone marrow with erythropoietin is being investigated.

Renal dysfunction

Most patients with HF have some renal dysfunction, and the prevalence increases with age.[34,35] There is a high prevalence of renal artery stenosis (RAS) in this population, as might be expected in patients with widespread vascular disease. However, the relationship between RAS and renal dysfunction is quite poor. Renal dysfunction is progressive, will limit the effectiveness of diuretics, and is associated with a worse prognosis. Renal dysfunction is associated with hyperuricaemia that may precipitate gout.

Diabetes mellitus

About 25% of patients have diabetes, mainly type 2.[1,2] About half of these patients develop diabetes only after the onset of HF. It is likely that many of these patients had insulin resistance before developing HF and that the metabolic stress of and treatment for HF made the disease overt. Overall, patients with diabetes and HF have a worse prognosis but this may be predominantly in patients treated with insulin whose diabetes preceded the onset of HF.

Liver disease

Patients, especially those with acute HF, may develop hepatic dysfunction. This prevents them degrading aldosterone, which contributes to retention of sodium and loss of potassium. It may also cause hypoalbuminaemia, which exacerbates oedema.

Valve disease, dyssynchrony, and pulmonary hypertension

Secondary to LVSD, many patients have mitral regurgitation that will be moderate or severe in 20%.[36] About 25–40% of patients with LVSD will have a QRS duration exceeding 120 ms and many of these will have ventricular dyssynchrony that should be considered for bi-ventricular pacing.[17,37] Chronic left-atrial hypertension may lead to pulmonary hypertension in 16%.

Hypotension

A low arterial pressure is an ominous sign in HF. Since most treatments, with the exception of bi-ventricular pacing, reduce arterial pressure, it also becomes an important factor in deciding what therapy a patient can tolerate. It is also an important determinant of renal function.

Heart failure co-morbidities

Many patients with HF will have respiratory, cerebrovascular, or peripheral vascular disease.[1,2,7] Major cognitive impairment is probably present in about 10% of patients.

Epidemiology of severe HF

The problem with trying to quantify the epidemiology of severe HF is that patients usually die or, at least for a while, get better. Stable severe HF is to some extent a contradiction in terms that implies that the care team are not trying very hard! Severe HF is not and should not be a stable state. It is clear that patients who have had an episode of severe HF despite treatment have a poor outcome both in terms of relapses and mortality, even if their symptoms can be temporarily controlled. However, it is difficult to predict prognosis of HF until the terminal few days. Studies suggest that patients, relatives, and their carers are often in disagreement about whether an individual should be resuscitated.[38,39] They also suggest that patients hospitalized with HF who indicate that they do not want to be resuscitated have often changed their mind when they recover. Just as failure to prevent a depressed person committing suicide is usually considered poor medical practice, accepting a sick but treatable patient's wish to die may not be in their best interest (see the discussion on advance directives in Chapter 22).

Most patients with worsening HF will be admitted to hospital. The discharge rate for HF has been reported as about 600 events per 100,000 population per year but this is probably a serious underestimate due to failure of adequate diagnostic coding at discharge.[40] There are about 1000 discharges per 100,000 population on loop diuretics, few of which are for renal failure. About one-third of these will represent repeat admission so the number of patients involved is probably 600 and a third or more of these will be first-time admissions. These data suggest that perhaps 10% of the prevalent pool of patients have or have recently had, and will soon again have, severe symptomatic HF. These patients consume a great deal of health-care resources over a relatively short period of time.

One long-term study (COMET) has described the patient journey in some detail.[41] The COMET trial recruited patients with LVSD and predominantly mild to moderate symptoms and randomly assigned them to carvedilol or metoprolol. Survival was substantially greater with carvedilol. Despite the greater longevity on carvedilol, an effect that is likely to be greatest in sicker patients, well-being also appeared to improve. Throughout the study, a fairly constant proportion of patients reported they felt their health to be poor (~10%) or very poor (~3%). Although such patients had a high mortality, these losses were replenished by the deterioration of new patients to more symptomatic classes. Analysis of patients who had severe symptoms at baseline (NYHA Class IV) showed that over 4 years of follow-up, almost 40% of days were lost to death but only about 2% were spent in hospital. Assuming that the quality of life of even a very sick patient is about two-thirds of one spent in full health, then about 25% of surviving days were lost to ill-health.

Summary

HF is common, complex, deadly, and treatable. The epidemiology of HF is often over-simplified. Proper understanding, in absolute terms, of the numbers of patients and the type of HF that requires management should assist in the better planning of diagnosis and management.

References

1. Cleland JGF, Swedberg K, Follath F *et al.* for the Study Group on Diagnosis of the Working Group on Heart Failure of the European Society of Cardiology (2003). The EuroHeart Failure Survey Programme: survey on the quality of care among patients with heart failure in Europe. Part 1: Patient characteristics and diagnosis. *Eur Heart J* **24**: 422–63.

2. Cleland JGF, Cohen-Solal A, Cosin-Aguilar J *et al.* for the IMPROVEMENT of Heart Failure Programme Committees and Investigators and the Study Group on Diagnosis of the Working Group on Heart Failure of the European Society of Cardiology (2002). An international survey of the management of heart failure in primary care. The IMPROVEMENT of Heart Failure Programme. *Lancet* **360**: 1631–9.

3. Cowie MR, Mosterd A, Wood DA *et al.* (1997). The epidemiology of heart failure. *Eur Heart J* **18**: 208–23.

4. Cleland JGF, Tendera M, Adamus J, Freemantle N, Polonski L, Taylor J on behalf of PEP-CHF Investigators (2006). The perindopril in elderly people with chronic heart failure (PEP-CHF) study. *Eur Heart J* **27**: 2338–45.

5. Doust JA, Pietrzak E, Dobson A, Glasziou P (2005). How well does B-type natriuretic peptide predict death and cardiac events in patients with heart failure: systematic review. *Br Med J* **330**: 625–34.

6. Shelton RJ, Clark AL, Goode K, Rigby AS, Cleland JGF (2006). The diagnostic utility of N-terminal pro-B-type natriuretic peptide for the detection of major structural heart disease in patients with atrial fibrillation. *Eur Heart J* **27**: 2353–61.

7. Brown A, Cleland JGF (1998). Influence of concomitant disease on patterns of hospitalisation in patients with heart failure discharged from Scottish hospitals in 1995. *Eur Heart J* **19**: 1063–9.

8. Cleland JGF, Nasir M, Tageldien A (2007). Cardiac resynchronization therapy or atriobiventricular pacing—what should it be called? *Nature Clin Prac Cardiovasc Med* **4**: 90–101.

9. Johansson S, Wallander M-W, Ruigomez A, Rodriguez LAC (2001). Incidence of newly diagnosed heart failure in UK general practice. *Eur J Heart Fail* **2**: 225–31.

10. Cleland JGF, Khand A, Clark AC (2001). The heart failure epidemic: exactly how big is it? *Eur Heart J* **22**: 623–6.

11. McDonagh TA, Morrison CE, Lawrence A *et al.* (1997). Symptomatic and asymptomatic left-ventricular systolic dysfunction in an urban population. *Lancet* **350**: 829–33.

12. McDonagh T, Robb SD, Murdoch DR *et al.* (1998). Biochemical detection of left-ventricular systolic dysfunction. *Lancet* **351**: 9–13.

13. Davies MK, Hobbs FDR, Davis RC *et al.* (2001). Prevalence of left-ventricular systolic dysfunction and heart failure in the Echocardiographic Heart of England Screening study: a population based study. *Lancet* **358**: 439–44.

14. Cleland JGF, Gemmel I, Khand A, Boddy A (1999). Is the prognosis of heart failure improving? *Eur J Heart Fail* **1**: 229–41.

15. Khand A, Gemmel I, Clark A, Cleland JGF (2000). Is the prognosis of heart failure improving? *J Am Coll Cardiol* **36**: 2284–6.

16. Lloyd-Jones DM, Larson MG, Leip MS *et al.* (2002). Lifetime risk for developing congestive heart failure – The Framingham Heart Study. *Circulation* **106**: 3068–72.

17. Khan NK, Goode KM, Cleland JGF *et al.* for the EuroHeart Failure Survey Investigators (2007). Prevalence of ECG abnormalities in an international survey of patients with suspected or confirmed heart failure at death or discharge. *Eur J Heart Fail* **9**: 491–501.

18. McDonagh T, Morrison CE, McMurray JJ *et al.* (1996). Global left ventricular systolic dysfunction in north Glasgow. *J Am Coll Cardiol* **27**: 106A.

19. Kober L, Torp-Pedersen C, Jorgensen S, Eliasen P, Camm AJ on behalf of the TRACE study (1998). Changes in absolute and relative importance in the prognostic value of left ventricular systolic function and congestive heart failure after acute myocardial infarction. *Am J Cardiol* **81**: 1292–7.

20. Yusuf S (1991). Effect of enalapril on survival in patients with reduced left ventricular ejection fractions and congestive heart failure. *New Engl J Med* **325**: 293–302.

21. The SOLVD Investigators (1992). Effect of enalapril on mortality and the development of heart failure in asymptomatic patients with reduced left ventricular ejection fraction. *New Engl J Med* **327**: 685–91.

22. Cleland JGF, Massie BM, Packer M (1999). Sudden death in heart failure: vascular or electrical? *Eur J Heart Fail* **1**: 41–5.

23. Cleland JGF, Pennell DJ, Ray SG *et al.* on behalf of the CHRISTMAS (Carvedilol Hibernating Reversible Ischaemia Trial: marker of success) investigators (2003). Myocardial viability as a determinant of the ejection fraction response to carvedilol in patients with heart failure (CHRISTMAS trial): randomised controlled trial. *Lancet* **362**: 14–21.

24. Richardson P, McKenna W, Bristow M *et al.* (1996). Report of the 1995 World Health Organization/International Society and Federation of Cardiology Task Force on the Definition and Classification of Cardiomyopathies. *Circulation* **93**: 841–2.

25. Hallstrom AP, Anderson JL, Carlson M *et al.* (1995). Time to arrhythmic, ischemic, and heart failure events: exploratory analyses to elucidate mechanisms of adverse drug effects in the Cardiac Arrhythmia Suppression Trial. *Am Heart J* **130**: 71–9.

26. MERIT-HF Study Group (1999). Effect of metoprolol CR/XL in chronic heart failure: Metoprolol CR/XL Randomised Intervention Trial in Congestive Heart Failure (MERIT-HF). *Lancet* **353**: 2001–7.

27. Banerjee P, Banerjee T, Khand A, Clark AL, Cleland JGF (2002). Diastolic heart failure – neglected or misdiagnosed? *J Am Coll Cardiol* **39**: 138–41.

28. Caruana L, Petrie MC, Davie AP, McMurray JV (2000). Do patients with suspected heart failure and preserved left ventricular systolic function suffer from 'diastolic heart failure' or from misdiagnosis? A prospective descriptive study. *Br Med J* **321**: 215–18.

29. Bhatia RS, Tu JV, Lee DS *et al.* (2006). Outcome of heart failure with preserved ejection fraction in a population-based study. *New Engl J Med* **355**: 260–9.

30. Owan TE, Hodge DO, Herges RM, Jacobsen SJ, Roger VL, Redfield MM (2006). Trends in prevalence and outcome of heart failure with preserved ejection fraction. *New Engl J Med* **355**: 251–9.

31. Yusuf S, Pfeffer MA, Swedberg K *et al.* for the CHARM Investigators and Committees (2003). Effects of candesartan in patients with chronic heart failure and preserved left-ventricular ejection fraction: the CHARM-Preserved Trial. *Lancet* **362**: 771–81.

32. Khand A, Rankin AC, Kaye GC, Cleland JGF (2000). Systematic review of the management of atrial fibrillation in patients with heart failure. *Eur Heart J* **21**: 614–32.

33. de Silva R, Rigby AS, Witte KKA *et al.* (2006). Anemia, renal dysfunction and their interaction in patients with chronic heart failure. *Am J Cardiol* **98**: 391–8.

34. De Silva R, Nikitin NP, Witte KK *et al.* (2006). Incidence of renal dysfunction over 6 months in patients with chronic heart failure due to left ventricular systolic dysfunction: contributing factors and relationship to prognosis. *Eur Heart J* **27**: 569–81.

35. de Silva R, Nikitin NP, Bhandari S, Nicholson A, Clark AL, Cleland JGF (2005). Atherosclerotic renovascular disease in chronic heart failure: should we intervene? *Eur Heart J* **26**: 1596–605.

36. Yiu SF, Enriquez Sarano M, Tribouilloy C, Seward JB, Tajik J (2000). Determinants of the degree of functional mitral regurgitation in patients with systolic left ventricular dysfunction: a quantitative clinical study. *Circulation* **102**: 1400–6.

37. Cleland JGF, Daubert J-C, Erdmann E *et al.* for the Cardiac Resynchronisation – Heart Failure (CARE-HF) Study Investigators (2005). The effect of cardiac resynchronization on morbidity and mortality in heart failure. *New Engl J Med* **352**: 1539–49.

38. Freeborne N, Lynn J, Desbiens NA (2000). Insights about dying from the SUPPORT Project. *J Am Geriatr Soc* **48**: S199–205.

39. Puchalski CM, Zhong Z, Jacobs MM *et al.* (2000). Patients who want their family and physician to make resuscitation decisions for them: observations from SUPPORT and HELP. *J Am Geriatr Soc* **48**: S84–S90.

40. Khand A, Shaw M, Gemmel I, Cleland JG (2005). Do discharge codes underestimate hospitalisation due to heart failure? Validation study of hospital discharge coding for heart failure. *Eur J Heart Fail* **7**: 792–7.

41. Cleland JGF, Charlesworth A, Lubsen J *et al.* (2006). A comparison of the effects of carvedilol and metroprolol on 'well-being', morbidity and mortality (the patient journey) in patients with heart failure: a report from the Carvedilol or Metoprolol European Trial (COMET). *J Am Coll Cardiol* **47**: 1603–11.

Chapter 3

Heart failure: pathophysiology

Yasuhiro Ikeda, Takeshi Yamamoto,
Masafumi Yano, and Masunori Matsuzaki

Introduction

In healthy subjects, the heart is an indefatigable muscular pump that uses two atria and ventricles to receive blood from the veins and pump it out through the arteries. The right-side pump supports pulmonary circulation to oxygenize the blood; while the left-side pump maintains the systemic circulation to meet the metabolic demands of the body. The valvular architecture between the atrium and ventricle, or between the ventricle and arterial outflow tract, controls the unidirectional blood flow to ensure proper cardiac output. The periodical contraction–relaxation rhythm of the heart is governed by the sequence of electrical excitation from the cardiac pacemaker cells at the right upper atrium toward ventricular myocytes through the atrioventricular conduction system. Proper oxygen supply to the heart through the right and left coronary arteries ensures the synergistic motion of these four chambers. A variety of heart disorders involving these components impede the heart from its normal contraction and relaxation, leading to cardiac pump dysfunction.

Heart failure (HF) is a complex clinical syndrome that arises from the above disorders and leads to an inability to maintain adequate cardiac output to meet systemic metabolic needs. The term 'heart failure' should not be confused with 'cessation of the heartbeat', which is also known as cardiac arrest or asystole. HF should also be distinguished from circulatory failure that displays defects of other components of the circulation, including loss of circulating blood volume or decreased concentration of oxygenated hemoglobin in the red blood cells. Most patients with HF have excessive volume retention at either the lungs or systemic veins, and HF of this type is known as congestive HF.

HF is the leading cause of death in developed countries.[1] The morbidity and mortality rates remain high despite recent significant progress in medical and surgical therapies. Currently, heart transplantation is the only curative procedure, although its availability is very limited due to the small number of donor hearts. In addition, even in transplant recipients, chronic mortality remains considerably high due to the enhanced progression of atherosclerosis. With respect to these clinical situations, appropriate medical therapy is essential to improve both the quality of life and long-term mortality of HF patients.

HF occurs not only in human beings but also in other mammals;[2] therefore, similar clinical characteristics and pathophysiology can also be observed in experimentally conditioned animals.[3] Over the past several decades, analyses using these experimental animal models have revealed not only the precise hemodynamic characteristics of HF but also the molecular basis of HF and the systemic response. In particular, the use of genetically engineered animal models has highlighted several pivotal molecular pathways that promote cardiac hypertrophy and adverse ventricular remodeling, and eventually lead to HF.[4] In this chapter, we will summarize the pathophysiological characteristics of HF, and discuss the link between these features and recent advances in the molecular basis of HF.

Clinical characteristics of HF

Classification of HF

The features of HF can be classified into several categories according to their pathophysiological characteristics: acute or chronic HF; systolic or diastolic failure; right-sided or left-sided HF; and high output or low output failure. These characteristics are discussed in detail below.

Acute or chronic HF

When symptoms of HF manifest with an acute onset secondary to acute coronary syndrome (ACS) or cardiac inflammation, patients are diagnosed as having acute HF and usually require intensive care in a cardiac (coronary) care unit in a hospital, whereas chronic ongoing cardiac (either right- or left-ventricular) dysfunction, or inappropriate cardiac output, that leads to chronic congestion of the circulating blood in either the lungs or veins is diagnosed as chronic HF.

Right-sided or left-sided HF

Left-sided HF is characterized by low cardiac output associated with left-ventricular (LV) dysfunction, pulmonary congestion, increased LV end-diastolic pressure (EDP), impaired LV fluid filling, and hypotension. Physical examination often reveals increased moist rales in the lung field. Symptoms include dyspnea, easy fatigability, orthopnea or paroxysmal nocturnal dyspnea (dyspnea worsening upon lying down). Right-sided HF is characterized by a pump dysfunction of the right ventricle with peripheral edema, liver congestion, and jugular venous distension. Symptoms of right-sided HF include easy fatigability, loss of appetite, and abdominal fullness. Right-sided HF can be caused by isolated lung or right-heart disorders; importantly, the most frequent cause of right-sided HF is the advance of left-sided HF; therefore, HF is also diagnosed as biventricular failure in such cases.

Systolic failure and diastolic failure

Systolic HF is characterized by severely impaired LV systolic function and enlarged LV chamber size, accompanied by elevated ventricular filling pressure and pulmonary congestion. Usually, the ejection fraction (EF) of the left ventricle is 45% or less, and the pressure–volume relationship is shifted rightward (Fig. 3.1a,b), accompanied by an increased LV end-diastolic volume (EDV), a reduction of stroke volume (SV), and a decrease in the slope of the end-systolic pressure–volume relationship (Emax),[5] while the compliance of the LV, i.e. the distensibility of the LV, is relatively preserved. Consequently, LVEDP increases according to the same diastolic pressure–volume curve as in the normal heart (Fig. 3.1b).[5] When the LV pressure–volume loop shifts rightward accompanied by a decreased slope of Ees, any given change (the arrow in Fig. 3.1b) in the effective arterial resistance (Ea), an index of arterial resistance (afterload) normalized by heart rate, will yield a larger change in SV than in the normal heart (the arrow in Fig. 3.1a). Therefore, SV in the patients with systolic HF is largely afterload-dependent.[6]

In contrast, HF is caused not only by systolic dysfunction but also by isolated relaxation abnormality of the LV.[7–10] In fact, about 40% of patients with HF in the general population display increased LVEDP and associated pulmonary congestion with normal systolic function, and therefore are diagnosed as diastolic HF (see also Chapter 2). Diastolic HF may be caused by the hypertrophied ventricle wall, restriction of infiltrative cardiomyopathies, and/or tachycardia that limits the time of diastolic filling, resulting in an increase in ventricular filling pressure. The pressure–volume curve is only affected at the diastolic portion shifts upward (Fig. 3.1c) due to the decreased LV compliance. Accordingly, the diseased heart with diastolic dysfunction is unable to increase in SV and EDV in response to a given change in preload, thereby leading to an increase in LVEDP. Moreover, when the afterload, Ea, is increased in the diseased heart as indicated in Fig. 3.1(c), SV prominently decreases and pulmonary congestion eventually occurs.[5] Diagnosis of diastolic HF is not easy unless a direct measurement of LVEDP is performed at the period of the decompensated stage of HF, but recent advances in echocardiographic technology have improved the diagnosis of diastolic HF significantly, revealing the alteration of ventricular filling without the requirement for an invasive catheter technique. In this regard, assessment of the movement velocity of the mitral

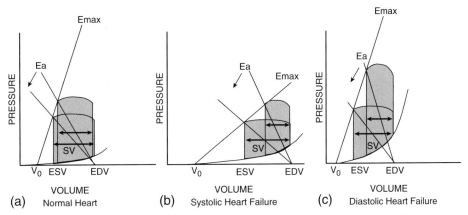

Fig. 3.1 Pressure–volume relationship in the normal heart (a), systolic heart failure (b), and diastolic heart failure (c). ESV, end systolic volume; EDV, end diastolic volume; SV, stroke volume; Emax, slope of end systolic pressure–volume relationship; Ea, effective arterial elastance; V_0, volume intercept.

valvular annulus (E velocity) and the peak velocity of transmitral flow (E velocity) at the early diastolic period provides a good clue for detecting elevated LVEDP.[11] When LVEDP increases in diastolic HF, the value of E/E', which is calculated by dividing the E velocity by the E^1 velocity, is more than 15, whereas it is less than 8 in the normal heart. Elderly women with hypertension or diabetes mellitus appear to show an increase in morbidity due to diastolic HF,[12,13] which perhaps is associated with a lack or cessation of gonadotropic hormonal regulation. It is not precisely clear why elderly women with hypertension or diabetes mellitus show a predisposition to developing LV hypertrophy and diastolic HF (see Chapter 17).

In either case of HF, individuals are sensitive to small shifts in their intravascular volume (i.e. the amount of fluid in their circulatory system). Increasing the volume in their circulatory system can cause symptoms and signs of decompensated HF, while decreasing the volume in the circulatory system can cause significant hypotension.

Low-output and high-output HF

Since the status of HF is determined by the balance between cardiac output and metabolic demand of the body, HF occurs even when the cardiac pump function is normally preserved. In this regard, HF is classified as a low-output or high-output failure. Low-output failure represents reduced cardiac pump function, accompanied by reduced or normal oxygen consumption in peripheral organs. Typical etiologies of low-output HF are as summarized in Table 3.1. In contrast, high-output failure denotes manifestation of HF despite a normal or higher cardiac output, which is associated with an arterio-venous shunt or exaggerated increase in oxygen uptake in peripheral organs. In particular, when a patient has organic shunt disease, pregnancy, anemia, infection, vitamin B_1 deficiency, or any of these conditions in combination with cardiac dysfunction, high-output failure eventually occurs.

Table 3.1 Etiology of HF

1. Mechanical overload	Volume overload (regurgitant valvular disease, arterial value regurgitation, mitral value regurgitation, arterio-venous shunt disease) Pressure overload (aortic stenosis) Overload due to systemic disease (beriberi, anemia, hyperthyroidism)
2. Myocardial abnormality associated with primary and secondary myocardial disease	Primary myocardial disease: hypertrophic cardiomyopathy; dilated cardiomyopathy; restrictive cardiomyopathy Secondary myocardial disease: acute and chronic myocarditis (viral, parasite associated); drug-induced cardiomyopathy
3. Cardiac rhythm abnormality	Tachycardia induced (atrial flutter and fibrillation) Bradycardia induced (sinoatrial and atrioventricular conduction abnormality)
4. Myocardial ischemia and reperfusion injury	Post-myocardial infarction Hibernation and myocardial stunning Ischemic cardiomyopathy

AR,; MR,

Table 3.2 NYHA classification

Class I	Patients with cardiac disease but without resulting limitations of physical activities. Ordinary physical activity does not cause undue fatigue, palpitation, dyspnea, or anginal pain
Class II	Patients with cardiac disease resulting in slight limitation of physical activity. These patients are comfortable at rest. Ordinary physical activity results in fatigue, palpitation, dyspnea, or anginal pain
Class III	Patients with cardiac disease resulting in marked limitation of physical activity. These patients are comfortable at rest. Less than ordinary physical activity causes fatigue, palpitation dyspnea, and anginal pain
Class IV	Patients with cardiac disease resulting in inability to carry on any physiological activity without discomfort. Symptoms of cardiac insufficiency or of the anginal syndrome may be present even at rest. If any physical activity is undertaken, discomfort is increased

Evaluating the severity of HF

To evaluate the severity of HF, a classification system by the New York Heart Association (NYHA) has been used over the years (Table 3.2). This classification is advantageous for simply expressing symptomatic severity in HF patients; however, the drawback of this classification is that the estimated severity class does not always correlate with the disease severity. Determination of the NYHA class largely depends on the subjective interpretation of individual physicians, and thus lacks precision. For example, it changes over the short term in response to treatment, and therefore it may not be suitable for establishing the long-term effects of various therapeutic strategies in HF patients. In consideration of this problem, the NYHA classification is currently being used to express the therapeutic efficacy before and after treatment.

Alternatively, a new classification system from the American College of Cardiology/ American Heart Association Guideline Committee is now being used (Table 3.3).[14,15] This classification more precisely describes the disease progression status in conjunction with the corresponding strategy for prevention and treatment. Stage A includes patients who are at risk of developing HF but who have no structural heart disease at present. This includes patients with hypertension, diabetes mellitus, coronary artery disease,

Table 3.3 ACC/AHA classification of chronic HF (2001)

Stage	Description
A: High risk for developing HF	Hypertension, diabetes mellitus, CAD, family history of cardiomyopathy
B: Asymptomatic HF	Previous myocardial infarction, LV dysfunction, valvular heart disease
C: Symptomatic HF	Structural heart disease, dyspnea and fatigue, impaired exercise tolerance
D: Refractory end-stage HF	Marked symptoms at rest despite maximal medical therapy

use of cardiac toxins, and familial history of cardiomyopathy. Strategies to prevent ventricular remodeling, including angiotensin-converting enzyme (ACE) inhibitors in selected cases, are advised. Stage B includes patients with structural heart disease but no symptoms. The use of ACE inhibitors and β-blockers is recommended. Stage C includes patients with structural heart disease and symptomatic HF. Diuretics, digoxin, and aldosterone antagonists may be added to ACE inhibitors and β-blockers depending upon the severity of symptoms (see Chapter 4). Cardiac resynchronization therapy may also be considered in selected patients (see Chapter 5). Stage D includes patients with severe refractory HF. Physicians are urged to consider either end-of-life care or high-tech therapies such as cardiac transplantation, based on individual cases (see Chapter 23).

Etiology of HF

As summarized in Table 3.1, there are four main mechanisms that cause HF; these are discussed below.

Mechanical overload and HF

Mechanical overload is classified into volume overload or pressure overload. Volume overload includes regurgitant valvular heart diseases, anemia, vitamin B_1 deficiency, hyperthyroidism, and large vascular shunt diseases. Pressure overload is typically represented by aortic stenosis and arterial hypertension. These mechanical overloads, caused by defects of the heart architecture or induced by systemic diseases, are initially compensated by a variety of adaptation mechanisms, including alteration of metabolic energy production, changes of myocardial architecture, and activation of neurohormonal peptide secretions. In this regard, volume overload usually triggers eccentric LV hypertrophy as a myocardial adaptive mechanism, whereas pressure overload evokes concentric LV hypertrophy. In consequence, these adaptive mechanisms activate various pathophysiological pathways, and lead to cardiac dysfunction, chamber dilation, and finally HF.[16]

Cardiomyopathy and HF

Myocardial abnormality caused by primary functional defects in cardiomyocytes leads to cardiomyopathy with overt HF. There are three subcategories in primary myocardial disease, namely hypertrophic cardiomyopathy (HCM), dilated cardiomyopathy (DCM), and restrictive cardiomyopathy (RCM) (for review, see Morita et al.[17] and Ahmad et al.[18]).

Hypertrophic cardiomyopathy is characterized by increased cardiac mass with a thickened ventricular wall and normal or reduced chamber volume accompanied by enlarged cardiomyocytes and myofibrillar disarray. Genetic abnormalities are often documented as mutations in myofibrillar component genes (in more than 50% of the patient population), including β-myosin heavy chain, ventricular myosin 1 and 2, cardiac troponin T, α-tropomyosin, myosin-binding protein C, α-cardiac actin, and so forth (Table 3.4).[17,18] The hypertrophic phenotype is frequently associated with impaired diastolic

Table 3.4 Genetic abnormality reported in hypertrophic cardiomyopathy (HCM) (adapted from Ahmad et al.[18])

Cardiac troponin T2	Beta myosin heavy chain
Titin	Alpha myosin heavy chain
Essential myosin light chain	Cardiac actin
Cardiac troponin C	Alpha tropomyosin
Cardiac myosin-binding protein C	Cardiac troponin I
Regulatory myosin light chain	

function and HF; however, some gene mutations, which occur in about 10% of HCM patients, cause progressive chamber dilation and severely impaired contractility, leading to systolic HF.

Dilated cardiomyopathy is characterized by impaired systolic and diastolic function, marked dilation of the LV chamber, and thinning of the ventricular wall. In about 25% of dilated cardiomyopathy cases the structural and functional defects seem to be attributable to hereditary gene mutations in the cardiomyocytes. At present, more than 10 gene mutations have been reported to be responsible for dilated cardiomyopathy.[17–19] These include mutations in cardiac actin, dystrophin, desmin, δ-sarcoglycan, lamin A/C, phospholamban, and others (Table 3.5).

Restrictive cardiomyopathy, a rare case of myocardial abnormality, is characterized by a decreased myocardial compliance and elevated LV filling pressure. Diastolic dysfunction is remarkable and leads to progressive pulmonary congestion and overt HF. Although genetic analysis is rather limited due to the infrequent nature of this type of cardiomyopathy (occurring in fewer than 5% of patients with genetic cardiomyopathy), mutations have been reported in an intermediate fiber gene, desmin,[20] which encodes a mutant protein that has been shown to cause abnormal protein deposition and marked decline in LV compliance. Another causative gene for RCM is cardiac troponin I,[21] although this gene mutation is also known to cause HCM as well.

Some gene defects induce a hypertrophic response, while others directly cause ventricular dilation without showing a hypertrophic phenotype, and still others show the restrictive physiology of the LV without showing hypertrophy. Presumably, the primary gene function that governs cellular homeostasis determines these different phenotypes. In this regard, mutations in sarcomeres (contractile apparatus) tend to cause hypertrophic cardiomyopathy, whereas genetic mutations in cytoskeleton, mitochondria, and the Ca^{2+} handling regulatory protein are often associated with the dilated phenotype. Importantly, however, it has been reported that certain gene mutations can cause one of two distinct types of cardiomyopathy. That is, mutations of cardiac actin[7] or other HCM-related genes, such as myosin heavy chain and cardiac troponin T,[19] can induce DCM and HCM, while cardiac troponin I mutation[21] can lead to RCM and HCM, as

Table 3.5 Genetic abnormality reported in dilated cardiomyopathy (DCM) (adapted from Towbin and Bowles[19])

Lamin A/C	Cardiac myosin-binding protein C
Cardiac troponin T2	Cardiac muscle LIM protein
Titin	ATP-sensitive potassium channel
Desmin	Beta myosin heavy chain
Delta-sarcoglycan	Cardiac actin
Desmoplakin	Alpha tropomyosin
Phospholamban	Cardiotropin I
EYA4	Dystrophin
Metavinculin	Tafazzin
Cypher/ZASP	

mentioned above. These overlaps in cardiomyopathic phenotype may be attributable to the protein domain function of the mutant allele, or additional genetic and environmental factors.

Moreover, these cardiomyopathy phenotypes are also observed in myocardial disease secondary to inflammation and subsequent fibrous changes, or abnormal protein deposition. Chronic myocarditis-induced, drug-induced, and alcohol intake-induced cardiomyopathies are frequent causes of secondary cardiomyopathy. Systemic diseases such as sarcoidosis or amyloidosis are also frequently accompanied by cardiac involvement which leads to progressive cardiomyopathy and resultant HF.

Cardiac rhythm abnormality and HF

Abnormalities in cardiac rhythm, such as tachycardia or bradycardia, often induce low cardiac output with overt HF.[22] Even tachycardia *per se*, such as atrial flutter, limits ventricular filling initially, and ultimately causes chronic ventricular systolic dysfunction. In particular, elderly patients with hypertension or cardiac hypertrophy are predisposed to suffer from atrial fibrillation and flutter, resulting in reduced diastolic filling time and pulmonary congestion. Defects in the heart conduction system, which includes sinoatrial and atrioventricular node disease, frequently occur in the elderly, leading to bradycardia-induced low cardiac output.[23] Treatment of these cardiac arrhythmias is also clinically important to avoid the formation of atrial thrombus and subsequent cardiogenic embolic events.

Myocardial ischemia/reperfusion and HF

HF associated with ischemia and reperfusion injury is a major cause of morbidity in the HF population in developed countries.[16] Increased prevalence of coronary artery disease and improved survival after the onset of acute myocardial infarction due to recent advances in percutaneous coronary intervention technologies are significant factors in the increased number of patients with HF secondary to ischemic heart disease. In the United States, approximately 5 million people have been diagnosed with chronic HF, and the majority of these patients have HF associated with myocardial ischemia/reperfusion.

Epidemiological factors and HF

HF etiology has been reported to be affected by a variety of specific social factors, such as nutrition and situations endemic to either a particular era or region. For instance, approximately 100 years ago in Japan, HF morbidity was considerably high both in young and elderly populations, due to a deficiency of vitamin B1.[24,25] At that time, people had been eating polished white rice as their major energy source, and polished rice lacks bran, which is rich in vitamin B_1. Another example is so-called Chagas disease in South America, an infectious disease-related cardiomyopathy[26] caused by infection with *Trypanosoma cruzi*. Infection by this parasite causes chronic myocarditis that eventually leads to dilated cardiomyopathy and HF. Therefore, in addition to the precise clinical evaluation of myocardial architecture, anatomy, and contractile/relaxation function, it is important to know details about where the patient lives, their dietary habits, and their lifestyle for appropriate diagnosis and planning of HF therapy.

The molecular basis of HF

The renin–angiotensin–aldosterone system and HF

Before the 1970s, based on the definition of HF as pump failure, patients were treated with diuretics and inotropic agents, including digitalis, catecholamines, and phosphodiesterase III inhibitors, to enhance the impaired cardiac pump function. However, administration of these agents, particularly milrinone, a phosphodiesterase III inhibitor, was shown to reduce the survival of patients with HF.[27,28] Accordingly, treatment of HF patients with vasodilators, which do not have any inotropic effects on cardiac function, were initiated by using a combination of nitrate and hydralazine to reduce afterload in HF patients, thereby increasing cardiac output.[29] Similarly, ACE inhibitors, recognized as vasodilators that act on both the arteries and veins in a balanced manner, have been utilized to provide a vasodilator effect in HF patients. Importantly, treatment with ACE inhibitors was found to extend the long-term survival of HF patients.[30–32] However, another vasodilator therapy using an α-blocker, prazosin, failed to improve the long-term outcome of HF patients,[29] although prazosin exhibited similar vasodilator effects with ACE inhibitors. These findings have suggested that, in addition to their vasodilator effects, ACE inhibitors may have other benefits for the treatment of HF patients. Thereafter, a number of studies were performed to investigate this possibility, and have shown that the renin–angiotensin–aldosterone system plays a pivotal pathophysiological role during the development of HF, with respect to angiotensin receptor signaling in the heart, vessel walls, and other important organs.[33,34] Moreover, the renin–angiotensin–aldosterone system is also intimately associated with other aspects of neurohormonal regulation, namely secretion of arginine-vasopressin through the pituitary gland and release of norepinephrine from the peripheral nerve endings. Inappropriate activation of the renin–angiotensin–aldosterone system in HF is often accompanied by an exaggerated secretion of vasopressin and excessive release of norepinephrine. These neurohormonal abnormalities have been known not only to provoke salt and water retention and an increase in systemic vascular resistance, but also to promote pathophysiological cardiac hypertrophy, tissue inflammatory response, and interstitial fibrosis in the heart. These features are in contrast to the essentially adaptive hypertrophic mechanism of α-adrenergic signaling in the heart that has also been experimentally demonstrated by Simpson and colleagues.[35]

The introduction of pharmacological treatment with ACE inhibitors has thus led to new paradigms of HF pathophysiology over the last two decades. Although the beneficial effect of ACE inhibitors has been attributed to an action that blocks the production of angiotensin II from its precursors and also subsequently blocks the downstream event, i.e. aldosterone secretion, chronic administration of ACE inhibitors[36–41] has been shown to cause a paradoxical increase in angiotensin II and subsequent secretion of aldosterone, which is known as the 'escape phenomenon'. Further investigation has revealed that this phenomenon arises from an additional enzymatic pathway in the heart that produces angiotensin II, i.e. a chymase system.[42,43] Therefore it seems to be important to use specific angiotensin receptor blockers (ARBs) in combination with ACE inhibitors to ensure blocking of the renin–angiotensin–aldosterone system in HF. In this regard, several ARB compounds have been developed to achieve more specific inhibition of the angiotensin type 1 receptor. According to a number of large randomized clinical trials, ARBs appear to be equally effective for improving the long-term outcome of patients with HF. However, candesartan[36–39] is the only ARB that has been shown to have an additive effect when administered in conjunction with an ACE inhibitor; the fact that other ARBs did not show such an effect[40,41] suggests that there are differential class effects among the ARBs. It has also been reported that blockade of aldosterone by spironolactone or eplerenone has additional beneficial effects on the long-term outcome in HF patients.[44,45] These benefits are attributed to the direct inhibitory effect of aldosterone, which provokes interstitial inflammation and fibrosis in the diseased heart (See also Chapter 4).[46]

β-Adrenergic regulation and Ca^{2+} cycling in HF

One of the hallmarks of HF pathophysiology is hyperactivation of the sympathetic nervous system and increased secretion of norepinephrine into the circulating blood from peripheral nerve endings.[47] Indeed, patients with increased serum norepinephrine levels exhibit a worse outcome than patients with lower levels.[47] Although an increase in serum catecholamines is initially an adaptive mechanism in response to the decreased cardiac performance, and has a favorable effect due to its adjustment of cardiac output over the short term,[27] it has been shown to be detrimental over the long term because it causes LV hypertrophy that increases myocardial oxygen consumption and induces progressive LV remodeling and fatal cardiac arrhythmias.[48] Therefore the plasma norepinephrine level serves as a good diagnostic tool to predict the outcome of patients with HF. Furthermore, chronic administration of β-receptor blockers has been shown to be largely beneficial in preventing progression of HF and improving patient mortality. These findings have highlighted β-adrenergic receptor signaling as a common underlying mechanism in HF (Fig. 3.2).[49]

In the normal heart, sympathetic activation causes activation of β-adrenergic receptors, which in turn activate adelylate cyclase and enhance intracellular cyclic AMP, thereby causing the activation of protein kinase A (PKA).[50] Activated PKA phosphorylates intracellular targets, including ryanodine receptors and phospholamban, a key phosphoprotein in the regulation of intracellular Ca^{2+} cycling.[50] In failing cardiomyocytes, β-receptor signaling through activation of the sympathetic nervous system is blunted due to the downregulation of β-receptor density, i.e. desensitization of β-adrenergic receptors in the failing heart,[51] which leads to an impaired contractility in the failing cardiomyocytes. Accordingly, for years, it was thought that intracellular downstream signals of β-adrenergic receptors, i.e. phosphorylation of the target protein, are decreased in the failing heart. Conversely, phosphorylation of one of the downstream targets, the ryanodine receptor, has been shown to be hyperphosphorylated at the PKA phosphorylation site, leading to leaky channel gating and increased Ca^{2+} concentration at diastole, and finally to increased cellular damage, as independently reported by Marks and colleagues,[52] and by our group.[53] In a related context, the phosphorylation status of phospholamban is decreased in the same experimental setting,[54] suggesting that regulation of intracellular phosphorylation through β-adrenergic signaling in HF depends on the local regulation of the corresponding microdomain.[50,55] There are also reports describing increased protein phosphatase 1 activity[56–60] and decreased sarcoplasmic reticulum (SR) phosphodiesterase 4D activity in the failing heart,[61] implying that such altered function of phosphorylation modifiers contributes to the progression of HF. These abnormal balances in intracellular phosphorylation and defective regulation in SR Ca^{2+} cycling are also involved in the onset of fatal cardiac arrhythmia and thus may provide a good therapeutic target. On the other hand, diastolic Ca^{2+} uptake is also impaired due to the decreased expression of SR Ca^{2+} ATPase and increased phosphorylation in phospholamban at Ser16, a PKA-dependent phosphorylation site. In an experiment using small rodents, overexpression of the SERCA gene[62,63] or inhibition of phospholamban[64–66] suppressed the progression of progressive HF, suggesting another therapeutic target involving intracardiomyocyte regulation of Ca^{2+}. Although this molecular intervention is recognized as a promising molecular therapy that increases cardiac contractility in the failing heart, it should be distinguished from classic inotropic therapy by β-stimulant or phosphodiesterase inhibitors because it does not enhance intracellular cyclic AMP production.

As mentioned above, oscillation of Ca^{2+} concentration in cardiomyocytes is a key factor that determines cardiomyocyte contractility; on the other hand, another important aspect is that changes in intracellular Ca^{2+} concentration trigger cardiac hypertrophy

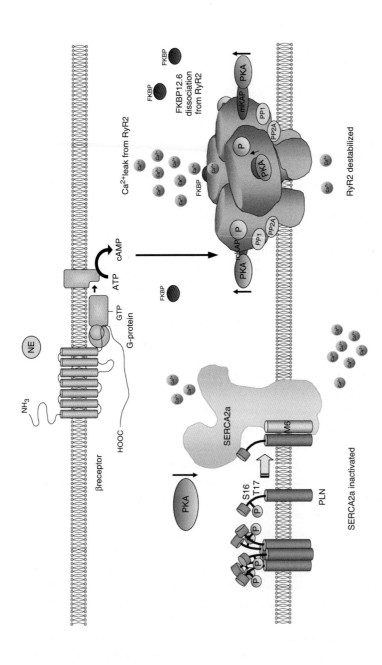

Fig. 3.2 The intracellular signaling pathway that is important for the failing myocardium. Abbreviations: βAR, β-adrenergic receptor; αAR, α-adrenergic receptor; AT1R, angiotensin type 1 receptor; ET-1R, endothelin 1 receptor; IGFs, insulin-like growth factors; FGF, fibroblast growth factors; IL-6, interleukin-6; CT-1, cardiotrophin-1; GC, guanylate cyclase; Gs, Gs-protein; Gq/11, Gq/11 protein; TYK, tyrosine kinase; PLC, phospholipase C; Ras, rat sarcoma virus oncogene; JAK, Janus tyrosine kinase; PKG, protein kinase G; PKA, protein kinase A; CaMK, calmodulin-dependent kinase; MAPK, mitogen-activated kinases; STAT, signal transducer and activator of transcription; NFAT, nuclear factor of activated T cells; GATA-4, GATA-binding protein 4; MEF-2, myocyte enhancing factor 2.

through activation of Ca^{2+}-dependent kinases[67–69] and calcineurin phosphatases.[70] Until recently, it was not clear how intracellular Ca^{2+} simultaneously regulates the beat-by-beat contractility and cardiomyocyte hypertrophy in the diseased condition. Recently, a landmark study by Bers and colleagues[71] has reported that local Ca^{2+} control at the nuclear membrane via inositol,4,5-triphosphate receptors plays a pivotal role in transcriptional activation during cardiac hypertrophy. Thus intracellular Ca^{2+} regulation in cardiomyocytes is important not only for maintaining normal cardiac function but also for preventing pathophysiological cardiac hypertrophy.

Heart dysfunction, cardiac hypertrophy, and ventricular remodeling

Cardiac hypertrophy is initially an adaptive mechanism in response to the increased mechanical load when the heart is exposed to any given stress; however, prolonged exposure to stress induces a certain metabolic transition in the heart muscle—basic energy production in cardiomyocytes using a fatty acid oxidation system switches to glycolytic energy production, as is seen during development of the fetal heart. Consequently, a variety of fetal gene programs, including atrial natriuretic peptide production and alteration in the isoform of myosin heavy chain and cardiac actin, occur in hypertrophied cardiomyocytes.[72,73] This altered gene regulation in the hypertrophied heart seems to be well correlated with the deterioration of cardiac contractile function, adverse ventricular remodeling, and chamber dilatation, thereby eventually leading to the manifestation of HF. Numerous studies have been conducted to decipher the principal molecular mechanisms during the development of cardiac hypertrophy and to seek novel molecular interventions that directly prevent pathological hypertrophy. Under certain stress conditions either hypertrophy or apoptotic cell death is induced in cardiomyocytes. The balance between myocyte hypertrophy and apoptosis appears to be a major determinant for the transition from cardiac hypertrophy to ventricular dilation.[74] Currently, it is thought that a variety of neurohormonal stimulations or biomechanical stretch activations evoke cardiomyocyte hypertrophy through the activation of β-receptor and Gq agonist coupled receptors, such as angiotensin II and endothelin receptors. The stimulation of these receptors triggers the activation of intracellular second messengers, such as cyclic AMP and Ca^{2+}, thereby activating the downstream signaling pathway (Fig. 3.3). Among these signaling pathways, an increase in Ca^{2+} concentration drives the activation of Ca^{2+}-dependent phosphatase calcineurin[70] and Ca^{2+}-dependent protein kinases including protein kinase C (PKC), calmodulin-dependent kinase (CaMK), and mitogen-activated protein kinase (MAPK), while cyclic AMP activates protein kinase A. These signaling pathways ultimately cause subsequent activation of transcriptional factors such as NFAT, GATA-4, MEF-2, and so on,[75] thereby activating the cardiac hypertrophic gene program. In contrast, guanylyl cyclase-mediated protein kinase G signaling, a natriuretic peptide-associated intracellular signaling process, has been shown to be a mechanism that inhibits these hypertrophic transcriptional activations.[76] Furthermore, phosphorylation of a subclass of histone deacetylase (Class II), a chromatin-modifying enzyme, has been shown to modulate these hypertrophic signals, and also appears to

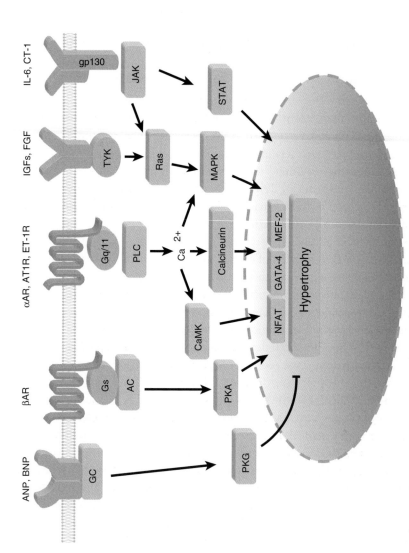

Fig. 3.3 Intracellular signaling associated with cardiomyocyte hypertrophy. Abbreviations: SERCA2a, sarcoendoplasmic reticulum calcium ATPase; RyR2, ryanodine receptor type 2; FKBP12.6, FK506-binding protein 12.6; PLN, phospholamban; PP1, protein phosphatase 1; PP2A, protein phosphatase 2A; mAKAP, muscle A-kinase anchoring protein.

negatively regulate cardiomyocyte hypertrophy.[77] Disruption or dominant negative inhibition of these pathways has been reported to inhibit either the hypertrophic phenotype or the eventual HF phenotype in experimental settings.[69,78,79] The modifiers of these signaling pathways are currently being examined to determine whether they will be useful for treatment of HF.[80] Future study in this field is warranted for the development of novel molecular therapies against pathological cardiac hypertrophy and HF.

Mitochondrial dysfunction and abnormal energy metabolism

Energy deprivation in the failing cardiomyocytes is another important aspect in understanding the abnormal intracellular signaling. In the failing heart it has been reported that an increase in reactive oxygen species (ROS) causes accelerated oxidative stress signaling in the heart.[81] Since in the normal heart the intracellular environment is physiologically maintained in a reduced condition to promote appropriate cellular signaling, these increases in oxidative stress signaling injure the appropriate protein folding and trigger DNA damage in the nucleus and mitochondria. Damage to mitochondrial DNA further causes a vicious cycle of increased oxidative stress and subsequent cellular damage.[82] Hence, mitochondrial energy production and regulation of ROS are also potential therapeutic targets in HF.[83]

Other neurohormonal regulators in HF

A large number of neurohormones have been found to circulate in abnormal quantities in HF. The natriuretic peptides—atrial natriuretic peptide (ANP), brain natriuretic peptide (BNP), and C-type natriuretic peptide–are thought to act as physiological counter-regulatory mechanisms against increased activity in the sympathetic nervous and renin–angiotensin–aldosterone systems,[84] because they decrease atrial pressure, promote urinalysis, reduce systemic vascular resistance, aldosterone secretion, sympathetic nerve activation and hypertrophy of the cardiomyocytes, and can promote sodium excretion. These natriuretic hormones are secreted in response to the elevated atrial and ventricular pressure, and play an important role in maintaining the complex circulatory integrity together with other hormones, including norepinephrine, the arginine-vasopressin system, and the renin–angiotensin–aldosterone system. Endothelins (ETs) are a family of vasoconstrictive peptides produced by vascular endothelial cells. Although the physiological role of ET is not yet precisely understood, serum ET levels are increased in HF patients. A drug that blocks ET receptor signaling, bosentan, has been tested to determine whether it is useful for treatment of HF; however, chronic ET blockade failed to improve the long-term outcome of HF patients.[85] These results suggest that the role of ET is not simply that of a vasospastic deleterious hormone in the complex circulatory homeostasis in HF, although its blockade seems to be beneficial in primary pulmonary hypertension.

Circulating tumor necrosis factor alpha (TNF-α), a proinflammatory cytokine, is increased in cachetic patients with HF. Additionally, interleukin 1 (IL-1) and IL-6 have also been reported to be increased in HF. Since inflammation may aggravate the outcome of patients with HF, blockade of TNF-α has been studied for the treatment of patients with late-stage HF; however, these trials have failed to demonstrate a survival benefit (see Chapter 13).[86]

Factors that aggravate HF

Factors that aggravate HF include increased uptake of water or sodium, infection, stress, poor blood pressure control, non-compliance with oral medication, transient cardiac arrhythmia including atrial fibrillation and tachycardia, anemia, and renal dysfunction, advanced aging, sleep apnea syndrome, lethal cardiac arrhythmia, and myocardial disease secondary to systemic disease such as amyloidosis or sarcoidosis. Appropriate adjunctive therapy, for example oxygen therapy for sleep apnea syndrome and anti-arrhythmic medicine for serious and paroxysmal arrhythmia, can mitigate the effects of HF.

Future clinical and research implications

Recent progress in molecular cardiology makes it possible to conceive a new therapeutic approach to HF targeting key molecules involved in intracellular Ca^{2+} handling (such as RyR, SERCA2a, PLN) and cardiac hypertrophy (i.e. anti-hypertrophic molecules). Controlling these molecular functions has been found to be beneficial in certain experimental conditions. However, it is not yet sufficient to set up a blueprint to apply these molecular characteristics of HF to treatment in clinical settings. This is because the heterogeneous nature of human HF as examined in these various studies (i.e. different stages and etiologies) may not be simply applied to the clinical settings. Clearly, further research is needed to determine whether these molecular approaches might be generally applicable for the treatment of HF. Such translational research could lead to novel therapeutic strategies for the treatment of HF.

Finally, from the clinical viewpoint, proper evaluation of HF pathophysiology as well as recognition of its background etiology is essential to structure a realistic therapeutic plan for the management of HF. In this regard, optimal care of the outpatient during everyday life, for example the assistance of non-physician clinicians in telephone support to check daily activities and proper compliance with medication in patients with HF,[87] may also be important to improve both the quality of life and long-term mortality.

References

1. American Heart Association (2005). *Heart Disease and Stroke Statistics 2005 Update*. Dallas: American Heart Association.
2. Sisson DD (2004). Neuroendocrine evaluation of cardiac disease. *Vet Clin North Am Small Anim Pract* **34**: 1105–26.
3. Chien KR (2000). Genomic circuits and the integrative biology of cardiac diseases. *Nature* **407**: 227–32.
4. Chien KR, Olson EN (2002). Converging pathways and principles in heart development and disease: CV@CSH. *Cell* **110**: 153–62.

5. Sagawa K, Maughan L, Suga H, Sunagawa K (1988). *Cardiac Contraction and the Pressure Volume Relationship*. New York: Oxford University Press.

6. Ross J, Jr (1976). Afterload mismatch and preload reserve: a conceptual framework for the analysis of ventricular function. *Prog Cardiovasc Dis* **18**: 255–64.

7. Chen J, Chien KR (1999). Complexity in simplicity: monogenic disorders and complex cardiomyopathies. *J Clin Invest* **103**: 1483–5.

8. Vasan RS, Benjamin EJ, Levy D (1995). Prevalence, clinical features and prognosis of diastolic heart failure: an epidemiologic perspective. *J Am Coll Cardiol* **26**: 1565–74.

9. Vasan RS, Benjamin EJ, Levy D (1996). Congestive heart failure with normal left ventricular systolic function. Clinical approaches to the diagnosis and treatment of diastolic heart failure. *Arch Intern Med* **156**: 146–57.

10. Gaasch WH, Zile MR (2004). Left ventricular diastolic dysfunction and diastolic heart failure. *Annu Rev Med* **55**: 373–94.

11. Galderisi M (2005). Diastolic dysfunction and diastolic heart failure: diagnostic, prognostic and therapeutic aspects. *Cardiovasc Ultrasound* **3**: 9.

12. Vasan RS, Larson MG, Benjamin EJ, Evans JC, Reiss CK, Levy D (1999), Congestive heart failure in subjects with normal versus reduced left ventricular ejection fraction: prevalence and mortality in a population-based cohort. *J Am Coll Cardiol* **33**: 1948–55.

13. Ahmed A (2004). Management of diastolic heart failure in older adults. *Br Med J* **328**: 1114.

14. Hunt SA, Baker DW, Chin MH *et al.* (2001). ACC/AHA guidelines for the evaluation and management of chronic heart failure in the adult: executive summary. A report of the American College of Cardiology/American Heart Association Task Force on Practice Guidelines (Committee to Revise the 1995 Guidelines for the Evaluation and Management of Heart Failure): developed in collaboration with the International Society for Heart and Lung Transplantation; endorsed by the Heart Failure Society of America. *Circulation* **104**: 2996–3007.

15. Hunt SA, Baker DW, Chin MH *et al.* (2001). ACC/AHA guidelines for the evaluation and management of chronic heart failure in the adult: executive summary. A report of the American College of Cardiology/American Heart Association Task Force on Practice Guidelines (committee to revise the 1995 guidelines for the evaluation and management of heart failure). *J Am Coll Cardiol* **38**: 2101–13.

16. Opie LH, Commerford PJ, Gersh BJ, Pfeffer MA. (2006). Controversies in ventricular remodelling. *Lancet* **367**: 356–67.

17. Morita H, Seidman J, Seidman CE (2005). Genetic causes of human heart failure. *J Clin Invest* **115**: 518–26.

18. Ahmad F, Seidman JG, Seidman CE (2005). The genetic basis for cardiac remodeling. *Annu Rev Genomics Hum Genet* **6**: 185–216.

19. Towbin JA, Bowles NE (2002). The failing heart. *Nature* **415**: 227–33.

20. Zhang J, Kumar A, Stalker HJ *et al.* (2001). Clinical and molecular studies of a large family with desmin-associated restrictive cardiomyopathy. *Clin Genet* **59**: 248–56.

21. Mogensen J, Kubo T, Duque M *et al.* (2003). Idiopathic restrictive cardiomyopathy is part of the clinical expression of cardiac troponin I mutations. *J Clin Invest* **111**: 209–16.

22. Umana E, Solares CA, Alpert MA (2003). Tachycardia-induced cardiomyopathy. *Am J Med* **114**: 51–5.

23. Chien KR, Karsenty G (2005). Longevity and lineages: toward the integrative biology of degenerative diseases in heart, muscle, and bone. *Cell* **120**: 533–44.

24. Paul O (1989). Background of the prevention of cardiovascular disease. I. Nutritional, infectious, and alcoholic heart disease. *Circulation* **79**: 1361–8.

25. Paul O (1989). Background of the prevention of cardiovascular disease. II. Arteriosclerosis, hypertension, and selected risk factors. *Circulation* **80**: 206–14.

26. Rassi A, Jr, Rassi A, Little WC (2000). Chagas' heart disease. *Clin Cardiol* **23**: 883–9.

27. Packer M (1992). The neurohormonal hypothesis: a theory to explain the mechanism of disease progression in heart failure. *J Am Coll Cardiol* **20**: 248–54.

28. Cruickshank JM (1993). Phosphodiesterase III inhibitors: long-term risks and short-term benefits. *Cardiovasc Drugs Ther* **7**: 655–60.

29. Cohn JN, Archibald DG, Ziesche S *et al.* (1986). Effect of vasodilator therapy on mortality in chronic congestive heart failure. Results of a Veterans Administration Cooperative Study. *New Engl J Med* **314**: 1547–52.

30. The CONSENSUS Trial Study Group (1987). Effects of enalapril on mortality in severe congestive heart failure. Results of the Cooperative North Scandinavian Enalapril Survival Study (CONSENSUS). *New Engl J Med* **316**: 1429–35.

31. The SOLVD Investigators (1991). Effect of enalapril on survival in patients with reduced left ventricular ejection fractions and congestive heart failure. *New Engl J Med* **325**: 293–302.

32. The SOLVD Investigators (1992). Effect of enalapril on mortality and the development of heart failure in asymptomatic patients with reduced left ventricular ejection fractions. *New Engl J Med* **327**: 685–91.

33. Varagic J, Frohlich ED (2002). Local cardiac renin-angiotensin system: hypertension and cardiac failure. *J Mol Cell Cardiol* **34**: 1435–42.

34. Re RN (2004). Mechanisms of disease: local renin-angiotensin-aldosterone systems and the pathogenesis and treatment of cardiovascular disease. *Nature Clin Pract Cardiovasc Med* **1**: 42–7.

35. O'Connell TD, Swigart PM, Rodrigo MC *et al.* (2006). Alpha1-adrenergic receptors prevent a maladaptive cardiac response to pressure overload. *J Clin Invest* **116**: 1005–15.

36. Yusuf S, Pfeffer MA, Swedberg K *et al.* (2003). Effects of candesartan in patients with chronic heart failure and preserved left-ventricular ejection fraction: the CHARM-Preserved Trial. *Lancet* **362**: 777–81.

37. Granger CB, McMurray JJ, Yusuf S *et al.* (2003). Effects of candesartan in patients with chronic heart failure and reduced left-ventricular systolic function intolerant to angiotensin-converting-enzyme inhibitors: the CHARM-Alternative trial. *Lancet* **362**: 772–6.

38. McMurray JJ, Ostergren J, Swedberg K *et al.* (2003). Effects of candesartan in patients with chronic heart failure and reduced left-ventricular systolic function taking angiotensin-converting-enzyme inhibitors: the CHARM-Added trial. *Lancet* **362**: 767–71.

39. Pfeffer MA, Swedberg K, Granger CB *et al.* (2003). Effects of candesartan on mortality and morbidity in patients with chronic heart failure: the CHARM-Overall programme. *Lancet* **362**: 759–66.

40. Cohn JN, Tognoni G (2001). A randomized trial of the angiotensin-receptor blocker valsartan in chronic heart failure. *New Engl J Med* **345**: 1667–75.

41. Pitt B, Segal R, Martinez FA *et al.* (1997). Randomised trial of losartan versus captopril in patients over 65 with heart failure (Evaluation of Losartan in the Elderly Study, ELITE). *Lancet* **349**: 747–52.

42. Urata H, Hoffmann S, Ganten D (1994). Tissue angiotensin II system in the human heart. *Eur Heart J* **15**(Suppl. D): 68–78.

43. Fleming I (2006). Signaling by the angiotensin-converting enzyme. *Circ Res* **98**: 887–96.

44. Pitt B, Williams G, Remme W *et al.* (2001). The EPHESUS trial: eplerenone in patients with heart failure due to systolic dysfunction complicating acute myocardial infarction. Eplerenone Post-AMI Heart Failure Efficacy and Survival Study. *Cardiovasc Drugs Ther* **15**: 79–87.

45. Pitt B, Zannad F, Remme WJ *et al.* (1999). The effect of spironolactone on morbidity and mortality in patients with severe heart failure. Randomized Aldactone Evaluation Study Investigators. *New Engl J Med* **341**: 709–17.

46. Rocha R, Funder JW (2002). The pathophysiology of aldosterone in the cardiovascular system. *Ann NY Acad Sci* **970**: 89–100.

47. Cohn JN, Levine TB, Olivari MT *et al.* (1984). Plasma norepinephrine as a guide to prognosis in patients with chronic congestive heart failure. *New Engl J Med* **311**: 819–23.

48. Dorn GW, 2nd (2002). Adrenergic pathways and left ventricular remodeling. *J Card Fail* **8**: S370–S373.

49. Bristow M (2003). Antiadrenergic therapy of chronic heart failure: surprises and new opportunities. *Circulation* **107**: 1100–2.

50. Bers DM (2002). Cardiac excitation–contraction coupling. *Nature* **415**: 198–205.

51. Rockman HA, Koch WJ, Lefkowitz RJ (2002). Seven-transmembrane-spanning receptors and heart function. *Nature* **415**: 206–12.

52. Marx SO, Reiken S, Hisamatsu Y *et al.* (2000). PKA phosphorylation dissociates FKBP12.6 from the calcium release channel (ryanodine receptor): defective regulation in failing hearts. *Cell* **101**: 365–76.

53. Yano M, Ono K, Ohkusa T *et al.* (2000). Altered stoichiometry of FKBP12.6 versus ryanodine receptor as a cause of abnormal Ca(2$^+$) leak through ryanodine receptor in heart failure. *Circulation* **102**: 2131–6.

54. Doi M, Yano M, Kobayashi S *et al.* (2002). Propranolol prevents the development of heart failure by restoring FKBP12.6-mediated stabilization of ryanodine receptor. *Circulation* **105**: 1374–9.

55. Sim AT, Scott JD (1999). Targeting of PKA, PKC and protein phosphatases to cellular microdomains. *Cell Calcium* **26**: 209–17.

56. Boknik P, Fockenbrock M, Herzig S *et al.* (2000). Protein phosphatase activity is increased in a rat model of long-term beta-adrenergic stimulation. *Naunyn Schmiedebergs Arch Pharmacol* **362**: 222–31.

57. Huang B, Wang S, Qin D, Boutjdir M, El-Sherif N (1999). Diminished basal phosphorylation level of phospholamban in the postinfarction remodeled rat ventricle: role of beta-adrenergic pathway, G(i) protein, phosphodiesterase, and phosphatases. *Circ Res* **85**: 848–55.

58. Gupta RC, Mishra S, Rastogi S, Imai M, Habib O, Sabbah HN (2003). Cardiac SR-coupled PP1 activity and expression are increased and inhibitor 1 protein expression is decreased in failing hearts. *Am J Physiol Heart Circ Physiol* **285**: H2373–H2381.

59. Neumann J, Eschenhagen T, Jones LR *et al.* (1997). Increased expression of cardiac phosphatases in patients with end-stage heart failure. *J Mol Cell Cardiol* **29**: 265–72.

60. Yamada M, Ikeda Y, Yano M *et al.* (2006). Inhibition of protein phosphatase 1 by inhibitor-2 gene delivery ameliorates heart failure progression in genetic cardiomyopathy. *FASEB J* **20**: 1197–9.

61. Lehnart SE, Wehrens XH, Reiken S *et al.* (2005). Phosphodiesterase 4D deficiency in the ryanodine-receptor complex promotes heart failure and arrhythmias. *Cell* **123**: 25–35.

62. del Monte F, Hajjar RJ (2003). Targeting calcium cycling proteins in heart failure through gene transfer. *J Physiol* **546**: 49–61.

63. Hajjar RJ, del Monte F, Matsui T, Rosenzweig A (2000). Prospects for gene therapy for heart failure. *Circ Res* **86**: 616–21.

64. Minamisawa S, Hoshijima M, Chu G *et al.* (1999). Chronic phospholamban-sarcoplasmic reticulum calcium ATPase interaction is the critical calcium cycling defect in dilated cardiomyopathy. *Cell* **99**: 313–22.

65. Hoshijima M, Ikeda Y, Iwanaga Y *et al.* (2002). Chronic suppression of heart-failure progression by a pseudophosphorylated mutant of phospholamban via in vivo cardiac rAAV gene delivery. *Nature Med* **8**: 864–71.

66. Iwanaga Y, Hoshijima M, Gu Y *et al.* (2004). Chronic phospholamban inhibition prevents progressive cardiac dysfunction and pathological remodeling after infarction in rats. *J Clin Invest* **113**: 727–36.

67. Zhang T, Maier LS, Dalton ND *et al.* (2003). The deltaC isoform of CaMKII is activated in cardiac hypertrophy and induces dilated cardiomyopathy and heart failure. *Circ Res* **92**: 912–19.

68. Zhang T, Brown JH (2004). Role of Ca^{2+}/calmodulin-dependent protein kinase II in cardiac hypertrophy and heart failure. *Cardiovasc Res* **63**: 476–86.

69. Braz JC, Gregory K, Pathak A *et al.* (2004). PKC-alpha regulates cardiac contractility and propensity toward heart failure. *Nature Med* **10**: 248–54.

70. Molkentin JD, Lu JR, Antos CL *et al.* (1998). A calcineurin-dependent transcriptional pathway for cardiac hypertrophy. *Cell* **93**: 215–28.

71. Wu X, Zhang T, Bossuyt J *et al.* (2006). Local InsP3-dependent perinuclear Ca^{2+} signaling in cardiac myocyte excitation-transcription coupling. *J Clin Invest* **116**: 675–82.

72. Rockman HA, Ross RS, Harris AN *et al.* (1991). Segregation of atrial-specific and inducible expression of an atrial natriuretic factor transgene in an in vivo murine model of cardiac hypertrophy. *Proc Natl Acad Sci USA* **88**: 8277–81.

73. Olson EN, Schneider MD (2003). Sizing up the heart: development redux in disease. *Genes Dev* **17**: 1937–56.

74. Hunter JJ, Chien KR (1999). Signaling pathways for cardiac hypertrophy and failure. *New Engl J Med* **341**: 1276–83.

75. Olson EN (2004). A decade of discoveries in cardiac biology. *Nature Med* **10**: 467–74.

76. McFarlane SI, Winer N, Sowers JR (2003). Role of the natriuretic peptide system in cardiorenal protection. *Arch Intern Med* **163**: 2696–704.

77. Zhang CL, McKinsey TA, Chang S, Antos CL, Hill JA, Olson EN (2002). Class II histone deacetylases act as signal-responsive repressors of cardiac hypertrophy. *Cell* **110**: 479–88.

78. Vega RB, Bassel-Duby R, Olson EN (2003). Control of cardiac growth and function by calcineurin signaling. *J Biol Chem* **278**: 36981–4.

79. Zhang R, Khoo MS, Wu Y *et al.* (2005). Calmodulin kinase II inhibition protects against structural heart disease. *Nature Med* **11**: 409–17.

80. McKinsey TA, Olson EN (2005). Toward transcriptional therapies for the failing heart: chemical screens to modulate genes. *J Clin Invest* **115**: 538–46.

81. Giordano FJ (2005). Oxygen, oxidative stress, hypoxia, and heart failure. *J Clin Invest* **115**: 500–8.

82. Russell LK, Finck BN, Kelly DP (2005). Mouse models of mitochondrial dysfunction and heart failure. *J Mol Cell Cardiol* **38**: 81–91.

83. Huss JM, Kelly DP (2005). Mitochondrial energy metabolism in heart failure: a question of balance. *J Clin Invest* **115**: 547–55.

84. McGrath MF, de Bold ML, de Bold AJ (2005). The endocrine function of the heart. *Trends Endocrinol Metab* **16**: 469–77.

85. Kirchengast M, Luz M (2005). Endothelin receptor antagonists: clinical realities and future directions. *J Cardiovasc Pharmacol* **45**: 182–91.

86. Muller-Ehmsen J, Schwinger RH (2004). TNF and congestive heart failure: therapeutic possibilities. *Expert Opin Ther Targets* **8**: 203–9.

87. GESICA Investigators (2005). Randomised trial of telephone intervention in chronic heart failure: DIAL trial. *Br Med J* **331**: 425.

Chapter 4

Heart failure—optimal pharmacological therapy

J. Paul Rocchiccioli and John J. V. McMurray

Introduction

The treatment of heart failure (HF) continues to be refined and improved.[1] Our greater understanding of the pathophysiology and natural history of HF has allowed the development of targeted therapy to achieve symptom control, reduce hospital admissions, and prolong life. On the basis of large and robust randomized controlled trials, drugs are the established mainstay of treatment for patients with HF, particularly those with reduced left-ventricular function. These benefits appear to have been translated to the greater unselected population, with observational studies demonstrating improvements in outcome which temporally correlate with the emergence of evidenced-based therapy.[2,3]

The health-care professional treating patients with HF faces several challenges in implementing optimal therapy. Studies of prescribing patterns show delays in uptake of evidence-based therapy in both hospitals and primary care.[4,5] This under-treatment denies patients the benefits of these proven treatments. Delays may be due to the unfamiliarity of physicians with the evidence, concern over adverse effects, or to the perceived problems of polypharmacy. This is certainly a problem in a predominantly elderly population with associated co-morbidities. In contrast, other therapies have been embraced more rapidly and, at times, inappropriately. This is best illustrated with the aldosterone antagonist spironolactone. Inappropriate use of this drug has been associated with an unacceptable rate of serious adverse events related to hyperkalaemia.[6] This further reinforces the need for appropriate awareness of practical clinical guidelines for all health-care professionals treating patients with HF.

The best-accepted approach is to use proven agents in their proven dosing regimens and not to simply assume a 'class effect'. Current guidelines accept the potential difficulties in implementing optimal practice and advise us that some drug is better than none.[7] These treatment combinations are nevertheless complicated and best managed in a structured care setting. A standard of optimal care with staged, disease-modifying therapy has been established for all patients with left-ventricular dysfunction. For patients with persisting symptoms, a stepwise approach of additional therapy provides both symptomatic and prognostic benefits.

Diuretics

Diuretics were amongst the first therapies to be used in the treatment of HF. They are needed in virtually all patients with dyspnoea or evidence of salt and water retention.[8] They provide rapid relief of these symptoms and signs and are best used in the minimum dose needed to maintain euvolaemia. Although highly effective in this way, diuretics themselves are not a sufficient treatment for HF and should be co-administered with a proven disease-modifying agent. Indeed, need for a diuretic indicates the need, unless there is a contraindication or proven intolerance, for an ACE inhibitor and β-blocker (and possibly other treatments).

Mechanism of action

The different diuretics exert their pharmacological actions within different parts of the nephron.[9] A ubiquitous feature is the blockade of sodium reabsorption within the renal tubules, thus enhancing sodium excretion with associated water loss. This sodium loss is often associated with the loss of other metabolically important electrolytes and may interfere with the renal handling of organic solutes such as uric acid.

The diuretic effect of the thiazides (e.g. bendroflumethiazide) is relatively weak. They act by blockade of the sodium/chloride transporter in the distal renal convoluted tubule. Loop diuretics (e.g. furosemide, bumetanide) act by blocking the sodium/potassium/chloride transporter in the thick ascending limb of the loop of Henle. In contrast to these drugs, which are associated with 'bystander' loss of potassium, the potassium-sparing diuretics (e.g. amiloride) decrease sodium reabsorption and potassium excretion by antagonism of a sodium/potassium transporter in the distal tubule and may thus be associated with an elevation of plasma potassium. Aldosterone antagonists are also potassium sparing, and because of their other benefits (see below) have largely rendered other potassium-sparing diuretics redundant.

Clinical benefits

Although not proven to improve mortality and morbidity in randomized controlled trials, the clinical use of diuretics is well established and widespread.[8] No other treatment provides such rapid relief of symptoms and clinical fluid overload. The rapid relief of symptoms may be explained by a reduction in left-ventricular filling pressure in the initial stages of therapy. Once initiated, most patients will require diuretic therapy indefinitely to maintain euvolaemia.

Adverse effects and interactions

Hypokalaemia, hyponatraemia, hypocalcaemia, and hypomagnesaemia are common features of long-term therapy. There is also a tendency to hypochloraemic metabolic alkalosis. Of particular concern is the increased risk of arrhythmias associated with hypokalaemia and hypomagnesaemia in an already high-risk population.

The renal handling of uric acid is adversely affected by diuretics, leading to a propensity for gout. Less common effects include elevated serum glucose and lipids in thiazide therapy and ototoxicity with high-dose loop diuretics.

In a predominantly elderly patient population, the rapid onset and intense diuresis these agents provoke may cause significant social inconvenience, particularly in those with history of bladder weakness or incontinence.

Combination diuretic therapy (e.g. a loop and thiazide) will intuitively increase the risk of renal dysfunction and electrolyte imbalance. Particular caution and monitoring must be undertaken, with co-administration of an aldosterone antagonist and potassium supplementation as needed. Co-administration with non-steroidal anti-inflammatory drugs (NSAIDs), either non-specific or specific COX-2 inhibitors, impairs the natriuretic effect of diuretics and may reduce glomerular filtration rate, further compromising renal function.[10] This group of drugs should generally be avoided in patients with HF.

Practical use (Table 4.1)

Diuretics should be prescribed flexibly, and at the minimum dose required to maintain euvolaemia whilst avoiding electrolyte imbalance or metabolic effects. These electrolyte abnormalities may be partly offset by co-administration of ACE inhibitors, potassium-sparing agents, or electrolyte replacement therapy. Temporary dose increases may be necessary during periods of fluid overload and should be appropriately reduced if there are any signs or symptoms of hypovolaemia. In some patients with very mild HF symptoms, a small dose of thiazide diuretic may suffice.

Table 4.1 Practical diuretic use

Drug class	Initial dose (mg)		Maximum recommended daily dose (mg)	
Loop diuretics				
Furosemide	20–40		250–500	
Bumetanide	0.5–1.0		5–10	
Torasamide	5–10		100–200	
Thiazide diuretics				
Bendroflumethiazide	2.5		10	
Hydrochlorothiazide	25		50–75	
Indapamide	2.5		2.5	
Metolazone	2.5		10	
Potassium-sparing diuretics	+ACEi	−ACEi	+ACEi	−ACEi
Amiloride	2.5	5	20	40
Triamterene	2.5	500	100	200
Spironolactone	12.5–25	50	50	100–200
Cautions/seek specialist advice in:	Hypo/hyperkalaemia Renal dysfunction (glomerular filtration rate <30ml min⁻¹) Diabetes mellitus Hyperlipidaemia Gout			

However, with increasing severity of HF and associated renal dysfunction, loop diuretics are usually necessary. They produce a more potent and rapid diuresis than thiazides. The oral bioavailability of furosemide is around 50% with higher absorption of bumetanide or torasamide of the order of 80–100%.

Advanced HF and long-term use of a loop diuretic may be associated with a loss of clinical efficacy. This is known as diuretic resistance. The precise mechanism remains unclear, but probably reflects reduced bioavailability through impaired intestinal absorption, hypotension, and renal perfusion as well as maladaptive changes in the nephron promoting sodium reabsorption. Higher doses may be required, or the combination with a thiazide or thiazide-like diuretic (e.g. metolazone) to produce a synergistic 'double nephron blockade' and temporary improvement in diuresis.[11] Close biochemical monitoring is mandatory when such combinations are used.

Angiotensin-converting enzyme inhibitors

Angiotensin-converting enzyme (ACE) inhibitors are considered the first-line therapy in the management of HF with reduced left-ventricular systolic function. This premise is supported by multiple randomized clinical trials and almost two decades of use in wider clinical practice. These agents were initially used for their vasodilatory properties. However, our greater understanding of the pathophysiology of HF suggests that there are probably additional beneficial effects of blockade of the adverse neurohormonal cascade associated with the HF syndrome.[12]

Mechanism of action

These drugs act by inhibiting the enzyme that converts the inactive angiotensin I to the active angiotensin II. The neurohormonal response to HF includes excessive production of angiotensin II which exerts its adverse effects through the angiotensin II receptor subtype-1 (AT_1R). These maladaptive processes include excessive vasoconstriction, left-ventricular remodelling, activation of the sympathetic nervous system and promoting a hypercoagulable state. Angiotensin II promotes retention of water and sodium through augmentation of arginine vasopressin and aldosterone release as well as exerting a direct effect in the renal tubule. These effects are antagonized by ACE inhibition. Some of the biological effects of ACE inhibition may be secondary to the reduced breakdown of the vasodilator bradykinin (ACE inhibitors also inhibit kininase II). In addition to its vasodilatory properties, the increase of biologically active bradykinin may inhibit pathological growth and remodelling and exert an anti-thrombotic action.

Clinical benefits

The potential value of ACE inhibition was first suggested by studies demonstrating improved haemodynamics and symptom control. In the landmark Cooperative North Scandinavian Enalapril Survival (CONSENSUS) study, 253 patients with severe (NYHA class IV) HF were randomized to receive placebo or enalapril at a target dose of 20 mg twice daily.[13] There was a 40% ($p = 0.003$) relative risk reduction of the principal endpoint of mortality with further improvements in hospital admissions and recorded symptoms. In the largest study, the treatment arm of the Studies of Left Ventricular Dysfunction (SOLVD-T), 2569 patients with mild to severe HF were randomized to receive placebo or enalapril at a target dose of 10 mg twice daily.[14] There was a 16% ($p = 0.0036$) relative risk reduction of the primary endpoint of mortality. There were similar substantial improvements in hospital admissions.

The remarkable clinical benefits of ACE inhibitors have been further demonstrated in both symptomatic and asymptomatic patients, with reduced left-ventricular systolic function, after acute myocardial infarction.[15–17] These agents have also been shown to reduce the risk of myocardial infarction, diabetes, stroke, and atrial fibrillation.[18,19] Whilst a class effect may be assumed, the best clinical approach is to use proven agents in the dosing regimens supported by clinical trials (Figure 4.1).

The use of 'high'-dose ACE inhibition has been investigated by the ATLAS trial which compared a low dose (2.5–5.0 mg) with a high dose (32.5–35mg) of lisinopril. There was no significant difference in the primary endpoint of death from any cause between the low- and high-dose regimens. Patients in the high-dose group, however, had a lower

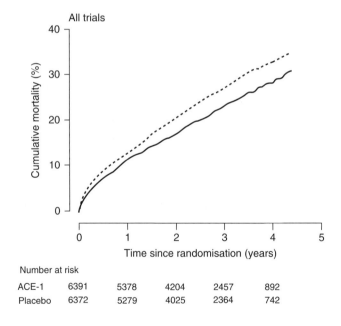

Number at risk					
ACE-1	6391	5378	4204	2457	892
Placebo	6372	5279	4025	2364	742

Fig. 4.1 Mortality curve from the meta-analysis of long term (>1 year) placebo-controlled trials (>1000 patients) of ACE inhibitors in chronic HF or left-ventricular dysfunction after a recent myocardial infarction. (Reprinted from Flather MD, Yusuf S, Kober L et al. Long-term ACE-inhibitor therapy in patients with heart failure or left-ventricular dysfunction: a systematic overview of data from individual patients. ACE-inhibitor myocardial infarction collaborative group. *Lancet* **355**: 1575–81. Copyright ©2000, with permission from Elsevier.)

risk of the composite outcomes of death or admission to hospital ($p = 0.002$) and cardiovascular death or cardiovascular admission ($p = 0.03$); they also had a lower risk of cardiovascular admission ($p = 0.04$) and chronic HF admission (relative risk reduction 24%, $p < 0.001$) than patients in the low-dose lisinopril group.[20]

Adverse effects and interactions

The reduced bioactivity of angiotensin II may result in hypotension, a decrease in renal perfusion, and a reduction in the glomerular filtration rate. Patients should be carefully monitored for excessive hypotension, hyperkalaemia, or renal dysfunction. Serum creatinine may increase by 10–15% from baseline irrespective of prior renal dysfunction. Changes in serum potassium are usually small (< 0.2 mmol L^{-1}). These effects may be exacerbated by co-administration of blood-pressure lowering (e.g. calcium channel blockers) or nephrotoxic agents (e.g. NSAIDs) and potassium supplements or potassium-sparing diuretics.

Bradykinin accumulation is associated with a dry non-productive cough, which occurs in up to 15% of patients. This occasionally necessitates a switch to angiotensin receptor blocking agents (ARBs). This may also be associated with troublesome rash or, rarely, angioedema. In the latter case, ACE inhibitor should be stopped and an ARB substituted with caution.

Practical use

Therapy should be started with a low initial dose and doubled slowly, aiming for the target dose or the highest tolerated dose. Dose increments were previously advised at not less than 2-weekly intervals, but in a stable patient with a satisfactory blood pressure and renal function more rapid titration is possible, provided the patient can be monitored appropriately. An ACE inhibitor should be used cautiously in the presence of significant hypotension (systolic blood pressure (BP) <90 mmHg) and is contraindicated in a patient with bilateral renal artery stenosis. The previously unrecognized presence of the latter may also be indicated by a precipitous deterioration in renal function. Moderate renal dysfunction (creatinine up to 221 μmol L^{-1}/2.5 mg dl^{-1}) is not a contraindication to therapy but does indicate the need for close monitoring. Serum electrolytes and renal function should be monitored 1–2 weeks following treatment initiation and each dose increment. A rise in creatinine of up to 50% of baseline or to 266 μmol/3 mg dl^{-1}, whichever is the lower, is acceptable. A potassium of ≤ 5.5 mmol L^{-1} is acceptable (Table 4.2).

Patients who develop symptomatic hypotension should be carefully evaluated for evidence of hypovolaemia, and if necessary diuretic therapy should be reduced. With derangement of renal function or excessive hyperkalaemia, firstly one should consider obvious drug interactions; thereafter, consider halving ACE inhibitor dose whilst monitoring blood chemistry and considering investigation for underlying renovascular disease. It is rarely necessary to stop an ACE inhibitor, and doing so may risk clinical deterioration. Thus, specialist advice should be sought before therapy is discontinued.

Table 4.2 Practical ACE inhibitor use

Drug	Initial dose (mg)	Target dose (mg)
Captopril	6.25 thrice daily	50 thrice daily
Enalapril	2.5 twice daily	10–20 twice daily
Lisinopril	2.5–5 once daily	20–35 once daily
Ramipril	2.5 once daily	10 once or 5 twice daily
dailyTrandolapril	0.5 once daily	4 once daily
Cautions/seek specialist advice:	Significant hyperkalaemia (K$^+$ >5.0 mmol L^{-1}) Significant renal dysfunction (creatinine >221µmol L^{-1} or >2.5 mg dl^{-1}) Symptomatic or severe asymptomatic hypotension (systolic BP < 90 mmHg)	
Dose titration:	Double at not less than 2-weekly intervals Monitor blood pressure and blood chemistry 1–2 weeks after initiation and at each increment Aim for target dose, or highest tolerated dose	

Angiotensin receptor blockers

Angiotensin receptor blockers (ARBs) are the most recent class of drugs to be shown to be of benefit in HF. The recent and evolving evidence base for this drug group has been controversial, not least because of difficulties in trial design and the ethics of comparison with drugs of proven benefit such as ACE inhibitors. Nonetheless, there is now robust evidence that an ARB provides similar benefits to an ACE inhibitor but, much more importantly, additional benefits in patients already treated with standard neurohormonal therapy including an ACE inhibitor and β-blocker.

Mechanism of action

ARBs prevent the binding of angiotensin II to its type 1 receptor and provide an alternative means of blocking the renin–angiotensin system (RAS). It is recognized that angiotensin II is produced by enzymes other than ACE, and thus ACE inhibitors may, in theory, be less effective at blocking the harmful effects of angiotensin II than ARBs.[21] Angiotensin type-1 receptor blockade also makes more angiotensin II available to stimulate the unblocked type 2 receptor (and perhaps other subtypes) which may have beneficial actions in reducing disease progression.[22] ARBs do not inhibit breakdown of kininase II and bradykinin, and are thus not associated with cough, and rarely with angioedema. On the other hand, inhibition of bradykinin breakdown may also be beneficial in HF as bradykinin has vasodilator, anti-mitotic, and fibrinolytic actions. The net benefit of an ARB compared with an ACE inhibitor may, therefore, reflect more complete blockade of the actions of angiotensin with an ARB but additional effects of bradykinin accumulation with an ACE inhibitor. Arguably, the use of both types of agent together might give the best overall effect ('the best of both worlds').

Clinical benefits

Several trials have been undertaken in an attempt to overcome the difficulties in comparing this new drug class with ACE inhibitors which have established and incontrovertible
benefits. The first approach involved a head-to-head comparison with an established
ACE inhibitor. The ELITE-II (Evaluation of Losartan in the Elderly) study compared the
tolerability and efficacy of losartan 50 mg once daily, with captopril 50 mg three times
daily in 3152 patients with NYHA Class II–IV HF.[23] Although there was no significant
difference in all-cause mortality, there was a strong trend in favour of captopril. Losartan
appeared to be significantly better tolerated, with fewer discontinuations, perhaps
suggesting the dose was too low—an ARB should probably not cause less hypotension or
renal dysfunction than an ACE inhibitor.

The second approach has been to examine the role of ARBs versus placebo, added to an
ACE inhibitor. In the Val-HeFT (Valsartan Heart Failure Trial) trial, 5010 patients were
randomized to placebo or valsartan at target dose of 160 mg twice daily. The majority
(93%) of patients were on standard background therapy, including an ACE inhibitor.

There was no effect on all-cause mortality but a significant reduction in the
composite endpoint of mortality or morbidity (mainly HF hospitalizations)
(hazard ratio (HR) 0.87; $p = 0.009$).

In a retrospective analysis, valsartan improved the combined endpoint of mortality
and morbidity alone in a small subgroup of patients not receiving an ACE inhibitor.[24,25]
Meta-analyses show similar efficacy of ARBs on mortality and morbidity and have

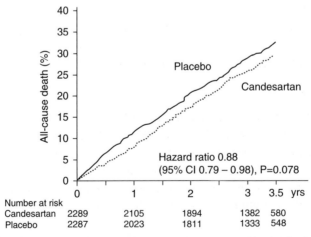

Fig. 4.2 Mortality curve from the pooling of CHARM-Alternative and CHARM-Added trials
(Reproduced from Young JB, Dunlap ME, Pfeffer MA (2004). Mortality and morbidity reduction
with candesartan in patients with chronic heart failure and left-ventricular systolic dysfunction:
results of the CHARM low-left-ventricular ejection fraction trials. *Circulation* **26**: 110(17):
2618–26, with permission from Lippincott, Williams & Wilkins.)

recently been supported by another randomized trial in patients with HF, left-ventricular systolic dysfunction, or both complicating acute myocardial infarction.[26]

These findings have been confirmed and extended by the CHARM (Candesartan in Heart Failure: Assessment of Reduction in Mortality and Morbidity) programme. The CHARM-Alternative trial randomized 2028 patients who were previous intolerant to ACE inhibitor to placebo or candesartan at target dose of 32 mg once daily.[27] The risk of death from a cardiovascular cause or hospitalization for HF was reduced by 23% ($p = 0.0004$). The benefits of candesartan were consistent across a range of subgroups irrespective of background therapy. These benefits were of a similar magnitude as those seen in previous ACE inhibitor trials (Figure 4.2).

The CHARM-Added trial has identified an important role for ARBs in the larger population of HF patients already on standard neurohormonal therapy.[28] In this study, 2548 patients, all treated with an ACE inhibitor (and in 55% of cases a β-blocker), were treated with candesartan at a target dose of 32 mg once daily. There was a 15% reduction in relative risk in the primary endpoint of death from a cardiovascular cause or hospitalization for HF (HR 0.85; $p = 0.011$). Candesartan was also effective when added to either 'high' or 'lower' dose ACE inhibitor treatment.[29] These findings are consistent with recent favourable effects of 'triple therapy' on left-ventricular remodelling.[30] Consequently, the addition of an ARB to both an ACE inhibitor and β-blocker should be considered in any patient with persisting symptoms, i.e. in NYHA Class II–IV.

Adverse effects and interactions

Blockade of the effects of angiotensin II generally produces the same adverse reactions as during ACE inhibitor therapy. Effects such as hypotension, hyperkalaemia, and renal dysfunction are encountered as frequently and similar treatment initiation and monitoring is advocated (see above).

Use of multiple inhibitors of the RAS requires even more diligent monitoring, especially in those with higher baseline risk (i.e. patients aged ≥75 years or with a systolic blood pressure < 100 mmHg, diabetes, or renal impairment).

Practical use

As with an ACE inhibitor, the specific agents, dosing regimens, and target doses used in clinical trials demonstrating benefits are recommended (Table 4.3). Those trials demonstrating most clinical benefit used large target doses (candesartan 32 mg once daily in CHARM-Added and CHARM-Alternative; valsartan 160 mg twice daily in Val-HeFT). This suggests that higher doses are required to achieve maximal benefit. There is also evidence of incremental benefits of high-dose ARBs beyond those achieved with an ACE inhibitor alone.

β-Blockers

The detrimental effects of an activated sympathetic nervous system in HF have been known for several decades. Despite this, few considered β-blockade as a therapy in HF and many considered them contraindicated. β-Blockers are considered the greatest

Table 4.3 Practical angiotensin receptor blocker use

Drug	Initial dose (mg)	Target dose (mg)
Candesartan	4 or 8 once daily	32 once daily
Valsartan	40 twice daily	160 twice daily
Cautions/seek specialist advice:	Significant hyperkalaemia (K^+ > 5.0 mmol L^{-1}) Significant renal dysfunction (creatinine > 221 µmol L^{-1} or > 2.5 mg dl^{-1}) Symptomatic or severe asymptomatic hypotension (systolic BP < 90 mmHg)	
Dose titration:	Double at not less than 2-weekly intervals Monitor blood pressure and blood chemistry 1–2 weeks after initiation and at each increment Aim for target dose, or highest tolerated dose	

advance in the treatment of HF since ACE inhibitors and lead to a further substantial reduction in mortality and morbidity. The beneficial effects have been consistently observed across all subgroups and irrespective of HF aetiology. These benefits were identified early with the three landmark trials terminating prematurely after around 1-year follow-up. With ACE inhibition, β-blockade is considered the first line and foundation of HF therapy (see also Pathophysiology, Chapter 3).

Mechanism of action

β-Blockers counteract the harmful effects of sympathetic activation in HF by antagonizing the effects of norepinephrine and epinephrine. In the short term, conventional doses of β-blockers have an adverse haemodynamic effect as they reduce heart rate, force of contraction, and cardiac output and increase systemic vascular resistance.[31] The key is therefore to start with a very small dose and subsequently increase the dose in a slow, step-wise fashion. With chronic therapy, reduction in cardiac dimensions, improved myocardial contractility, and stabilization of cardiac rhythm (which may reduce the risk of lethal arrhythmia and sudden cardiac death) are observed.

Clinical benefits

Each of the three landmark randomized controlled trials produced an approximately 33% relative reduction in the risk of death and similarly substantial and impressive reductions in hospital admissions. The effective agents used were a slow-release preparation of metoprolol (succinate) in MERIT-HF (Metoprolol CR/XL Randomised Intervention Trial in Congestive Heart Failure), bisoprolol in CIBIS-2 (Cardiac Insufficiency Bisoprolol Study), and carvedilol in the COPERNICUS (Effect of Carvedilol on Survival in Severe Chronic Heart Failure) study.[32–34] In the recent SENIORS (Study of the Effects of Nebivolol Intervention on Outcomes and Re-hospitalisation in Seniors

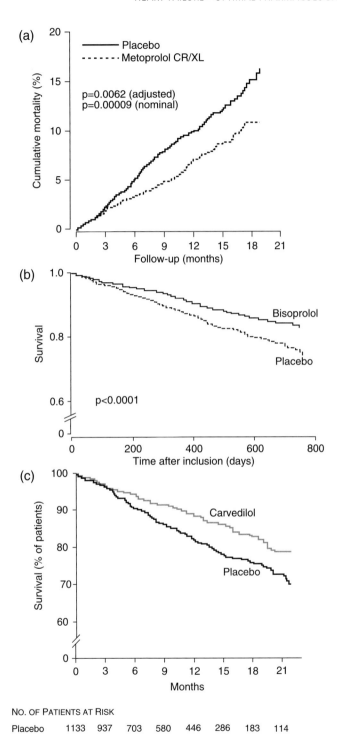

Fig. 4.3 Kaplan–Meier curves of the three major survival studies with beta blocker therapy: (a) MERIT-HF; (b) CIBIS-II; (c) COPERNICUS. (Reprinted from CIBIS Investigators[33], Copyright (c)1999 with permission from Elsevier.)

with Heart Failure) study, nebivolol, a β-blocker with vasodilating properties, was shown to be an effective and well-tolerated treatment in very elderly patients, with a 25% relative risk reduction in the primary morbidity-mortality endpoint.[35] In other studies the non-selective β-blocker bucindolol was ineffective in clinical studies, and in a direct comparison, carvedilol was superior to metoprolol tartrate.[36,37] Overall, the evidence base supports the use of proven agents in their proven dosing regimens and one can simply not assume a class effect.

Adverse effects and interactions

Recognized adverse effects include bradycardia, symptomatic hypotension, fatigue or tiredness, and bronchoconstriction. Contrary to popular belief, each of these is uncommon and rarely leads to treatment discontinuation. Temporary symptomatic fluid retention is less common. It is also important to consider potential drug interactions, including with other blood pressure-lowering agents (e.g. nitrates) and negatively chronotropic drugs (e.g. verapamil, digoxin, amiodarone).[38]

Practical use

The major contraindications to using a β-blocker in HF are asthma, second- or third-degree atrioventricular block, and untreated acute HF (Table 4.4). As with ACE inhibitors, β-blockers should be introduced as early as possible in the course of the disease.

Table 4.4 Practical β-blocker use

Drug	Initial dose (mg)	Target dose (mg)
Bisoprolol	1.25 once daily	10 once daily
Carvedilol	3.25 twice daily	25–50 twice daily
Metoprolol CR/XL	12.5–25 once daily	200 once daily
Nebivolol	1.25 once daily	10mg once daily
Cautions/seek specialist advice:	Severe (NYHA Class IV) HF Current or recent (< 4 weeks) exacerbation of HF, e.g. hospital admission Atrioventricular block or heart rate < 60 min⁻¹ Persisting signs of sodium and water overload, e.g. marked peripheral oedema Symptomatic or severe asymptomatic hypotension (systolic BP < 90 mmHg) Suspicion of bronchial asthma or severe pulmonary disease	
Dose titration:	Double at not less than 2-weekly intervals Monitor heart rate, blood pressure, clinical status (especially body weight if fluid overloaded) Monitor blood chemistry 1–2 weeks after initiation and at each increment	

A 'start low, go slow' approach should be adopted with dose increments at not less than 2-weekly intervals aiming for the target or highest tolerated dose. Patients should be checked for symptomatic hypotension and excessive bradycardia after each dose increment. Both are uncommon and are potentially resolved by reviewing the need for interacting drugs. Patients should be informed of expected benefits and that symptomatic improvement may develop slowly after starting treatment, taking as long as 3–6 months to occur. They should be advised to report deterioration. To detect deterioration, patients should be encouraged to weigh themselves daily and to increase their diuretic dose should their weight increase, persistently (>2 days) by 1.5–2.0 kg. This approach usually suffices and avoids discontinuation of the β-blocker. If there is serious deterioration, the β-blocker dose should be halved or (rarely) stopped. This may have significant detrimental effects on myocardial function and remodelling and should be discussed with a specialist.

Aldosterone antagonists

Aldosterone is a steroid hormone which facilitates sodium retention and potassium loss. It activates the sympathetic nervous system and has a detrimental effect on vascular and myocardial function by stimulating fibrosis, further increasing the risk of myocardial remodelling and sudden death. Even with standard neurohormonal therapy including an ACE inhibitor, the production of aldosterone continues through the phenomenon of 'aldosterone escape' and plasma levels of aldosterone correlate with increased mortality.[39] Unlike ACE inhibitors, ARBs and β-blockers, which were studied across the range of severity of HF, aldosterone blockade has only been investigated in studies in more severe symptomatic HF. Whether blockade is advantageous in milder or even asymptomatic HF remains unclear but is under investigation in a large randomized trial.

Mechanism of action

Aldosterone receptors antagonize the effects of aldosterone at its specific receptor and also act as potassium-sparing diuretics. The non-selective antagonist spironolactone shares some affinity for progesterone and testosterone receptors and is thus associated with endocrine side-effects.

Clinical benefits

Aldosterone antagonism was evaluated in the RALES (Randomised Aldactone Investigators) study where 1633 patients with NYHA Class III–IV HF received spironolactone (25–50 mg once daily) or placebo (Figure 4.4). Ninety-five per cent of patients were also treated with an ACE inhibitor therapy but only 11% with a β-blocker (the value of β-blockers had not been shown at the time RALES was conducted). There was a 30% relative risk reduction in mortality ($p < 0.001$) attributed to a lower risk of death from both progressive HF and sudden cardiac death.[40]

Further support for the co-administration of both an ACE inhibitor and aldosterone blocker was demonstrated from the more recent EPHESUS (Eplerenone Post-Acute

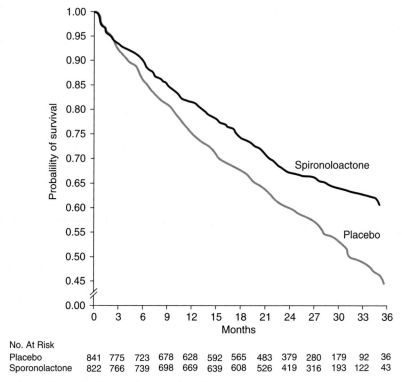

Fig.4.4 Kaplan–Meier survival curve showing the effect of spironolactone in severe chronic HF: findings from RALES. (Reproduced from Pitt *et al.*[40], Copyright ©1999 Massachusetts Medical Society. All rights reserved.)

Myocardial Infarction Heart Failure Efficacy and Survival Study) study. In this trial, 6632 patients with left-ventricular systolic dysfunction and clinical or radiological HF (or diabetes) after acute myocardial infarction were randomized to receive eplerenone 50 mg once daily or placebo, in addition to standard therapy. There was a 15% relative risk reduction in all-cause mortality ($p = 0.008$) with further benefits in reducing hospital admissions. The mortality benefit was associated with a 21% relative risk reduction in sudden cardiac death ($p = 0.03$). These benefits were achieved despite high baseline use of ACE inhibitors and β-blockers, demonstrating the incremental advantage for these high-risk post-infarct patients.[41]

Adverse effects

As with other antagonists of the RAS, renal dysfunction and, especially, hyperkalaemia are the adverse effects of greatest concern. An aldosterone antagonist should not be given to patients with a serum potassium concentration of >5.0 mmol L^{-1}, serum creatinine > 221 mmol L^{-1} or other evidence of markedly impaired renal function. Painful gynaecomastia occurred in up to 10% of male patients receiving spironolactone in RALES but in a much smaller (0.5%) proportion with the selective aldosterone antagonist eplerenone in EPHESUS. Therapy should be used cautiously in conjunction with diuretics, potassium supplements, and any potentially nephrotoxic agent.

Practical use

An aldosterone antagonist should be considered in patients who remain in severe HF despite standard therapy with a diuretic, ACE inhibitor (or ARB), and β-blocker and should be given indefinitely. Treatment should be initiated with a very low dose and serum electrolytes and renal function monitored closely with a check within a week of starting treatment. Symptom improvements are expected within a few weeks or months of initiation. Patients should be advised to stop their medication should they develop diarrhoea and/or vomiting which could lead to hypovolaemia and renal dysfunction.

The major practical concern is hyperkalaemia, and this risk is higher in a patient receiving an ACE inhibitor or ARB. This risk is emphasized by reports of a higher incidence of serious hyperkalaemia in community practice settings than anticipated from the clinical trials.[6] Expert advice recommends close monitoring and dose reduction should potassium rise above 5.5 mmol L^{-1} and complete cessation at >6.0 mmol L^{-1} or significant renal dysfunction (see Table 4.5).

Dose titration is best managed in a structured care network which may include community HF nurses for close biochemical monitoring. At present, the combination of an ACE inhibitor, ARB, and aldosterone antagonist has not been adequately evaluated and can therefore not be recommended.

Table 4.5 Practical aldosterone antagonist use

Drug	Initial dose (mg)	Target dose (mg)
Spironolactone	25 once daily or on alternate days	25–50 once daily
Eplerenone	25 once daily	50 once daily
Cautions/seek specialist advice:	Significant hyperkalaemia (K^+ > 5.0 mmol L^{-1}) Significant renal dysfunction (creatinine > 221 μmol L^{-1} or > 2.5 mg dl^{-1})	
Dose titration:	Increase dose at 1 month if tolerated Check blood chemistry at 1, 4, 8, and 12 weeks; 6, 9, 12, months; 6-monthly thereafter If K^+ rises 5.5 mmol L^{-1} or creatinine rises > 221 μmol L^{-1} (2.5 mg dl^{-1}) reduce to initial dose on alternate days and monitor blood chemistry closely If K^+ rises 6.0 mmol L^{-1} or creatinine rises > 310 μmol L^{-1} (3.5 mg dl^{-1}) stop immediately and seek specialist advice	

Hydralazine and isosorbide dinitrate

Vasodilator therapy directed at augmenting the nitric oxide system may be an alternative or supplemental approach to slow or reverse progressive HF. The combination of the vasodilators hydralazine and isosorbide dinitrate (H-ISDN) was the first treatment shown to improve survival in HF. Subsequent studies suggested inferiority to ACE inhibitors. Recently, however, the same combination was shown to reduce mortality and morbidity in African-American patients already treated with standard therapy including an ACE inhibitor, β-blocker, and spironolactone. Although the combination of hydralazine and isosorbide dinitrate is beneficial, there is no evidence that either agent used alone is beneficial.

Mechanism of action

Isosorbide dinitrate is a nitrosovasodilator and dominant venodilator. It causes smooth muscle cell relaxation by stimulating production of endothelial nitric oxide and cyclic GMP. Therapy is limited, however, by the rapid development of pharmacological tolerance which is thought to be secondary to the production of vascular superoxide species.[42] In contrast, the mechanism of action of hydralazine is poorly understood. It appears to be a dominant arterial vasodilator and may act by promoting the generation of cyclic nucleotides. It also appears to reduce the effect of nitrate tolerance and may do so through an antioxidant effect.[43]

Clinical benefits

The first V-HeFT (Vasodilator in Heart Failure) study randomized 642 men with mild to moderate HF to receive placebo, prazosin, or H-ISDN in addition to diuretics and digoxin. There was a significant survival benefit in the H-ISDN group at 2 years.[44] With the advent of ACE inhibitors, a second V-HeFT trial compared H-ISDN with enalapril in 804 patients. This trial showed that mortality was significantly lower in the enalapril group than in the H-ISDN group.[45]

A retrospective analysis of these trials suggested that self-identified Black patients had a particular clinical response to the vasodilator combination. The A-HeFT (African American Heart Failure) trial recruited 1050 patients who were randomized to a fixed dose combination of H-ISDN three times daily. This was in addition to standard therapy. This trial demonstrated a 43% ($p = 0.01$) relative risk reduction in all-cause death and similar impressive reductions in HF admissions.[46] It is widely believed that incremental benefits of hydralazine nitrate are also likely to be obtained in non-Black patients.

Adverse effects and interactions

The main dose-limiting adverse effects with H-ISDN are headache and dizziness. A rare adverse effect of higher doses of hydralazine (especially in slow acetylators) is a systemic lupus erythematosus-like syndrome.[47]

Practical use

Other than for Black patients, the main indication for H-ISDN is as a substitute in patients truly intolerant of ACE inhibitors or ARBs, especially if due to renal dysfunction (e.g. bilateral renal artery stenosis) or angioedema. H-ISDN should be used as additional treatment in African-American patients and considered for others that remain symptomatic on other proven therapies. A fixed combination (hydralazine 75 mg/ISDN 60 mg three times daily) was used in the trials and was initiated in a low dose (hydralazine 37.5 mg/ISDN 20 mg three times daily), and gradually increased according to tolerability.

Cardiac glycosides

The most commonly used cardiac glycosides are digoxin and digitoxin. They have similar pharmacodynamic effects but distinct pharmacokinetics. Digoxin is eliminated renally; digitoxin is metabolized by the liver. Both may improve symptom control in HF and have a role in the control of ventricular rate in patients with atrial fibrillation.

Mechanism of action

Cardiac glycosides inhibit the cell membrane sodium–potassium adenosine triphosphatase pump and thus increase intracellular calcium and myocardial contractility. In addition to its inotropic effects, digoxin has autonomic, neurohormonal, and diuretic actions, including inhibition of renin release and suppression of the sympathetic nervous system.

Clinical benefits

The DIG (Digitalis Investigation Group) trial investigated the value of digoxin in 6800 patients with HF and sinus rhythm receiving diuretic and ACE inhibitor therapy. Digoxin had no effect on survival but there was a reduction in hospitalizations for worsening HF.[48] In a recent *post hoc* analysis of the DIG trial, the relationship between serum digoxin concentration (SDC) and outcome was examined. This suggested that there was an increased risk of death when the SDC exceeded 1 ng ml^{-1}. Although no firm conclusions can be drawn from this retrospective study, it does revive interest in this therapy.[49]

Adverse effects

Intolerance to digoxin is mostly due to nausea, anorexia, and visual disturbances, although conduction disturbances and arrhythmias are also a concern. Toxicity is more likely with higher doses, especially if the SDC is >2.0 ng ml^{-1}, and is increased by hypokalaemia.

In the light of the above analysis of the DIG trial, a lower therapeutic range of 0.5–0.9 ng ml^{-1} is recommended. The dose of digoxin should be reduced in the elderly and those with renal dysfunction. SDC may be increased by the co-administration of other drugs, including amiodarone and, possibly, atorvastatin. Monitoring of SDC is recommended because of its narrow therapeutic window, particularly in those with documented renal dysfunction and the elderly.

Practical use

Digoxin is recommended only in patients in sinus rhythm with persisting symptoms and signs of HF, despite treatment with an ACE inhibitor, β-blocker, and ARB or aldosterone antagonist, i.e. it is a 'fourth-line' disease-modifying agent (patients will usually also be taking a diuretic). Contraindications include second- and third-degree atrioventricular block and sick sinus syndrome.

In patients with atrial fibrillation, digoxin may be used at an earlier stage if a β-blocker fails to control the ventricular rate (ideally < 70 min^{-1} at rest and < 100 min^{-1} during exercise). There is also a role for digoxin to control the ventricular rate when β-blocker therapy is being initiated or up-titrated. The usual dose of digoxin is 0.125–0.25 mg daily (or 0.065–0.125 mg in the elderly or those with renal dysfunction). Steady-state concentration is usually achieved within 7–10 days. Blood should be taken for therapeutic monitoring at least 6 h following the last dose. There is evidence that the rapid withdrawal of digoxin can lead to worsening of HF, thus this should be discussed with a specialist.[50]

HF with preserved ejection fraction

There is still little evidence from clinical trials or observational studies on how to treat HF with preserved left-ventricular ejection fraction (HF-PEF). Furthermore, there is much debate as to the true prevalence of this type of HF. This population may have a distinct aetiology and better survival expectation than those with impaired left-ventricular function (see discussions in Chapters 2 and 3).[51] Whatever the underlying pathophysiology, evidence suggests that this is a common and important syndrome.[52] Most of the randomized controlled trials discussed above excluded these patients. This makes an evidence-based direction of optimal therapy difficult. However, there has been a drive to conduct such trials in this type of HF and the results are keenly awaited. These studies have been fraught by statistical difficulties. Patients with heart failure in HF-PEF trials demonstrate a trend towards lower mortality and morbidity rates than one would anticipate from epidemiological studies, and when compared to patients with LVSD.[53] This translates to smaller number of event rates, which, when combined with a higher proportion of non-cardiovascular events, may lead to a considerable loss of statistical power to show a treatment effect. These issues may only be addressed with larger adequately powered and robustly designed trials specifically designed to investigate the treatment effects in this rather heterogeneous patient population

The potential cause of HF should be identified and treated appropriately. This includes myocardial ischaemia, hypertension, myocardial/pericardial constriction, and arrhythmias.

Other significant co-morbidity such as diabetes mellitus or anaemia should be managed appropriately.[54] Diuretics are used empirically to treat symptoms of fluid retention, using the same principles as in HF with low ejection fraction. However, care must be taken not to excessively lower pre-load and thus stroke volume and cardiac output. In patients with atrial fibrillation, control of ventricular rate with a β-blocker or rate-limiting calcium channel blocker, or indeed restoration of sinus rhythm, may be particularly beneficial.

Ventricular relaxation and diastolic filling are probably affected, adversely, by angiotensin and aldosterone which promote myocardial fibrosis and ventricular hypertrophy. Drugs blocking the action of these hormones may improve relaxation and diastolic filling and may lead to regression of ventricular hypertrophy and fibrosis. The most persuasive evidence to date comes from the CHARM-Preserved trial.[55] Whilst the ARB candesartan did not reduce the risk of the primary outcome, there was a 15% reduction in patients admitted with heart failure (p=0.017) and a 29% reduction in total hospitalisations (p=0.014) reported by the investigators. The effect of another ARB on mortality and morbidity in HF-PEF is being evaluated further in the Irbesartan in Heart Failure with Preserved Systolic Function (I-PRESERVE) trial. The potential value of an ACE inhibitor has also been investigated in the recently reported Perindopril for Elderly People with Chronic Heart Failure (PEP-CHF) trial. This large study of elderly patients (mean age 76y) was troubled by poor recruitment and low-event rates which resulted in a considerable reduction in statistical power. Treatment with perindopril failed to reduce the primary composite end-point of death or heart failure hospitalisation. However, there was a trend toward improvement at 1-year, particularly heart failure hospitalisations and this was supported by complementary data demonstrating improved functional status and exercise capacity. This, and the aforementioned studies, supports the hypothesis that modulation of the renin-angiotensin system could be beneficial in patients with HF-PEF. Expanding on this premise, the potential benefits of aldosterone receptor blockade are currently under investigation in the TOPCAT (Treatment of Preserved Cardiac Function Heart Failure with Aldosterone Antagonist) trial, which is expected to publish in 2011.

Smaller studies support the use of the calcium channel blocker verapamil which has been shown to improve symptoms and exercise capacity, possibly by increasing the duration of left-ventricular diastole and by directly enhancing myocardial relaxation, though the effect of this agent on mortality and morbidity has not been evaluated.[56,57] Insights into the potential efficacy of beta-blockers in patients with HF-PEF have been drawn from the Study of the Effects of Nebivolol Intervention on Outcomes and Rehospitalisation in Seniors (SENIORS) trial, which included patients with "preserved" LV systolic function (LVEF>35%).[35] This study demonstrated safety and efficacy of Nebivolol in an elderly (mean age 76y) population with heart failure (pooled results). However, the treatment effect of Nebivolol was only modest when compared with that of the other cardinal beta-blocker studies. This, in part, could relate to the inclusion of patients with HF-PEF in whom event rates were lower, thus diluting the statistical power. It therefore, remains to be proven if beta-blockade provides convincing mortality and morbidity benefits in HF-PEF. This needs to be prospectively evaluated in adequately powered randomised trials.

Digoxin has been investigated as a potential therapy in HF-PEF. There is some evidence from the DIG trial that these patients benefits from digoxin with regard to death or hospitalisation from heart failure and this has been reaffirmed by the recent post-hoc analysis.[49] Contrary to this, in a recent randomised controlled trial in patients with LVEF >45%, digoxin (in addition to ACE inhibitor and diuretic) failed to impact significantly on outcome, although showed a trend towards reduced hospitalisations for heart failure (p=0.061).[58] Consequently, digoxin should currently be considered primarily as a rate-controlling strategy in patients with atrial fibrillation and HF-PEF whom are inadequately controlled with a betablocker or rate-limiting calcium channel antagonist. A role as specific disease modifying therapy has not yet been demonstrated.

The treatment of patients with HF and preserved systolic function therefore remains difficult and at times frustrating. This is partly reflected by the diverse aetiology of this syndrome and the lack of controlled data for guidance. Therapy must be tailored at an individual level with an emphasis on symptom control and prevention of disease progression.

Other pharmacological therapies

Cardiovascular risk factors should be targeted with a standard secondary prevention approach. Therapies of proven value for cardiovascular conditions underlying, or associated with, HF should be aggressively treated. Many of these have not been specifically investigated in HF patients. Anti-platelet therapy is generally recommended in patients with cardiovascular disease, although the role of aspirin remains controversial and greatly debated.[59] The major trials of statins generally excluded patients with HF, but two studies of the effect of statins on outcomes in HF are now under way.[60,61] Warfarin, unless contraindicated, should be used in patients with atrial fibrillation or those with intracardiac thrombus detected on echocardiography. Warfarin interacts with many other drugs, including some statins and amiodarone and the dietary supplement St John's wort. Care must be taken when initiating warfarin therapy or indeed adding a new drug in a patient already receiving warfarin.[62]

Co-morbidities, for example anaemia, are now considered therapeutic targets in their own right. There is growing interest in the use of erythropoietic agents to treat anaemia in HF, and outcome trials are awaited.[63] Vaccination against influenza and pneumoccocal infection is recommended in patients with HF, in whom infection may lead to life-threatening deterioration.

Drugs to use with caution

Patients with HF, particularly if severe, may have renal and/or hepatic dysfunction. Any drug excreted predominantly by the kidneys or liver may accumulate in patients with HF. Extreme caution should be taken with drugs with a narrow therapeutic index (e.g. digoxin) in these patients.[62]

The list of drugs which, if possible, should be avoided in HF is not exhaustive. Nevertheless, health-care professionals should be aware of the potential risks. These include most anti-arrhythmic drugs (with the exception of amiodarone and dofetilide) which are associated with an increased risk of death, most calcium channel blockers (with the exception of amlodipine and felodopine), corticosteriods, non-steroidal anti-inflammatory drugs, and many antipsychotics and antihistamines which may be associated with prolongation of the QT interval and arrhythmia. In patients with type-2 diabetes, metformin should be prescribed with caution because of the risk of lactic acidosis and the newer thiazolidinediones because of the risk of fluid retention.[64]

Conclusion

The pharmacological management of heart failure has improved exponentially in the last decade and is supported by the most robust evidence base in clinical medicine. These results require the combination of a variety of neurohormonal antagonists, diuretics, and vasodilating agents and can be complex and confusing. There is evidence that under-prescribing and under-dosing of some treatments is a persistent problem, thus denying patients the resultant benefits. The adoption of a stratified, staged therapeutic ladder (Figs 4.5 and/or 4.6) will help guide health-care professionals on how to best tailor optimal therapy.

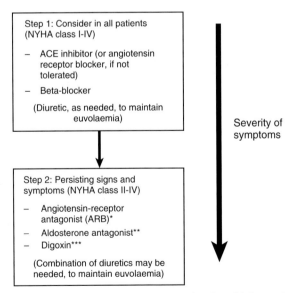

Fig. 4.5 Treatment algorithm for patients with HF and reduced left-ventricular systolic function. *ARBs have been evaluated in patients with NYHA Class II–IV HF. **Spironolactone has been evaluated in patients with NYHA Class III and IV HF. Note that an ACE inhibitor, ARB, and spironolactone should *not* be used together. ***In patients in sinus rhythm, an ARB or aldos-terone antagonist should be used before digoxin.

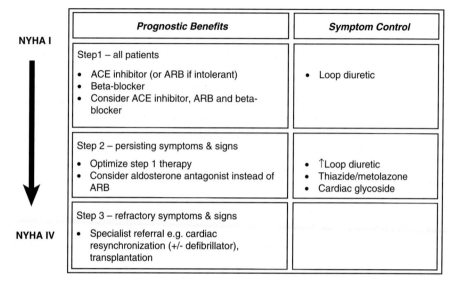

	Prognostic Benefits	**Symptom Control**
NYHA I	**Step1 – all patients** • ACE inhibitor (or ARB if intolerant) • Beta-blocker • Consider ACE inhibitor, ARB and beta-blocker	• Loop diuretic
	Step 2 – persisting symptoms & signs • Optimize step 1 therapy • Consider aldosterone antagonist instead of ARB	• ↑Loop diuretic • Thiazide/metolazone • Cardiac glycoside
NYHA IV	**Step 3 – refractory symptoms & signs** • Specialist referral e.g. cardiac resynchronization (+/- defibrillator), transplantation	

Fig. 4.6 Treatment algorithm for patients with HF and reduced left-ventricular systolic function.

Using this practical and problem-solving approach, health-care professionals will be empowered with the ability to maximize the potential benefits to their patients.

Despite the impressive therapeutic armamentarium, patients with HF continue to experience progressive symptoms and shorter life expectancy. Superior therapeutic agents are needed rather than simply adding to an already extensive polypharmacy. Tailoring pharmacological therapy and targeting treatment on the basis of pathophysiology, or even genomics, are attractive approaches that remain unproven. However, the rate of generation of potential therapeutic targets is remarkable and offers a realistic hope of sustained future advancement.

References

1. MacIntyre K, Capewell S, Stewart S (2000). Evidence of improving prognosis in heart failure: trends in case fatality in 66547 patients hospitalized between 1986 and 1995. *Circulation* **102**: 1126–31.
2. Mosterd A, Reitsma JB, Grobbee DE (2002). Angiotensin converting enzyme inhibition and hospitalisation rates for heart failure in the Netherlands, 1980 to 1999: the end of an epidemic? *Heart* **87**: 75–6.
3. Schaufelberger M, Swedberg K, Koster M (2004). Decreasing one-year mortality and hospitalization rates for heart failure in Sweden: data from the Swedish Hospital Discharge Registry 1988 to 2000. *Eur Heart J* **25**: 300–7.
4. Bungard TJ, McAlister FA, Johnson JA, Tsuyuki RT (2001). Underutilisation of ACE inhibitors in patients with congestive heart failure. *Drugs* **61**: 2021–33.
5. Komajda M, Follath F, Swedberg K *et al.* (2003). The EuroHeart Failure Survey programme – a survey on the quality of care among patients with heart failure in Europe. Part 2: treatment. *Eur Heart J* **24**: 464–74.
6. Juurlink DN, Mamdani MM, Lee DS (2004). Rates of hyperkalemia after publication of the Randomized Aldactone Evaluation Study. *New Engl J Med* **351**: 543–51.

7. McMurray J, Cohen-Solal A, Dietz R (2001). Practical recommendations for the use of ACE inhibitors, beta-blockers and spironolactone in heart failure: putting guidelines into practice. *Eur J Heart Fail* **3**: 495–502.

8. Faris R, Flather M, Purcell H (2002). Current evidence supporting the role of diuretics in heart failure: a meta analysis of randomized controlled trials. *Int J Cardiol* **82**: 149–58.

9. Brater DC (1998). Diuretic therapy. *New Engl J Med* **339**: 387–95.

10. Mackay IG, Muir AL, Watson ML (1984). Contribution of prostaglandins to the systemic and renal vascular response to frusemide in normal man. *Br J Clin Pharmacol* **17**: 513–19.

11. Channer KS, McLean KA, Lawson-Matthew P, Richardson M (1994). Combination diuretic treatment in severe heart failure: a randomised controlled trial. *Br Heart J* **71**: 146–50.

12. Packer M (1995). Evolution of the neurohormonal hypothesis to explain the progression of chronic heart failure. *Eur Heart J* **16**(Suppl. F): 4–6.

13. CONSENSUS Trial Study Group (1987). Effects of enalapril on mortality in severe congestive heart failure: results of the Cooperative North Scandinavian Enalapril Survival Study (CONSENSUS). *New Engl J Med* **316**: 1429–35.

14. (1991). Effect of enalapril on survival in patients with reduced left ventricular ejection fractions and congestive heart failure. The SOLVD Investigators. *New Engl J Med* **325**: 293–302.

15. Pfeffer MA, Braunwald E, Moye LA *et al.* (1992). Effect of captopril on mortality and morbidity in patients with left ventricular dysfunction after myocardial infarction. Results of the survival and ventricular enlargement trial. The SAVE Investigators. *New Engl J Med* **327**: 669–77.

16. (1993). Effect of ramipril on mortality and morbidity of survivors of acute myocardial infarction with clinical evidence of heart failure. The Acute Infarction Ramipril Efficacy (AIRE) Study Investigators. *Lancet* **342**: 821–8.

17. Kober L, Torp-Pedersen C, Carlsen JE *et al.* (1995). A clinical trial of the angiotensin-converting-enzyme inhibitor trandolapril in patients with left ventricular dysfunction after myocardial infarction. Trandolapril Cardiac Evaluation (TRACE) Study Group. *New Engl J Med* **333**: 1670–6.

18. Yusuf S, Sleight P, Pogue J, Bosch J, Davies R, Dagenais G (2000). Effects of an angiotensin-converting-enzyme inhibitor, ramipril, on cardiovascular events in high-risk patients. The Heart Outcomes Prevention Evaluation Study Investigators. *New Engl J Med* **342**: 145–53.

19. Finkielstein D, Schweitzer P (2004). Role of angiotensin-converting enzyme inhibitors in the prevention of atrial fibrillation. *Am J Cardiol* **93**: 734–6.

20. Packer M, Poole-Wilson PA, Armstrong PW *et al.* (1999). Comparative effects of low and high doses of the angiotensin-converting enzyme inhibitor, lisinopril, on morbidity and mortality in chronic heart failure. ATLAS Study Group. *Circulation* **100**: 2312–18.

21. Petrie MC, Padmanabhan N, McDonald JE, Hillier C, Connell JM, McMurray JJ (2001). Angiotensin converting enzyme (ACE) and non-ACE dependent angiotensin II generation in resistance arteries from patients with heart failure and coronary heart disease. *J Am Coll Cardiol* **37**: 1056–61.

22. Siragy HM, Xue C, Abadir P, Carey RM (2005). Angiotensin subtype-2 receptors inhibit renin biosynthesis and angiotensin II formation. *Hypertension* **45**: 133–7.

23. Pitt B, Poole-Wilson PA, Segal R *et al.* (2000). Effect of losartan compared with captopril on mortality in patients with symptomatic heart failure: randomised trial–the Losartan Heart Failure Survival Study ELITE II. *Lancet* **355**: 1582–7.

24. Cohn JN, Tognoni G and the Valsartan Heart Failure Trial Investigators (2001). A randomized trial of the angiotensin-receptor blocker valsartan in chronic heart failure. *New Engl J Med* **345**: 1667–75.

25. Maggioni AP, Anand I, Gottlieb SO, Latini R, Tognoni G, Cohn JN (2002). Effects of valsartan on morbidity and mortality in patients with heart failure not receiving angiotensin-converting enzyme inhibitors. *J Am Coll Cardiol* **40**: 1414–21.

26. Pfeffer MA, McMurray JJ, Velazquez EJ (2003). Valsartan, captopril, or both in myocardial infarction complicated by heart failure, left ventricular dysfunction, or both. *New Engl J Med* **349**: 1893–906.

27. Granger CB, McMurray JJ, Yusuf S (2003). Effects of candesartan in patients with chronic heart failure and reduced left-ventricular systolic function intolerant to angiotensin-converting-enzyme inhibitors: the CHARM-Alternative trial. *Lancet* **362**: 772–6.

28. McMurray JJ, Ostergren J, Swedberg K (2003). Effects of candesartan in patients with chronic heart failure and reduced left-ventricular systolic function taking angiotensin-converting-enzyme inhibitors: the CHARM-Added trial. *Lancet* **362**: 767–71.

29. McMurray JJ, Young JB, Dunlap ME *et al.* (2006). Relationship of dose of background angiotensin-converting enzyme inhibitor to the benefits of candesartan in the Candesartan in Heart failure: Assessment of Reduction in Mortality and morbidity (CHARM)-Added trial. *Am Heart J* **151**: 992–8.

30. McKelvie RS, Rouleau JL, White M (2003). Comparative impact of enalapril, candesartan or metoprolol alone or in combination on ventricular remodelling in patients with congestive heart failure. *Eur Heart J* **24**: 1727–34.

31. Andersson B, Lomsky M, Waagstein F (1993). The link between acute haemodynamic adrenergic beta-blockade and long-term effects in patients with heart failure. A study on diastolic function, heart rate and myocardial metabolism following intravenous metoprolol. *Eur Heart J* **14**: 1375–85.

32. (1999). Effect of metoprolol CR/XL in chronic heart failure: Metoprolol CR/XL Randomised Intervention Trial in Congestive Heart Failure (MERIT-HF). *Lancet* **353**: 2001–7.

33. (1999). CIBIS Investigators. The Cardiac Insufficiency Bisoprolol Study II (CIBIS-II): a randomised trial. *Lancet* **353**: 9–13.

34. Packer M, Fowler MB, Roecker EB (2002). Effect of carvedilol on the morbidity of patients with severe chronic heart failure: results of the carvedilol prospective randomized cumulative survival (COPERNICUS) study. *Circulation* **106**: 2194–9.

35. Flather MD, Shibata MC, Coats AJ (2005). Randomized trial to determine the effect of nebivolol on mortality and cardiovascular hospital admission in elderly patients with heart failure (SENIORS). *Eur Heart J* **26**: 215–25.

36. The Beta-Blocker Evaluation of Survival Trial Investigators (2001). A trial of the beta-blocker bucindolol in patients with advanced chronic heart failure. *New Engl J Med* **344**: 1659–67.

37. Poole-Wilson PA, Swedberg K, Cleland JG *et al.* (2003). Comparison of carvedilol and metoprolol on clinical outcomes in patients with chronic heart failure in the Carvedilol Or Metoprolol European Trial (COMET): randomised controlled trial. *Lancet* **362**: 7–13.

38. McMurray J, Cohen-Solal A, Dietz R *et al.* (2001). Practical recommendations for the use of ACE inhibitors, beta-blockers and spironolactone in heart failure: putting guidelines into practice. *Eur J Heart Fail* **3**: 495–502.

39. Swedberg K, Eneroth P, Kjekshus J, Wilhelmsen L (1990). Hormones regulating cardiovascular function in patients with severe congestive heart failure and their relation to mortality. CONSENSUS Trial Study Group. *Circulation* **82**: 1730–6.

40. Pitt B, Zannad F, Remme WJ (1999). The effect of spironolactone on morbidity and mortality in patients with severe heart failure. Randomized Aldactone Evaluation Study Investigators. *New Engl J Med* **341**: 709–17.

41. Pitt B (2003). Eplerenone, a selective aldosterone blocker, in patients with left ventricular dysfunction after myocardial infarction. *New Engl J Med* **348**: 1309–21.

42. Ignarro LJ, Napoli C, Loscalzo J (2002). Nitric oxide donors and cardiovascular agents modulating the bioactivity of nitric oxide: an overview. *Circ Res* **90**: 21–8.

43. Munzel T, Kurz S, Rajagopalan S *et al.* (1996). Hydralazine prevents nitroglycerin tolerance by inhibiting activation of a membrane-bound NADH oxidase. A new action for an old drug. *J Clin Invest* **98**: 1465–70.

44. Cohn JN, Archibald DG, Ziesche S, Franciosa JA, Harston WE, Tristani FE (1986). Effect of vasodilator therapy on mortality in chronic congestive heart failure. Results of a Veterans Administration Cooperative Study. *New Engl J Med* **314**: 1547–52.

45. Cohn JN, Johnson G, Ziesche S, Cobb F, Francis G, Tristani F (1991). A comparison of enalapril with hydralazine-isosorbide dinitrate in the treatment of chronic congestive heart failure. *New Engl J Med* **325**: 303–10.

46. Taylor AL, Ziesche S, Yancy C *et al.* (2004). Combination of isosorbide dinitrate and hydralazine in blacks with heart failure. *New Engl J Med* **351**: 2049–57.

47. Richardson B (2003). DNA methylation and autoimmune disease. *Clin Immunol* **109**: 72–9.

48. Digitalis Investigation Group (1997). The effect of digoxin on mortality and morbidity in patients with heart failure. *New Engl J Med* **336**: 525–33.

49. Ahmed A, Rich MW, Love TE *et al.* (2006). Digoxin and reduction in mortality and hospitalization in heart failure: a comprehensive post hoc analysis of the DIG trial. *Eur Heart J* **27**: 178–86.

50. Packer M, Gheorghiade M, Young JB, Radiance S (1993). Withdrawal of digoxin from patients with chronic heart failure treated with angiotensin-converting enzyme inhibitors. *New Engl J Med* **329**: 1–7.

51. Zile MR, Brutsaert DL (2002). New concepts in diastolic dysfunction and diastolic heart failure: Part II: causal mechanisms and treatment. *Circulation* **105**: 1503–8.

52. Smith GL, Masoudi FA, Vaccarino V, Radford MJ, Krumholz HM (2003). Outcomes in heart failure patients with preserved ejection fraction: mortality, readmission, and functional decline. *J Am Coll Cardiol* **41**: 1510–18.

53. McMurray, J (2006). Renin Angiotensin Blockade in Heart Failure with Preserved Ejection Fraction: The Signal Gets Stronger. *Eur Heart J* **27**(19):2257–9.

54. Aurigemma GP, Gaasch WH (2004). Clinical practice: diastolic heart failure. *New Engl J Med* **351**: 1097–105.

55. Yusuf S, Pfeffer MA, Swedberg K (2003). Effects of candesartan in patients with chronic heart failure and preserved left-ventricular ejection fraction: the CHARM-Preserved Trial. *Lancet* **362**: 777–81.

56. Setaro J, Zaret BL, Schueman D (1990). Usefulness of verapamil for congestive heart failure associated with abnormal left ventricular diastolic performance. *Am J Cardiol* **66**: 981–6.

57. Hung MJ, Cherng WJ, Kuo LT, Wang CH (2002). Effect of verapamil in elderly patients with left ventricular diastolic dysfunction as a cause of congestive heart failure. *Int J Clin Pract* **56**: 57–62.

58. Shibata MC, Flather MD, Bohm M *et al.* (2002). Study of the Effects of Nebivolol Intervention on Outcomes and Rehospitalisation in Seniors with Heart Failure (SENIORS). Rationale and design. *Int J Cardiol* **86**: 77–85.

59. Cleland JG, Findlay I, Jafri S, Sutton G, Falk R, Bulpitt C (2004). The Warfarin/Aspirin Study in Heart failure (WASH): a randomized trial comparing antithrombotic strategies for patients with heart failure. *Am Heart J* **148**: 157–64.

60. Kjekshus J, Dunselman P, Blideskog M *et al.* (2005). A statin in the treatment of heart failure? Controlled rosuvastatin multinational study in heart failure (CORONA): study design and baseline characteristics. *Eur J Heart Fail* **7**: 1059–69.

61. Tavazzi L, Tognoni G, Franzosi MG (2004). Rationale and design of the GISSI heart failure trial: a large trial to assess the effects of n-3 polyunsaturated fatty acids and rosuvastatin in symptomatic congestive heart failure. *Eur J Heart Fail* **6**: 635–41.

62. Amabile CM, Spencer AP (2004). Keeping your patient with heart failure safe; a review of potentially dangerous medications. *Arch Intern Med* **164**: 709–20.

63. Katz SD (2004). Mechanisms and treatment of anemia in chronic heart failure. *Congest Heart Fail* **10**: 243–7.

64. Tang WH, Francis GS, Hoogwerf BJ, Young JB (2003). Fluid retention after initiation of thiazolidinedione therapy in diabetic patients with established chronic heart failure. *J Am Coll Cardiol* **41**: 1394–8.

Chapter 5

Device therapy for heart failure patients

Sarah J. Goodlin and Mandeep R. Mehra

Introduction

Several decades of research and clinical experience in cardiac care have improved clinical outcomes, patient functional status, and annual mortality. These advances in medical therapy for heart failure (HF) have occurred on the basis of targeting neurohormonal aberrations. However, a ceiling effect has been observed with universally applied stack-on neurohormonally directed therapy with little or no benefit beyond that provided by the judicious use of angiotensin-converting enzyme inhibition, angiotensin receptor blockade, and β-blockade.[1] Some therapeutic targets that initially appeared promising have even yielded negative outcomes, as in the case of cytokine antagonism, endothelin receptor blockade, and centrally acting sympatholytic drugs. Recent studies of patients recruited from within hospitalized settings have demonstrated high morbidity and mortality despite otherwise 'optimum medical therapy' (see Chapter 4).[2] Thus, attention has been diverted to the non-pharmacological management of otherwise 'optimally treated' HF with the use of devices such as cardiac resynchronization therapy (CRT), designed to favorably influence pump dysfunction, and implantable cardioverter defibrillators (ICD), designed to abrogate sudden arrhythmic death. Surgical interventions and surgically implanted devices have also gained support in investigational settings (see Chapter 6). This chapter will review the indications for, and the management of, ICD and CRT in HF.

Implantable cardioverter defibrillators

ICDs are small sophisticated devices implanted under the chest wall with leads into the myocardium through the venous system to detect and terminate arrhythmias with electroshock and/or pacing. A titanium can about the size of a matchbook houses a microprocessor, capacitor, and battery. The microprocessor interprets rhythms, records the rhythm and intervention any time the ICD discharges, and can be programmed to modify both detection and output. Back-up pacing is set at a rate of 40 min or more. Similar to a pacemaker, data can be retrieved from an ICD to evaluate its function and heart rhythms periodically.

Early ICDs delivered electroshocks to cardiovert rhythms detected as lethal, but newer devices also deliver anti-tachycardia pacing and varying voltage shocks.[3] Anti-tachycardia pacing cardioverts some episodes of ventricular tachycardia without delivering a shock and thus decreases discomfort from cardioversion. Earlier versions of ICDs paced only the right ventricle; however, newer devices have dual pacing capacity (with leads in the right atrium and right ventricle) that provide sequential atrial and ventricular contraction. The ICD only treats potentially lethal ventricular tachycardia or fibrillation, and does not improve cardiac function or provide other benefit. ICDs do not treat all lethal rhythms, so do not effectively prevent all sudden cardiac deaths (SCDs).

Initial use of ICDs in the 1980s was limited to persons with documented symptomatic ventricular arrhythmias or survivors of SCD. This 'secondary prevention' of SCD by ICDs was more effective than medical anti-arrhythmic therapy in persons with documented lethal ventricular arrhythmias. Studies demonstrated a relative reduction in total mortality or SCD, although the mortality rate in those who received ICDs was still high (18.4% in ICD recipients compared to 25.4% to control subjects in the Anti-arrhythmic versus Implantable Defibrillator (AVID) trial).[4] The reduction of death with ICDs is greatest in persons with reduced left-ventricular function and in certain conditions such as long-QT syndrome with recurrent syncope or SCD despite β-blocker therapy. ICD therapy is therefore considered appropriate to prevent SCD for anyone with a prior lethal arrhythmia or SCD unless they are known to have a high likelihood of dying soon from their heart disease or from other conditions. In advanced HF with a limited survival (<1 year) and little option for alteration of its natural history (CRT, heart transplantation), concerns have been raised that the ratio of risks to benefit from ICD cannot be supported.[5] As discussed later, when the clinical condition in HF transitions to palliative care, responsible clinical decisions regarding cessation of ICD therapy must be entertained to minimize end-of-life discomfort (see Chapter 24).

Ventricular arrhythmias and sudden cardiac death

About half of episodes of SCD occur in persons without known heart disease. As HF evolves from cardiac injury to cardiac repair to cardiac scarring, the nidus for ventricular arrhythmias becomes manifest. Thus, early after cardiac injury, such as an acute myocardial infarction, ventricular arrhythmias occur as a consequence of metabolic cellular abnormalities. These episodes are not associated with poor prognosis when they occur within 48 h of the event. Subsequently, as cardiac repair sets in, neurohormonal activation is heightened, and in this setting aggressive neurohormonal blockade with aldosterone antagonists, in combination with ACE inhibitors and β-blockers, has been shown to lower mortality.[6] Later after scarred myocardium appears in areas of infarction, re-entrant circuits can propagate which predispose to ventricular ectopy and arrhythmias. This is why persons with HF and reduced left-ventricular ejection fraction (LVEF) are at higher likelihood than the rest of the population to suffer SCD. Many patients may have ventricular tachycardia that is asymptomatic and that terminates spontaneously, independently of an intervention. In persons with HF, the risk of lethal ventricular arrhythmias increases when the LVEF is low. This risk is moderate when

LVEF is <40% and higher when LVEF is <30%. Severe HF, elevated neurohormone levels, and conduction delays (associated with prolongation of the QRS complex on the electrocardiogram) also carry a high risk of SCD. It is clear that appropriate medical management significantly reduces the incidence of SCD in persons with HF (see Chapter 4). Recent studies have evaluated the use of ICD therapy, using LVEF ≤ 30% or 35% as a marker for those at risk of SCD, in whom the risk–benefit ratio of ICD therapy as prophylaxis is most favorable to device insertion.

Benefits of ICDs in HF patients

Thirteen trials since the mid-1990s have addressed the use of the ICD to prevent life-threatening arrhythmias. Some of these trials were performed prior to current consensus about optimal medical management of HF, and thus did not include β-blockers in the armamentarium. However, current beliefs and guidelines for ICD use are based on the cumulative evidence from these studies. The Multicenter Automatic Defibrillator Implantation (MADIT) trials evaluated the ICD in persons after a myocardial infarction with LVEF ≤ 35% in MADIT-I and to ≤ 30% in MADIT-II. MADIT-I enrolled subjects in whom an electrophysiologic study showed inducible but non-suppressible ventricular tachyarrhythmias, and ICDs reduced all-cause mortality by 54% relative to control subjects or an absolute reduction in mortality of 18% over 2 years.[7] The MADIT-II trial enrolled subjects without documenting a history of arrhythmia and demonstrated a 31% relative reduction and a 5.6% absolute reduction in all-cause mortality over 2 years with an ICD compared to medical therapy. Special points about these two trials include an imbalance of greater β-blocker therapy in the ICD arm in MADIT I (which may have driven the higher absolute benefits) while the benefits of an ICD did not surface until after the first year in MADIT II.

The Multicenter Unsustained Tachycardia Trial (MUSTT) also enrolled subjects with previous myocardial infarction and reduced LVEF (<40%), but stratified their risk using electrophysiologic study. In patients with inducible ventricular tachycardia ICDs reduced mortality.[8] The Defibrillator in Acute Myocardial Infarction Trial (DINAMIT) enrolled patients 4–40 days following an acute myocardial infarction, and failed to show benefit from defibrillator implantation, suggesting that an ICD is inappropriate soon after the acute event.

Subsequently, the Sudden Cardiac Death in Heart Failure Trial (SCD-HeFT) randomized subjects with HF from any cause and LVEF ≤ 35% to an ICD, amiodarone, or placebo. Over 5 years, patients with either ischemic or non-ischemic cardiomyopathy had similar relative risk reduction in overall mortality. Post hoc analysis raised concerns about the absolute benefits in non-ischemic patients, those with New York Heart Association (NYHA) Class III HF at entry and those intolerant to a β-blocker (perhaps indicating more advanced disease). The mortality benefit from ICDs became apparent after 12–18 months following insertion. Overall the ICD was superior to both amiodarone and placebo therapy; though the impact of ICDs on mortality was a 23% relative reduction from the other groups, the absolute numbers are less impressive. ICDs led to an absolute 7.3% fewer deaths in patients with ischemic cardiomyopathy, and

6.5% absolute reduction in patients with non-ischemic cardiomyopathy. For every 100 patients receiving an ICD over 2.5 years, 14 died despite the device, 4 who would have died with either amiodarone or placebo lived through the study period, and 7 more persons survived with an ICD than without. Some subjects who survived a SCD event with an ICD went on to die from progressive HF. Those who survived with an ICD had progression of their HF and required more HF hospitalizations than the control groups.[9]

In the Defibrillators in Non-Ischemic Cardiomyopathy Treatment Evaluation (DEFINITE) trial, subjects with NYHA Class I–III HF, no evidence of coronary disease, and LVEF <36% had a reduction in arrhythmic death with ICD and total mortality between groups trended to decrease with an ICD but was not significant. ICDs provided the greatest benefit in persons with NYHA Class II HF (avoiding 12 SCD events per 100 patients over 5 years versus other groups), and in persons with recently diagnosed cardiomyopathy. In DEFINITE the use of ACE inhibitors and β-blockers exceeded 85%, and was probably responsible for overall reduced deaths and SCD events.

Adverse outcomes

Concerns have surfaced that ICD use is associated with worsening HF. Pacing of the right ventricle with an ICD is associated with the development of HF in persons with asymptomatic reduced LVEF, possibly explaining one mechanism of worsening HF with ICDs.[10] Worsening of quality of life score and exercise duration and no change in NYHA class were seen in subjects who received an ICD without resynchronization therapy in the Multicenter InSync ICD Randomized Clinical Evaluation (MIRACLE ICD) trial. Side-effects or undesired effects from ICDs also include anxiety and depression,[11] multiple shocks, and inappropriate shocks (shocks delivered without evidence of a lethal arrhythmia when the ICD is interrogated). A small number of persons also suffer with phantom shocks—perceived ICD discharges that are not documented when the device is interrogated.

Appropriate ICD shocks associated with a record of ventricular tachycardia are followed by a decline in function or a three-fold worsening of prognosis over the subsequent year. ICD shocks for ventricular fibrillation are followed by a five-fold increased death rate over a year.[12] It may be that ventricular fibrillation or tachycardia are markers of worsening underlying disease. In fact, in patients on a waiting list for cardiac transplantation and with severe HF, these rhythms and SCD are common. ICDs are used for ventricular arrhythmias in about 35% of these patients.[13] In this very ill group awaiting transplant, the number of ICD discharges correlated with the number of SCD events in patients without ICDs. However, in other studies, many appropriate ICD discharges appear to be for rhythms that terminate spontaneously in controls.[14,15]

Several studies of single-center populations of ICD recipients shed light on complications of ICDs. Infections and inappropriate shocks are more common in patients with prior atrial fibrillation and in persons with asymptomatic (NYHA Class I) reduced LVEF.[16] Rates of inappropriate shocks vary in studies. In SCD-HeFT the rate of inappropriate shocks was 2.4% per year. In series at individual centers, the rate of inappropriate shocks ranged from 11–24% per year, and was highest in patients with symptoms of advanced HF.[17]

Complications of ICDs occurred in nearly one-third of patients over 4 years in one series, including adverse events during implantation, generator malfunction, lead problems, ICD system infections, stroke, and inappropriate shocks.[18] Recent device malfunctions have required large numbers of persons to have existing ICDs replaced.

Other data

With increased use of ICDs, registries of patients receiving ICDs will evaluate aspects of the indications and outcomes of this therapy. Funding by the Centers for Medicare and Medicaid Services (CMS) for ICDs is contingent on participation in a data registry that is part of the 'Coverage with Evidence' initiative. A registry currently collects data that identify features of the implantation and patient characteristics. A longitudinal data base is also in development. The Triggers of Ventricular Arrhythmia (TOVA) study collects data in 31 centers in the United States for patients receiving ICD for secondary prevention of SCD. Forty-four per cent of subjects had HF at enrollment (others had familial conditions, cardiac arrest or spontaneous ventricular tachycardia and syncope, or prior myocardial infarction or coronary artery disease). Of subjects with HF in this study, just under 20% had an appropriate ICD discharge in under a year. ICD shocks for ventricular tachycardia or fibrillation were more common in persons with NYHA Class III HF and with LVEF <20%.[19]

For whom is an ICD indicated?

Summaries of the data from ICD trials and recommendations for their use are presented in the American Heart Association/American College of Cardiology Guidelines for Evaluation and Management of Chronic Heart Failure,[20] and in the Heart Failure Society of America Heart Failure Guidelines.[21] When a patient survives a SCD event or has a documented lethal ventricular arrhythmia, an ICD is felt to be appropriate to prevent subsequent SCD ('secondary prevention').

Table 5.1 ICD indications, contraindications and cautionary conditions in persons with HF

Indications for ICD	Contraindications to ICD	Cautions
Survivor of SCD, syncope due to ventricular arrhythmia, or prolonged symptomatic ventricular tachycardia	Life expectancy of 1 year or less from any condition	Patients with atrial fibrillation have higher rates of both inappropriate and appropriate shocks than those in sinus rhythm
LVEF ≤ 35% and mild to moderate HF after 3 months of optimal medicines	Advanced, refractory HF despite optimal medications, or NYHA Class IV symptoms (except for patients awaiting heart transplantation)	Average age of patients in trials was 60 or younger. Age over 80 has been less well studied
Conditions known to have high risk of SCD (long-QT syndrome, Brugada syndrome)	Placement less than 40 days after myocardial infarction	Ejection fraction should be assessed once medical therapy optimized for at least 3 months before ICD is considered

Prophylactic ICD placement is appropriate for persons with reduced LVEF ($\leq$ 35%) with NYHA Class II–III HF, or mild to moderate HF symptoms. The trials of ICDs for primary prevention suggest that no benefit is achieved within the first year after implantation, thus ICDs are felt to be appropriate only when the patient is likely to live longer than a year. Studies excluded persons with severe advanced HF, thus ICD implantation is not indicated for persons with severe refractory HF when there is no expectation of improvement. Randomized trials did not include persons of advanced age, thus the benefit of an ICD is uncertain for persons over the age of about 75 years.

What should patients know about an ICD?

Patient comprehension of what an ICD accomplishes is inaccurate; when queried, many HF patients with ICDs as well as those without ICD expect the device to prevent SCD in as many as half of persons who receive it, rather than the 7% demonstrated in SCD-HeFT.[22] Patients may also not understand that the ICD may lead to worsened HF and at the end of life that ICDs might preclude sudden, painless death and lead to death from progressive organ failure. Thus, the ICD should be presented as a device that treats certain abnormal rhythms and somewhat reduces the likelihood of a SCD event. Patients should understand that ICDs may never fire in some individuals, and that about 5–14% of persons may receive an inappropriate shock for a rhythm that is not dangerous. Many episodes receiving ICD pacing or shock as programmed would have terminated spontaneously in the absence of an ICD.[23]

In order to talk about SCD, the discussion about an ICD implantation should include a discussion about dying from HF. The course of HF and progression to advanced HF over time must be acknowledged. Patient preferences for management of SCD should be elicited in the conversation. Clearly those persons who prefer to allow natural death for a SCD event should not receive an ICD. Persons who would want an attempt at cardiopulmonary resuscitation should discuss the option of an ICD with their clinician.

When patients want numerical information about their likelihood of death, data from clinical trials provides an estimate (recognizing that clinical trial subjects differ from the general HF population). Data from a recent secondary analysis of the COMPANION trial provides one frame of reference: over 1 year, 5% patients with moderately severe HF (1/20) died suddenly, 5% died from problems not related to their HF, and another 8% (1/12) died from worsened HF.[24] Patients need to be aware that the device may effectively prolong life, particularly for persons in whom HF medications are optimized and whose HF is only moderately symptomatic. Patients with advanced HF (NYHA Class III and blood urea nitrogen BUN greater than 25 mg dl^{-1}) are more likely to die with HF than those with less severe disease. The SCD-HeFT data suggest that these individuals benefit less from an ICD than those with less symptomatic disease; however, an analysis of MADIT II data found that ICDs conferred similar benefit to NYHA Class III patients with elevated BUN and prior myocardial infarction as to subjects with less severe HF.[25]

The conversation about ICDs should be framed to provide information that permits patients to make an informed decision about the ICD, but information should be delivered so that patients have the opportunity to dictate how much data they receive in what format (see Chapter 22). Decision-making about an ICD with a patient will be easiest if the patient already understands the nature and course of HF, and the ICD conversation occurs as one in a series of discussions.

Patients receiving ICDs and their families should also be made aware that the device may be deactivated in the future at their discretion. Recent lay press has given increased attention to the hazard of ICD shocks at the end of life that might be painful or prolong life when HF or other illness has progressed to a stage that natural death is preferred. The devices can be programmed to not deliver shocks, but this requires intervention by either a clinician or manufacturer's representative who is familiar with the device. Thus, the option of device deactivation in the future should be made available, and when death is near, a plan for elective deactivation should be developed and implemented.

Management of ICDs

Ongoing care for individuals with ICDs requires regular interrogation of the device. Patients are also expected to complete a log and notify their physicians when the device fires. New technology permits some ICDs to be interrogated via wireless or dial-up internet connections. Newest devices may also include the ability to monitor venous impedance to assess volume status or central venous pressure and feed back data from a wireless antenna in the device over the internet to clinical staff. Other equipment for some devices includes measurement of weight via a scale with wireless connection or modem to report to the patient's clinician. Such additional data may facilitate HF management. The delivery of inappropriate shocks can be addressed by the electro-physiologist's adjustment of device sensitivity and response. Batteries must be replaced every 4 to 7 years. As devices have become more sophisticated, some clinicians offer an 'upgrade' to a newer device at the time of battery replacement. Both battery replacement and device upgrade should be accompanied by a review of the indications for the ICD and the patient's preferences regarding the device. If HF or other conditions have progressed since the initial device placement, some patients might elect to not replace the battery or the device.

Discontinuation of ICDs

Defibrillators may be discontinued for several reasons. Repeated distressing shocks, either warranted or inappropriate, may lead a patient to elect to discontinue their ICD. A percentage of patients, as high as 25% in some studies, have significant anxiety and psychological distress associated with their ICD whether or not it has fired.[26,27] This anxiety may be severe enough to lead the patient to elect to discontinue defibrillator therapy. Alternatively, a recommendation to discontinue ICD function may come from the clinician when HF becomes end-stage.

The ethical issues surrounding withdrawal of an existing therapy are discussed in detail in Chapter 24. Although the withdrawal of a therapy may feel more active than deciding not to initiate it, these are ethically equivalent and acceptable ethical decisions when the goals of care and burdens and benefits of a therapy are weighed.

Decision-making about discontinuing defibrillator therapy should begin by considering the patient's current status and likely course with or without the therapy. Identifying their status, options for care, and likely course for the patient at a given point can begin with an invitation to the patient to review the goals of their care. Clarifying goals as to 'live as long as possible' or to 'maximize comfort until the time comes when your heart or breathing stop' then allows the clinician to review how to manage each therapy the patient is receiving and how it might help or hinder the goals. When HF is advanced, the option of allowing the patient to die naturally when their heart or breathing stop is consistent with deactivating the defibrillator function (see also Chapter 22).

Clinicians should clarify how defibrillators will be deactivated in advance of the need to do so for a given patient. Although a device can be deactivated when death is imminent, organizing a plan in advance of this point reduces pressure and anxiety for all involved. Either the electrophysiologist or their staff or a representative from the device manufacturer should be identified as the person to contact when a decision is made to deactivate a device.

Cardiac resynchronization therapy

Prolongation of electrical conduction through the heart, characterized by left bundle branch block, is associated with a higher rate of death in HF patients than normal conduction.[28,29] The lack of synchronous left ventricle and right ventricle contraction leads to increased stroke work, altered mitral valve leaflet tethering and decreased left-ventricular ejection. This 'dyssynchrony' (also called 'dyssynergy') results in as much as 20% of the work of contraction being spent in translocation of blood due to differential septal and lateral wall activation times rather than forward ejection. Dyssynchrony may also adversely affect left anterior descending artery flow and cause perfusion abnormalities in the septum that are interpreted as 'false positives' since they occur in the absence of obstructive coronary artery disease.

CRT is achieved with a pacemaker-sized device that is implanted with three leads into: (1) the atrium, (2) the right ventricle, and (3) via the coronary sinus into a vein on the lateral free wall of the left ventricle. Resynchronization of right and left-ventricular contraction, accomplished by simultaneous impulses to both ventricle walls, improves dyssynchrony in 50–70% of those in whom a CRT device is placed. Placement of a lead in the left ventricle is complex and sometimes cannot be accomplished except with minimally invasive thoracic surgery. The left-ventricular pacemaker lead is also subject to displacement or malfunction more readily than right ventricular leads.

CRT has been evaluated with and without ICD capability in persons with NYHA Class III or IV symptoms and QRS prolongation (greater than 120 ms) on the electrocardiogram. In the Multicenter InSync Randomized Clinical Evaluation (MIRACLE) trial CRT resulted in improved symptoms, quality of life scores, 6-min walk test distance, and maximal oxygen consumption (VO_2max) and echocardiographic assessment of left-ventricular end diastolic volume. Subsequently the Comparison of Medical Therapy, Pacing and Defibrillation in Heart Failure (COMPANION) and Cardiac

Resynchronization-Heart Failure (CARE-HF) trials demonstrated a reduction in all-cause mortality with CRT (not significant in COMPANION).[30,31] In COMPANION and in the MIRACLE ICD trial CRT was evaluated with ICD. MIRACLE ICD demonstrated efficacy of ICD in the presence of CRT. COMPANION demonstrated a mortality benefit of CRT with ICD over medical therapy alone. CRT reduced HF hospitalization more significantly when left bundle branch block (rather than right bundle branch block or intraventricular conduction delay) was present, when QRS interval was greater than 148 ms, and when patients received β-blockers. CARE-HF demonstrated reduction in N-terminal pro-brain natriuretic peptide (BNP) levels and ventricular remodeling with CRT. In this trial, echocardiographic parameters depicting mechanical dyssynchrony were used for patient enrollment when the QRS interval was narrow (in the 120–149 ms range).

For whom is CRT indicated?

Resynchronization therapy has been primarily evaluated in patients with advanced HF with reduced LVEF who have refractory symptoms despite optimal medical management and prolonged QRS greater than 120 ms. While CRT can be accomplished in atrial fibrillation (usually with ablation of atrial-ventricular conduction), sinus rhythm is recommended. Studies have not yet identified how to predict which patients will benefit from CRT; however, evidence of dyssynchrony on echocardiography has been proposed as one criterion. In COMPANION, patients with a QRS duration less than 147ms did not benefit from CRT. In CARE-HF, patients with a QRS duration less than 150 ms were required to have echocardiographic evidence of dyssynergy for study enrollment. This additional criterion in CARE-HF may explain its better outcomes than COMPANION for CRT without defibrillation. A series of patients undergoing CRT in one institution found that over approximately 2 years HF death or rehospitalization due to HF was most common in patients who were NYHA Class IV prior to insertion; non-HF death was most common in NYHA Class III patients but on multivariate analysis, death from any cause was statistically associated with NYHA Class IV status prior to CRT.[32]

Resynchronization therapy should be considered only when medical therapy has been optimized, as both symptoms and left-ventricular function improve significantly with the combination of medications, exercise, diet and sleep-disorder management indicated for HF due to systolic dysfunction. Complications of CRT include infection, bleeding (including cardiac tamponade), and stroke or myocardial infarction.

No data currently support the use of CRT for patients with mild to moderate HF symptoms, and concern exists about hazards associated with a device, including infection, generation of arrhythmias, or ventricular irritability as well as considerable expense. Also, the trials of CRT are shorter in duration than the average life-expectancy of persons with optimally managed mild to moderate chronic HF, thus the impact on longevity is uncertain except in persons with advanced disease. In an extension of the CARE-HF trial, CRT had a small but significant impact on death from either progressive HF or SCD. Rates of HF death diverged between the CRT and medical management groups after about 2.5 years, and SCD rates were equivalent until about 4.5 years, after which there was a benefit from CRT. In this series only 37% of persons with NYHA Class IV HF survived or avoided rehospitalization, compared to 64% in Class III and 70% in NYHA Class II prior to CRT implantation.[33]

Management of resynchronization devices

Similar to other electrical devices, CRT devices require regular follow-up and interrogation. An uncertain percentage of persons with CRT lose the benefit from the device after a period of time. This may be due to loss of lead placement, and, if so, effect can be regained with replacement of the lead but there is a definite morbidity associated with this procedure. Similarly, the presence of an ICD in combination with CRT (CRT-D), results in early depletion of the battery and it is estimated that for responders, most will require at least one device replacement in their lifetime. These issues should be discussed with patients at the time a primary CRT implant is advocated.

Decision-making with patients about CRT

Fewer data inform decisions about CRT than ICDs. The discussion with patients about CRT (with or without ICD) should include a review of the patient's clinical status and the likely course of their HF. Approximately three to four out of five patients in whom resynchronization can be achieved with CRT have improvement in quality of life and HF symptoms. When effectively implanted, CRT also appears to prolong life with or without a defibrillator, though this benefit is least evident in persons with NYHA Class IV or very advanced HF.

   When patients desire an attempt at life-prolongation and meet clinical criteria for CRT, they should be informed that device placement fails in 10% of patients, and that even when placement is achieved as many as one in three patients do not receive benefit from CRT. CRT alone may prolong life, but given that ICD criteria are met by patients qualifying for CRT, many clinicians feel that defibrillator capacity should be offered with CRT. Patients must be informed of potential defibrillator shocks and the option to deactivate the defibrillator function in the future.

Conclusions

Implantable devices bring the opportunity to decrease SCD in HF patients, and in the case of CRT also to improve function and quality of life in moderate to advanced disease. Both ICD and CRT should be implanted after careful review with the patient of device actions, potential benefits, and burdens. When an ICD is implanted, the option of device deactivation in the future should be acknowledged. The deactivation of ICDs should be organized and planned by centers or physicians who implant ICDs to minimize anxiety associated with the decision to deactivate.

References

1. Mehra MR, Uber PA, Francis GS (2003). Heart failure therapy at a crossroad: are there limits to the neurohormonal model? *J Am Coll Cardiol* **41**: 1606–10.

2. Konstam MA, Gheorghiade M, Burnett JC, Jr *et al.* and the Efficacy of Vasopressin Antagonism in Heart Failure Outcome Study With Tolvaptan (EVEREST) Investigators (2007). Effects of oral tolvaptan in patients hospitalized for worsening heart failure: the EVEREST Outcome Trial. *J Am Med Assoc* **297**: 1319–31.

3. Wathen MS, Sweeney MO, DeGroot PJ *et al.* (2001). Shock reduction using antitachycardia pacing for spontaneous rapid ventricular tachycardia in patients with coronary artery disease. *Circulation* **104**: 796–801.

4. The AVID Investigators (1997). A comparison of antiarrhythmic-drug therapy with implantable defibrillators in patients resuscitated from near-fatal ventricular arrhythmias. *New Engl J Med* **337**: 1576–83.

5. Cesaria DA, Dee GW (2006). Implantable cardioverter-defibrillator therapy in clinical practice. *J Am Coll Cardiol* **47**: 1507–17.

6. Pitt B, Remme W, Zannad F, *et al.* (2003). Eplerenone, a selective aldosterone blocker, in patients with left ventricular dysfunction after myocardial infarction. *New Engl J Med* **348**: 1309–21.

7. Moss AJ, Hall WJ, Cannom DS *et al.* (1996). Improved survival with an implanted defibrillator in patients with coronary disease at high risk for ventricular arrhythmia. *New Engl J Med* **335**: 1933–40.

8. Buxton AE, Lee KL, Fisher JD *et al.* (1999). A randomized study of the prevention of sudden death in patients with coronary artery disease. *New Engl J Med* **341**: 1882–90.

9. Bardy GH, Lee KL, Mark DB *et al.* for the Sudden Death in Heart Failure Trial (SCDHeFT) Investigators (2005). Amiodarone or an implantable cardioverter-defibrillator for congestive heart failure. *New Engl J Med* **352**: 225–37.

10. Smit MD, Van Dessel PF, Nieuwland W *et al.* (2006). Right ventricular pacing and the risk of heart failure in implantable cardioverter-defibrillator patients. *Heart Rhythm* **3**: 1397–403.

11. Hegel MT, Griegel LE, Black C, Goulden L, Ozahowski T (1997). Anxiety and depression in patients receiving implanted cardioverter-defibrillators: a longitudinal investigation. *Int J Psychiat Med* **27**: 57–69.

12. Moss AJ, Greenberg H, Case RB *et al.* for the Multicenter Automatic Defibrillator Implantation Trial-II (MADIT-II) Research Group (2004). Long-term clinical course of patients after termination of ventricular tachyarrhythmia by an implanted defibrillator. *Circulation* **110**: 3760–5.

13. Saba S. Atiga WL, Barrington W *et al.* (2003). Selected patients listed for cardiac transplantation may benefit from defibrillator implantation regardless of an established indication. *J Heart Lung Transplant* **22**: 411–15.

14. Kadish A, Dyer A, Daubert JP *et al.* (2004). Prophylactic defibrillator implantation in patients with nonischemic dilated cardiomyopathy. *New Engl J Med* **350**: 2151–8.

15. Sweeney MO, Wathen MS, Volosin K *et al.* (2005). Appropriate and inappropriate ventricular therapies, quality of life, and mortality among primary and secondary prevention implantable cardioverter defibrillator patients: results from the Pacing Fast VT REduces Shock ThErapies (PainFREE Rx II) trial. *Circulation* **111**: 2898–905.

16. Nanthakumar K, Dorian P, Paquette M *et al.* (2003). Is inappropriate implantable defibrillator shock therapy predictable? *J Interv Card Electrophysiol* **8**: 215–20.

17. Hreybe H, Ezzeddine R, Barrington W *et al.* (2006). Relation of advanced heart failure symptoms to risk of inappropriate defibrillator shocks. *Am J Cardiol* **97**: 544–6.

18. Alter P, Waldhans S, Plachta E, Moosdorf R, Grimm W (2005). Complications of implantable cardioverter defibrillator therapy in 440 consecutive patients. *Pacing Clin Electrophysiol* **28**: 926–32.

19. Whang W, Mittleman MA, Rich DO *et al.* for the TOVA Investigators, Heart Failure and the Risk of Shocks inpatients With Implantable Cardioverter Defibrillators (2004). Results from the Triggers of Ventricular Arrhythmias Study. *Circulation* **109**: 1386–91.

20. Hunt SA, Abraham WT, Chin MH *et al.* (2005). ACC/AHA 2005 guideline update for the diagnosis and management of chronic heart failure in the adult: a report of the American College of Cardiology/American Heart Association Task Force on Practice Guidelines. *Circulation* **112**: e154–e235.

21. (2006). HFSA 2006 Comprehensive Heart Failure Practice Guideline. *J Card Fail* **12**: e1–e122.

22. Weintraub JR, Semigran MJ, Tsang S *et al.* (2006). What do patients know about ICDs? *Heart Rhythm* **3**: S139.

23. Ellenbogen KA, Levine JH, Berger RD *et al.* for the Defibrillators in Non-Ischemic Cardiomyopathy Treatment Evaluation (DEFINITE) Investigators (2006). Are implantable cardioverter defibrillator shocks a surrogate for sudden cardiac death in patients with nonischemic cardiomyopathy? *Circulation* **113**: 776–82.

24. Carson P, Anand I, O'Connor C *et al.* (2005). Mode of death in advanced heart failure: the Comparison of Medical, Pacing, and Defibrillation Therapies in Heart Failure (COMPANION) trial. *J Am Coll Cardiol* **46**: 2329–34.

25. Zareba W, Piotrowicz K, McNitt S, Moss AJ, MADIT II Investigators (2005). Implantable cardioverter-defibrillator efficacy in patients with heart failure and left ventricular dysfunction (from the MADIT II population). *Am J Cardiol* **95**: 1487–91.

26. Rozanski A, Blumenthal JA, Kaplan J (1999). Impact of psychological factors on the pathogenesis of cardiovascular disease and implications for therapy. *Circulation* **99**: 2192–217.

27. Sears SF, Conti JB (2003). Understanding ICD shocks and storms: Medical and psychosocial considerations for research and clinical care. *Clin Cardiol* **26**: 107–11.

28. Shamin W, Francis DP, Yousufuddin M *et al.* (1999). Intraventricular conduction delay: a prognostic marker in chronic heart failure. *Int J Cardiol* **70**: 171–8.

29. Baldesseroni S, Opasich C, Gorini M *et al.* (2002). Left bundle-branch block is associated with increased 1-year sudden and total mortality rate in 5517 outpatients with congestive heart failure. *Am Heart J* 398–405.

30. Bristow MR, Saxon LA, Boehmer J *et al.* (2004). Cardiac-resynchronization therapy with or without an implantable defibrillator in advanced chronic heart failure. *New Engl J Med* **350**: 2140–50.

31. Cleland JG, Daubert JC, Erdmann E *et al.* (2005). The effect of cardiac resynchronization on morbidity and mortality in heart failure. *New Engl J Med* **352**: 1539–49.

32. De Sisti A, Toussaint J-F,Lavergne T *et al.* (2005). Determinants of mortality in patients undergoing cardiac resynchronization therapy: baseline clinical, echocardiographic, and angioscintigraphic evaluation prior to resynchronization. *PACE* **28**: 1260–70.

33. Cleland JF, Daubert J-C, Erdmann E *et al.* for the CARE-HF Study Investigators (2006). Longer-term effect of cardiac resynchronization therapy on mortality in heart failure [the Cardiac Resynchronization-Heart Failure (CARE-HF) trial extension phase]. *Eur Heart J* **27**: 1928–32.

Chapter 6

Advanced heart failure: the role of the surgeon

Stephen Westaby and Gabriele B. Bertoni

The clinical syndrome of congestive heart failure (HF) is the final pathway for many diseases that affect the myocardium. The debilitating symptoms of advanced HF stem from two major pathophysiological processes: raised left-ventricular end diastolic pressure (LVEDP) results in pulmonary congestion and breathlessness and decreased systemic blood flow triggers numerous vascular cytokine and humoral responses, which cause salt and water retention and fatigue.

In Western countries coronary artery disease is responsible for about 75% of HF cases.[1] In the Italian SEOSI study 70% of patients had a previous myocardial infarction, whereas 15% had hypertension-related restrictive cardiomyopathy.[2] Idiopathic dilated cardiomyopathy and valvular heart disease accounted for 15% of patients. Ten per cent of the HF population are Stage D (New York Heart Association (NYHA) Class IV) and 20% of these patients are under 65 years of age.[3] They have advanced structural heart disease with symptoms at rest, despite detailed medical or resynchronization therapy. They become progressively more dependent on hospital admissions for symptomatic stabilization and outpatient nursing for palliative care. Despite improvements in medical management, Stage D HF carries a grim prognosis. In the Consensus Trial half of the patients in the control arm had died within 6 months.[4] In the Rematch Study only 8% of patients in the medically treated group were alive at 2 years.[5] Stage D HF affects between 300,000 and 800,000 patients in the United States and approximately 100,000 patients in the United Kingdom. This generates a massive economic burden without gaining substantial symptomatic benefit or prognostic improvement. Nevertheless most societies are prepared to invest in both drugs and devices to palliate symptoms and improve quality of life within reasonable limits. These limits are largely set by age considerations and economics rather than the ethical dilemmas surrounding a particular intervention.

For end-stage patients cardiac transplantation provides the benchmark for increased longevity and symptomatic relief.[6] However, the vast majority of Stage D patients are over 65 years of age or are referred with established co-morbidity which precludes transplantation. For these patients the goal of surgical treatment is to reverse the remodelling process. Left-ventricular shape and volume are important predictors of survival. Patients with a left-ventricular ejection fraction (LVEF) of <30% have a 5-year survival of only 54% when the left-ventricular end systolic volume index (LVESVI) exceeds 150 ml m^{-2}.[7] In both ischaemic and idiopathic dilated cardiomyopathy, increased chamber sphericity and the onset of mitral regurgitation are markers of worse prognosis (1-year mortality 54–70%).[8] Mitral regurgitation occurs with altered left-ventricular geometry, papillary muscle dysfunction, and annular dilatation. Progressive volume overload results in left-ventricular dilatation, worsened mitral regurgitation, and decreased survival. Myocardial hypertrophy and ventricular dilatation are responses to increased ventricular pressure or volume stress. In the early stages both are reversible by relieving the causes of increased stress. In contrast, there is no evidence that a reduction in wall stress arrests the myopathic process in large uncompensated ventricles that are continuing to dilate. Accordingly, surgery for HF is best performed before decompensation with the aim of reducing ventricular strain (stretch) and wall stress in order to arrest stretch-induced cardiomyopathy. Given the remarkable developments in circulatory support technology and non-transplant HF operations over the past 10 years there is a clear requirement to redefine the surgeon's role in treating Stage C/D disease.

Cardiologists have yet to be persuaded that non-transplant surgical alternatives are beneficial and safe. The UK National Institute for Health and Clinical Excellence (NICE) has published a 'best practice' document for the management of chronic HF. Remarkably, it mentions surgery in only two sentences. The first states that 'coronary revascularisation should not be routinely considered in HF due to systolic left-ventricular impairment unless the patient has refractory angina'. The second states that 'specialist referral for transplantation should be considered in patients with refractory symptoms or refractory cardiogenic shock'. This lack of insight into the role of surgery in HF is balanced by the comment that 'Heart failure care should be delivered by a multi-disciplinary team with an integrated approach across the health care community'. Given that it is preferable to repair rather than replace the diseased heart, the role of emerging procedures needs further definition. As the treatment options increase there is an imperative to decide whether to treat, how to treat, and when to treat.

Currently there are few guidelines as to which operation best suits an individual patient or pathological process. Detailed clinical assessment is needed to identify the pathology and extent of structural and functional abnormalities. The object of investigation is to determine whether there are lesions amenable to surgical repair, whether dysfunctional myocardium is potentially recoverable, or, in the event of neither of these, whether long-term circulatory assist is feasible (Fig. 6.1).

How does the HF patient reach the surgeon?

There are often three tiers of medical care before surgical assessment. A patient with the symptoms and clinical signs of HF first presents to the primary-care physician who may instigate medical therapy. It can be difficult to determine the cause of left-ventricular dysfunction. In one study in Glasgow (UK), 95% of symptomatic and 71% of asymptomatic patients with definite left-ventricular systolic dysfunction had evidence of coronary artery disease.[1] Those with symptomatic HF were more likely to have a previous

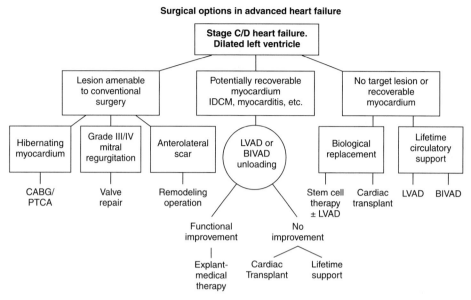

Fig. 6.1 Decision-making algorithm in advanced HF.

myocardial infarction (50% vs 14%) and concurrent angina (62% vs 43%). Hypertension was also present in 80% of those with symptomatic HF.

Age has a varying influence in different health-care systems. In the elderly further referral may not be considered unless a murmur (valvular heart disease) is detected or the patient has angina. Patients under 75 years of age are generally referred to a local cardiologist to define the aetiology and the extent of left-ventricular dysfunction. Echocardiography and coronary angiography are usually performed at this stage to differentiate between ischaemic, restrictive, or idiopathic dilated cardiomyopathy.

The local cardiologist determines further management by tertiary referral to an interventional cardiologist, surgeon, or a transplant centre if the patient is severely symptomatic (and conventionally less than 65 years of age). The patient may proceed to percutaneous coronary intervention or receive either an implantable defibrillator or cardiac resynchronization therapy. In ischaemic heart disease hibernating myocardium, anterolateral or septal scar, and mitral regurgitation are each amenable to surgical repair.[9] Patients with idiopathic dilated cardiomyopathy, a remodelled ventricle, and worsening mitral regurgitation may benefit from mitral valve repair or external constraint. In the absence of a target lesion or transplant eligibility some patients can now be considered for long-term mechanical circulatory support either as definitive treatment or to reverse the remodelling process sufficient to allow removal of the device.[10]

Given these potential surgical strategies, all Stage C and D patients should be assessed by a multidisciplinary HF team with access to state-of-the-art investigational facilities. Allocation to the appropriate intervention needs very detailed definition of coronary anatomy, myocardial structure, dynamic dimensions, ventricular function, viability, and the potential for improvement. Age and significant co-morbidity must be taken into consideration before deciding upon a particular procedure. The surgeon's role is to determine which operation or combination of surgical procedures best suits an individual and whether the operation can be performed with acceptable risk and likelihood of benefit given the overall condition of the patient. The time to operate is before the heart dilates, not afterwards. High-risk procedures should not be considered until optimization of medical treatment has provided the best setting for recovery. Non-transplant options should always be considered first and carried out in such a way that a cardiac transplant or mechanical circulatory support remains feasible in the future.

How to determine the surgical strategy

At the time of surgical referral most patients are Stage C or D with a dilated left ventricle and impaired cardiac output. For those who present in cardiogenic shock with either acute or decompensated chronic HF, urgent mechanical circulatory support may be necessary before further investigation and definitive treatment (Fig. 6.2). A bank of clinical investigations including coronary angiography, echocardiography, magnetic resonance imaging, and assessment of myocardial viability together with functional assessment by 6-min walk test and measurement of mixed venous oxygen content on exercise (MVO_2) provide the required information about cardiac pathophysiology and

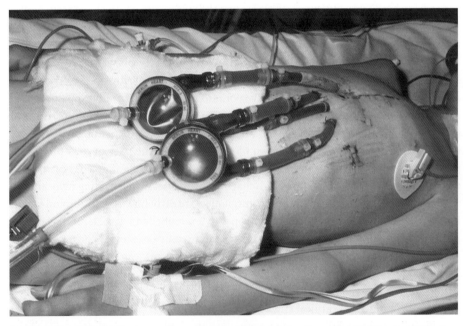

Fig. 6.2 Child with a Berlin heart. (Reproduced with permission from Fig. 35.37 on p. 674 of *Heart Failure: Pathogenesis and Treatment* by J Narula, R Virmani, M Ballester, I Carrio, S Westaby, O Frazier, and J Willerson, Martin Dunitz, 2002.)

functional status.[11] Cardiac assessment is supported by a careful determination of other risk factors including respiratory, vascular, renal, and hepatic dysfunction. On the basis of these findings the multidisciplinary team should decide whether there is a lesion amenable to conventional surgery, or potentially recoverable myocardium (stunning, hibernation, idiopathic dilated cardiomyopathy or myocarditis). If there is no conventional surgical option a cardiac transplant or long-term circulatory support are the remaining possibilities (Fig. 6.1). Eligibility for cardiac transplantation is determined during the course of medical assessment but committal to a transplant waiting list should only occur when other avenues have been exhausted.

The potential surgical procedure, its risks, and likely benefit can then be discussed with the patient.

Decision-making in patients with ischaemic cardiomyopathy

Impairment of left-ventricular function at rest may be the result of myocardial scar, stunning or hibernation, and is most commonly a combination of these entities.[12] The ventricle in ischaemic cardiomyopathy contains microenvironments of irreversibly injured myocytes with necrosis or scar tissue, together with viable myocardial cells in varying proportions. These changes are self-aggravating because of the restrictive effects on blood flow to the subendocardial layer. Repeated infarction cause more scarring. Eventually, left-ventricular systolic and diastolic dysfunction result in congestive HF. Alternatively, patients with ischaemic myocardium die suddenly from infarction or ventricular fibrillation triggered by electrical instability.

The relationship between the extent of infarction, degree of left-ventricular dysfunction, and late mortality was defined by Yoshida and Gould.[13] A myocardial infarction greater than 23% of the left-ventricular circumference causes impaired LVEF (<45%) and a 3-year mortality rate exceeding 40% (Table 6.1). This contrasts with less extensive infarction, which carries a 3-year mortality rate of around 5%. Nevertheless, LVEF alone is a poor predictor of mortality if the patient has hibernating myocardium.

Table 6.1 Relationship between infarct size and mortality (from Yoshida and Gould[4])

	Three-year mortality (%)	P-value
Myocardial infarction or scar ≥ 23%	43	0.014
Myocardial infarction or scar < 23%	5	
EF < 43%	38	0.029
EF > 43%	6	
EF ≤ 43% without viable myocardium	63	0.059
EF ≤ 43% with viable myocardium[a]	13	

[a]For all patients with viable myocardium the 3-year mortality rate was 8% [80% had coronary artery bypass graft (CABG)]. For patients with only fixed scar >23% mortality rate was 50% (P = 0.018, only 40% had CABG).

EF, ejection fraction.

Viable myocardium is an independent predictor of survival and a marker for those with impaired LVEF who are likely to benefit from revascularization. Accordingly, the 3-year mortality rate in those with a LVEF of <43% and no viable myocardium was 63% in contrast with 13% mortality for those with viable myocardium submitted for revascularization. For patients with only scar in the territory at risk from coronary occlusion, a 3-year mortality rate of 50% with or without revascularization, suggests no benefit from intervention in this subgroup.

The components of post-infarction remodelling include infarct expansion, myocardial hypertrophy, and global left-ventricular dilatation resulting in a more spherical contour. Increased wall stress results in lengthening and thinning of the left-ventricular wall through lateral slippage of myocardial planes. The changes in ventricular geometry, local wall tension, and filling pressures combine to increase the metabolic requirements of the non-ischaemic myocardium, which maintains cardiac output. Working segments undergo compensatory hypertrophy. Whilst a low LVEF (<30%) indicates that the ventricle has remodelled, a dilated chamber with low LVEF can eject virtually the same stroke volume as a normal ventricle. Exercise capacity has a poor relationship with left-ventricular function, although LVEF is an important determinant for survival. Patients with a LVEF > 40% have modest annual mortality rate (<10%) whereas those with a LVEF < 30% have annual mortality rates >25%.[8] In patients with LVEF of 15–40% there is an almost linear relationship between LVEF mortality.

In most patients with extensive coronary disease abnormalities of left-ventricular diastolic function can be demonstrated during stress.[6] These are manifest by a reduced peak left-ventricular filling rate and increased time-to-peak filling rate. Hypoxia also impairs relaxation of the papillary muscles during early diastole because this is an active energy-dependent process. Ischaemic abnormalities of left-ventricular systolic and diastolic function during stress may cause substantially elevated LVEDP. Some patients have moderately increased LVEDP at rest with considerably reduced exercise capacity, but only mildly increased cardiac size on chest radiography. These patients often have moderate scarring and marked ischaemic dysfunction in non-scarred parts of the ventricles, and may be helped by revascularization. Others have moderate or severe cardiomegaly, reduced cardiac index, and substantial elevation of right atrial pressure with hepatomegaly and fluid retention. This latter group usually have extensive myocardial scarring and are unlikely to be improved by revascularization alone.

The relationship between myocardial stunning, hibernation, and HF remains complex. Some patients with coronary disease do not stun, whereas others suffer repeated clinically silent episodes of stunning during normal daily activities. If such episodes are frequent with incomplete recovery of contractile function before the next insult, then chronic ventricular dysfunction may ensue. Repetitive stunning may trigger the development of myocardial hibernation, which is associated with changes in myocyte metabolism and structure.[6] Structural changes depend on the time that myocardial blood supply remains jeopardized during demand ischaemia. Thus, myocardium may progress through a phase of functional hibernation (without changes in the contractile protein apparatus) to a phase of structural hibernation with morphological abnormalities within the myocyte, including loss of myofibrillar material and accumulation of glycogen.[12]

In structural hibernation, functional recovery after revascularization is more prolonged and dependent on new protein synthesis and myocyte repair. In the absence of revascularization, repetitive ischaemia may progress to myocyte necrosis or apoptosis, indicating that hibernating myocardium is not fully adapted to chronic hypoperfusion. Cellular degeneration and myocyte loss are accompanied by reparative fibrosis. They combine to cause degeneration in the structural and functional integrity of the left ventricle, even in the absence of myocardial infarction. Consequently, if revascularization is to succeed, it must be applied early before functional hibernation progresses to structural hibernation. Hibernating myocardium is present in about 78% of patients after myocardial infarction treated by thrombolysis.[7] As many as 50% of coronary patients referred for transplantation have hibernating myocardium.[14] Cardiac events including death, non-fatal myocardial infarction, or unstable angina occur in 33% of patients with hibernation, versus only 8% for those with scar.[12]

Testing for myocardial viability

Evidence that segmental and global left-ventricular function will improve after revascularization is obtained using imaging methods that show the presence of myocardial viability. The techniques with the greatest evidence base for predicting recovery are those that detect preserved metabolic activity, cell membrane integrity, or contractile reserve in dysfunctional regions. Positron emission tomography (PET), single photon emission tomography (SPECT) with thallium-210 or technetium-99m perfusion tracers and low-dose dobutamine stress echocardiography have emerged as accurate and accepted methods for viability assessment, particularly when taken in combination.[14] Contrast-enhanced magnetic resonance imaging (MRI) also holds great promise in this area by providing very accurate information about left-ventricular volume indices, myocardial wall thickness, and valve function.[15] Patients who benefit from viability testing include those with suspected coronary disease or dilated cardiomyopathy who are being considered for cardiac transplantation, and those with coronary disease and left-ventricular dysfunction (LVEF <35%) who are asymptomatic or have breathlessness with only mild angina. Viability testing is redundant in patients with unstable angina, post-infarction angina, and those with severe chronic stable angina because revascularization is indicated for symptomatic relief. For ischaemic HF patients without angina, the combination of good target vessels and >25% myocardial viability suggests the potential to benefit from revascularization. For those with <25% viability, poor target vessels, or in re-operative candidates, surgery is unlikely to produce improvement.[16] Other unfavourable patient characteristic include advanced aged, female gender, severity of coronary artery disease, presence of pre-operative dysrhythmias, and renal failure. Table 6.2 provides guidelines supporting the use of coronary artery bypass grafting (CABG) in preference to cardiac transplantation in patients with advanced ischaemic cardiomyopathy.[17]

Table 6.2 Guidelines for coronary bypass versus transplantation in end-stage coronary artery disease

CABG	Transplant
Prevailing hibernation	Prevailing scar
Short duration of heart failure	Prolonged heart failure
Low dose diurectics	High dose diuretics
No right ventricular failure	Chronic R.V. failure
Stable cardiac output	Chronic low output
CI > 2.0 Lmin^{-1}m^{-2}	CI < 2.0 Lmin^{-1}m^{-2}
LVEDP ≤ 24mm Hg	LVEDP > 24mm Hg
Good target vessels	Poor Vessels
First operation	Previous revascularisation

Outcome after non-transplant surgery for ischaemic cardiomyopathy

Useful data regarding patient selection and outcome for high-risk revascularization have emerged from centres where transplant candidates were selected out for CABG instead. Hausmann *et al.*[17] in Berlin compared 225 potential transplant candidates who underwent CABG with 231 others who received a donor organ. This was not a randomized trial. Differences between the groups were the longer duration of symptoms, the presence of right-heart failure, and a greater incidence of previous CABG in the heart transplant recipients. Operative risk in the CABG group was significantly higher for those with a greatly increased LVEDP (>24 mmHg), a low pre-operative cardiac index (< 2.0 L min^{-1} m^{-2}) and for patients in NYHA Class IV. Hospital mortality was 7.1% for the CABG patients versus 18.2% in the transplant group. There was no significant difference in hospital mortality in patients with LVEF between 10% and 20% versus those between 20% and 30%. Survival for the CABG group was 78.9% after 6 years versus 68.9% for the transplant group. Reinvestigation of CABG patients showed a significant decrease in mean pulmonary artery pressure from 28.2 mmHg to 21.2 mmHg ($p < 0.01$). Pulmonary capillary wedge pressure fell from 19.2 mmHg to 13.1 mmHg ($p < 0.01$) and LVEF improved from a mean of 0.24 to 0.39 ($p < 0.0001$). Others have reported similar findings.[18]

Observational studies have documented substantial improvement in left-ventricular regional and global function following revascularization of hibernating myocardium.[19] Relief from HF symptoms, improved quality of life, and survival benefit have been demonstrated in these patients. The advantages of viability assessment in patient selection were demonstrated by Haas *et al.*[20] in a series of 69 patients with three vessels disease and LVEF < 35%. Thirty-five patients were operated on the basis of angiographic findings alone whereas 34 were selected on the basis of PET-documented hibernating myocardium and favourable target vessels. The hibernating myocardium group had a lower hospital mortality (0% vs 11.4%, $p = 0.04$), a lower incidence of post-operative complications (33% vs 67%, $p = 0.05$), and fewer patients with low cardiac output syndrome (3% vs 17%, $p = 0.05$). Furthermore, the 1-year survival rate was better ($97 \pm 8\%$ vs $79 \pm 8\%$, $p < 0.01$). The LVEF increased from 26% to 35% ($p = 0.003$) in those with myocardial viability but was unchanged in those without. Similarly, in a retrospective review of 70 ischaemic cardiomyopathy patients undergoing CABG, Pagley et al.[21] demonstrated an improved short- and long-term cardiac event-free survival in patients with hibernating myocardium. In those who were similar with regard to age, gender, presenting clinical syndrome, haemodynamical variables, number of diseased coronary arteries, and LVEF, the myocardial viability index was the only independent predictor of event-free survival. Tjan et al.[22] compared the outcome in 51 potential transplant candidates (all LVEF < 20%) who underwent CABG instead, with 163 others who were transplanted. The survival analysis was performed on the basis of intention to treat independent of subsequent transplantation. Groups were comparable with regard to left-ventricular function, pulmonary capillary wedge pressure, and serum creatinine. Patients in the CABG group were older (63 ± 8 years) and included a higher percentage of females. One-year survival was similar in both groups (CABG 71.9% vs transplant 66.3%). In CABG patients, hospital survival was 88.2%. Pre-operative serum creatinine and the non-usage of the left internal thoracic artery were predictors of adverse outcome. The authors concluded that up to 50% of transplant candidates could be redirected towards CABG after assessing myocardial viability and general risk factors such as age, peripheral vascular disease, history of hypertension, and suitability of the target vessels. In contrast, selection according to pre-operative LVEF was not useful. Only the degree of myocardial viability was predictive of outcome. The authors recommended pre-operative insertion of an intra-aortic balloon pump and left-ventricular assist device (LVAD) stand-by during the operation.

With worsening donor availability, many centres now support high-risk revascularization as a transplant alternative, though the benefits may be time-limited. Luciani et al.[23] showed only 47% of patients with advanced pre-operative left-ventricular dysfunction to be free from HF symptoms 5 years after CABG, despite 75% survival at this time. CABG appears to influence the mode of death, however. Mortality occurs predominantly through left-ventricular failure and not dysrhythmias which otherwise accounts for more than 60% of deaths in unoperated ischaemic cardiomyopathy.

Improvement in myocardial function

Irrespective of the symptomatic and survival benefits afforded by revascularization, the functional response is unpredictable. In detailed studies of regional perfusion, glucose usage, and contractile function, Bax et al.[24] showed functional improvement in only 70% of stunned myocardial segments and 31% of hibernating segments by 3 months. Whilst there was no further improvement in stunned segments, 61% of hibernating segments manifest gradual improvement in wall motion score by 14 months. Haas et al.[20] studied the time course of functional recovery in relation to the histology (intraoperative biopsy) from dysfunctional areas. PET was used to distinguish stunned from hibernating myocardium. Stunning was identified in 70% of 240 dysfunctional segments and hibernation in 24%. Hibernation was associated with more severe depression of wall motion and incomplete post-operative recovery. One year after revascularization, only 31% of stunned segments and 18% of hibernating segments showed complete functional recovery. Failure to improve was associated with more severe degenerative ultrastructural changes in the myocyte. The authors concluded that myocardial stunning was more prevalent than hibernation and that myocardial morphology determined the time course and extent of functional improvement after revascularization.

The observation that only 31% of stunned myocardial segments attained complete functional recovery challenges the definition of 'stunning' from which complete recovery is expected over time. In this population with severe long-lasting coronary artery disease, previous infarction, and a history of congestive HF it is likely that other factors such as the degree of left-ventricular remodelling and persistent elevated wall stress may preclude myocardial recovery.[25] Myocardial histology in these patients suggests a continuum between stunning and hibernation, with structural hibernation representing the limit of viability. Kim and colleagues,[26] using enhanced contrast MRI, found that 78% of dysfunctional segments identified as completely viable showed improvement in contractility after revascularization. In contrast, 90% of the regions with 50–75% of wall thickness scar did not improve. These regions would be considered entirely non-viable according to wall motion criteria, even though a substantial epicardial rim of viable tissue remains. Maes et al.[27] showed the degree of fibrosis within the myocardial segment to be a determinant of improvement. Others have shown severely hypokinetic or akinetic segments to have a 2.4-fold increase in α-receptor density with a concomitant 50% decrease in β-receptor density compared with normal segments.[28] Graded reciprocal changes in α- and β-adrenergic receptor density in hibernating myocardium may account in part for the depression in resting myocardial function, and confirms that alterations in β-receptor density are associated with hibernating myocardium.

Clearly, in many cases of ischaemic cardiomyopathy no conservative option is possible. These patients have advanced left-ventricular remodelling with LVESVI > 100 ml m^{-2}, suffer breathlessness with no angina, and have no reversible ischaemia on viability testing. This combination is often associated with a degree of right-ventricular failure and pulmonary hypertension with a right atrial pressure exceeding 20 mmHg. For these patients, cardiac transplantation or a 'lifetime' LVAD implant are the only options. Mitral regurgitation is not a contraindication to LVAD use but mitral stenosis clearly is.

Left-ventricular restoration surgery

Ventricular restoration surgery is the successor to left-ventricular aneurysmectomy, now that thrombolysis usually arrests myocardial infarction before it reaches the transmural stage. Substantial improvement in left-ventricular systolic function is uncommon after reperfusion therapy. With healing of infarcted myocardium, scar is maximal in the subendocardial region, though the epicardial surface may appear normal because of a rim of reperfused muscle. This contrasts with the leather-like appearance of full thickness myocardial scar in a dyskinetic left-ventricular aneurysm. MRI studies by Bogaert et al.[25] demonstrated epicardial viability but loss of between 80% and 90% of contractile muscle in the endocardium and mid-myocardium after thrombolysis. The veneer of epicardial salvage is insufficient to prevent dilatation of the ischaemic segment and increased sphericity. When more than 40% of the left-ventricular circumference becomes non-functional, the normal LVESVI of 25 ml m^{-2} increases to >60 ml m^{-2}. This is a threshold likely to be associated with subsequent cardiac mortality.

As left-ventricular size increases, the progressive left-ventricular hypertrophy and systolic wall stress produce worsening ischaemic symptoms. Stroke volume and global left-ventricular function gradually decline as ischaemia progresses in the non-aneurysmal segments. Once decompensation begins, functional deterioration occurs rapidly with an increase in the risk of surgical mortality. For this reason left-ventricular restoration surgery should be considered in patients with LVEF < 30%, mean pulmonary artery pressure > 25 mmHg, left-ventricular akinesia or dyskinesia > 60% and left-ventricular end-diastolic volume (LVEDV) > 250ml (LVEDVI > 140 ml m^{-2}).[29] Most of these patients are already NYHA Class III or IV with medical treatment.

Ventricular aneurysmectomy improves symptoms by lowering left-ventricular wall stress, but the linear amputation of a discrete dyskinetic scar commonly deforms the left-ventricular cavity into a box-like shape. Cooley[30] and Jatene[31] decreased surgical mortality by introducing intracavity patch reconstruction techniques to recreate an elliptical shape. Dor et al.[32] further refined these methods and translated the application from well-defined dyskinetic scar to akinetic myocardial segments with normal epicardium. At operation, the epicardium of the infarcted zone may appear normal, but the endocardial scar prevents improvement in wall motion by revascularization alone.

Details of the Dor procedure are presented elsewhere.[33] The overall effect is to reduce left-ventricular chamber size, restore the natural elliptical left-ventricular shape, and globally decrease wall stress (Fig. 6.3). This also enhances function in myocardial regions remote from the repair. The operation is usually supplemented by surgical revascularization of suitable target vessels and mitral valve repair when necessary. Grade 3 and 4 mitral regurgitation are best addressed by standard mitral annuloplasty techniques. Grade 2 mitral regurgitation can be treated satisfactorily using the Alfieri stitch via the left ventriculotomy (Fig. 6.4).[34]

In contrast to the somewhat slow and unpredictable recovery after revascularization, left-ventricular restoration surgery produces an immediate result. Dor et al.[29] studied a cohort of 781 ventricular restoration patients (age 57 ± 7 years) with mean LVEF 17 ± 3%. All were NYHA Class III or IV before surgery. Hospital mortality was 19.3%, but ejection fraction improved from 17 ± 3% to 37 ± 10% ($p < 0.0001$). By multivariate analysis, factors that influenced early mortality were the presence of critical narrowing in the circumflex coronary artery and the duration of cardiopulmonary bypass. At 1-year

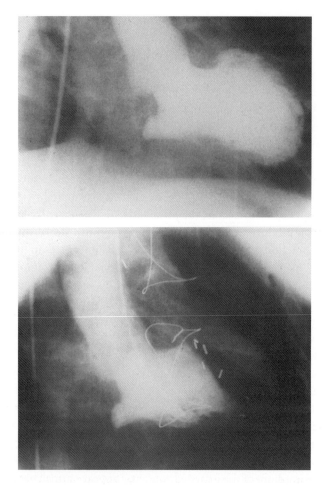

Fig. 6.3 Dor angiogram. (Reproduced with permission from Fig. 34.15 on p. 625 of *Heart Failure: Pathogenesis and Treatment* by J Narula, R Virmani, M Ballester, I Carrio, S Westaby, O Frazier, and J Willerson, Martin Dunitz, 2002.)

follow-up, a significant improvement in NYHA class was observed with no patients remaining in NYHA Class IV. Improvement in LVEF was maintained (39 ± 11%) as well as the reduction in inducible and spontaneous ventricular tachycardia. Late mortality was 10% at 5 years. Athanasulas *et al.*[35] applied left-ventricular restoration to a series of elderly patients (mean age 77 years, all NYHA Class IV) with a history of multiple admissions for congestive HF and gross left-ventricular enlargement. Pre-operatively, the mean LVEF was 20% (±8.5%), LVEDV was 300 ± 105 ml, and LVESV was 243 ± 81 ml (LVEDVI 169 ± 55 ml m^{-2} and LVESVI 132 ± 41 ml m^{-2}). After surgery LVEF increased from 20% to 35%. The average LVEDV was reduced by 80 ml (from 300 ml to 220 ml), an average of 28%. LVESV was reduced from 243 ml to 149 ml, an average of 49%. LVEDVI was

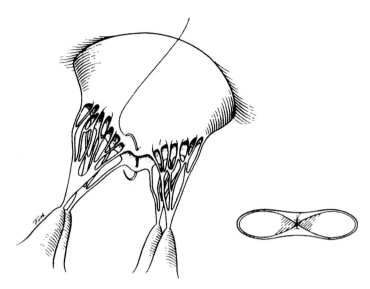

Fig. 6.4 Alfieri stitch. (Reproduced with permission from Fig. 33.18 on p. 611 of *Heart Failure: Pathogenesis and Treatment* by J Narula, R Virmani, M Ballester, I Carrio, S Westaby, O Frazier, and J Willerson, Martin Dunitz, 2002.)

reduced by 48 ml m^{-2} (from 170 ml m^{-2} to 121 ml m^{-2}) and the LVESVI was reduced by 45 ml m^{-2} (from 132 ml m^{-2} to 81 ml m^{-2}).

An additional benefit of volume reduction may be the shape alteration that realigns muscle fibre orientation to allow optimal ejection. Spotovitz *et al.*[36] have described transmural shearing planes on cross-sections of the myocardium. Contractile fibres run perpendicular to these planes and thickening of contracting heart muscle is produced by torsion or deformation of these fibres. This change in myocardial thickening is responsible for left-ventricular ejection and is evident during MRI of the left-ventricular wall. The torsion is related to the angle of fibre orientation with a conical formation towards the apex. The Dor procedure restores elliptical fibre orientation and improves wall thickening during left-ventricular contraction. Shape restoration produces a more normal orientation of sinubulbar and circular muscle around the left ventricle and re-establishes an ellipsoid form to improve systolic twisting compression.

In 1998, Buckberg and Dor initiated an international cooperative study to investigate the results of surgical left-ventricular restoration on a multicentre basis.[37] Nine centres reported on 449 patients with mean age of 63 ± 10 years with a baseline LVEF of 28 ± 10% and median LVESVI of 110 ml m^{-2}. Anterolateral akinesia was present in 67% and left-ventricular aneurysm (dyskinesia) in 33%. Ninety-six per cent of the patients had CABG and 23% had mitral valve repair. Only 7% required intra-aortic balloon pump support. Hospital mortality was 5.7%, estimated 1.5-year mortality was 10% and rehospitalization for congestive HF was 5%. LVEF increased to 39 ± 12.6% (an increase of 10.5%) with a median LVESVI of 68 ml m^{-2} (a decrease of 35.4 ml m^{-2}). The 88% late survival for those who underwent left-ventricular restoration and CABG suggest that this strategy is safe and at least equivalent to CABG alone. Whether left-ventricular restoration added to CABG improves outcome can only be answered by a randomized trial of these surgical options (as is currently under way in the STICH trial).

Mitral valve repair in ischaemic cardiomyopathy

There are now a number of clinical situation where mitral valve repair with or without revascularization improves outlook for the HF patient.[9] These include:

1. Ischaemia manifest by angina and variable mitral regurgitation, which becomes significantly worse during an acute ischaemic episode, causing dyspnoea at rest or left-ventricular failure with pulmonary oedema.

2. Acute myocardial ischaemia or infarction located inferobasally (right coronary or dominant circumflex distribution), which causes sudden posteromedial papillary muscle dysfunction and mitral regurgitation.

3. Acute catastrophic pulmonary oedema caused by papillary muscle rupture (inferobasal in 75% of the cases) several days after acute myocardial infarction.

4. Chronic progressive dyspnoea (NYHA Class III or IV) associated with previous myocardial infarction, and enlarged dysfunctional left ventricle and various degrees of pulmonary hypertension. This comprises the largest group.

The recommended threshold for mitral repair in ischaemic regurgitation is a LVESVI > 18 ml m^{-2} or a calculated regurgitant fraction > 50% of the forward LVEF. Patients with angina, good target vessels, mild to moderate mitral regurgitation, and reversible ischaemia posterolaterally on the PET scan can be treated by revascularization alone. Should valve replacement prove necessary, as much of the subvalvular apparatus as possible should be conserved to maintain left-ventricular geometry and function. Division of all chordae tendineae is accompanied by a 47% reduction in LVEmax.

Ischaemic mitral regurgitation is a functional problem of unsuccessful coordination of the entire mitral apparatus rather than simple failure of a single papillary muscle (Fig. 6.5). Mitral annuloplasty with significant undersizing of the valve ring greatly increases leaflet coaptation.[38] Systolic anterior motion (SAM) is avoided because of widening of the aorto-mitral angle and increased left-ventricular size. The undersized valve ring acutely remodels the base of the myopathic heart, helping to re-establish an ellipsoid shape to the left ventricle. Somewhat simpler, but controversial, is the Alfieri stitch.[34] This can be performed either centrally or towards the side of the ischaemic papillary muscle.

The role of stem cells

Collectively, most surgical studies suggest that, in ischaemic cardiomyopathy patients stable enough to undergo elective surgery, repair is better than replacement. This policy

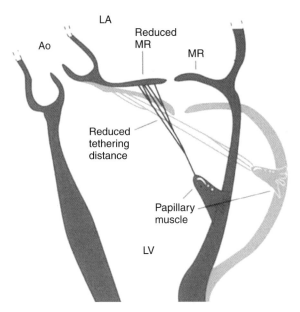

Fig. 6.5 Mitral failure in ICD. (Reproduced with permission from Fig. 34.29 on p. 638 of *Heart Failure: Pathogenesis and Treatment* by J Narula, R Virmani, M Ballester, I Carrio, S Westaby, O Frazier, and J Willerson, Martin Dunitz, 2002.)

may soon be reinforced by the introduction of autologous stem cell therapy whereby bone marrow stem cells are harvested from the iliac crest at the beginning of an open operation, processed in the laboratory, and than injected directly into ischaemic myocardium during coronary bypass surgery.[39] Alternatively, catheter-based delivery can be applied through the endocardium using an electromechanical mapping (EMM) system.[40] This locates ischaemic but viable myocardium and allows the injection catheter to be directed to the intraventricular target site. Around 30 million stem cells are introduced with the aim of inducing vasculogenesis and possibly generating new cardiac myocytes. The Texas Heart Institute have performed more than 500 such procedures with an excellent safety record and positive outcomes including clinical improvement and objective evidence of enhanced myocardial perfusion and longer treadmill exercise performance. Although it is unclear whether the stem cells create new vascular or cardiac muscle cells, or stimulate the development of one of both types of cells, the treatment protocol has proven to be sufficiently safe and effective to allow the US Food and Drug Administration to approve a randomized clinical trial.

Which patients should be transplanted?

Since Barnard's landmark operation in 1967, cardiac transplantation has made an exciting and effective contribution for a small and highly selected group of patients.

Survival data and symptomatic benefits were reported by the Stanford group in 1976 and have only recently been subjected to critical analysis in the light of improved medical and non-transplant HF surgery.[41] Ongoing problems include the management of organ rejection, the development of coronary occlusive disease, and the susceptibility to cancer and infection through immunosuppressive therapy. The identification of heart transplant candidates is based on the expected gain in survival and quality of life when compared with non-transplant options.[42] There have been no prospective randomized trials. Hospital survival has improved from around 75% in the early 1980s to 85% by 2000. Ten-year survival is now virtually 50%.[43]

In parallel with improved outcome for transplantation, medical management has reduced HF mortality. Between 1990 and 2000 the waiting list mortality for patients receiving a LVAD or intravenous inotropes (Status 1) decreased by 63% and by 55% for outpatients waiting at home in a stable condition (Status 2). In fact, the United Network for Organ Sharing identifies the fact that 1-year mortality for Status 2 patients approximates to 1-year survival after transplantation (87 ± 1%), revealing no definite survival advantage for Status 2 transplant candidates.[44] Between 1990 and 1999, the waiting list death rate fell from 432.2/1000 patients per year to 172.4/1000 patients per year. Clearly, mortality rate varies with risk status. For Status 1a patients with profound haemodynamic instability requiring LVAD support or high-dose intravenous inotropes, waiting list mortality remains at 589 deaths/1000 patients per year. This contrasts with 204.7 deaths/1000 patients per year for Status 1b patients on low-dose intravenous inotropes and 130.7 deaths/1000 patients per year for Status 2 patients.

The German Transplant Society and Eurotransplant International Foundation studied all 899 adult patients listed for cardiac transplantation in Germany in 1997. In the Comparative Outcomes and Clinical Profiles In Transplantation (COCPIT) study, the patients were stratified into high-, medium-, and low-risk categories according to HF survival score.[45] Waiting list mortality was 32% in high-risk patients and 20% in each of the medium- and low-risk groups. At 18 months after transplantation, a clear survival advantage could only be shown in the group with highest risk of waiting list mortality. To refine risk stratification in ambulatory patients (Status 2), the University of Pennsylvania and the Colombia University, New York, independently validated prognostication based on HF survival score.[46] At 1 year, survival for high-risk patients was 43 ± 7%, medium-risk 72 ± 5, and low-risk 93 ± 2%. This shows that the event-free survival for high- and medium-risk waiting list patients was much worse than after transplantation, whereas the survival of low-risk patients was better than after transplantation. In fact, with modern medical management including cardiac resynchronization therapy and implantable defibrillators, the outlook for stable patients who did not require inotropic support was better without transplantation.

Clearly, cardiac transplantation is an irreversible operation and the very restricted number of donor organs should be reserved for those patients most likely to benefit in life expectancy and quality of life. The donor supply in the United States is approximately 2000 hearts annually, in contrast to an estimated 100,000 patients who could meet the transplant criteria.[51] Corresponding figures in the UK are 150 hearts and 12,000 end-stage patients under 65 years of age. Survival benefit is a function of patient specific survival probability with transplantation minus expectation of survival without a transplant during the same period. Absolute indications for transplantation include refractory cardiogenic shock, dependence on intravenous inotropic support (both Status 1), or persistent class 4 symptoms with peak oxygen consumption (MVO_2) < 10 ml kg^{-1} min^{-1}.[43] Haemodynamic or renal indications to discontinue angiotensin-converting enzyme (ACE) inhibition and intolerance of β-blockade reinforce the need for intervention in Status 2 patients. In the category above, benefit is the difference between a 1-year survival of less than 50% versus 83% after a transplant. In practice most patients awaiting transplantation are ambulatory, on oral medication with an MVO_2 between 11 and 14 ml kg^{-1} min^{-1}. Many of these patients actually improve symptomatically and prognostically with the detailed medical management provided by the transplant centre. Another reason for improvement is the more rigorous selection of less ill patients (by excluding those with renal impairment and co-morbidities). As many as 30% of Status 2 candidates can be removed from the waiting list with excellent early survival. Shah et al.[48] showed that survival at 1 and 3 years for Status 2 patients removed from the transplant waiting list after 6 months of optimized treatment was 100% and 92%, respectively. Patients with idiopathic dilated cardiomyopathy had better outcomes than those with ischaemic cardiomyopathy. Accordingly, patients are deemed too well for transplantation if they are clinically stable with the sustained improvement of MVO_2 by >2 ml kg^{-1} min^{-1}. There is therefore a need for constant re-evaluation of Status 2 candidates by repeated measurement of MVO_2.

For the reasons above, the evidence base for transplantation is less secure than it was 20 years ago. Given the improved short-term survival of many Stage D HF patients there are continuous efforts to define which patients will gain maximum long-term benefit from transplantation. With the lack of secure information regarding risk-adjusted (patient-specific) time-related survival estimates for different aetiologies of HF, uniform agreement has not been achieved amongst transplant centres regarding the precise indications and timing of transplantation. Survival benefit margin is assessed by calculating the patient's specific survival probability with transplantation minus the survival expectation without transplantation during the same time period.[49] For instance, a patient with only 60% expected 1-year survival after transplant but with a 20% expected 1-year survival without would have a survival benefit margin of 40% in 1 year. In contrast, a patient with stable advanced HF may have a projected 1-year survival of 70% on medical therapy compared with 90% with transplantation. Such a patient would have a lower survival benefit margin (20%) but an improved use of the donor heart in terms of expected graft and patient survival. Currently, allocation of donor organs is governed by two axioms that are at times contradictory: equity (equal access of all patients to donor organs) with priority given to patients closest to death and utility (an allocation policy for organ that maximizes patient and graft survival). Application of these principles requires that a lower limit of acceptable expected post-transplant survival be determined, and that secure patient-specific information about mid-term survival with medical therapy for subsets of advanced HF is available. Irrespective of survival, the short- and long-term quality-of-life benefit is more difficult to quantify and is dependent upon the condition of other organ systems, which have been affected by the severity and chronicity of HF. Therefore, an important component of transplant evaluation is the assessment of co-morbid conditions that independently reduce duration or quality of life. In a study by Kirklin *et al.*[50] from the Cardiac Transplant Research Database (CTRD) of 7283 patients from 42 North American institutions (over 24,000 patient-years of follow-up) patients with multiple co-morbid conditions were shown to have significantly worse intermediate-term survival than those without co-morbidity. Patients were stratified low-risk when under the age of 65 with no other risk factors (insulin-dependent diabetes, peripheral vascular disease, chronic obstructive pulmonary disease, smoking within 6 months, gender mismatch, or congenital aetiology). A donor age of <40 years and an ischaemic time <240 min were associated with a low risk of complications. On the other hand, patients with significant co-morbidity, particularly those on a ventilator at the time of transplant and with a donor age >56 years or ischaemic time >360 min had much less satisfactory outcomes. Whereas patients categorized as low risk had 89% survival at 1 year and 80% 2-year survival, the corresponding figures for the high-risk group were 71% and 58% (see Chapter 17).

Table 6.3 General indications for cardiac transplantation (From Westaby S, Narula J. Surgical options in heart failure. *The Surgical Clinics of North America* 84(1): xv–xix. Copyright (c)2004, with permission from Elsevier.)

General indications for cardiac transplantation

Criteria for consideration of heart transplantation in advanced heart failure
Significant functional limitation (NYHA Class III–IV heart failure) despite maximum medical therapy
  that includes digitalis, diuretics, and vasodilators, preferably angiotensin-converting enzyme
  inhibitors, at maximum tolerated doses.
Refractory angina or refractory life-threatening arrhythmia
Exclusion of all surgical alternatives to transplantation, such as the following:
  Revascularization for significant reversible ischemia
  Value replacement for severe aortic value disease
  Valve replacement or repair for severe mitral regurgitation
  Appropriate ventricular remodelling procedures
Indications for cardiac transplantation determined by severity of heart failure despite optimal therapy
Definite indications
  Vo_2 max < 10 ml/kg/min
  NYHA Class IV
  History of recurrent hospitalization for congestive heart failure
  Refractory ischemia with inoperable coronary artery disease and left ventricular ejection fraction < 20%
  Recurrent symptomatic ventricular arrhythmias
Probable indications
  Vo_2 max <14 mg/kg/min (or higher with multiple other risk factors)
    NYHA Class III–IV
  Recent hospitalizations for congestive heart failure
  Unstable angina not amenable to coronary artery bypass grafting, percutaneous transluminal coro
    nary angioplasty with left ventricular ejection fraction < 0.25%

Table 6.4 Contraindications to cardiac transplantation (From Westaby S, Narula J. Surgical options in heart failure. *The Surgical Clinics of North America* **84**(1): xv–xix. Copyright © 2004, with permission from Elsevier.)

Contraindications to cardiac transplantation
General contraindications
Presence of any noncardiac condition that would itself shorten life expectancy or increase the risk of death from rejection or complications of immunosuppression
Specific Contraindications[a]
Age greater than about 65 years (program variability)
Active infection
Active ulcer disease
Severe diabetes mellitus with end-organ damage
Severe peripheral vascular or cerebrovascular disease
Coexisting neoplasm
Morbid obesity
Creatinine clearance <40–50 ml/min, effective renal plasma flow (ERPF) < 200 ml/min[b]
Bilirubin >2.5 mg/dl, transaminases >2 normal[c]
Severe pulmonary dysfunction with FVC and FEV1 <about 40% of predicated, especially with intrinsic lung disease
Pulmonary artery systolic pressure >60 mmHg, mean transpulmonary gradient >15 mmHg, or pulmonary vascular resistance >5 Wood units[d]
Acute pulmonary thromboembolism
Active diverticulitis
High risk of life-threatening non-compliance
Inability to make strong commitment to transplantation
Cognitive impairment severe enough to limit comprehension of medical regimen
Psychiatric instability severe enough to jeopardize incentive for adherence to medical regimen
History of recent smoking (within 6 months)
History of recurring alcohol or drug abuse
Failure of established stable address or telephone number
Previous demonstration of repeated noncompliance with medication or follow-up
Lack of independent family or social support system
History of marked depression or emotional instability

[a] May be relative or absolute, depending on severity or program philosophy.

[b] May be suitable for cardiac transplantation if inotropic support and hemodynamic management produce a creatinine < 2 mg% and creatinine clerarance >50 ml/min. Transplantation may also be advisable as combined heart-kidney transplant.

[c] Requires liver biopsy to exclude cirrhosis or other intrinsic liver disease.

[d] These apply only if the increased resistance is largely nonreactive (fixed).

General guidelines for transplant wait listing are shown in Table 6.3. In practice, it is easier to define contraindications to transplantation (Table 6.4). Age restriction is difficult to justify except on the ground of donor organ availability. Frazier (personal communication) has shown that transplantation provides very effective treatment for ischaemic cardiomyopathy patients in their 70s. In 2000 the average waiting time (869 days) for a group O blood type transplant recipient exceeded by far the projected life span of that patient at the time of being put on the waiting list.[51] Success was achieved only by mechanical bridging with a left-ventricular assist device (LVAD). In a prospective multicentre bridge to transplant trial undertaken with the ThermoCardio Systems Heartmate LVAD (Fig. 6.6) (1996–98) in the USA, the mean duration of support was 112 days.[52] Seventy-one per cent of patients survived to transplantation with an 84% 1-year survival. The others died before a donor organ became available. In contrast a more recent UK study (2002–04) using second-generation LVADs provided only 52% overall survival at 12 months because only 44% of patients received a donor heart[53] (again providing 84% 1-year survival). Given the progressive worldwide fall in donor availability, Adamson describes heart transplantation as an epidemiologically insignificant intervention. Nevertheless for a few fortunate patients a well-matched donor heart may provide good quality life for an extra 15–20 years.[54]

As it becomes socially less acceptable to discard patients at 65 years, indefinite mechanical circulatory support now provides an important off-the-shelf therapy with the potential to exceed transplant numbers by a factor of 50 to 1. The use of mechanical circulatory support as an alternative to maximum medical therapy has a strong evidence base in the REMATCH (Randomized Evaluation of Mechanical Assistance for the Treatment of Congestive Heart failure) trial (Fig. 6.7).[55] There are important differences between the application of mechanical support for acute HF versus chronic cardiac deterioration. Blood pumps implanted electively for chronic cardiomyopathy are usually placed in patients with long-standing HF who remain severely symptomatic or

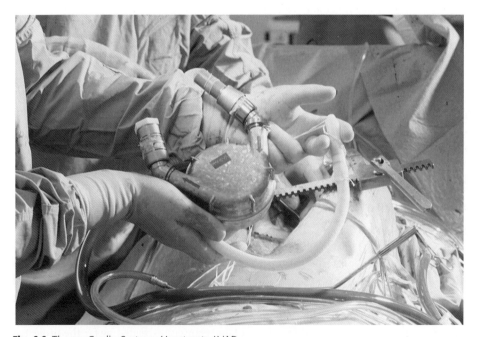

Fig. 6.6 ThermoCardio Systems Heartmate LVAD.

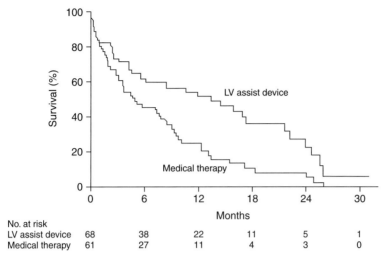

No. at risk					
LV assist device	68	38	22	11	5	1
Medical therapy	61	27	11	4	3	0

Fig. 6.7 REMATCH results. (From Westaby S, Narula J. Surgical options in heart failure. *The Surgical Clinics of North America* 84(1): xv–xix. Copyright (c)2004, with permission from Elsevier.)

decompensated on maximum medical therapy. In general, the end organs have been subjected to prolonged periods of low cardiac output and have adapted to this over time. Under these conditions, the majority of patients are well served with an implantable LVAD alone. Even in the presence of high pulmonary vascular resistance, the right ventri-cle rarely needs support (no more than 10% of patients).[56] On the other hand, patients with acute cardiogenic shock after massive myocardial infarction without pre-existing cardiomyopathy are subjected to profound low-flow states, which cause multiple organ failure if not promptly reversed (Fig. 6.8). Under these circumstances, biventricular support is particularly valuable, and in extreme cases biventricular replacement with the CardioWest total artificial heart may be required to sustain life (Fig. 6.9).[57] Patients with this device and a new portable power console are able to return home to wait for a donor heart (Fig. 6.10).

Decision-making in patients with idiopathic dilated cardiomyopathy

In dilated cardiomyopathy the projected mortality is directly related to the severity of systolic dysfunction. Increased chamber sphericity and the presence of mitral regurgitation are markers of worse prognosis (1-year mortality 54–70%). As the failing left ventricle dilates the papillary muscles are displaced, coaptation of the mitral valve leaflets is decreased, and a central jet of mitral regurgitation appears. Mitral regurgitation then leads to more volume overload of the already dilated chamber (see Fig. 6.5).

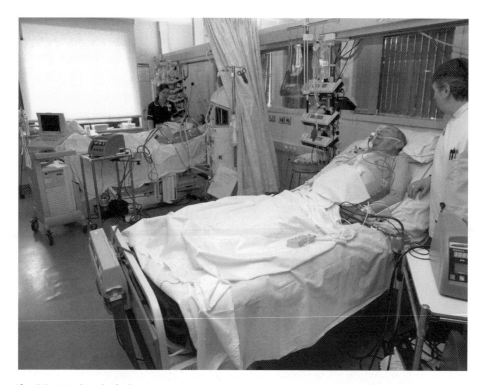

Fig. 6.8 A Levitronix device.

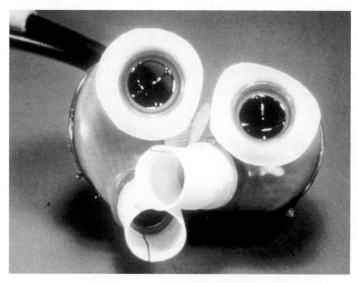

Fig. 6.9 CardioWest total artificial heart. (Reproduced with permission from Fig. 35.5 on p. 652 of *Heart Failure: Pathogenesis and Treatment* by J Narula, R Virmani, M Ballester, I Carrio, S Westaby, O Frazier, and J Willerson, Martin Dunitz, 2002.)

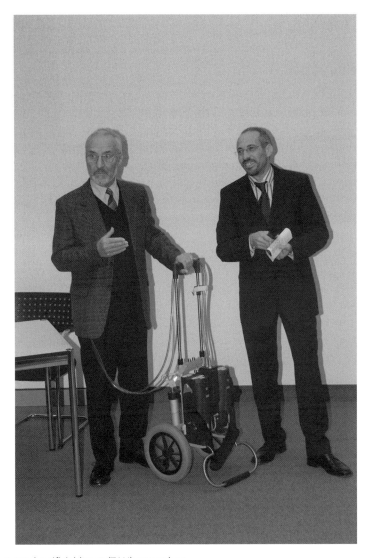

Fig. 6.10 A total artificial heart (TAH) outpatient.

The natural history of idiopathic dilated cardiomyopathy is less predictable than for ischaemic cardiomyopathy. Remission and prolonged survival are well documented in transplant-listed Stage D patients. In Shah's analysis of survival in patients removed from a heart transplant waiting list, survival 8 years after wait-listing exceeded 80% for idiopathic dilated cardiomyopathy, compared with around 30% for ischaemic patients.[48] In addition to improvement on medical management, left-ventricular unloading with a LVAD has the propensity to provide sustainable recovery in myocardial function in selected patients.[58] With increasing awareness of the mechanisms of ventricular recovery, together with the availability of other non-transplant surgical options, it is debatable whether cardiac transplantation should be undertaken as the primary treatment for this condition or for acute viral myocarditis.

Mitral valve repair

Reports of prohibitive operative mortality for mitral valve replacement in dilated cardiomyopathy patients in the early 1980s implied that the failing ventricle would deteriorate further if the 'blow-off' into the left atrium was removed. More recent information shows that mitral valve repair with preservation of the sub-valvular apparatus carries low perioperative mortality, good medium-term survival, and symptomatic relief through improvement in the cardiac index. Bolling et al.[38] have reported the effects of mitral repair in patients with very advanced disease. All had severe left-ventricular systolic dysfunction with pre-operative LVEF ranging from 8–25% (mean 16 ± 3%). The average duration of cardiomyopathy was 4 years (range 0–16). All patients underwent remodelling ring annuloplasty with an undersized flexible ring and half had tricuspid annuloplasty. Hospital mortality was less than 2% while 12- and 24-month survival were 82% and 72%, respectively. All patients were restored to NYHA Class I or II with mean post-operative LVEF of 26%. Peak MVO_2max rose from a mean of 14.5 to 18.6 ml kg^{-1} min^{-1}. Echocardiography 2 years post-operatively showed a pronounced reduction in sphericity, regurgitant volume, and regurgitant fraction. LVEF, end-diastolic and end-systolic volumes were all improved (Table 6.5).

External cardiac constraint

Following the disappointing results of dynamic skeletal muscle cardiomyoplasty, a much simpler concept has developed to arrest the progression of left-ventricular remodelling in dilated cardiomyopathy. Acorn Cardiovascular (Saint Paul, MN, USA) developed a passive constraint device of mesh-like polyester material to surround the left and right ventricle (Fig. 6.11).[59] The fabric has a unique bidirectional compliance that allows

Table 6.5

Variable	Pre-operative	Post-operative	Change (%)[a]	P-value
End-diastolic volume (ml)	335 ± 107	307 ± 103	−8 ± 9	0.06
End-systolic volume (ml)	277 ± 101	237 ± 98	−15 ± 14	0.03
Stroke volume (ml)	58 ± 13	70 ± 21	12 ± 10	0.02
Ejection fraction (%)	18 ± 5	24 ± 10	31 ± 24	0.03
Mitral inflow (L min^{-1})	12.4 ± 5.3	5.4 ± 0.5	−49 22	0.02
Forward cardiac output (L min^{-1})	3.2 ± 1.0	4.7 ± 0.9	52 ± 38	0.01
Regurgitant volume (L min^{-1})	9.2 ± 5.4	0.8 ± 0.6	88.6 ± 10.1	0.01
Regurgitant fraction (%)	70 ± 14	15 ± 11	−79 ± 15	< 0.001

[a]Percentage change from pre-operative study at 4–6 months post-operatively. The NYHA class fell significantly from 3.9 ± 0.4 to 1.8 ± 0.5 (P-value < 0.001); data modified from Bolling et al.[38]

the mesh to conform to the ellipsoid surface of the heart. The passive jacket is positioned around the ventricles and sutured posteriorly and laterally, slightly above or below the atrio-ventricular groove. This provides a slight and immediate reduction in the circumference of the heart. Animal models suggest reduction in left-ventricular volume and improved cardiac function compared with controls.[60] Obviously, the mesh does not improve cardiac contraction, but appears to prevent further deterioration. So far there is no evidence of constrictive physiology; the normal response to volume loading is preserved, left- and right-heart filling pressures do not equalize, and trans-mitral flow parameters do not change significantly. Myocardial biopsies from the animal models suggest a degree of reverse remodelling with the tendency towards less

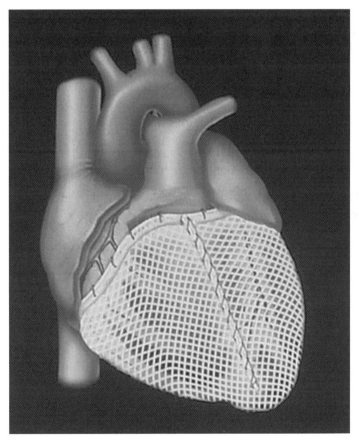

Fig. 6.11 Acorn Cardiovascular (Saint Paul, MN, USA) device. (Reproduced with permission from Fig. 34.34 on p. 643 of *Heart Failure: Pathogenesis and Treatment* by J Narula, R Virmani, M Ballester, I Carrio, S Westaby, O Frazier, and J Willerson, Martin Dunitz, 2002.)

myocyte hypertrophy, less interstitial fibrosis, and higher capillary density in the treated animals.

In clinical studies, application has been restricted to NYHA Class II or III patients, many of whom were also subject to mitral valve repair or replacement or left-ventricular restoration surgery. The Acorn device did not significantly improve left-ventricular end-diastolic dimensions, LVESV, peak oxygen consumption, or degree of mitral regurgitation when used in isolation. The safety and feasibility studies confirm that the device does not cause constrictive or restrictive physiology, has no effect on the epicardial coronary vessels, and can prevent progressive remodelling. In contrast, the effects on LVEF and cardiac output (independent from concomitant procedures) are limited. Important questions remain with the regard to patient selection process, potential long-term adverse effects, and the optimal timing for ventricular restraint.

It is possible that early ventricular compressive therapy after myocardial infarction could dramatically ameliorate the remodelling process. Whether external restraint will remain in the surgical armamentarium for dilated cardiomyopathy remains to be seen.

Partial left ventriculectomy (Batista operation)

The importance of wall stress and the Laplace principle is axiomatic in Batista's partial left ventriculectomy operation.[61] The procedure was developed in Brazil to treat young patients with Chagas' disease or idiopathic dilated cardiomyopathy. The concept that a dilated heart with thinned walls functions poorly because the myocytes are placed at a mechanical disadvantage was addressed by attempting to restore 'normal' left-ventricular geometry to reduce wall stress and improve contractile function. This was achieved in dilated cardiomyopathy patients by excising a large wedge of myocardium in the circumflex coronary territory with direct closure to produce a much smaller ventricular cavity (Fig. 6.12). The operation depends on the assumption that non-infarcted (but diseased) myocardium can contract normally if wall stress is reduced. The idea completely ignores the cellular and molecular changes in the failing heart, which account for the disappointing early and late results of this operation. Despite this, partial left ventriculectomy was widely adopted as an alternative to transplantation without guidelines or convincing information on sustainability and survival. The published hospital mortality was prohibitive, ranging from 1.8% to 27% with an average of 17.4%.[62] Acceptable hospital mortality was achieved by some centres with the aid of long-term LVAD support (20% of patients) and cardiac transplantation. In survivors, an immediate significant decrease in both end-diastolic and end-systolic volume indices was achieved. Whilst LVEF improved initially, some re-studies at 12 months failed to show significant differences from pre-operative LVEF in many patients.[12] There was an inverse relationship between the decrease of circumferential end-systolic stress and increase in LVEF.

In McCarthy's series, mean LVEF improved from 13% to 21% and peak oxygen consumption from 11 ml kg^{-1} min^{-1} to 16 ml kg^{-1} min^{-1} at 12 months.[63] Twelve-month

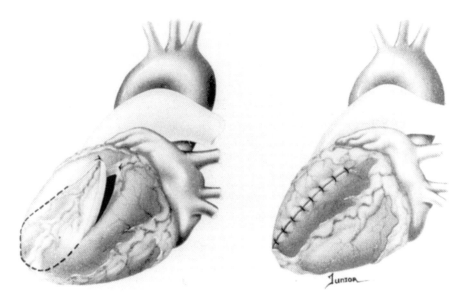

Fig. 6.12 Batista's partial left ventriculectomy operation. (Reproduced with permission from Fig. 34.20 on p. 630 of *Heart Failure: Pathogenesis and Treatment* by J Narula, R Virmani, M Ballester, I Carrio, S Westaby, O Frazier, and J Willerson, Martin Dunitz, 2002.)

survival at the Cleveland Clinic was 80%, but LVADs were required for bridge-to-transplantation in 16% of patients. Freedom from HF of any cause (including relisting for transplant, death, or NYHA Class IV symptoms) was only 50% by 12 months and 38% at 2 years. Though the reduced ventricular geometric dimensions may be sustained for up to 12 months, pump function began to deteriorate after 6 months. The discrepancy between geometry and sustainability of mechanical function was attributed to the fact that left-ventricular mass reduction caused changes in diastolic compliance.

Currently, most centres who adopted partial left ventriculectomy as a promising alternative to transplantation redirected this procedure to a small number of highly selected dilated cardiomyopathy patients. With emerging alternatives, the Batista operation has joined skeletal muscle cardiomyoplasty in the dustbin of HF operations. Even so, the author had some remarkably successful long-term results in very sick infants without alternatives (Fig. 6.13).

Mechanical left-ventricular unloading in dilated cardiomyopathy

The propensity for the idiopathic dilated cardiomyopathy heart to improve with a combination of ACE inhibition and β-blockade reflects the beneficial properties of preload and afterload reduction with reduced wall stress. This therapeutic effect on the

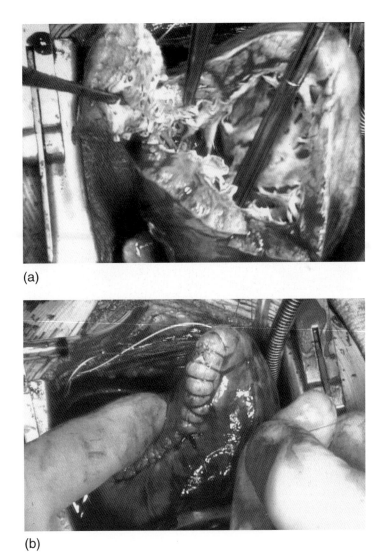

(a)

(b)

Fig. 6.13 The Batista operation as performed by one of the authors (SW). (Reproduced with permission from Fig. 34.21a and b on p. 630 of *Heart Failure: Pathogenesis and Treatment* by J Narula, R Virmani, M Ballester, I Carrio, S Westaby, O Frazier, and J Willerson, Martin Dunitz, 2002.)

remodelling process can be greatly amplified by mechanical unloading with a LVAD.[64] Pulsatile LVADs function in series with and completely offload the native left ventricle so that the aortic valve remains closed (Fig. 6.14). The improved systemic blood flow gradually reverses multi-organ failure, improves coronary blood flow, and increases physical activity. Serum aldosterone, plasma renin, atrial natriuretic peptide, and norepinephrine levels revert to normal as the HF syndrome disappears.[65]

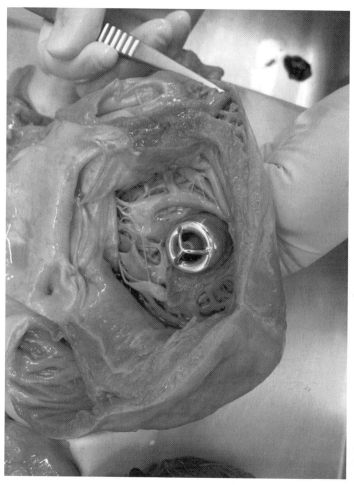

Fig. 6.14 Fusion of aortic cusps.

Until recently, transplantation was mandatory for all patients in the United States committed to LVAD. However, when the native heart was excised during transplantation, it became clear to Frazier and others that some ventricles with idiopathic dilated cardiomyopathy had reverted towards normal size and weight.[65] Comparison of myocardial biopsies taken first at LVAD implantation then during transplantation showed regression of myocyte hypertrophy, decreased myocytolysis, myocardial fibrosis, and apoptosis. Myocyte genetic expression and cellular metabolism reverted towards normal.[66] Realization that recovering hearts were being discarded by transplantation, led to the concept of a mechanical bridge to myocardial recovery. Complementary to this approach is the development of much smaller and more user-friendly axial flow and centrifugal blood pumps. In dilated cardiomyopathy patients, partial left-ventricular unloading with a continuous flow device provides a symbiotic relationship between the

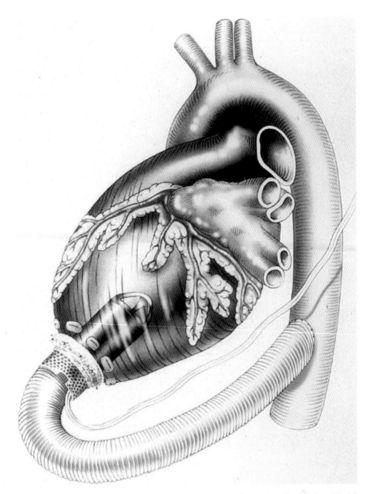

Fig. 6.15 Diagram of the Jarvik device. (Reproduced with permission from Fig. 35.18 on p. 662 of *Heart Failure: Pathogenesis and Treatment* by J Narula, R Virmani, M Ballester, I Carrio, S Westaby, O Frazier, and J Willerson, Martin Dunitz, 2002.)

improving native heart and the blood pump (Fig. 6.15). The majority of unloaded hearts show improvement in function and some LVADs can be removed with prolonged survival.[66]

The fact that LVAD use does not preclude transplantation but paradoxically improves post-transplant survival suggests that mechanical circulatory support should be used primarily for idiopathic dilated cardiomyopathy patients, leaving transplantation in reserve.[71] Since the REMATCH trial, blood pumps have been an accepted alternative to medical management in severely symptomatic patients not eligible for transplant.[55] With improved LVAD technology, the US Health Care Advisory Board predicts 100,000 'life-time' implants per year by 2010. There are early clues to the success of this approach. The

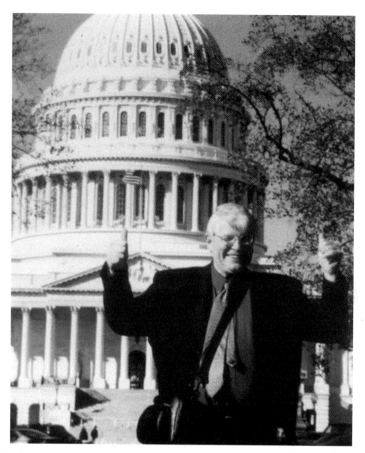

Fig. 6.16 The first permanent Jarvik 2000 patient 6 years after his operation. (From Westaby S, Narula J. Surgical options in heart failure. *The Surgical Clinics of North America* 84(1): xv–xix. Copyright (c)2004, with permission from Elsevier.)

first permanent Jarvik 2000 patient is NYHA Class II and leading a productive life 6 years after his operation (Fig. 6.16).[68]

Dilated cardiomyopathy and myocarditis patients have the potential for bridge-to-recovery but there are further requirements before this approach can be translated into clinical success. The first is a reliable LVAD for patients of all sizes. This should be relatively simple to implant and remove, and easy for the patient to control. The axial flow and centrifugal blood pumps are promising in this respect (Fig. 6.17).[69] Second, the LVAD should be employed before myocardial fibrosis renders reversal of ventricular remodelling unachievable. Strategies to promote myocardial recovery with drugs, growth factors, gene therapy, and inhibitors of apoptosis are under investigation and markers for sustainability of recovery are being explored. In this respect, the Berlin group has used the disappearance from the serum of the autoantibody against the β-adrenergic receptor.

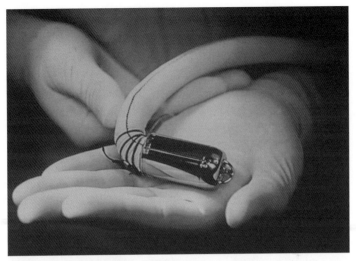

(a) Jarvik 2000 VAD

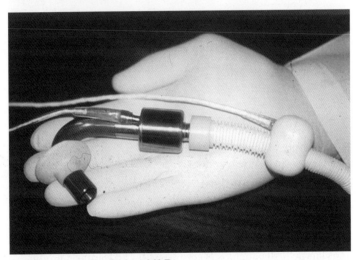

(b) Micromed De Bakey VAD

Fig. 6.17 (a)–(e) Axial flow pumps. (From Westaby S, Narula J. Surgical options in heart failure. *The Surgical Clinics of North America* 84(1): xv–xix. Copyright (c)2004, with permission from Elsevier.)

They speculate that this reflects abatement of the immune process, which causes functional impairment.[10]

Prospects for success with bridge-to-recovery are critically dependent on myocardial pathology. Patients with acute myocarditis or post-partum cardiomyopathy who are in terminal decline can be supported with a LVAD or biventricular assist device until resolution of the inflammatory process. Even those who require external cardiac massage and urgent cardiopulmonary bypass to sustain life before LVAD implantation can be restored to near normal cardiac function (Fig. 6.18).[70] In their study of weaning from

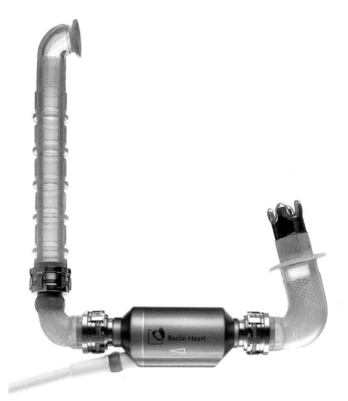

(c) Berlin Heart Incor I VAD

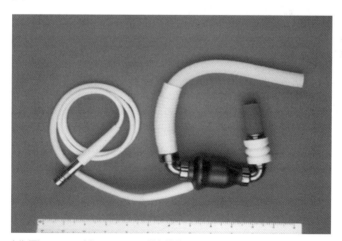

(d) Thoratec Heartmate II VAD

Fig. 6.17 (cont.)

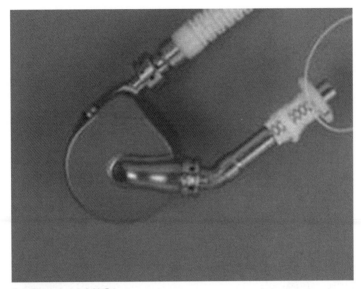

(e) Terumo L VAS

Fig. 6.17 (cont.)

chronic left-ventricular support, the Berlin group compared factors which distinguished those with well-sustained recovery from others who slipped back into HF.[10] Patients with long-lasting recovery were younger, had a shorter history of HF, had a more rapid improvement in cardiac performance, and needed a shorter duration of LVAD support before indices of cardiac volume and function justified device removal. The duration over which the autoantibody against the β-adrenergic receptors disappeared from the serum was shorter (8.8 weeks vs 9.7 weeks) in patients with sustainable recovery. Not different were mean age (41.5 years vs 50.3 years) mean left-ventricular end-diastolic diameter at the time of device placement (75.2 mm vs 78.7 mm), LVEF (14.8% vs 17.0%) and mean left-ventricular end-diastolic diameter 2 months after LVAD placement (53.7 mm vs 55.6 mm). The Berlin group concluded that a LVAD unloading period of between 8 and 10 weeks was optimal in patients destined for sustainable recovery and that longer support could lead to atrophy of myocytes. Others have reservations about this limited duration, and report success after much longer periods. However, Madigan *et al.*[75] explanted LVAD unloaded hearts between 8 and 155 days and found structural reverse remodelling to be complete in approximately 40 days. Both left-ventricular chamber size and myocyte size had stabilized during this period. Collagen content was significantly increased in hearts supported for more than 40 days, and this was consistent with a decrease in matrix metalloproteinase activity in these patients. Expression of sarcoplasmic endoreticular calcium ATPase (SERCA2a) increased to normal levels by approximately 20 days of LVAD support. This information is difficult to translate into clinical practice when trying to make a decision regarding device removal.[72] Nevertheless, all patients with idiopathic dilated cardiomyopathy who undergo LVAD implantation

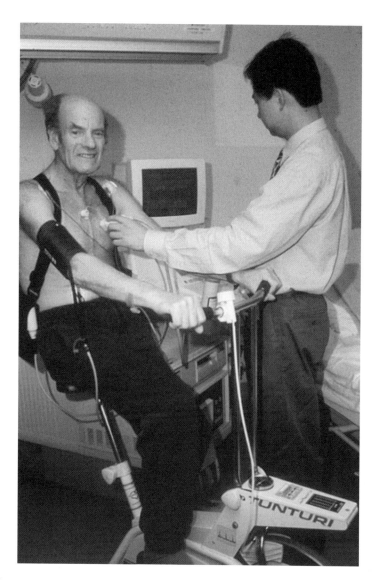

Fig. 6.18

should be regarded as potential candidates for weaning without any certainty of reaching this goal.

Many serum markers have been shown to be pathologically altered at the time of device implantation and are subsequently improved or normalized at the time of removal. These include TNFα, MMP-2 and -9, metallothionine, β-receptor density and responsiveness, apoptosis, atrial natriuretic factor, NO synthase, IL-6 and annexin-1, -2, -4, and –6.[72] However, none of these parameters are predictive in determining the reversibility of cardiac malfunction before LVAD implantation. Rather, they are markers of chronic overload, hyperactivity of the sympathetic nervous system, and, most likely, secondary phenomena of the disease. These parameters can, nevertheless, discriminate patients with reversed remodelling from those who remain dilated even during mechanical unloading with the LVAD.

Currently, the Berlin group considers the reversal of the inflammatory state in end-stage dilated cardiomyopathy as essential for reverse remodelling. To achieve this state they have treated dilated cardiomyopathy patients with immunoadsorption to remove the inflammatory autoantibodies. The Berlin treatment algorithm begins with optimal medical management. If this fails to improve cardiac status and pathological levels of β1 autoantibodies are demonstrated, immunoadsorption is employed. If cardiac function cannot be stabilized and heart transplant criteria are met, the patient is placed on the waiting list. In the event of further deterioration occurring before a donor is available then mechanical support is instituted with a hope of reversing the progressive cardiac impairment. If no improvement occurs, the LVAD functions as a bridge to transplantation. Given the potential for improvement, the decision to insert a LVAD should be made early since the prospect for reversal of the remodelling process deteriorates with time. Meanwhile, aggressive medical and antioxidative treatment of HF is pursued to enhance the chances of reverse remodelling. The patient is then followed by regular echocardiographic studies with the pump temporarily switched off to document LVEF and LV end-diastolic dimensions (LVEDD). Before considering device explantation, these must reach at least 50% and 55 mm respectively (Fig. 6.18).

Hetzer and colleagues have reported successful explantation of 33 LVADs in dilated cardiomyopathy or myocarditis patients since 1995. The mean duration since device removal for all 33 patients has been 6.5 years (range 1.3–9.3 years). Five-year survival after LVAD removal was 82%. Sustained improvement for more than 2 years after weaning occurred in 61% of the patients. The remainder relapsed into HF, resulting in cardiac transplantation or death. When comparing patients with long-term recovery (more than 3 years, $n = 17$) versus those who relapsed within 2 years of weaning ($n = 9$) there were no differences in regard to the mean age, mean LVEDD at the time of implantation, or mean LVEF. Sustainable recovery occurred in those with a shorter history of HF who required a shorter period of support to achieve improvement. The time to disappearance of the β1 autoantibody after LVAD placement was significantly shorter in patients with sustained recovery. Markers of myocardial fibrosis were greatly elevated before LVAD deployment and levels differed between successfully weaned and relapsing patients. Many end-stage patients had myocardial fibrosis, which already precluded reverse remodelling before LVAD implantation.

Whilst this pioneering work is promising, there are many further challenges. Can the repair mechanism be enhanced to provide predictable and sustained recovery? With newer more reliable LVADs, should earlier left-ventricular unloading be employed in order to improve the prospects for recovery? Can adjunctive pharmacological or stem cell treatment be used to promote recovery?

Yacoub and colleagues[73] have suggested the use of the anabolic β2-agonist Clenbuterol to induce so-called physiological myocardial hypertrophy during unloading. In rats the chronic administration of Clenbuterol (2 mg kg^{-1} day^{-1} vs placebo) produced significant hypertrophy and increased SERCA2a content with a prolonged action potential and increased oxidative carbohydrate utilization. In an uncontrolled study, the Harefield group combined LVAD unloading followed by administration of Clenbuterol to produce cardiac hypertrophy. With this regime the authors claim an increased likelihood of sustainable myocardial recovery after LVAD removal. Others have found Clenbuterol to have myotoxic effects which negatively influence cardiac function. Burniston et al.[74] found sub-endocardial and skeletal muscle necrosis and apoptosis in rats given 5 mg Clenbuterol kg^{-1}. Sleeper et al.[75] administered Clenbuterol (2.4 µg kg^{-1}) over 1 one week to 20 horses.[79] This resulted in a significant decrease in myocardial function and increased aortic root dimensions, suggesting the risk of aneurysm formation. Further evidence is required before this β2 agonist is adopted in clinical practice.

In the future, cells of extracardiac origin may have a role in myocardial repair and in prevention of remodelling in the infarcted heart.[76]

Lifetime circulatory support as a primary treatment for advanced HF

Three major developments have set the scene for long-term mechanical circulatory support (lifetime use or destination therapy) as a primary treatment for advanced HF. Firstly, considerable knowledge and expertise has been derived from long-term bridging to transplantation.[77] This experience with first-generation pulsatile LVADs has led to prolonged survival and fewer device-related complications. LVAD blood flow reverses the HF syndrome, whilst mechanical unloading improves native cardiac function. Secondly, the REMATCH trial has clearly demonstrated improved survival with LVAD use over medical management.[55] REMATCH provides the evidence base for widespread use of LVADs as an alternative treatment for patients not eligible for transplant. The fact that many transplant candidates die without receiving a donor organ, and that pre-transplant LVAD support improves transplant survival, suggest that more transplant-eligible patients should be offered circulatory support as a therapeutic option. Thirdly, the continuous-flow LVADs appear to be as effective as pumps which provide stroke volume and pulse pressure.[78] These miniaturized blood pumps are silent and less obtrusive, allowing early discharge from hospital and an active life in the community.[69]

As an off-the-shelf commodity, LVADs are destined to join the pacemaker, cardiac resynchronization therapy, and the implantable defibrillator as first-line treatment of the failing heart.[79] There are two major limitations to progress. The first is cost, which must fall as their application becomes more widespread. The second is the need for a major surgical procedure in a very sick patient. New developments in LVAD technology will address these issues so that circulatory support can be made available in all cardiac centres.

Patient selection for lifetime circulatory support

Analysis of mortality in LVAD patients shows that many die as a result of irreversible organ dysfunction or co-morbidities present at the time of implantation.[55] These cases have been seen too late. Until recently, patients considered for lifetime LVAD use have, by protocol, been ineligible for cardiac transplantation and in an advanced state of decompensation. Many have dual chamber pacing, an implantable defibrillator, or are already confined to a hospital with intravenous inotropes or an intra-aortic balloon pump. The REMATCH study showed that when a patient is considered unsuitable for transplantation, by the same argument they may already have an unreasonably high risk for any type of cardiac surgery.[55] The decision to proceed to lifetime circulatory support should therefore be made on an elective basis and not as a salvage procedure.[80] The patient should be a reasonable surgical candidate at acceptable risk. With safer, more user-friendly devices and less invasive operations, deployment of LVADs should be brought forward out of the end-stage arena.

With the expansion of information technology and increased patient awareness many HF patients now request LVAD therapy. A minority will require transplantation due to progressive right-heart failure. Paradoxically, many others who have been excluded from transplantation through renal impairment or increased pulmonary vascular resistance will improve sufficiently to achieve transplant status.

The process of evaluating and selecting patients for LVAD therapy directly affects outcome.[81] Identifying appropriate patients before the onset of advanced organ dysfunction improves survival and reduces the degree of post-operative morbidity. This is equivalent to the selection of transplant candidates. In contrast, significant organ dysfunction does not exclude patients from consideration if there is potential for organ recovery. The inclusion criteria for the REMATCH trial provide adequate guidelines for LVAD use.[82] These patients were in chronic end-stage HF (NYHA Class IV) initially for 90 days but later broadened to NYHA Class III or IV for 28 days but with recent requirement for intra-aortic balloon pump or inotrope support. The patient should have LVEF < 25% and peak exercise oxygen consumption <12 mg kg^{-1} min^{-1}. Whilst the great majority of REMATCH patient were inotrope or balloon pump dependent, it is widely recognized that lifetime LVAD should be performed electively before this pre-morbid state. Bridge-to-transplant selection criteria such as cardiac index ≤ 2 L min^{-1} m^{-2}, systolic blood pressure ≤ 80 mmHg, and pulmonary capillary wedge pressure ≥ 20 mmHg must not be requirements for a lifetime implant. Perhaps the best patients for long-term LVAD therapy are those with idiopathic dilated cardiomyopathy, NYHA Class III or IV, with multiple hospital admissions for medical stabilization and an unacceptable quality of life at home. The use of prognostic models such as the Heart Failure Survival Score, which relies on the use of non-invasive clinical variables, may prove useful in identifying a homogeneous group of high-risk patients in this category.[46]

In many respects it is easier to define contraindications to LVAD therapy (Table 6.6). Cognitive function plays an important role in the ability of the patient to manage a LVAD. Cognitive defects are common in advanced HF because of extended periods

Table 6.6 Indications/contraindications to LVAD therapy

Inclusion criteria (2 of 3 criteria must be present; non-transplant/eligible patients with a BSA between 1.2 and 2.3 m^2	Maximal oxygen uptake ≤ 16 ml kg^{-1} min^{-1} Ejection fraction ≤ 30%[a], ≤ 25%[b] Cardiac index ≤ 2.3 L min^{-1} m^{-2a}; ≤ 2 L min^{-1} m^{-2b}
Exclusion criteria (absolute criteria/*relative criteria*)	
Neurology, psychology	Intracranial bleed within 21 days s/p CPR for >5 min, neurology unknown Severe brain damage, no meaningful recovery High probability of non-compliance
Pulmonary	Fixed pulmonary vascular resistance ≥ 7 Wood units *Pulmonary vascular resistance 3–7 Wood units, FIO2 > 0.6*
Surgical/medical	Malignancy, life expectancy less than 18 months Aortic dissection or aneurysms requiring surgical treatment Previous cardiac surgery[b] Diabetes mellitus[b] Implanted mechanical heart valve *Aortic or mitral insufficiency grade 3–4*
Renal	Anuria, creatinine clearance ≤ 25 ml h^{-1} *Creatinine > 3.0, urine output < 30 cm^3 h^{-1} × 12 h*
Liver	Cirrhosis child c *Synthetic dysfunction (PT > 16, INR > 2)*
Infection	Severe infection present[a] *Sepsis or other severe infection[b]*
Haematology	Contraindication to heparin anticoagulation Thrombus in any cardiac chamber *History of thromboembolic events*
Gastrointestinal Tract	Ischaemic bowel necrosis Massive GI bleed (>6 UPRBCs) due to diffuse gastritis or colitis
Distance to hospital	Road journey to hospital > 180 min[a]
Risk score index[c]	Score > 5

[a]Criterion for German centres.

[b]Criterion for UK centres.

[c]Oz MC, Goldstein DJ, Pepino P *et al.* (1995) Screening scale predicts patients successfully receiving long-term implantable left-ventricular assist devices. *Circulation* 92(Suppl. II): 169–73.

Abbreviations: BSA, body surface area; FIO2, concentration of inspired oxygen; GI-bleed, gastrointestinal bleed; INR, international normalized ratio; LVEF, left-ventricular ejection fraction; MVO$_2$, maximal oxygen consumption per minute; PRBCs, packed red blood cells; PT, prothrombin time; s/p CPR, status post-cardiopulmonary resuscitation.

of cerebral hypoperfusion or prior cardiac arrest. Neuropsychological assessment is advisable before LVAD implantation through cognitive function may improve afterwards.[83] Candidates for a LVAD should have no major irreversible cognitive defects that would limit their understanding of LVAD maintenance or ability to troubleshoot LVAD alarms (see Chapter 14).

Previous stroke with motor impairment alone is not necessarily a contraindication if sufficient family support is available. Patients with chronic obstructive airways disease or pulmonary fibrosis are at increased risk of mortality, particularly in the presence of pulmonary hypertension that is not reversed by vasodilator therapy. LVAD therapy reduces right-ventricular afterload by reducing left-ventricular filling pressure. If the pulmonary vascular resistance is fixed, left-ventricular unloading may not produce a significant reduction in right-ventricular afterload and restrictive pulmonary blood flow may impair LVAD filling. Prolonged LVAD therapy may lower pulmonary vascular resistance and candidates are acceptable with resistance up to 7 Wood units. The possibility of pulmonary thromboembolic disease should be considered and eliminated. There are no absolute criteria for pulmonary function tests as these are unreliable in patients with pulmonary oedema or cardiogenic shock. Generally, when pulmonary function testing is feasible, a forced expiratory volume at 1 s of 50% of predicted or forced vital capacity of 50% of predicted, and diffusion capacity of the lung for carbon monoxide of 50% of predicted are adequate in patients for LVAD therapy.

Although renal insufficiency represents a significant risk factor for adverse LVAD outcome, careful evaluation must be performed in order not to exclude patients with the potential for recovery.[84] The effects of low cardiac output should be differentiated from diabetic nephropathy or hypertensive renal disease. In contrast, significant hepatic dysfunction (assessed by total serum bilirubin, international normalized ratio (INR), or both) is an important marker for adverse outcome. An INR exceeding 1.5, raised liver enzymes or bilirubin >5 times normal, established cirrhosis, or hepatic fibrosis with portal hypertension are all definite contraindications to LVAD therapy. Even mild elevation of serum bilirubin and liver enzymes, suggests the need for biventricular as opposed to left-ventricular support (see Chapter 17).

Significant right-heart failure is an infrequent but important obstacle to providing lifetime circulatory support with a LVAD alone. Risk factors for post-operative right-heart failure include elevated central venous pressure (>16 mmHg), significant tricuspid insufficiency, right-ventricular dysfunction despite low pulmonary artery pressure, low right-ventricular stroke work index, and myocardial infarction with significant right-ventricular and septal involvement. Patients at increased risk for RVAD support are an inappropriate group for destination therapy until better RVADs or total artificial hearts are available.

The heart valves must be carefully assessed before LVAD deployment. Aortic stenosis is not a contraindication to LVAD implant. In contrast, mild to moderate aortic regurgitation can have a catastrophic impact on LVAD haemodynamics. The reduction in left-ventricular pressure produced by the LVAD increases the pressure gradient across the aortic valve and exaggerates the aortic leak. Moderate aortic insufficiency becomes severe with the initiation of LVAD support, through a fall in end-diastolic pressure and an increase in aortic root pressure. Patients with a mechanical valve prosthesis in the aortic position must have this replaced with a bioprosthetic valve before LVAD implantation. Even so, a bioprosthesis in the aortic position is prone to thrombosis or cusp fusion during complete unloading of the left ventricle. Fusion of the native aortic valve leaflets can occur in patients with pusher-plate LVADs, which actively empty the ventricle and prevent ejection.

Patients with significant pre-existing mitral stenosis require valvuloplasty to ensure unobstructed filling of the LVAD, but mitral regurgitation does not have an impact on LVAD function. Elevation in pulmonary artery pressure may persist with severe mitral regurgitation and reverse remodelling of the left ventricle may be adversely affected. In situations where weaning from LVAD support might be anticipated, correction of the mitral regurgitation is necessary.

Adequate right-heart function is extremely important to maintain pulmonary blood flow early after LVAD implantation. Tricuspid regurgitation impairs the forward flow of blood through the lungs, particularly when pulmonary vascular resistance is elevated. Tricuspid regurgitation also contributes to elevated central venous pressure, hepatic congestion, and renal dysfunction. Severe tricuspid regurgitation may be present pre-operatively in the setting of volume overload and biventricular failure, but may also develop after LVAD insertion if right-ventricular dilatation occurs from leftward shift of the interventricular septum. Accordingly, tricuspid valve repair may be required to improve right-heart function.

Intracardiac shunts, such as patient foramen ovale or atrial septal defect, may cause important right-to-left shunting and systemic desaturation. These must be eliminated during the LVAD implant. Atrial flutter or fibrillation reduce right-ventricular filling but are reasonably well tolerated by LVAD patients. Even ventricular fibrillation may occur unnoticed in LVAD patients when pulmonary vascular resistance is low.

Conclusion

The scope of HF surgery has increased dramatically since the mid-1990s, largely in response to the demand for alternatives to cardiac transplantation. In turn, non-transplant operations are now regarded as preferable through avoidance of the complications of immunosuppressive therapy and competitive survival rates. The rapid evolution of circulatory assist technology holds great promise for the treatment of both acute and chronic HF in the future. Blood pumps relieve symptoms and prolong life with progressively less risk of surgical and device-related complications.

References

1. McMurray JJ, Stewart S (2000). Epidemiology, aetiology and prognosis of heart failure. *Heart* **83**: 596–602.
2. The SEOSI investigators (1997). Survey on heart failure in Italian hospital cardiology units. Results of the SEOSI study. *Eur Heart J* **18**: 1457–64.
3. ACC/AHA (2001). Guidelines for the evaluation and management of chronic heart failure in adults: executive summary. *J Am Coll Cardiol* **38**: 2101–13.

4. Yoshida F, Gould KL (1993). Quantitative relation of myocardial infarct size and myocardial viability by positron emission tomography to left ventricular ejection fraction and 3 year mortality with and without revascularization. *J Am Coll Cardiol* **22**: 984–97.

5. Adamson PB, Abraham WT, Love C *et al.* (2004). The evolving challenge of chronic heart failure management: a call for a new curriculum for training heart failure specialists. *J Am Coll Cardiol* **44**: 1354–7.

6. Rinaldi CA, Masani ND, Linka AZ *et al.* (1999). Effect of repetitive episodes of exercise induced myocardial ischemia on left ventricular function in patients with chronic stable angina: evidence for cumulative stunning or ischemic preconditioning? *Heart* **81**: 404–11.

7. Adams JN, Norton M, Trent R *et al.* (1996). Hibernated myocardium after acute myocardial infarction treated with thrombolysis. *Heart* **75**: 422–6.

8. Lee KS, Marvick TH, Cook SA *et al.* (1994). Prognosis of patients with left ventricular dysfunction, with and without viable myocardium after myocardial infarction. Relative efficacy of medical therapy and revascularization. *Circulation* **90**: 2687–94.

9. Westaby S (2000). Non-transplant surgery for heart failure. *Heart* **803**: 603–10.

10. Hetzer R, Muller J, Weng Y *et al.* (1999). Cardiac recovery in dilated cardiomyopathy by unloading with a left ventricular assist device. *Ann Thorac Surg* **68**: 742–9.

11. Di Carli MF, Maddhai J, Rockhsar S *et al.* (1998). Long term survival of patients with coronary artery disease and left-ventricular dysfunction: implication for the role of myocardial viability assessment in management decision. *J Thorac Cardiovasc Surg* **11**: 997–1004.

12. Westaby S (2004). Coronary revascularization in ischaemic cardiomyopathy. *Surg Clin North Am* **84**: 179–99.

13. Yoshida F, Gould KL (1993). Quantitative relation of myocardial infarct size and myocardial viability by positron emission tomography to left ventricular ejection fraction and 3 year mortality with and without revascularization. *J Am Coll Cardiol* **22**: 984–97.

14. Vanoverschelde JL, Berger BL, D'Handt AM *et al.* (1995). Preoperative selection of patients with severely impaired left ventricular function for coronary revascularization. Role of low dose dobutamine echocardiography and exercise redistribution-reinjection thallium SPECT. *Circulation* **92**(Suppl. II): 37–44.

15. Raymond JK, Edwin W, Allen R *et al.* (2000). The use of contrast-enhanced magnetic resonance imaging to identify reversible myocardial dysfunction. *New Engl J Med* **343**: 1445–53.

16. Mickleborough LL, Maruyama H, Yasushi T *et al.* (1995). Results of revascularization in patients with severe left-ventricular dysfunction. *Circulation* **92**(Suppl II): 73–9.

17. Hausmann H, Topp H, Siniawski H *et al.* (1997). Decision-making in end stage coronary artery disease: revascularization or heart transplantation. *Ann Thorac Surg* **64**: 1296–302.

18. Tjan TDT, Kondruweit M, Scheld HH *et al.* (2000). The bad ventricle – revascularization versus transplantation. *J Thorac Cardiovasc Surg* **48**: 9–14.

19. Arnese M, Cornel JH, Salustri A *et al.* (1995). Prediction of improvement of regional left ventricular function after surgical revascularization. A comparison of low-dose dobutamine echocardiography with 201Tl single-photon emission computed tomography. *Circulation* **91**: 2748–52.

20. Hass F, Jennen L, Heinzmann U *et al.* (2001). Ischemically compromised myocardium displays different time course of functional recovery: correlation with morphological alterations. *Eur J Cardiothorac Surg* **20**: 290–8.

21. Pagley PR, Beller GA, Watson DD *et al.* (1997). Improved outcome after coronary artery bypass surgery in patients with ischemic cardiomyopathy and residual myocardial viability. *Circulation* **95**: 793–800.

22. Tjan TDT, Kondruweit M, Scheld HH *et al.* (2000). The bad ventricle – revascularization versus transplantation. *J Thorac Cardiovasc Surg* **48**: 9–14.

23. Luciani GB, Faggani G, Razzaloni R *et al.* (1993). Severe ischemic left ventricular failure: coronary operation or heart transplantation? *Ann Thorac Surg* **55**: 719–23.

24. Bax JJ, Visser FC, Poldermans D *et al.* (2001). Time course of functional recovery of stunned and hibernating segments after surgical revascularization. *Circulation* **104**(Suppl. I): 314–18.

25. Bogaert J, Maes A, Van de Werf F *et al.* (1999). Functional recovery of subepicardial myocardial tissue in transmural myocardial infarction after successful reperfusion. *Circulation* **99**: 36–43.

26. Kim RJ, Wu E, Rafael A *et al.* (2000). The use of contrast-enhanced magnetic resonance imaging to identify reversible myocardial dysfunction. *New Engl J Med* **343**: 1445–53.

27. Maes A, Flameng W, Nuyts J *et al.* (1994). Histological alterations in chronically hypoperfused myocardium: correlation with PET findings. *Circulation* **90**: 735–45.

28. Shan K, Bick RJ, Poindexter BJ *et al.* (2000). Altered adrenergic receptor density in myocardial hibernation in humans. *Circulation* **102**: 2599–606.

29. Dor V, Sabatier M, Di Donato M *et al.* (1998). Efficacy of endoventricular patch plasty in large post infarction akinetic scar and severe left ventricular dysfunction: comparison with a series of large dyskinetic scars. *J Thorac Cardiovasc Surg* **116**: 50–9.

30. Cooley DA (1989). Ventricular endoaneurysmorrhaphy: a simplified repair for extensive post-infarction aneurysm. *J Card Surg* **4**: 200–5.

31. Jatene AD (1985). Left ventricular aneurysmectomy resection or reconstruction. *J Thorac Cardiovasc Surg* **89**: 321–31.

32. Dor V, Kreitmann P, Jourdan J *et al.* (1985). Interest of 'physiological closure' (circumferential plasty on contractile areas) of left ventricle resection and endocardectomy for aneurysm of akinetic zone. Comparison with classical technique about a series of 209 left ventricular resections [abstract]. *J Cardiovasc Surg* **26**: 73.

33. Dor V (2004). Surgical remodelling of the left ventricle. *Surg Clin N Am* **84**: 27–43.

34. Maisano F, Torracca L, Alfieri O *et al.* (1998). The edge-to-edge technique: a simplified method to correct mitral insufficiency. *Eur J Cardiothorac Surg* **13**: 240–5.

35. Athanasulsas CL, Stanley AWH, Buckberg GD (1998). Restoration of contractile function in the enlarged left ventricle by exclusion of remodeled akinetic anterior segment. *J Card Surg* **13**: 418–28.

36. Spotovitz HM, Spotnitz WD, Cotrell TS *et al.* (1974). Cellular basis for volume related wall thickness changes in the rat left ventricle. *J Mol Cell Cardiol* **6**: 317–31.

37. Athanasuleas CL, Stanley AW, Jr, Buckberg GD *et al.* (2001). Surgical anterior ventricular endocardial restoration (SAVER) in the dilated remodeled ventricle after anterior myocardial infarction. RESTORE group. Reconstructive Endoventricular Surgery, returning Torsion Original Radius Elliptical Shape to the LV. *J Am Coll Cardiol* **37**: 1199–209.

38. Bolling SF, Pagani FD, Deeb GM *et al.* (1998). Intermediate term outcome of mitral reconstruction in cardiomyopathy. *J Thorac Cardiovasc Surg* **115**: 381–8.

39. Stamm C, Westphal B, Kleine HD *et al.* (2003). Autologous bone marrow stem call transplantation for myocardial regeneration. *Lancet* **361**: 45–6.

40. Perrin EC, Dohmann HF, Borojevic R *et al.* (2004). Improved exercise capacity and ischaemia 6 and 12 months after transendocardial injection of autologous bone marrow mononuclear cells for ischaemic cardiomyopathy. *Circulation* **110**: 11.213–11.218.

41. Hunt SA, Rider AK, Stinson EB *et al.* (1976). Does cardiac transplantation prolong life and improve quality? An updated report. *Circulation* **54**(Suppl. III): 56–60.

42. Hertz M, Mohacsi P, Boucek M *et al.* (2002). The registry of the International Society for Heart and Lung Transplantation: past, present and future. *J Heart Lung Transplant* **21**: 945.

43. Deng MC (2004). Orthotopic heart transplantation: highlights and limitations. *Surg Clin N Am* **84**: 243–55.

44. Yancy CW, Kaiser P, DiMaio JM *et al.* (2002). Improved outcome in patients awaiting heart transplantation: making the case that Status 2 patients should not undergo transplantation [abstract]. *J Heart Lung Transplant* **21**: 69.

45. Deng MC, De Meester JMJ, Smith JMA *et al.* on behalf of the COCPIT study group (2000). The effect of receiving a heart transplant: analysis of a national cohort entered onto waiting list, stratified by heart failure severity. *Br Med J* **321**: 540–5.

46. Aaronson KD, Schwartz JS, Chen TMC *et al.* (1997). Development and prospective validation of a clinical index to predict survival in ambulatory patients referred for cardiac transplantation evaluation. *Circulation* **95**: 2660–7.

47. Taylor DO, Edwards LB, Boucek MM, Trulock EP, Keck BM, Hertz MI (2004). The registry of the International Society for Heat and Lung Transplantation: twenty-first official adult heart transplant report–2004. *J Heart Lung Transplant* **23**: 796–803.

48. Shah NR, Rogers JD, Ewald GA *et al.* (2004). Survival of patients removed from the heart transplant waiting list. *J Thorac Cardiovasc Surg* **127**: 1481–5.

49. Kirklin JK, McGiffin DC, Pinderski LJ, Tallaj J (2004). Selection of patients and techniques of heart. transplantation. *Surg Clin N Am* **84**: 257–87.

50. Kirklin J, Miller L, Brown R *et al.* (2001). Who is the most likely to enjoy long-term survival after cardiac transplantation with stratification in 10-year multi-institutional experience [abstract]. *J Heart Lung Transplant* **20**:168.

51. Hosenpud JD, Bennett LE, Keck BM *et al.* (2000). Registry of the International Society for Heart and Lung Transplantation; 17th official report – 2000. *J Heart Lung Transplant* **19**: 909–31.

52. Frazier OH, Rose EA, Oz MC *et al.* (2001). Multicenter clinical evaluation of the HeartMate vented electric left ventricular assist system in patients awaiting heart transplantation. *J Thorac Cardiovas Surg* **122**: 1186–95.

53. Sharples LD, Buxton MJ, Caine N (2006). Evaluation of the ventricular assist device programme in the United Kingdom. *J Heart Lung Transplant* **25**(Suppl.): 80–1.

54. Adamson PB, Abraham WT, Love C *et al.* (2004). The evolving challenge of chronic heart failure management: a call for a new curriculum for training heart failure specialists. *J Am Coll Cardiol* **44**: 1354–7.

55. Rose EA, Gelijns AL, Moskowitz AL *et al.* (2001). Long term use of left ventricular assist device for end stage heart failure. *New Engl J Med* **345**: 435–43.

56. Farrar DJ (1994). Ventricular interactions during mechanical circulatory support. *Semin Thorac Cardiovasc Surg* **6**: 163–8.

57. Copeland JG, Smith RG, Arabia FA *et al.* CardioWest Total Artificial Heart Investigators (2004). Cardiac replacement with a total artificial heart as a bridge to transplantation. *New Engl J Med* **351**: 859–67.

58. Mueller J, Wallukat G, Weng Y *et al.* (2001). Predictive factors for weaning from a cardiac assist device. An analysis of clinical, gene expression and protein data. *J Heart Lung Transplant* **20**: 202.

59. Konertz WF, Kleber FX, Dushe S *et al.* (2001). Efficacy trends with the Acorn cardiac support device in patients with advanced heart failure. *J Heart Fail* **7**: 39.

60. Acker MA (2005). Clinical results with the Acorn Cardiac Restraint Device with and without mitral valve surgery. *Semin Thorac Cardiovasc Surg* **17**: 361–3.

61. Batista RJV, Verde J, Nery P *et al.* (1997). Partial left ventriculectomy to treat end-stage heart disease. *Ann Thorac Surg* **64**: 634–8.

62. Suma H, Isomura T, Horii T *et al.* (1999). Two-year experience of the Batista operation for nonischemic cardiomyopathy. *J Cardiol* **32**: 269–76.

63. McCarthy PM, Starling RC, Wong J *et al.* (1997). Early results with partial left ventriculectomy. *J Thorac Cardiovasc Surg* **114**: 755–63.

64. Loebe M, Muller J, Hetzer R (1999). Ventricular assistance for recovery of cardiac failure. *Curr Opin Cardiol* **14**: 234–48.
65. Frazier OH, Benedict CR, Radovancevic B *et al.* (1996). Improved left ventricular function after chronic left ventricular unloading. *Ann Thorac Surg* **62**: 675–82.
66. Bartling B, Milting H, Schumann H *et al.* (1999). Myocardial gene expression of regulators of myocyte apoptosis and myocyte calcium homeostasis during hemodynamic unloading by ventricular assist devices in patients with end-stage heart failure. *Circulation* **100**(Suppl. II): 216–23.
67. Frazier OH, Rose EA, McCarthy PM *et al.* (1995). Improved mortality and rehabilitation of transplant candidates treated with a long-term implantable left ventricular assist system. *Ann Surg* **222**: 327.
68. Westaby S, Frazier OH, Banning A (2006). Six years of continuous circulatory support. *New Engl J Med* **355**: 325–7.
69. Westaby S (2004). Ventricular assist devices as destination therapy. *Surg Clinc N Am* **84**: 91–123.
70. Westaby S, Katsumata T, Pigott D *et al.* (2000). Mechanical bridge to recovery in fulminant myocarditis. *Ann Thorac Surg* **70**: 278–82.
71. Madigan JD, Barbone A, Choudhri AF *et al.* (2001). Time course of reverse remodeling of the left ventricle during support with a left ventricular assist device. *J Thorac Cardiovasc Surg* **121**: 902–8.
72. Zhang J, Narula J (2004). Molecular biology of myocardial recovery. *Surg Clin N Am* **84**: 223–42.
73. Hon JK, Yacoub MH (2003). Bridge to recovery with the use of left ventricular assist device and clenbuterol. *Ann Thorac Surg* **75**: S36–S41.
74. Burniston JG, Ng Y, Clark WA *et al.* (2002). Myotoxic effects of clenbuterol in the rat heart and soleus muscle. *J Appl Physiol.* **93**:1824–32.
75. Sleeper MM, Kearns CF, McKeever KH (2002). Chronic clenbuterol administration negatively alters cardiac function. *Med Sci Sports Exerc* **34**: 643–50.
76. Ott HC, Davis BH, Taylor DA (2005). Cell therapy for heart failure – muscle, bone marrow, blood and cardiac derived stem cells. *Semin Thorac Cardiovasc Surg* **17**: 348–60.
77. Kherani AR, Oz MC (2004). Ventricular assistance to bridge to transplantation. *Surg Clin N Am* **84**: 75–89.
78. Westaby S, Banning A, Saito S *et al.* (2002). Circulatory support as long-term treatment for heart failure. Experience with an intraventricular continuous flow pump. *Circulation* **105**: 2588–91.
79. Baldwin T, Robbins RC (2005). Executive summary for the National Heart, Lung and Blood Institute Working Group on Next Generation Ventricular Assist Devices for Destination Therapy. *Semin Thorac Cardiovasc Surg* **17**: 369–71.
80. Stevenson LW, Shekar P (2005). Ventricular assist devices for durable support. *Circulation* **112**: e111–e115.
81. Deng MC, Weynard M, Hammel D *et al.* (1998). Selection and outcome of ventricular assist device patients: the Muenster experience. *J Heart Lung Transplant* **17**: 817–25.
82. Park SJ, Tector A, Piccioni W *et al.* (2005). Left ventricular assist devices as destination therapy: a new look at survival. *J Thorac Cardiovasc Surg* **129**: 9–17.
83. Petrucci RJ, Truesdell KC, Carter A *et al.* (2006). Cognitive dysfunction in advanced heart failure and prospective cardiac assist device patients. *Ann Thorac Surg* **81**: 1738–44.
84. Butler J, Geisberg C, Howser R *et al.* Relationship between renal function and left ventricular assist device use. *Ann Thorac Surg* **81**: 1745–51.

Chapter 7

Interdisciplinary care in heart failure

Tiny Jaarsma

The need for teamwork

Heart failure (HF) management aims at preventing disease progression, prolonging survival, and improving the quality of life of affected patients. Recent decades have seen improvements in pharmacological, device, and surgical therapy; however these developments have yet to significantly reduce the high mortality, morbidity, and readmission rates associated with chronic HF.[1]

Decompensated HF is a common cause of readmission and is often unavoidable. However, several other avoidable factors contribute to the risk of readmission and intervention may prevent this. These factors include instability at discharge, non-compliance with the treatment regimen, adverse reactions to medications, use of detrimental drug therapy [e.g. anti-arrhythmic agents, non-steroidal anti-inflammatory drugs (NSAIDs), first-generation calcium antagonists], and problems with caregivers or extended care facilities (e.g. nursing homes, old people's homes).[2,3]

Readmissions may be avoided if medication is properly reviewed and up-titrated, if rehabilitation is more adequate, if discharge is more carefully planned, if potential non-compliance problems with medications and diet are identified and solved, if patients are instructed to seek medical attention when symptoms first occur, and if informal care-givers are supported in caring for HF patients.[4]

Superficially, application of this advice seems rather simple, but in daily practice the health-care provider is faced with the complexity of managing HF in older, sometimes cognitively and psychologically affected patients who often suffer from several medical conditions requiring multiple medications and lifestyle changes.

Older patients

According to guidelines, the therapeutic approach to HF in the elderly should not differ significantly from that in younger patients. However, therapy should be offered more cautiously.[5] Sometimes reduced dosages are necessary due to age-related effects on pharmacokinetic and pharmacodynamic properties of cardiovascular drugs and renal dysfunction. Changing lifestyle can also be more complicated in elderly patients who often lack adequate social support to help motivate them. Introducing a complex and frequently altered medication regimen can be particularly difficult.[6] Adjusting dietary and exercise patterns may not only be challenging from a motivational point of view but should also be applied with care if it requires major changes since altering long-established nutritional habits of elderly patients can lead to reduced protein/calorie intake further complicating their situation.

Coping with complex lifestyle changes

Most patients with HF need a complex therapeutic regimen that consists of medication, diet and fluid restriction as well as advice on activity and rest.[5] In addition, patients are asked to monitor their responses and to take appropriate action in the case of unexpected weight changes or increasing symptoms. The individual patient often has to integrate these HF lifestyle changes with those required for pre-existing co-morbid diseases. Non-compliance with medication and other lifestyle recommendations in HF patients is recognized as a major hazard and can have important consequences in worsening symptoms sometimes leading to readmission.[7] Education and counseling by a multidisciplinary team, with specific team members addressing specific items, is important to facilitate compliance.

Impaired cognitive function, depression, and other psychosocial problems

Many HF patients suffer from cognitive dysfunction and depression[8,9] that will influence educational strategies and adoption of the medical regimen. Forgetfulness or disinterest can negatively influence compliance with therapy and appointment keeping. These complex problems need a broad-based patient-centered approach, involving input from physicians, nurses, psychologists, and other health-care providers (see Chapters 14 and 15).

Complexity of diagnosis and treatment of HF

The clinical definition of HF states that HF consists of a constellation of symptoms and signs that includes breathlessness, fatigue, and fluid retention resulting from cardiac dysfunction.[5] This definition already alludes to the potential complexity inherent in this condition. Co-morbidities, age, and other medical treatment may further complicate the diagnosis and care of HF.

The specific treatment of HF-itself has become increasingly complex, and includes several medications that prolong life, alleviate symptoms, and reduce the risk of admission to hospital.[5] In individual patients we aim to up-titrate drugs to the target dosages as advised in the guidelines rather than accepting a dose response based on symptomatic improvement alone. Up-titrating agents in the commonly encountered setting of polypharmacy can sometimes be time-consuming, requires precision, and may involve several clinical decisions. Other complex decisions in treatment can be related to surgery or device therapy: implantable cardioverter defibrillators, cardiac resynchronization therapy, heart transplantation, or ventricular assist devices. Thus a multidisciplinary expert team is required to diagnose, optimally manage, and coordinate HF care.

Co-morbidity

In most patients, a range of concomitant disorders accompanies HF that both contribute to the cause of the disease (e.g. hypertension, ischemia, diabetes mellitus) and have a key role in its progression and response to treatment.[9] Co-morbid disorders often necessitate a medical regimen that includes multiple medications, contributing to the risk of adverse drug interactions, as well as several other non-pharmacological interventions such as dietary and exercise prescriptions.

Cardiologists, pharmacists, internists, primary-care physicians, HF nurses, and dieticians may all have a role in selecting the appropriate regime for a patient with several such co-morbidities.

These complex issues mean that health-care professionals who treat HF patients often face the challenge of managing the medical requirements of several conditions in older, sometimes cognitively and psychologically affected individuals. Thus, an interprofessional team approach is needed to accurately diagnose, monitor, and maintain optimal care of HF patients and their families both at home and across a variety of health-care settings (see Chapter 17).

Models to deliver interprofessional care

In recent years, multidisciplinary HF disease management programs have been increasingly developed, tested, and implemented.[10] Several meta-analyses have confirmed the positive effects of these programs in improving HF-related mortality, reducing readmission rates, and achieving cost savings.[11–13] However, due to non-uniformity in the models of care studied, and the variety of health-care settings in which they were evaluated, it is difficult to extrapolate these results as a guide to structuring clinical practice.[13] The challenge in interpreting these positive findings is the lack of clarity about what constitutes the optimal model of care. The European Society of Cardiology (ESC) guidelines[5] have described the key characteristics of a HF management program as:

- the use of a multidisciplinary team approach
- providing discharge planning
- ensuring vigilant follow-up
- enhancing access to health care
- optimizing medical therapy according to guidelines
- prescribing a flexible diuretic regimen
- early intervention if signs and symptoms suggest clinical deterioration
- providing inpatient and outpatient (home-based) care
- paying attention to behavioral strategies
- addressing barriers to compliance
- using intensive education and counseling strategies.

There are several models that can be used to deliver these components of disease management. Models can be classified as appropriate for HF hospital outpatient clinics, for home-based management programs, or for a combination of primary and secondary care. Telemonitoring is also increasingly used in disease management, either as an independent model (e.g. with a call centre) or in combination with a HF clinic or home-based program.

HF outpatient clinic

In a 'HF clinic' model, the primary site of care delivery is the hospital outpatient clinic. In some clinics the disease management program starts while the patient is hospitalized. In-hospital counseling by a variety of allied health-care professionals is followed by pre-discharge education and follow-up. Health-care professionals can have several roles in the HF clinic and have a responsibility to bridge the gap between inpatient and outpatient care. For example in a HF clinic studied by Strömberg and colleagues,[14] the program consisted of education aimed at assisting patients to improve their self-care regimen, non-pharmacological treatment, protocol-led changes in medication, psychosocial support, and availability of nurse contact in case of problems. The first HF clinic visit was scheduled 2–3 weeks after discharge. When patients were stable and well informed they were referred back to their general practitioner in primary care. Some other HF clinics will keep the patients under regular follow-up, without referring them back to their general practitioner.

Although there is no direct comparison between an outpatient HF clinic and other models, it is recognized that such a clinic affords the opportunity to access a specialist cardiology consultation, medical equipment, laboratory facilities, and patients' medical charts. At the same time it is accepted that an outpatient HF clinic is often impractical for the elderly and less mobile patients with moderate-to-severe chronic HF.[15,16]

Home-based management programs

In a home-based model, care is delivered primarily in patients' homes and sometimes includes home health facilities instead of delivering the care in a clinic or outpatient department. Rather, the health-care provider comes to the home of the patient in person, calls on the telephone, or both.

For example in a study from a tertiary referral hospital in Glasgow, Scotland, study patients received multiple home visits by HF nurses who initiated and titrated pharmacotherapy according to pre-established guidelines. Home-based specialist nurses provided comprehensive education and counseling during an early home visit, and frequent follow-up visits and calls. The home-based specialist nurse was accessible in case of problems and facilitated communication among other health-care providers.[17]

Other models for home-based care may be less intensive but still include patient education, counseling, and assessment of the need for medication adjustments as per protocol, during a home visit.

The advantage of home-based models is that the health-care provider has the opportunity to reach vulnerable and frail patients who might be unable to come to a HF clinic. Care is delivered in a non-threatening familiar environment allowing realistic assessment of the social situation and identification of possible barriers to compliance. Also, patients may more readily accept education in the less stressful home setting.[16] At the same time it should be realized that home visits might be very time-consuming and inefficient depending on the geography of the area and constraints on the time of professional staff, and access to specialist consultation, patient records, and medical equipment will be limited.

Combination of models and integrated care programs

There are several options to combine components from a secondary-care-based HF clinic and a home-based program. An example of such a hybrid intervention has been described by Thompson and colleagues.[18] In this model, the intervention started at the ward where patients received general information on HF and treatment and an appointment was arranged for a home visit. At the home visit, a clinical examination was performed and patients (and their family if appropriate) received further education on HF, symptom management, and lifestyle issues. Patients were also invited to attend a monthly nurse-led outpatient HF clinic for at least 6 months post-discharge. During the clinic visits, education and advice were reinforced and a clinical examination was performed to assess cardiac status and fluid retention. Medication was reviewed and prescribed according to protocol.

Other models aim to integrate primary and secondary care. For example, the Auckland Heart Failure Management Study uses an integrated management approach involving primary and secondary care in patients with HF. Patients receive early clinical review, three group education sessions, a patient diary, and regular follow-up appointments alternating between the general practitioner and the HF clinic.[19]

Home telemonitoring

In its simplest form, follow-up by telephone may facilitate continuity of care between the hospital and the patient at home. More sophisticated telemonitoring can be defined as home monitoring of patients using special telecare devices in conjunction with a telecommunication system. With technological equipment in patients' homes, data can be collected on weight, blood pressure, ECG, respiratory rate, transcutaneous O_2 saturations, and body temperature. Telemonitoring can either be used alone or as part of a multidisciplinary approach. Early studies have suggested that telemonitoring may reduce hospitalizations and readmission rates in patients with HF; however more evidence of efficacy is required.[20]

Independent of the mode or model of delivery, there are certain components that have been shown to be required for an effective HF disease management program. Effective programs were recently described as providing comprehensive multifaceted care. They included an in-hospital phase of care, intensive patient education, a self-care supportive strategy, optimization of medical regimen, and ongoing surveillance and management of clinical deterioration. All effective programs incorporated a multidisciplinary approach.[16]

Roles of members of the multidisciplinary HF team

The words 'multidisciplinary' or 'interdisciplinary' can be interpreted differently. Some studies report on a multidisciplinary team if, in addition to a cardiologist, another medical specialist (e.g. an internist) is involved or if a medical specialist liaises with a general practitioner. In other studies a multidisciplinary team involves a cardiologist and HF nurse, while others speak of a full multidisciplinary approach only if other health-care professionals such as a physical therapist, dietician, and pharmacist are involved.

In a European survey of HF disease management programs we found that most heart failure programs involved both nurses and physicians (87%). The physician was most frequently a cardiologist, and in 47% of all programs general practitioners were involved. After nurses and physicians, dieticians (39%) and physiotherapists (33%) were most often involved in providing specialist care. Three other health-care professional groups contributing to HF care were social workers (23%), pharmacists (19%), and psychologists (10%). Extended multidisciplinary teams (with more than three different health-care providers) were involved in 51% of the HF programs. In 46% of the programs the multidisciplinary teams had regular meetings to address joint issues relating to optimizing patient management and outcomes.[10]

Cardiologists

A medical doctor is responsible for the correct diagnosis and treatment of the patient. In most programs this is the cardiologist; however, in other cases a geriatrician or internist may be the medical specialist involved in medical management of the HF patient. In a recent review aimed at identifying the characteristics of HF management programs that are crucial to improve outcomes of older people with HF, the roles of the cardiologists included: simplifying the pre-discharge medication regime, participating in care planning, titrating medications, providing follow-up care in the clinic, and developing a comprehensive treatment plan of medications, exercise, and diet. Cardiologists also provided more indirect care, which included supervising the care delivered by nurses, developing algorithms for drug titration, and participating in patient-initiated telephone consultations.[16]

HF nurses

The HF nurse plays an important role in education and counseling of patients and family and helping patients when they show signs or symptoms of deterioration. HF nurses can help the patient to learn to live with the consequences of the condition, which means: to comply with a regimen concerning medication, diet, and exercise, monitor symptoms, to seek assistance when symptoms occur, and take appropriate action in the case of exacerbation. The role of the HF nurse has evolved, allowing a more independent function in regard to protocol-driven drug titration, seeing referrals, and post-discharge follow-up review of patients. Most nurses make protocol-led changes in medications, such as up-titrating angiotensin-converting enzyme (ACE) inhibitors and β-blockers, terminating inappropriate treatment with interacting drugs (usually potassium-sparing drugs), and adjusting diuretic dosage.[10] HF nurses usually have extensive experience in cardiac care and a personal commitment to HF care and treatment. Many nurses also have extended responsibilities in ordering and interpreting the results of laboratory tests and echocardiography. For legal reasons, written delegation for tasks that represent extended practice may be needed. There are huge differences within and between countries in the education and competencies of registered nurses,[10] and there are also legal differences and constraints defining the scope of practice within the nursing license.

General practitioners

The role of the general practitioner (primary care or family physician) in HF management differs from country to country and even from region to region within a country. There are clear differences in the patient populations and practices of general practitioners and cardiologists. In general, general practitioners treat more women and more elderly patients, whereas cardiologists treat more men, their patients tend to be younger, and with more ischemic heart disease as a contributory condition. Patients treated by cardiologists are more likely to receive ACE inhibitors, β-blockers, spironolactone, and angiotensin-receptor antagonists, while more general practice patients receive a diuretic as monotherapy.[21]

General practitioners are involved in a patient's course of HF at several stages. This starts with the important role in prevention of HF through the early identification of potential etiological causes and the aggressive management of identified risk factors. Additionally, the primary-care physician has a crucial role in initial diagnosis, implementation of evidence-based treatment, and subsequent follow-up arrangements, where all activities are aimed at maximizing prognosis.[22]

Whatever the model of the HF program, close cooperation between primary care and the hospital team must be established.

Dieticians

Promoting balanced nutrition is an essential component of comprehensive disease management of HF patients. Patients with HF may have a reduced food intake and this is thought to be related to a blunted sense of hunger, nausea, dietary restrictions, fatigue, shortness of breath, anxiety, and depression.[23] Early satiety and altered digestive efficiency related to decreased absorption might lead to nutritional deficiency in patients with HF.[24] In addition, water-soluble vitamins and minerals can be lost due to the use of diuretics.

Both hospital-based and primary-care dieticians can have a role in evaluating dietary intake and formulating tailored advice in regard to individual patient needs; for example combining HF and diabetic diets. They can also help patients to adhere to dietary advice.

Another important aspect in dietary counseling is the promotion of a healthy body weight. Being either overweight or underweight are serious concerns in patients with HF. The presence of obesity is independently associated with HF and contributes to the development of additional HF risk factors.[24] However, extreme weight loss programs are inappropriate in HF patients, making weight reduction in obese patients a complex issue needing specialized guidance by a dietician and a physician.[24] An adequate nutritional intake with advice on healthy eating and possibly vitamin and mineral supplementation is essential for those with HF.

Specific dietary advice may also be needed in avoiding and treating cardiac cachexia. Cardiac cachexia is associated with intense activation of the cytokine TNFα, elevated in chronically low cardiac output states. Cachectic patients risk serious morbidity, hospitalization, and impaired wound healing (see Chapter 13).

A dietician may assist patients to achieve optimal nutritional health while complying with a low-sodium diet. A small randomized Canadian study found that two counseling sessions with a dietician resulted in a significant decrease in sodium intake at 3 months. In contrast, there was no change in sodium intake in the usual care group who received nutritional advice by way of self-help literature.[25]

Physical therapists

In rehabilitation programs, in both secondary and primary care, physical therapists can assist in the care of HF patients. In hospitals and primary care a physical therapist can advise the patient with HF on reconditioning training and also give practical advice on energy conservation. Patients who are seen at the HF clinic have often become deconditioned by prolonged bed rest or repeated hospitalizations. Others have been inactive because of fear of inducing symptoms or a fear of undertaking exertion. These patients may benefit from exercise programs, either in a cardiac rehabilitation centre or from hospital or home-based exercise programs. Low-intensity home walking exercise programs for patients with stable moderate HF are safe, well accepted, and effective in improving functional status (submaximal exercise capacity) and global perception of symptoms.[26]

Pharmacists

In general health care pharmacists have a well-established role in anticipating and preventing drug interactions and minimizing the potential for adverse events, particularly when new drugs are initiated. Although this is not a HF-specific activity, polypharmacy in these patients necessitates a good system of awareness of possible drug interactions. In some hospitals or disease management programs, pharmacists are actively involved to advise physicians in the choice of an appropriate drug regime and dosages. Pharmacists can also have a role in improving compliance and enhancing patient knowledge of HF. Studies show that patient education and goal setting by pharmacists can improve patient knowledge, appropriateness of prescribed medication, and patient compliance.[27]

Psychologists or other related professionals

In addition to the classical cardiovascular risk factors, psychosocial factors have been demonstrated to be independently predictive of morbidity and mortality in HF patients—notably anxiety, depression, a lack of social support, and poor quality of life.[28]

Depressive symptoms have been described in 11–25% of outpatients and in 35–77% of inpatients and these features are associated with an increase in health-care costs.[28] Depression is often overlooked in HF patients due to non-specific signs and symptoms, often interpreted merely as apathy or fatigue.

It is advocated that the possibility of depression and anxiety needs to be routinely assessed to facilitate adaptation and decrease patients' risk of decompensation or other cardiac events.[29] Additionally, patients can be trained in anxiety management by using relaxation techniques and cognitive behavioral therapy. Teaching relaxation and cognitive coping skills such as cognitive restructuring of negative cognitions can be helpful and empowering to patients adapting to HF (see Chapter 15).[24]

In several disease management programs psychosocial care is provided mainly by nurses, who might liaise with clinical psychologists, psychiatric nurse practitioners, or social workers. Other programs formally incorporate a psychologist within the HF team or consult a psychiatric nurse practitioner as required.[10,30] At present, the level of support is usually dictated by the local availability of those with expertise in these various disciplines, their involvement and experience with HF, and both local and national reimbursement policies. Psychologists or related professionals can help patients to cope with the effects of HF on their daily lives. Psychologists can also help doctors and HF specialist nurses specifically to look for and identify symptoms of depression in patients with HF at an early stage.

Potential reasons for infrequent assessment and treatment of psychosocial factors in HF include inadequate dissemination of research about the link between psychosocial factors and outcomes, insufficient training in heart–mind interactions, perceived problems with interventions, and concerns about how to assess psychosocial factors in clinical practice.[31] Increased interdisciplinary collaboration may improve acceptance of the notion of the influence of psychosocial aspects on cardiac outcomes and vice versa.

Other professionals involved in HF management

Depending on the specific needs of patients and the expertise of the team members, other health-care professionals might also be involved in the care of HF patients. As HF patients often face co morbidities like diabetes and pulmonary disease, other medical specialists might be involved in the comprehensive management plan. These may also include members of a palliative care team or a sexual counselor.

Palliative care team

Although health-care systems and legal regulations differ from country to country, issues relating to end-of-life care for patients with advanced HF need to be highlighted. Local practice guidelines for these patients should include the need to amend treatment decisions over the course of the illness and the development of policies for end-of-life care including the role of advanced directives. In some countries patients with advanced HF are considered for hospice services, while in other countries these services do not exist or are considered inapplicable.[32] In several HF management programs, formal collaboration with palliative care services is already established.

Sexual counselor

A considerable amount of HF patients report a marked decrease both in sexual interest and the frequency of sexual relations caused by their HF. Symptoms of dyspnea and fatigue may hinder sexual activity. Patients might avoid sexual activity because of anxiety that this might induce complications, including the possibility of death during intercourse. Health professionals in the multidisciplinary HF team are in key positions to provide reassurance, outlining the anticipated effects of this condition and its treatment on sexual function, and to encourage a successful return to sexual activity. Persistent or complicated problems might need the specialist advice of a sexual counselor or specialized clinic.

The optimal HF team

It seems obvious that a HF disease management program must be tailored to accommodate individual patients' needs and that there is no 'one-size-fits-all' model. Therefore, it is sometimes difficult for the health-care provider to offer an optimal evidence-based model of care delivery applicable to all patients across a practice. Decisions about who should be involved in a HF management program should be driven by evidence on patient outcomes and criteria for optimal care. Acknowledgment of professional boundaries and critical evaluation of professional and personal expertise are a prerequisite for a flexible HF management structure. In the meantime, more research is needed on the optimal staffing configuration for HF clinics and the multidisciplinary team enabling us to make rational and informed choices in the future and to maximize the impact of these resources on HF management.

References

1. McMurray JJ, Stewart S (2003). The burden of heart failure. *Eur Heart J* (Suppl. 5): 3–14.
2. Tsuyuki RT, McKelvie RS, Arnold JM, Avezum A, Jr, Barretto AC, Carvalho AC *et al.* (2001). Acute precipitants of congestive heart failure exacerbations. *Arch Intern Med* **161**: 2337–42.
3. McDonald K, Ledwidge M, Cahill J, Quigley P, Maurer B, Travers B *et al.* (2002). Heart failure management: Multidisciplinary care has intrinsic benefit above the optimization of medical care. *J Card Fail* **8**: 142–8.
4. Michalsen A, Konig G, Thimme W (1998). Preventable causative factors leading to hospital admission with decompensated heart failure. *Heart* **80**: 437–41.
5. Swedberg K, Cleland J, Dargie H, Drexler H, Follath F, Komajda M *et al.* (2005). Guidelines for the diagnosis and treatment of chronic heart failure: executive summary (update 2005): The Task Force for the Diagnosis and Treatment of Chronic Heart Failure of the European Society of Cardiology. *Eur Heart J* **26**: 1115–40.
6. van der Wal MH, Jaarsma T, van Veldhuisen DJ (2005). Non-compliance in patients with heart failure; how can we manage it? *Eur J Heart Fail* **7**: 5–17.
7. van der Wal MH, Jaarsma T, Moser DK, Veeger NJ, van Gilst WH, van Veldhuisen DJ (2006). Compliance in heart failure patients: the importance of knowledge and beliefs. *Eur Heart J* **27**: 434–40.
8. Havranek EP, Ware MG, Lowes BD (1999). Prevalence of depression in congestive heart failure. *Am J Cardiol* **8**: 348–50.
9. Freudenberger R, Cahn SC, Skotzko C (2004). Influence of age, gender, and race on depression in heart failure patients. *J Am Coll Cardiol* **44**: 2254–5.
10. Jaarsma T, Strömberg A, De Geest S, Fridlund B, Heikkila J, Mårtensson J *et al.* (2006). Heart failure management programmes in Europe. *Eur J Cardiovasc Nurs* **5**: 197–205.
11. McAlister FA, Stewart S, Ferrua S, McMurray JJ (2004). Multidisciplinary strategies for the management of heart failure patients at high risk for admission: a systematic review of randomized trials. *J Am Coll Cardiol* **44**: 810–19.
12. Gonseth J, Guallar-Castillon P, Banegas JR, Rodriguez-Artalejo F (2004).The effectiveness of disease management programmes in reducing hospital re-admission in older patients with heart failure: a systematic review and meta-analysis of published reports. *Eur Heart J* **25**: 1570–95.

13. Whellan DJ, Gaulden L, Gattis WA *et al.* (2001). The benefit of implementing a heart failure disease management program. *Arch Intern Med* **161**: 2223–8.

14. Stromberg A, Martensson J, Fridlund B, Levin LA, Karlsson JE, Dahlstrom U (2003). Nurse-led heart failure clinics improve survival and self-care behaviour in patients with heart failure. Results from a prospective randomised study. *Eur Heart J* **24**: 1014–23.

15. Ekman I, Andersson B, Ehnfors M, Matejka G, Persson B, Fagerberg B (1998). Feasibility of a nurse-monitored, outpatient program for elderly patients with moderate-to-severe, chronic heart failure. *Eur Heart J* **19**: 1254–60.

16. Yu DSF, Thompson DR, Lee DTF (2006). Disease management programmes for older people with heart failure: crucial characteristics which improve post-discharge outcomes. *Eur Heart J* **27**: 596–612.

17. Blue L, Strong E, Murdoch DR *et al.* (2002). Improving long-term outcome with specialist nurse intervention in heart failure: a randomized trial. *Br Med J* **323**: 1112–15.

18. Thompson DR, Roebuck A, Stewart S (2005). Effects of a nurse-led, clinic and home-based intervention on recurrent hospital use in chronic heart failure. *Eur J Heart Fail* **7**: 77–84.

19. Doughty RN, Wright SP, Pearl A *et al.* (2001). Randomised, controlled trial of integrated heart failure management: The Auckland Heart Failure Management Study. *Eur Heart J* **23**: 139–46.

20. Louis AA, Turner T, Gretton M, Baksh A, Cleland JG (2003). A systematic review of telemonitoring for the management of heart failure. *Eur J Heart Fail* **5**: 583–90.

21. Ruttten FH, Grobbee DE, Hoes AW (2003). Differences between general practitioners and cardiologists in diagnosis and management of heart failure: a survey in everyday practice. *Eur J Heart Fail* **5**: 337–344.

22. Hobbs FD (1999). Primary care physicians: champions of or an impediment to optimal care of the patient with heart failure? *Eur J Heart Fail* **1**: 11–15.

23. Lennie TA, Moser DK, Heo S, Chung ML, Zambroski CH (2006). Factors influencing food intake in patients with heart failure: a comparison with healthy elders. *J Cardiovasc Nurs* **21**: 123–9.

24. Heart Failure Society of America (2006). HFSA 2006 comprehensive heart failure practice guideline. *J Card Fail* **12**: e29–e37.

25. Arcand JA, Brazel S, Joliffe C *et al.* (2005). Education by a dietitian in patients with heart failure results in improved adherence with a sodium-restricted diet: a randomized trial. *Am Heart J* **150**: 716.e1–716.e5.

26. Corvera-Tindel T, Doering LV, Woo MA, Khan S, Dracup K (2004). Effects of a home walking exercise program on functional status and symptoms in heart failure. *Am Heart J* **147**: 339–46.

27. Gattis WA, Hasselblad V, Whellan DJ, O'Connor CM (1999). Reduction in heart failure events by the addition of a clinical pharmacist to the heart failure management team: Results of the Pharmacist in Heart Failure Assessment Recommendation and Monitoring (PHARM) study. *Arch Intern Med* **59**: 1939–45.

28. Konstam V, Moser DK, De Jong MJ (2005). Depression and anxiety in heart failure. *J Card Fail* **11**: 455–63.

29. Moser DK, Worster PL (2000). Effect of psychosocial factors on physiologic outcomes in patients with heart failure. *J Cardiovasc Nurs* **14**: 106–15.

30. van der Wal MH, van Voorst R, Jaarsma T (2005). Psychiatric nurse; member of the HF management team? *Eur J Cardiovasc Nurs* **4**: 99–100.

31. Moser DK (2001). Psychosocial factors and their association with clinical outcomes in patients with heart failure: why clinicians do not seem to care. *Eur J Cardiovasc Nurs* **1**: 183–8.

32. Zambroski CH, Moser DK, Roser L, Heo S, Chung M (2005). Patients with heart failure who die in hospice. *Am Heart J* **149**: 558–64.

Part 2

Patient symptomatic burden

Chapter 8

Quality of life in heart failure

Corrine Jurgens, Jom Suwanno, and Barbara Riegel

Chronic illnesses such as heart failure (HF) are known to impair quality of life. HF, in particular, is associated with unpleasant symptoms, limitations in activities of daily living, and increased risk of hospitalization for symptom management.[1] The effects of chronic illness on symptoms, functioning, and the risk of hospitalization decrease quality of life in persons with HF.

Clinicians, patients, and their families know that living longer is not necessarily desirable if quality of life is poor. Thus, quality of life has emerged as an important factor in both the delivery of health care and in health-care research. In health-care research, quality of life measures are often included when assessing the effectiveness of interventions or therapies. These measures are integral, because testing new therapies includes evaluating efficacy *and* patients' subjective judgments of whether their lives are improved.

A controversy within the HF field is the effectiveness of interventions in improving quality of life. For example, some believe that disease management improves quality of life,[2] while others disagree.[3] This controversy is probably related to the lack of a universally accepted definition of quality of life, which has hampered both measurement and comparisons among studies.[4–6] Often, in studies of quality of life, a definition is omitted, related concepts are substituted, or measurement is limited to one or more components of the construct.[7] The purpose of this chapter is to lend some clarity to the discussion of quality of life in HF. To do so, we will explore definitions of quality of life, review the literature on the effect of HF on quality of life, and end by summarizing what is known about the effect of interventions on quality of life in persons with HF.

Defining quality of life

Widespread multidisciplinary use of the term quality of life[5] and its complexity[6] have been suggested as reasons for the lack of a consensus on a definition of quality of life. Initially only objective social indicators like type of housing and educational level were thought to influence quality of life. However, these factors accounted for only 15% of the variance in quality of life for an individual. Subjective indicators such as satisfaction with life, happiness, and well-being are now believed to be important dimensions; these psychological factors account for over 50% of the variance in quality of life.[8] In one study of quality of life in HF, the subjective variables perceived health status and perception of symptom status influenced quality of life more than objective measures of functional status.[9]

Concept analysis has been used in an effort to further clarify the construct of quality of life.[4–6] In one such concept analysis, Meeberg[4] defined quality of life as:

> ... a feeling of overall life satisfaction, as determined by the mentally alert individual whose life is being evaluated. Other people from outside that person's living situation must also agree that the individual's living conditions are not life-threatening and are adequate in meeting that individual's basic needs. [p. 37]

Not everyone includes both subjective and objective indicators and some do not limit the definition to those able to provide self-report data. For example, Haas[6] defined quality of life as:

> ... a multidimensional evaluation of an individual's current life circumstances in the context of culture and value systems in which they live and the values they hold. Quality of life is primarily a subjective sense of well-being encompassing physical, psychological, social, and spiritual dimensions. In some circumstances, objective indicators may supplement or, in the case of [people] unable to subjectively perceive, serve as a proxy assessment of quality of life.[p. 219]

In this definition, subjective indicators are weighted heavily and quality of life is not limited to the mentally alert. An important contribution of this definition is Haas' differentiation of quality of life from the related concepts of well-being, satisfaction with life, and functional status. Table 8.1 shows some other definitions of quality of life using variations of the components reflecting physical, emotional, and social function.

Health-related quality of life is more restrictive than global quality of life, conceptually limiting the components or factors to those related to health and health care. Other factors such as income and education may be indirectly related to health but are not included in the definition.[10,11] Health-related quality of life measures are useful in health-care research because they reflect patient experiences and health status resulting from health care.

Although quality of life has been defined in numerous ways, generally most agree on the following. Quality of life as a construct is complex, multidimensional, and dynamic. Subjective self-report of quality of life by individuals is preferred over the views of others or objective measures alone.[12,13] The complexity and multidimensional characteristics are reflected in the physical, psychological, and social domains cited both explicitly and implicitly in several models of quality of life.[6,11,12,14,15]

Models of quality of life

Domains of quality of life have been identified and models explaining their relationships have been proposed. Although terminology varies from author to author, the domains are similar and incorporate both subjective and objective indicators.[6,11,12,14,15] Three models were chosen for discussion; one is a global quality of life model and the other two are health-related quality of life models.

The model by Haas[6] reflects a global perspective where subjective well-being is considered the primary indicator of quality of life. The objective component is functional status. Functional status is not limited to physical functioning, but refers to all

Table 8.1 Definitions of quality of life

Author	Definition
World Health Organization (1993)[57]	'... individuals' perception of their position in life in the context of the culture and value systems in which they live and in relation to their goals, expectations, standards, and concerns. It is a broad ranging construct affected in a complex way by the person's physical health, psychological state, level of independence, social relationships, and their relationships to salient features of their environment.'
Ferrans and Powers (1985)[58]	'satisfaction of needs' where satisfaction is defined as the 'perceived discrepancy between aspiration and achievement, ranging from the perception of fulfillment to that of deprivation' and need was defined as 'the amount of a particular reward that a person may require.'
Meeberg (1993)[4]	'... a feeling of overall life satisfaction, as determined by the mentally alert individual whose life is being evaluated. Other people from outside that person's living situation must also agree that the individuals living conditions are not life- threatening and are adequate in meeting that individual's basic needs.'
Guyatt (1993)[10]	'Health-related negatively valued aspects of life, including death, to more positively valued aspects of life such as role function or happiness.'
Osoba (1994)[59]	'A multidimensional construct encompassing perceptions of both positive and negative aspects of physical, emotional, social, and cognitive functions, as well as the negative aspects of somatic discomfort and other symptoms produced by a disease or its treatment.'
Wilson and Cleary (1995)[11]	'Subjective well-being related to how happy or satisfied someone is with life as a whole.'
Haas (1999)[6]	'... a multidimensional evaluation of an individual's current life circumstances in the context of culture and value systems in which they live and the values they hold. Quality of life is primarily a subjective sense of well-being encompassing physical, psychological, social, and spiritual dimensions. In some circumstances, objective indicators may supplement or, in the case of [people] unable to subjectively perceive, serve as a proxy assessment of quality of life.'

dimensions of life—physical, psychological, and social dimensions—common to several models, plus a spiritual dimension. The indicators of quality of life (subjective well-being and objective functional status) are interrelated with all of the dimensions.

A health-related quality of life model useful for testing the effects of HF and medical care on patients' lives was proposed by Rector (Fig. 8.1).[15] In this model 'symptoms, functional status, and psychological distress are distinct, but interrelated phenomena that mediate the effects of HF pathophysiology on a patient's quality of life' [p. 173]. Symptoms are abnormal states produced by the pathophysiology and are subjectively perceived by the patient. Functional status is broadly defined to include physical, social, and emotional functioning. Psychological distress refers to negative psychological responses to illness and is related to symptoms and functional status.

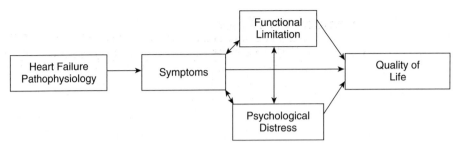

Fig. 8.1 Rector's model of quality of life (Reprinted from Rector[15], copyright ©2005 Elsevier Inc. With permission from Elsevier.)

Wilson and Cleary[11] integrated clinical and social science models in their health-related quality of life model depicted as a continuum that begins with biological and physiological variables sequentially leading to symptom status, functional status, general health perceptions, and quality of life. Each preceding component is thought to influence the subsequent one, culminating in overall health-related quality of life. Characteristics of the individual and the environment are included in the model but were not discussed by the authors. Similar to Rector's definition, symptoms were defined as the patient's subjective perception of abnormal physical, emotional, or cognitive states. Functional status was defined as the ability to perform tasks in multiple domains (physical, social, role, psychological).

In a revision of Wilson and Cleary's model, Ferrans and colleagues[14] described characteristics of the individual and environment omitted in the original publication of the model. Characteristics of the individual were defined as demographic, developmental, psychological, and biological factors that influence health. Environmental characteristics were categorized as social or physical. Social environmental characteristics acknowledge the influence of family, friends, and health-care providers on health. Physical environmental characteristics such as the home, neighborhood, or workplace factors can influence health. Arrows from characteristics of the individual and environment to biological function were added to demonstrate their influence on that domain.

A major limitation of these models of quality of life and other published taxonomies is the use of several terms with similar meanings. Conceptually unique terms like life satisfaction, subjective well-being, health status, and satisfaction of needs are used synonymously and interchangeably with quality of life. Cultural considerations further complicate the quest to identify a universal definition of quality of life. Culture contributes in important ways to quality of life,[16] but only Spilker's model[17] (Fig. 8.2) illustrates how patient values, including those influenced by culture, influence relationships between medical treatments and quality of life.

Effect of HF on quality of life

The common dimensions of quality of life in all the models reviewed are physical, emotional, and social function. In this section, we describe the effect of HF on each of these dimensions. The physical dimension includes biological or illness characteristics, symptoms, and functional status. The emotional dimension includes the psychological response to HF. Social functioning includes sociodemographic factors, including cultural and environmental aspects.

Effect of HF on physical function

In persons with HF, symptom burden and functional limitations are the most significant predictors of quality of life.[18,19] Common and bothersome symptoms include lack of energy, fatigue, shortness of breath, swelling, difficulty breathing while sleeping supine, and coughing.[20,21] Patients with HF experience an average of 3 to 13 symptoms.[22] In one study, more than 90% of 139 patients had multiple symptoms; 15% had every symptom queried about. An average of 7.2 symptoms was identified on admission and 4.2 symptoms 6 weeks after a HF hospitalization. Initially, shortness of breath was the primary symptom but by 6 weeks, fatigue was most common and troubling. Low vigor scores were similar to those with cancer.[22]

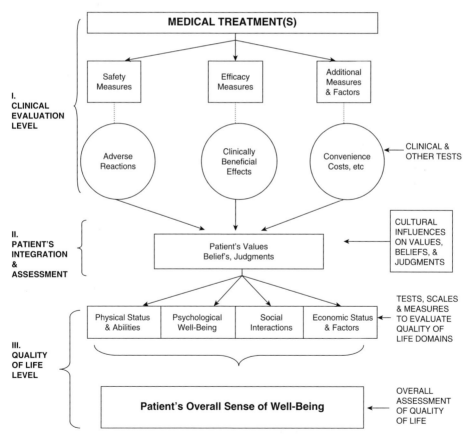

Fig. 8.2 Model of how clinical aspects of efficacy (i.e. benefits), safety (e.g. adverse reactions) or other factors are integrated through the patient's values, beliefs, and judgments to influence his or her quality of life. (Reprinted from Spilker[17] with permission from Lippincott, Williams, and Wilkins.)

HF patients who are asymptomatic [New York Heart Association (NYHA) functional Class I] have better quality of life than those with symptoms and impaired functioning (NYHA Class II–IV).[23] Patients with less severe symptoms have a better mood and higher life satisfaction than those with more severe symptoms.[24] Those with poor physical functioning have worse health outcomes, including quality of life.[25] These symptomatic, functionally compromised patients frequently delay returning to normal daily, work, and social activities.[26]

Effect of HF on emotional function

HF causes anxiety, depression, and overall emotional distress (for a detailed discussion see Chapter 15). In a recent study of 100 outpatients with systolic HF drawn from a community HF program in the United Kingdom, the prevalence of anxiety was 18.4% by clinical diagnostic interview.[27] Whether or not anxiety is higher in persons with HF than other cardiac populations or the general population is unclear. One study found mean anxiety scores in HF patients to be only slightly higher than the general population[28] but another study found that anxiety was similar in the patient groups but higher than healthy older adults.[29] Predictors of anxiety include a history of mental illness, co-morbid physical illness (diabetes and angina), and NYHA class. Specifically, anxiety is probably higher in patients who are relatively more functionally compromised (NYHA Class III/IV) compared with those without as much functional compromise.[28]

The prevalence of depression has been estimated to range from 13% to 77% in patients with HF, depending on the timing and manner in which depression is measured.[30,31] Patients with HF in whom depression is assessed during hospitalization have higher rates of major depression than those assessed in an outpatient setting (30% to 75% of hospitalized patients[22,30] vs 24% to 42% in outpatient settings[32]). Depression in HF is associated with the severity of illness, functional capacity, and symptom severity. Carels[33] suggests that depressive symptoms may have a greater impact on quality of life than severity of cardiac dysfunction or functional impairment.

Effect of HF on social function

Some investigators have suggested that women with HF have worse quality of life than men,[34] but other investigators have found few clinically significant gender differences.[35] In another study, women with HF had significantly better health perceptions and constructed meaning than men.[36] Age of onset may explain this discrepancy. In one study, women under the age of 65 years had poorer quality of life compared with their male counterparts in the same age group.[37] The authors suggested that the interaction of age and gender in relationship to quality of life may be related to baseline psychological state or the burden of other illnesses. For example, young women may have family and work responsibilities that have already stretched their coping abilities. Diabetes and hypertension are common causes of HF in younger women. When HF is added to existing social burdens and/or other chronic conditions, a measurable influence on quality of life may become evident.

Social functioning encompasses the ability to maintain social and work activities. Few investigators have specifically examined these outcomes in persons with HF. Carels et al.[38] found a link between physical symptoms and psychosocial functioning, including social conflict. Friedman and King[24] found that HF patients with higher levels of emotional support had higher life satisfaction than those with lower levels of emotional support. Others have found that changes in perceived social support significantly predicted changes in quality of life.[39] Again, in this study, there was a significant interaction of gender by age, with younger men (<65 years) perceiving less support than older men (≥65 years) and women in general. It should be noted, however, that the link between social support and quality of life is neither strong nor consistent.[40]

Surprisingly few investigators have studied the effect of cultural factors on quality of life. We have[41] illustrated that quality of life improved significantly more following an acute HF hospitalization in Hispanics compared with a matched sample of non-Hispanic Whites. No other comparisons of ethnic cultural groups were located in the literature. Cultural aspects of care are reviewed in Chapter 25.

Even fewer investigators have assessed return to work in persons with HF. It is known that HF outcomes are poorer in patients in the low socioeconomic status groups.[42] Research on the influence of return to work on quality of life in persons with HF is greatly needed.

Quality of life measures

Several HF-specific quality of life instruments have been developed and tested in response to the need for clinically relevant measures which are sensitive to clinical change. The most commonly used instruments are the Chronic Heart Failure Questionnaire, the Minnesota Living with Heart Failure Questionnaire, and the Kansas City Cardiomyopathy Questionnaire.[10,43,44] These instruments differ on their clinical responsiveness and the range of clinical domains addressed.

The Chronic Heart Failure Questionnaire tests the domains of dyspnea, fatigue, and emotional function.[10] Patients identify five frequent activities associated with shortness of breath that are important in their daily lives. These activities are used to evaluate their effect on the three domains of social, emotional, and physical quality of life using a seven-point scale.

The Minnesota Living with Heart Failure Questionnaire is the most commonly used quality of life measure in patients with HF.[44] This instrument is a 21-item scale focusing on patients' perceptions of the effects of HF on their lives. It has two subscales testing physical and emotional domains of quality of life using a six-point scale. The social domain is evident in specific items.

The Kansas City Cardiomyopathy Questionnaire is a 23-item instrument that tests physical limitations, symptoms, social interference, and self-efficacy. Symptoms are independently quantified in relation to frequency, severity, and stability.

All of these instruments are reported to be more sensitive to clinical change than generic quality of life measures. The Chronic Heart Failure Questionnaire may be particularly useful in small samples because a smaller change in score is needed to detect a clinically important improvement than that of the Minnesota Living with Heart Failure Questionnaire.[45] The Kansas City Cardiomyopathy Questionnaire is substantially more sensitive to clinical change than generic quality of life measures or the Minnesota Living with Heart Failure Questionnaire.[43]

Increasingly, providers are administering one of these HF-specific measures to patients in their clinical practices and tracking their quality of life over time. Others who want to avoid the burden of scale completion simply ask their patients to rate their overall quality of life on a scale from poor to excellent. Regardless of the approach used, some assessment of this penultimate indicator of treatment effectiveness is needed.

Effectiveness of interventions in improving quality of life in HF

In this section we briefly review studies of the effectiveness of various medications and disease management approaches on quality of life. Most studies of the effect of angiotensin-converting enzyme (ACE) inhibitors found an improvement in quality of life associated with this medication.[46] It should be noted, however, that in most of those studies, quality of life was defined as physical functioning (e.g. symptoms, functional class). Some studies have found little or no specific benefit of ACE inhibitors on quality of life.[47,48]

The data on the effect of β-blockers on quality of life is also inconclusive. In a review of 10 studies that measured quality of life with one of two specific instruments (Quality of Life Questionnaire in Severe Heart Failure; Minnesota Living with Heart Failure Questionnaire), only three reported significant improvements in quality of life. Using a single-question global assessment, improved quality of life was found in five of seven studies.[49]

Recent meta-analyses summarizing the effect of disease management have been unconvincing about its effect on quality of life. Six of the 18 studies reviewed by Phillips et al.[50] assessed quality of life and all six found improvements. The pooled effect showed a 13.5% improvement in quality of life. McAlister et al.[51] reviewed 29 studies, 18 of which assessed quality of life. Seven of those 18 studies found significant improvements in quality of life and two more found a 'trend' toward improvement. A trend toward improved quality of life was also noted by the authors of another meta-analysis reviewing eight trials, four of which assessed quality of life.[52] Two of these four found a significant improvement in quality of life. Finally, Whellan et al.[2] reviewed 19 trials and concluded that there was 'consistent improvement in quality of life'; the number of trials on which this conclusion was based was not specified and no data were provided.

It should be noted that a publication bias could be in effect with the disease management literature. We have examined quality of life in each of our HF disease management studies, but rarely included these data in our results.[53–55] In each trial we found a consistent picture; as shown in Fig. 8.3, quality of life improved over time after hospital discharge when measured using the Minnesota Living with Heart Failure Questionnaire, regardless of the group (intervention or usual care) to which the patient was assigned. This consistent result may reflect a relatively insensitive measure[56] or a true

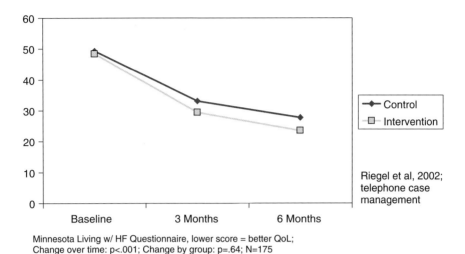

Minnesota Living w/ HF Questionnaire, lower score = better QoL;
Change over time: p<.001; Change by group: p=.64; N=175

Fig. 8.3 Changes in quality of life over time by group.

observation that disease management is not sufficiently powerful to influence quality of life. Others have substantiated this finding of a lack of effect on quality of life with disease management.[3] A meta-analysis of the effect of HF disease management on quality of life would be an extremely valuable contribution to the literature.

Conclusion

In this chapter we have described various models and definitions of quality of life. Quality of life was defined as a complex, multidimensional, and dynamic construct. Most models specify the domains of physical, emotional, and social functioning. Health-related quality of life was differentiated from the global concept as those aspects of quality of life specific to health. The extant literature was used to support our conclusion that HF has a negative influence on all aspects of quality of life, although more research is needed on social functioning.

Some evidence suggests that optimal medical therapy and perhaps disease management can improve quality of life, but many of the studies are limited by failure to define the construct and measure it in its complexity. A publication bias may be evident, with negative trials going unreported. Although quality of life has been measured relatively more commonly in recent years, trials are still conducted that fail to include this essential outcome. Further research is greatly needed to identify interventions that effectively improve the quality of life for persons with HF.

References

1. Bennett SJ, Cordes DK, Westmoreland G, Castro R, Donnelly E (2000). Self-care strategies for symptom management in patients with chronic heart failure. *Nurs Res* **49**: 139–45.
2. Whellan DJ, Hasselblad V, Peterson E, O'Connor CM, Schulman KA (2005). Meta-analysis and review of heart failure disease management randomized controlled clinical trials. *Am Heart J* **149**: 722–9.

3. Smith B, Forkner E, Zaslow B *et al.* (2005). Disease management produces limited quality-of-life improvements in patients with congestive heart failure: evidence from a randomized trial in community-dwelling patients. *Am J Manag Care* **11**: 701–13.

4. Meeberg GA (1993). Quality of life: a concept analysis. *J Adv Nurs* **18**: 32–8.

5. Farquhar M (1995). Definitions of quality of life: a taxonomy. *J Adv Nurs* **22**: 502–8.

6. Haas BK (1999). A multidisciplinary concept analysis of quality of life. *West J Nurs Res* **21**: 728–42.

7. King LA, Napa CK (1998). What makes a life good? *J Pers Soc Psychol* **75**: 156–65.

8. Day H, Jankey SG (1996). Lessons from the literature: toward a holistic model of quality of life. In: *Quality of Life in Health Promotion and Rehabilitation* (ed. R Renwick, I Brown, M Nagler), pp. 39–62. Thousand Oaks, CA: Sage.

9. Heo S, Moser DK, Riegel B, Hall LA, Christman N (2005). Testing a published model of health-related quality of life in heart failure. *J Card Fail* **11**: 372–9.

10. Guyatt GH (1993). Measurement of health-related quality of life in heart failure. *J Am Coll Cardiol* **22**: 185A–191A.

11. Wilson IB, Cleary PD (1995). Linking clinical variables with health-related quality of life. A conceptual model of patient outcomes. *J Am Med Assoc* **273**: 59–65.

12. Ferrans CE (1996). Development of a conceptual model of quality of life. *Sch Inq Nurs Pract* **10**: 293–304.

13. Vallerand AH (2003). The use of long-acting opioids in chronic pain management. *Nurs Clin North Am* **38**: 435–45.

14. Ferrans CE, Zerwic JJ, Wilbur JE, Larson JL (2005). Conceptual model of health-related quality of life. *J Nurs Scholarship* **37**: 336–42.

15. Rector TS (2005). A conceptual model of quality of life in relation to heart failure. *J Card Fail* **11**: 173–6.

16. Cella DF (1992). Quality of life: the concept. *J Palliat Care* **8**: 8–13.

17. Spilker B (1996). Introduction. In: *Quality of Life and Pharmacoeconomics in Clinical Trials* (ed. B Spilker), pp. 1–10. Philadelphia: Lippincott-Raven.

18. Friedman M (1997). Older adults' symptoms and their duration before hospitalization for heart failure. *Heart Lung* **26**: 169–76.

19. Todero CM, LaFramboise LM, Zimmerman LM (2002). Symptom status and quality-of-life outcomes of home-based disease management program for heart failure patients. *Outcomes Manag* **6**: 161–8.

20. Nordgren L, Sorensen S (2003). Symptoms experienced in the last six months of life in patients with end-stage heart failure. *Eur J Cardiovasc Nurs* **2**: 213–17.

21. Horowitz CR, Rein SB, Leventhal H (2004). A story of maladies, misconceptions and mishaps: effective management of heart failure. *Soc Sci Med* **58**: 631–43.

22. Friedman MM, Griffin JA (2001). Relationship of physical symptoms and physical functioning to depression in patients with heart failure. *Heart Lung* **30**: 98–104.

23. Gorkin L, Norvell NK, Rosen RC *et al.* (1993). Assessment of quality of life as observed from the baseline data of the Studies of Left Ventricular Dysfunction (SOLVD) trial quality-of-life substudy. *Am J Cardiol* **71**: 1069–73.

24. Friedman M, King K (1994). The relationship of emotional and tangible support to psychological well-being among older women with heart failure. *Res Nurs Health* **17**: 433–40.

25. Gott M, Barnes S, Parker C *et al.* (2006). Predictors of the quality of life of older people with heart failure recruited from primary care. *Age Ageing* **35**: 172–7.

26. De Jong M, Moser DK, Chung ML (2005). Predictors of health status for heart failure patients. *Prog Cardiovasc Nurs* **20**: 155–62.

27. Haworth JE, Moniz-Cook E, Clark AL, Wang M, Waddington R, Cleland JG (2005). Prevalence and predictors of anxiety and depression in a sample of chronic heart failure patients with left ventricular systolic dysfunction. *Eur J Heart Fail* **7**: 803–8.

28. Majani G, Pierobon A, Giardini A *et al.* (1999). Relationship between psychological profile and cardiological variables in chronic heart failure. The role of patient subjectivity. *Eur Heart J* **20**: 1579–86.

29. Moser DK, Zambroski CH, Lennie TA *et al.* (2004). Aging with a broken heart: The effect of heart disease on psychological distress in the elderly [abstract]. *Circulation* **110**(Suppl.): 416.

30. Vaccarino V, Kasl SV, Abramson J, Krumholz HM (2001). Depressive symptoms and risk of functional decline and death in patients with heart failure. *J Am Coll Cardiol* **38**: 199–205.

31. Thomas SA, Friedmann E, Khatta M, Cook LK, Lann AL (2003). Depression in patients with heart failure: physiologic effects, incidence, and relation to mortality. *AACN Clin Issues* **14**: 3–12.

32. Murberg T, Aarsland T, Svebak S (1998). Functional status and depression among men and women with congestive heart failure. *Int J Psychiat Med* **28**: 273–91.

33. Carels RA (2004). The association between disease severity, functional status, depression and daily quality of life in congestive heart failure patients. *Qual Life Res* **13**: 63–72.

34. Riedinger MS, Dracup KA, Brecht ML, Padilla G, Sarna L, Ganz PA (2001). Quality of life in patients with heart failure: do gender differences exist? *Heart Lung* **30**: 105–16.

35. Riegel B, Moser DK, Carlson B *et al.* (2003). Gender differences in quality of life are minimal in patients with heart failure. *J Card Fail* **9**: 42–8.

36. Evangelista LS, Kagawa-Singer M, Dracup K (2001). Gender differences in health perceptions and meaning in persons living with heart failure. *Heart Lung* **30**: 167–76.

37. Hou N, Chui MA, Eckert GJ, Oldridge NB, Murray MD, Bennett SJ (2004). Relationship of age and sex to health-related quality of life in patients with heart failure. *Am J Crit Care* **13**: 153–61.

38. Carels RA, Musher-Eizenman D, Cacciapaglia H, Perez-Benitez CI, Christie S, O'Brien W (2004). Psychosocial functioning and physical symptoms in heart failure patients: a within-individual approach. *J Psychosom Res* **56**: 95–101.

39. Bennett SJ, Perkins SM, Lane KA, Deer M, Brater DC, Murray MD (2001). Social support and health-related quality of life in chronic heart failure patients. *Qual Life Res* **10**: 671–82.

40. Luttik ML, Jaarsma T, Moser D, Sanderman R, van Veldhuisen DJ (2005). The importance and impact of social support on outcomes in patients with heart failure: an overview of the literature. *J Cardiovasc Nurs* **20**: 162–9.

41. Riegel B, Carlson B, Glaser D, Romero T (2003). Changes over 6-months in health-related quality of life in a matched sample of Hispanics and non-Hispanics with heart failure. *Qual Life Res* **12**: 689–98.

42. Blair AS, Lloyd-Williams F, Mair FS (2002). What do we know about socioeconomic status and congestive heart failure? A review of the literature. *J Fam Pract* **51**: 169.

43. Green CP, Porter CB, Bresnahan DR, Spertus JA (2000). Development and evaluation of the Kansas City Cardiomyopathy Questionnaire: a new health status measure for heart failure. *J Am Coll Cardiol* **35**: 1245–55.

44. Rector T, Kubo S, Cohn J (1987). Patient's self-assessment of their congestive heart failure. Part 2: Content, reliability and validity of a new measure, The Minnesota Living with Heart Failure Questionnaire. *Heart Fail* **1**: 198–209.

45. Bennett SJ, Oldridge NB, Eckert GJ *et al.* (2003). Comparison of quality of life measures in heart failure. *Nurs Res* **52**: 207–16.

46. Nasution SA (2006). The use of ACE inhibitor in cardiovascular disease. *Acta Med Indones* **38**: 60–4.

47. Jenkinson C, Jenkinson D, Shepperd S, Layte R, Petersen S (1997). Evaluation of treatment for congestive heart failure in patients aged 60 years and older using generic measures of health status (SF-36 and COOP charts). *Age Ageing* **26**: 7–13.

48. Wolfel EE (1998). Effects of ACE inhibitor therapy on quality of life in patients with heart failure. *Pharmacotherapy* **18**: 1323–34.

49. Reddy P, Dunn AB (2000). The effect of beta-blockers on health-related quality of life in patients with heart failure. *Pharmacotherapy* **20**: 679–89.

50. Phillips CO, Wright SM, Kern DE, Singa RM, Shepperd S, Rubin HR (2004). Comprehensive discharge planning with postdischarge support for older patients with congestive heart failure: a meta-analysis. *J Am Med Assoc* **291**: 1358–67.

51. McAlister FA, Stewart S, Ferrua S, McMurray JJJV (2004). Multidisciplinary strategies for the management of heart failure patients at high risk for admission: a systematic review of randomized trials. *J Am Coll Cardiol* **44**: 810–19.

52. Gwadry-Sridhar FH, Flintoft V, Lee DS, Lee H, Guyatt GH (2004). A systematic review and meta-analysis of studies comparing readmission rates and mortality rates in patients with heart failure. *Arch Intern Med* **164**: 2315–20.

53. Riegel B, Carlson B, Glaser D, Hoagland P (2000). Which patients with heart failure respond best to multidisciplinary disease management? *J Card Fail* **6**: 290–9.

54. Riegel B, Carlson B, Kopp Z, LePetri B, Glaser D, Unger A (2002). Effect of a standardized nurse case-management telephone intervention on resource use in patients with chronic heart failure. [see comment]. *Arch Intern Med* **162**: 705–12.

55. Riegel B, Carlson B, Glaser D, Romero T (2006). Randomized controlled trial of telephone case management in Hispanics of Mexican origin with heart failure. *J Card Fail* **12**: 211–19.

56. Spertus J, Peterson E, Conard MW *et al.* (2005). Monitoring clinical changes in patients with heart failure: a comparison of methods. *Am Heart J* **150**: 707–15.

57. World Health Organization, Division of Mental Health (1993). *WHO-QOL study protocol: the development of the world health quality of life assessment instruments*. Geneva: World Health Organization.

58. Ferrans CE, Powers MJ (1985). Quality of life index: development and psychometric properties. *ANS Adv Nurs Sci* **8**: 15–24.

59. Osoba D (1994). Lessons learned from measuring health-related quality of life in oncology. *J Clin Oncol* **12**: 608–16.

Chapter 9

Dyspnoea

Patricia M. Davidson, Phillip J. Newton, and
Peter S. Macdonald

Objectives for this chapter

Supportive care in heart failure (HF) management is the multidisciplinary holistic care
of patients and their families from the time of diagnosis, during treatment aimed
at prolonging life, through to the end of life when palliative care is provided.[1] The
management of dyspnoea is a key consideration in supportive care of HF. This chapter
will describe the physiological basis of dyspnoea, present a conceptual model for perceiving and managing dyspnoea, outline pharmacological and non-pharmacological strategies, and summarize key considerations for clinicians, patients, and their families to
manage this debilitating symptom. In spite of the frequency and severity of dyspnoea,
sparse information exists on symptom management in a supportive model of HF care.
However, from experience obtained in other clinical conditions, interventions such as
self-management techniques and the prescribing of anxiolytic and opiate medications
can be expected to reduce the symptomatic burden of dyspnoea in addition to
HF-specific treatments.[2,3] A supportive approach to care in HF requires a change as the
disease progresses from a focus on one of prolongation of life to symptom management
and promotion of quality of life.[1] A useful but limited armamentarium is available for
the clinician to treat dyspnoea in HF. In spite of the burden and prevalence of dyspnoea,
the pathophysiological processes remain poorly understood, not just in HF but across a
range of conditions. As the reader works through this chapter it is important to consider
recommendations within the paradigm of supportive care. Supportive care involves
recognizing and caring for the side-effects of active therapies, patients' co-morbidities,
psychological, social, and spiritual concerns, as well as addressing family needs.[4]

In this chapter we aim to: (1) describe the physiological basis of dyspnoea; (2) discuss a
conceptual model for the patient's perception and management of dyspnoea; (3) outline
useful pharmacological and non-pharmacological strategies; and (4) summarize key
considerations for patients, their families, and clinicians to manage this complex symptom.
Dyspnoea (breathlessness) is defined as the sensation and/or perception of shortness of
breath. Breathlessness impacts upon the individual's quality of life by reducing the ability
of the person to sustain their normal activities. This limitation can range from dyspnoea on
exertion [New York Heart Association (NYHA) Class II], which is mildly troublesome,
through to being breathless at rest (NYHA Class IV), which is severely debilitating.

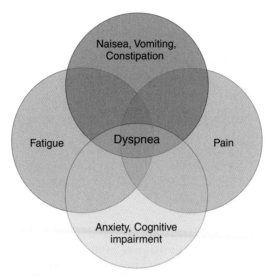

Fig. 9.1 Interrelationship of symptoms with dyspnoea.

Dyspnoea and fatigue are the most common reasons given by patients with HF for limiting their activities.[5] Symptoms rarely occur alone, but tend to cluster. In particular, the sensation and manifestation of dyspnoea is closely linked with other symptoms, such as fatigue and anxiety, as illustrated in Fig. 9.1. These symptoms are interrelated and impact upon each other. For example constipation can cause distress, nausea, and bloating. These symptoms can increase both physiological and psychological distress and worsen the sensation of dyspnoea. Therefore the management plan for dyspnoea should not be a unifocal approach but rather a multifaceted approach taking into account the interaction and influence of co-morbid conditions, additional symptom burden, and concomitant therapeutic approaches. Given the complexity of this interaction the information in this chapter should not be considered in isolation but within the context of other chapters in this book.

What is dyspnoea?

Dyspnoea is the sensation and/or perception of shortness of breath and is one of the most burdensome symptoms for people with HF.[6,7] Dyspnoea may reflect deconditioning of cardiac or pulmonary disease and in many instances a combination of both.[8,9] It is noteworthy that patients with HF report dyspnoea with similar frequency and intensity as those with chronic obstructive pulmonary disease (COPD).[10] The importance of this symptom in HF management is illustrated by the NYHA, one of the most common systems of classification of functional class which is based upon the impact of the sensation of dyspnoea on the activities of daily living.[11] Although it is often assumed that an increase in the sensation of dyspnoea is related to an increase in physical activity, people with both advanced cardiovascular and pulmonary disease find that the experience of dyspnoea can occur with no or limited activity.[7] It is of particular significance that the symptom of dyspnoea has both a physiological and psychological dimension and is mediated by numerous pathophysiological mechanisms as well as environmental, cognitive, behavioural, psychological, and spiritual aspects.[7] Pressure and volume overload as well as activation of neurohormonal and inflammatory pathways can impact upon the myocardial substrate which affects the processes that cause dyspnoea.[3,7,12,13] It is increasingly recognized that HF is a diverse and heterogeneous clinical condition that is characterized by a range of co-morbid conditions all of which increase the complexity of clinical management.[14] It is often important to differentiate breathlessness in HF from other causes of dyspnoea, such as asthma, COPD, and also deconditioning.[15] Health-care professionals should understand that studies in both people with normal and abnormal physical function have identified that manifestation of the symptom can affect the perception of the intensity of the symptom.[16] As many people with HF have experienced the terrifying and suffocating sensation associated with acute pulmonary oedema,[17] it is hardly surprising that dyspnoea continues to be a troublesome, distressing, and dreaded manifestation of HF across the illness trajectory.

Pathophysiology of dyspnoea

While the exact mechanisms of dyspnoea are not fully understood, it is likely that more then one mechanism is involved.[13,18] Research has shown that the qualitative descriptors used by dyspnoeic patients can correlate with the underlying disease and physiological mechanism.[19,20] The terms used to describe dyspnoea can provide the first clue for the clinician about possible causes of the sensation. In HF some common terms used by patients to describe their dyspnoea include 'shortness of breath', 'gasping', and 'cannot get enough air'.[10] Whilst these terms are a useful starting place for understanding the mechanism behind the sensation, due to the multidimensional nature of the sensation, the same terms may be used to describe a range of pathophysiological and adaptive processes.

A common misconception is that the perception of dyspnoea in HF is purely related to fluid overload. Table 9.1 summarizes a variety of pathophysiological factors that may contribute to the symptom of dyspnoea in HF and these processes are discussed briefly below.

Chemoreceptor activation

Located in the carotid and aortic bodies, peripheral chemoreceptors respond to changes in arterial oxygen and carbon dioxide levels. Central chemoreceptors are located in the medulla and respond to changes in carbon dioxide and arterial pH.[21] Whilst the precise physiological mechanism is unclear, hypercapnia is thought to mediate dyspnoea through changes in pH at central chemoreceptors which respond to changes in PCO_2 and acidity.[18] Hypercapnia has been shown to have an independent effect on dyspnoea, though it may not be the sole cause.[18] Hypoxia, which may have an indirect effect on dyspnoea by altering nerve discharge in the cerebral cortex, results in respiratory muscle

Table 9.1 Summary of factors responsible for dyspnoea in heart failure

Factor	Impact
Respiratory	Increased lung stiffness
	Increased dead space due to tachypnoea
	Increased physiological dead space due to diminished apical ventilation
	Ventilation perfusion mismatch
	Impairment of ventilation, through diaphragmatic splinting, due to hepatic congestion and ascites
	Increased work of breathing
	J receptors are nerve endings of C-fibres located on the alveolar wall
Central chemoreceptors	Chemoreceptors respond to changes in carbon dioxide and arterial pH
Muscle changes	Skeletal muscle wasting
Psychological and social	Fear and anxiety
	Compliance and adherence
Myocardial	Ischaemia

weakness and thus an increased sense of respiratory effort.[18] Respiratory muscle fatigue has also been documented during exercise in HF patients and is thought to contribute to dyspnoea in these patients.[22,23]

Mechanoreceptors

Multiple receptors that contribute to the sensation of breathlessness are found throughout the airways.[21]

Upper airway receptors

The intensity of dyspnoea can decrease by sitting in front of a window or fan, suggesting that sensory receptors in the distribution of the trigeminal nerve can influence the intensity of dyspnoea. In some COPD patients, breathing cold air increases exercise tolerance, though the mechanisms are unclear.

Lung receptors

Pulmonary stretch receptors respond to lung inflation and therefore participate in termination of inspiration. Irritant receptors respond to chemical and mechanical stimuli to mediate bronchoconstriction. Dynamic airway compression can cause dyspnoea due to mechanical distortion of airways during exhalation. Pursed lipped breathing can redistribute transmural pressures along the airway reducing compression and therefore dyspnoea. Afferent information from the lung is transmitted via the vagus nerve, and stimulation of vagal irritant receptors increases the sensation of dyspnoea and chest tightness, though stimulation of pulmonary stretch receptors may decrease the sensation of dyspnoea.

Chest wall receptors

Mechanoreceptors are present in the joints, tendons, and muscles of the chest wall, contributing to proprioception and kinaesthesia. Muscle spindles in the intercostal muscles contribute to the sense of dyspnoea by sensing chest wall expansion.[7] The application of a physiotherapeutic vibrator over the parasternal intercostals muscles can reduce dyspnoeic sensations.[7,18]

Afferent mismatch

A change in lung volume is thought to precipitate dyspnoea when there is an afferent mismatch caused by a disparity between the length and tension of the respiratory muscles. The disparity causes a displacement between the spindles in the intercostal muscles which are responsible for the transmission of the afferent signal. This change causes a conscious awareness of the rate and depth of breathing.[7,18] Given a certain set of conditions, if a deviation from the 'expected' respiration pattern occurs, dyspnoea results. For example, such a deviation may include a mismatch between minute ventilation and end-tidal carbon dioxide.

The activation of neural pathways is one of the most common hypotheses for the sensation of dyspnoea. J-receptors are nerve endings of C-fibres located on the alveolar wall that respond to increased interstitial congestion.[13,18] When stimulated, these receptors cause a rapid, shallow breathing pattern.[18] It is possible that stimulation of these receptors may be a cause of dyspnoeic sensations in HF.[13,24]

Impaired sense of effort/increased motor command

The ability of the lungs to change in response to increased pressure is diminished in HF due to increased lung stiffness.[25] Greater strain is placed on the respiratory muscles which must increase the negative pressure required to expand the lungs thereby increasing the sense of effort.[25] Sense of effort refers to an increased degree of motor neurosignalling where patients become consciously aware of the outgoing motor command. This is distinct from the sensation directly associated with changes to muscle length or tension. The 'sense' of effort is due to a corollary discharge sent from the motor to the sensory cortex and can be relieved by muscle training.[18] The normal physiological response of the heart to muscle respiratory fatigue is to increase cardiac output by increasing stroke volume rather then heart rate.[25] However, the ability to increase stroke volume with HF is greatly diminished and therefore an early onset of tachycardia occurs, causing fatigue earlier and probably contributing to diminished exercise capacity.[25] Regardless of the cause, dyspnoea can be a disabling symptom and is a key symptom of HF of all aetiologies. This reflects the complex interplay between physiological factors, such as ventricular dilatation, the status of the alveolar capillary membrane, and neurohormonal activation.

Dyspnoea is a common and troublesome symptom in HF

Dyspnoea is a recurrent symptom in the HF trajectory from diagnosis to death and is estimated to affect up to 90% of patients.[26] Although fatigue, dyspnoea, and peripheral oedema are typical symptoms and signs of HF, there is a poor relationship between symptoms and the severity of HF. Equally there is not always a close correlation between symptoms and prognosis.

An important observation in determining management strategies is that patients may experience severe dyspnoeic episodes without documented hypoxia or hypercapnia.[3,12] Dyspnoea is a common and defining symptom in HF in patients with both preserved and impaired systolic function. Dyspnoea is a trigger to alert the patient and clinician that something is 'not right'. Dyspnoea is commonly a driver for patients to seek medical care and a frequent reason for rehospitalization, reflecting poor symptom control.[16] The sensation of dyspnoea is a common feeling for the HF patient, although individual perceptions and responses may vary. The patient's severity of dyspnoea depends both on the level of physiological disturbance and the patient's self-management strategies. The sensation of dyspnoea can be as minor as the marker of a 'bad day' through to the intense suffocating sensation of impending doom associated with a life-threatening episode of pulmonary oedema. Equally, symptom responses can vary between some individuals who have developed effective self-management strategies in response to increased dyspnoea or at the other extreme where the sensation of dyspnoea can introduce fear and panic. It is important to consider that no matter how effective self-management strategies are, if the physiological disturbance is severe enough or symptom management is inadequate, patients will experience dyspnoea. As HF advances dyspnoea therapy should be tailored to improve the patient's subjective sensation rather than to amend physiological anomalies. Yet it is important to remember that drugs, such as β-blockers, commonly associated with mortality benefits, are also pivotal in achieving symptom management.

Barriers to effective dyspnoea management

It is important to appreciate that key management strategies, such as neurohormonal blockade, play an important role across the HF trajectory. Understanding the ranges of physiological and psychological responses is critical to being able to minimize the distress associated with dyspnoea and applying effective management strategies.

As described above, in spite of the prevalence of this troubling symptom, the causal mechanisms of dyspnoea are still not fully understood and there has been little research on how to manage this symptom in people with HF. Most information available to clinicians is derived from other clinical conditions and/or clinical trials in stable populations.[13] In particular, dyspnoea research is made difficult by the subjectivity of the symptom, the heterogeneity of patient populations, and the complex interplay between physiological and psychological responses that can influence the sensation and manifestation of dyspnoea. These challenges notwithstanding, dyspnoea is a fertile area for further research as we face a global epidemic of chronic conditions that are likely to be accompanied by dyspnoea.

Importantly, the successful management of dyspnoea depends upon a comprehensive assessment and diagnostic approach (Fig. 9.2). Taking a comprehensive clinical history and assessment will help the clinician determine whether the manifestation or exacerbation of dyspnoea is due to factors such as disease progression and/or treatment failure, an intercurrent problem such as infection, or issues related to treatment adherence, poor social support, and functional decline.[27] A range of problems associated with HF, such as anaemia and atrial fibrillation, can worsen the sensation of dyspnoea. Factors including the introduction of medications such as non-steroidal anti-inflammatory agents can precipitate HF decompensation and subsequent dyspnoea. Anaemia has been documented to be present in 10–60% of patients with advanced HF. This occurs due to factors such as disruption to erythropoietin function, dietary inadequacies, and haemodilution. These factors can cause fatigue and a decrease in exercise tolerance, worsening the sensation of dyspnoea.[28] It is notable that many of these factors can be readily treated and decrease symptom burden.

As HF progresses pleural effusions may develop due to changes in both plasma and hydrostatic oncotic pressure.[29] It is mandatory that an astute clinical assessment is

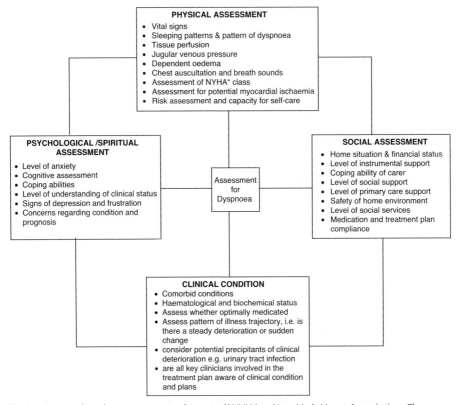

Fig. 9.2 Comprehensive assessment schemata (*NYHA = New York Heart Association Class: Kossman CE (ed.) (1964). *Diseases of the Heart and Blood Vessels; Nomenclature and Criteria for Diagnosis*, 6th edn, p. 112. Boston: Little Brown). Figure modified from Davidson *et al.*[65]

undertaken, together with clarification of the goals of treatment, as this will determine the management strategy for the HF patient. We recommend a 10-step plan that may be of use to clinicians in developing a management plan and this is detailed in Fig. 9.3. In undertaking this assessment, it is also important for clinicians to consider the frequency of problems such as cognitive difficulties and metabolic changes among older people, which can increase the difficulty of assessment, diagnosis, and management.[30] The high rate of HF in the elderly underscores the need for a complex cardiogeriatric assessment approach, rather than one focused entirely on the cardiorespiratory system (see also Chapter 17).[31]

Sleep-disordered breathing occurs commonly in people with HF, with at least 50% of people with HF having either central sleep apnoea or obstructive sleep apnoea (see also Chapter 10).[32] Central sleep apnoea results from a reduction in the central respiratory drive. It is known that the presence of central sleep apnoea is associated with higher mortality, but it is not known whether higher mortality is the result of poor myocardial contractility or if sleep apnoea independently contributes to mortality.

Obstructive sleep apnoea occurs as a result of an obstruction causing a narrowing of the pharynx.[32] This narrowing is usually associated with obesity, with a layer of fatty tissue next to the pharynx narrowing the lumen. Obstructive sleep apnoea usually

---

10 Step approach for assessment and management approach to dyspnea

Step 1: Undertake a comprehensive clinical assessment and appraisal of psychological, social and spiritual issues

Step 2: Clarify the goals of treatment and the wishes of patient and family

Step 3: Determine the place of clinical care and related health professional competencies

Step 4: Appraise the previous experiences of dyspnoea and level of psychosocial supports

Step 5: Address reversible causes such as anaemia, ischaemia and arrhythmia

Step 6: Carefully weight the risks and benefits of treatment and management approaches

Step 7: Adopt a risk management approach to avoid iatrogenesis and avoidable adverse events

Step 8: Develop an action plan anticipating deterioration and crisis aversion

Step 9: Regularly appraise the goals of treatment and efficacy and modify plans accordingly

Step 10: Ensure communication with all members of the health team, patients and family members.

Fig. 9.3 Ten-step scheme for developing a dyspnoea management plan.

produces snoring and repeated oxygen desaturation resulting in a range of physiological responses including mechanical, haemodynamic, chemical, neural, and inflammatory responses. Oedema and increased pulmonary pressures can aggravate this sensation.

The physiological consequences of sleep-disordered breathing are paroxysmal nocturnal arousal and excessive daytime sleepiness.[33,34] It would appear that improving cardiac output should be a major goal of clinicians in managing sleep-disordered breathing in the setting of HF.[35] Continuous positive airway pressure (CPAP) can relieve the perception of dyspnoea and fatigue as well as improving haemodynamics. The link between sleepiness and cognitive dysfunction in HF is increasingly being established.[36,37]

Diagnosis and physical assessment of dyspnoea and HF

Diagnostic testing can be used in HF to: (1) confirm the clinical diagnosis; (2) identify a cause and/or exacerbating factors; and (3) provide an empirical baseline to guide therapy and monitor the severity and disease progression. A range of both invasive and non-invasive therapies is available to assess cardiac function.[38,39] The echocardiogram is the key investigation for confirming the diagnosis of HF, determining its pathophysiological basis and likely cause. The echocardiogram provides important information about left- and right-ventricular systolic function, integrity of the pericardium, regional wall motion function as well as valvular structure and function.[38,40,41] As dyspnoea may be a manifestation of ischaemia this should be considered in a diagnostic work-up. Nuclear imaging is also useful in providing information about the presence of inducible ischaemia, as well as the extent of viable myocardium.[42] A coronary angiogram may be considered in the patient with regional wall motion anomalies to assess for the presence of potentially obstructive coronary artery disease. The type and nature of diagnostic tests needs to be considered carefully within a context of risks and benefits, particularly in the advanced stages of HF. HF is often associated with a range of co-morbid conditions, such as COPD and renal dysfunction, and an assessment of these co-morbid conditions needs to be considered in the diagnosis and management of HF and the impact on the sensation and management of dyspnoea. It is often necessary to differentiate whether the primary cause of dyspnoea is related to pulmonary or cardiac disease. The use of respiratory function tests such as spirometry may be useful.

In the dynamic and labile status of the HF trajectory it is important to consider that management of complications and exacerbating factors may improve the perception of dyspnoea and decrease symptom burden. For example, treating an undetected urinary tract infection in an elderly person can improve the patient's dyspnoea.[43] Table 9.2 provides a summary of diagnostic tests and rationale for assessment. Although measurement of plasma B-type natriuretic peptides (BNP) shows promise for diagnosing HF and monitoring therapy and determining prognosis, its role in the assessment and treatment paradigm is evolving. It is important to recognize that factors such as body mass index, age, gender, and renal function need to be considered in the interpretation of an individual result.[44]

Table 9.2 Diagnostic and assessment tests in the supportive care of HF management

Investigation	Rationale and utility
Electrocardiogram (ECG)	A comparison with previous ECGs may reveal new ST segment changes which may be indicative of ischaemia
	New onset atrial fibrillation can precipitate breathlessness. Strategies to improve rate control can improve symptom perception
Chest X-ray	Interstitial oedema may be present, particularly in the peri-hilar region suggesting the need for increased diuresis
	Pleural effusions obscuring the costo-phrenic angles
	Kerley B lines, indicative of lymphatic oedema due to raised left atrial pressure are indicative of fluid overload
Biochemistry	Renal function often declines as HF progresses, with a rise in serum creatinine and urea. Adjustment of diuretics and ACE inhibitors may be necessary
	Dilutional hyponatraemia, exacerbated by high-dose diuretic therapy which can be treated by free water restriction
	Hyperkalaemia in the presence of impaired renal function or as a result of the use of potassium-retaining diuretics or ACE inhibitors
	Hypokalaemia is more common and is often secondary to diuretic therapy (both thiazide and loop diuretics) and responds to dietary changes and supplementation
	Serum magnesium levels may be reduced due to the effects of diuretic therapy. Magnesium replacement to normal levels reduces ectopy and helps normalize potassium levels
	Hypoalbuminaemia may reflect markers of impaired albumin synthesis, cardiac cachexia, and is a marker of adverse prognosis
	Thyroid function should be assessed, particularly in the elderly
Haematology	Anaemia is often present and may worsen as the severity of HF progresses
	Severe anaemia, in itself, may worsen dyspnoea and can be treated
	The erythrocyte sedimentation rate may be elevated due to the presence of infection
Urinalysis	Proteinuria is common and is a marker of worsening condition and/or urinary tract infection
	Leukocytes are suggestive of urinary tract infection
Respiratory function setting	Spirometry—the forced expiratory volume (FEV_1) is often reduced
	The gas transfer will be reduced in moderate HF, generally as low as 50% of predicted function
	Sleep tests may be indicated particularly if the patient is likely to be compliant with therapy.
Natriuretic peptides	Atrial natriuretic peptides (ANP) and B-type natriuretic peptides (BNP) relate to the severity of HF, risk of hospitalization, and survival
	A BNP level of >200 pg ml^{-1} is highly sensitive and specific for the presence or absence of left-ventricular dysfunction determined by echocardiography and for differentiating HF from respiratory diseases
Functional evaluation	The 6-min walk test is a simple, safe, and non-invasive measure of the distance covered in consecutive 25-m laps, over a 6-min period

Following an initial diagnosis of HF and confirmation of aetiological factors, diagnostic tests in HF management should be undertaken within a context of 'manage what you measure'. Particularly in end-stage HF, diagnostic tests should only be undertaken on the basis of 'intention to treat' rather than 'nice to know'. This approach not only minimizes patient burden but is also fiscally responsible. In end-stage HF it is anticipated and highly probable that there will be biochemical and physiological dysfunction. For example, as the patient deteriorates and requires increased diuretics it is inevitable that renal function will decline and azotaemia is highly indicative of imminent death.[45]

The importance of physical assessment

It is well recognized that effective clinical assessment is critical in HF management.[46] Figure 9.3 outlines a schema that may assist in the assessment and management of dyspnoea. Grady et al.[26] have developed a model for haemodynamic assessment that can be useful in guiding therapeutic interventions in the context of the presence and absence of congestion.

In HF management the physical examination is important to monitor symptom status and therapeutic interventions. Assessment of jugular venous pressure and chest auscultation are important to identify fluid overload. Crepitations may be heard in the bases of the lung fields, and the rate and depth of breathing as well as the presence or absence of cough or expectorant needs to be assessed. Pleural effusions can be identified on the basis of decreased lung sounds and dull percussion. Intercurrent chest infections require prompt treatment. As HF advances or in times of decompensation, patients may be tachypnoeic at rest and need to sit in an upright position to obtain symptomatic relief. The draining of pleural effusions may provide benefit in very symptomatic cases.[47] However, the management of pleural effusions is usually more effectively managed by treating the underlying HF. In people with HF, sleeping patterns may be disrupted by orthopnoea. This disruption to sleep can have an adverse impact on quality of life. Assessment of the jugular venous pressure is important in the prescription of diuretics.[26] In left-ventricular dilatation, the apex beat will be displaced laterally and a third heart sound is typically heard in more advanced left-ventricular dysfunction or during periods of symptomatic decompensation. In advanced HF, liver engorgement may result in the liver being palpable below the costal margin. This enlargement may cause discomfort to the patient due to stretching of the liver capsule. Fluid retention is a key problem in HF and may manifest as peripheral oedema, especially in dependent areas such as the ankles and, in recumbent patients, the sacral area. Ascites may also occur and be a source of discomfort and pain for the patient. The patient's level of consciousness and cognition should also be assessed.

A conceptual framework to guide treatment and management decisions

Prior to discussing management strategy, and in view of the complexity of the aetiology and manifestation of dyspnoea discussed above, it is useful to have a conceptual framework to inform interventions in symptom management. Carrieri-Kohlman and Stulbarg[50] have developed a model in which antecedent personal illness and situational factors are seen to influence therapeutic strategies. Notably, this model explains the impact of the individual's reaction and capacity to cope with the sensation of dyspnoea. Although primarily developed for people with chronic respiratory disease the model demonstrates some utility in management of dyspnoea in people with HF. McCord and Cronin-Stubbs[49] have identified a framework for consideration of dyspnoea which we consider to be useful in planning the management of dyspnoea. Key elements of this model are *antecedents* (physiological and psychological events or stimuli preceding the manifestation of dyspnoea); *mediators* (characteristics of individuals or the environment influencing the response to dyspnoea and outcome); *reactions* to the perceived sensation of dyspnoea; and *outcomes* that result once the individual has reacted to a stimulus. This model, as illustrated in Fig. 9.4, allows for interventions in the antecedent, mediator, and reaction responses to the dyspnoea sensation. It is likely that unless each of these aspects is addressed, significant symptom burden will persist. As a consequence multifaceted interventions addressing each of these dimensions are likely to be the most successful.

Monitoring the dyspnoea sensation

Monitoring dyspnoea is important for the clinician to be able to track the severity and intensity of symptoms to inform management strategies. The subjective experience of breathlessness makes communication of intensity and severity difficult. Further, the conceptual model in Fig. 9.4 and the assessment methods outlined in Fig. 9.3 and described above indicate that the impact of dyspnoea is a complex, multifaceted phenomenon. Empirical measures, of both a discriminative and evaluative function, are available to assist clinicians, although their application can be problematic. A number of questionnaires can also assess the multidimensional impact of dyspnoea.[50] Although valuable, the use of psychometric measurements in the advanced stages of illness can be problematic due to responder burden. A range of validated assessments are available such as the Baseline Dyspnoea Transitional Dyspnoea Index (BDI/TDI) and the Modified Borg Questionnaire which can assist with patient management when these are not overly burdensome. Of note, the visual analogue scale (VAS) has demonstrated significant utility not only for its simplicity but also its reliability and validity.[51] The VAS is a continuous scale of 100 mm on either a horizontal or vertical axis. Descriptors such as *no breathlessness* or *greatest breathlessness* are anchors at each end of the continuum. It is useful for the clinician, patient, and family members to each have reference points and anchors and, importantly, 'speak the same language'. Implementing the use of the VAS early in the HF trajectory can assist in teaching the patient to self-assess their level of dyspnoea. People can then point to a place on a ruler. Benchmarking dyspnoea against a predetermined common activity such as walking to the corner or bathing/showering can also help the clinician to assess treatment efficacy as well as help

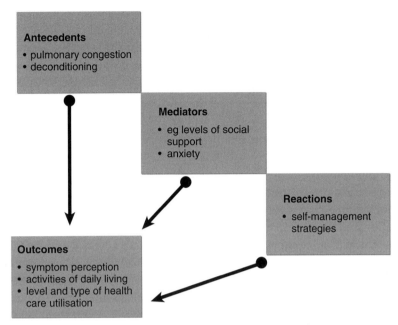

Fig. 9.4 Conceptual model to inform dyspnoea management interventions.

the patient to monitor symptoms. Evaluating the patient's sleeping patterns is another useful approach to explore the clinical status. Asking the patient: 'How have you been sleeping?' can alert the clinician to a range of factors from orthopnoea to fear and anxiety.

Management of dyspnoea in HF

The dyspnoea management strategy is as complex and multifaceted as the pathophysiology described above. Beyond core HF therapies[37,38] much of the information we have to manage dyspnoea, particularly in end-stage disease, is derived from people with malignant and respiratory diseases as well as expert opinion. In spite of this sparse evidence base it is clear that a unimodal treatment path is not sufficient but rather a combination of pharmacological and non-pharmacological strategies is required. The management of dyspnoea is a fundamental element of supportive care and should be tailored to the individual's co-morbidities, psychological, social, and spiritual concerns, as well as addressing family needs

Management of dyspnoea across the HF trajectory

A range of strategies can assist the person with HF in diminishing the sensation of dyspnoea. Assessment for reversible causes such as ischaemia and anaemia are important as well as implementation of a disease management approach to care.[52]

Evidence-based pharmacotherapy should be the platform for reducing symptoms. Non-pharmacological strategies, including exercise therapy, dietary sodium and fluid restrictions, can also assist in diminishing the sensation of dyspnoea. A number of randomized controlled clinical trials have demonstrated physiological benefits of exercise, at least in the short term.[53] Exercise therapy can also promote an individual's sense of control and can also relieve the sensation of anxiety. In spite of the limited evidence base for non-pharmacological strategies, these are important consideration in HF management. Clearly, the coordination of these therapies in a coordinated disease management strategy underpinned by a supportive care philosophy can improve patient outcomes.[54] Some of these treatment strategies are expanded on below.

Oxygen therapy in the supportive management of dyspnoea in HF

The use of oxygen therapy to manage dyspnoea in HF is controversial, and the absence of evidence prohibits access to this therapy in spite of anecdotal evidence of benefit. An appraisal of the evidence clearly indicates a state of equipoise. The reported benefits of oxygen therapy may relate to promoting a sense of control in the management of dyspnoea and/or the stimulation of facial nerve fibres. The potential benefit of oxygen administration to patients with HF is currently being examined in randomized controlled clinical trials.[55] Currently, supplemental oxygen is indicated when it can be shown that the patient's disability is related to arterial hypoxaemia which can be reversed by oxygen administration. Home oxygen relieves dyspnoea and adds to the comfort and quality of life of patients in whom reversible hypoxaemia is the cause of discomfort. The objective is to provide a resting PaO_2 of 60 mmHg using the lowest flow rate that will achieve this, usually at 2 L min^{-1}. When indicated, the flow rate should be increased by 1 L min^{-1} during exercise and during sleep to maintain an oxygen saturation of 90%. In the home setting, safety issues such as the importance of avoiding combustion due to exposure to naked flames needs to be stressed to patients and their families. In particular it should be stressed that people should not smoke in the vicinity of the oxygen supply.

The use of oxygen may reverse hypoxia and allow increased activity. As there may be a significant placebo response with administration of oxygen, it is important to determine whether the patient requires oxygen continuously or only during exacerbations of their symptoms. In some instances portable oxygen cylinders may be considered to promote and maintain physical and social activities. It is important to consider that the prescription of long-term oxygen without demonstrated hypoxaemia may render the patient unnecessarily immobile, leading to further functional decline. The potential for carbon dioxide retention in some patients who may be dependent on hypoxia to drive respiration should also be considered. Even in this group of patients, low-flow oxygen (<3 L min^{-1}) via a controlled mask at 28% oxygen can be administered with close supervision.[56] Generally nasal cannulae are preferred to masks as they allow the patient to converse and eat while still receiving therapy. Importantly, in patients with HF, nasal administration avoids drying of the mucous membranes and stimulation of thirst. As outlined above, in spite of the reports of the beneficial effects of oxygen therapy in HF, and its frequent use, there is limited clinical trial evidence to support its use. Clearly there is an urgent need for systematic evaluation in randomized controlled trials, particularly given the significant placebo response to oxygen therapy.[57]

Psychological and social aspects in dyspnoea management

Undeniably, psychological responses have a significant impact on the manifestation of dyspnoea. Some important considerations relate to management of this dimension. Firstly, it is very important to understand prior experiences of dyspnoea. Strategies to promote control of circumstances for both the patient and their family can be effective. Carrieri-Kohlman and colleagues[58] have developed techniques for desensitization and guided mastery in patients with COPD which may be useful. In this technique teaching strategies to manage dyspnoea can increase the sense of self-efficacy and control. This increased sense of control and minimization of anxiety may dampen the perception of intensity of dyspnoea.[58] Therefore negotiation of an action plan, incorporating strategies such as breathing exercises and relaxation, can promote a sense of control over the dyspnoea sensation for patients and their families. Other strategies, such as access to a clinician who is readily contactable, can also alleviate anxiety and prevent escalation of the sympathetic response which can be deleterious in escalating myocardial oxygen demand. It is often difficult to differentiate psychological symptoms that have pathological sequelae from those that are purely reactive and responsive. A careful clinical history can provide evidence of a history of depression and anxiety. Assessment using validated instruments early in the illness trajectory can provide important baseline data to anticipate future problems (see also Chapter 15).

The role of social support in influencing the outcomes of people with HF is well described and it is in the advanced stages of the disease when this is of increased importance. Social isolation is a predictor of adverse outcome, and as the patient's condition worsens and their need for assistance with daily living increases, mobilization of additional social services and home help needs to be considered.[59] If the patient wishes to die at home, the coordination of community and family resources is often complex. At this time it is often family members who require considerable support and strategies to manage the care of their family member. Effective dyspnoea management minimizes distress equally to the patient and their family. With the assistance of community-based palliative care teams, family members can be instructed on the administration of subcutaneous morphine and/or scopolamine in times of emergency. Recommendations on these strategies are often dependent on local protocols and procedures.

Pharmacological management

The pharmacological management of HF focuses on treating the adverse impact of neuro-hormonal activation. β-Blockers, angiotensin-converting enzyme (ACE) inhibitors, angiotensin receptor blockers, and spironolactone are key therapies. Whilst the optimal doses of these agents is well documented,[60,61] dyspnoea can still persist in spite of optimal pharmacotherapy. Adjuvant therapies such as nitrates, diuretics, and digoxin are used to achieve symptomatic benefit. It is important to remember that as well as improving mortality, pharmaceutical agents such as ACE inhibitors and β-blockers significantly improve symptoms and reduce the frequency of hospitalization for HF exacerbations. Therefore these drugs should only be withdrawn in the context of adverse side-effects and/or difficulties in swallowing at the end of life. It is important for clinicians to remember that overall these drugs are well tolerated in all stages of HF (see also Chapter 4).[61,62]

As a consequence we recommend a layered and additive approach to dyspnoea management in HF, where the foundation is evidence-based therapies. This is illustrated in Fig. 9.5. This foundation should be built upon using adjunctive therapies. Figure 9.5 illustrates the complexity of this management regimen and illustrates the complexity of a supportive approach to HF management. As HF progresses and co-morbid conditions worsen, particularly renal dysfunction, pharmacotherapy can become increasing complex. The following pharmacological strategies targeting dyspnoea management are based

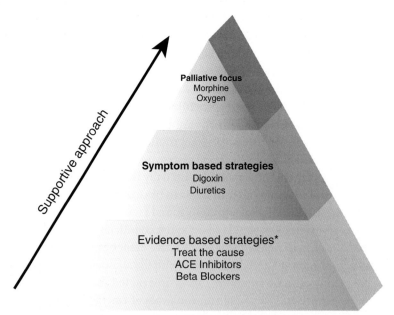

Fig. 9.5 Layered approach to HF management. (*American College of Cardiology/American Heart Association 2005 Guideline Update for the Diagnosis and Management of Chronic Heart Failure in the Adult (http://www.americanheart.org/); European Society of Cardiology Chronic Heart Failure Guidelines (http://www.escardio.org/); National Heart Foundation/Cardiac Society of Australia and New Zealand Guidelines on the Contemporary Management of the Patient with Chronic Heart Failure in Australia (http://www.heartfoundation.org.au/).)

upon the assumption that reversible causes of dyspnoea have been assessed and medical therapy for HF has been optimized or intolerance demonstrated.

Diuretic therapy in HF

In spite of the paucity of clinical trial evidence supporting their use, diuretics remain an important strategy for managing the burden of congestion. Within the context of diuretic requirements it is also important to emphasize the importance of fluid and salt restriction. Strategies such the use of ice chips infused with lemon juice and fresh mint can assist in maintaining moist mucous membranes and eliminating thirst. Vigilant mouth care should also be undertaken if the patient is unable to take care of activities of daily living. Achieving euvolaemia is an important strategy in the management of HF. There are minimal data to support diuretic use other than for symptomatically treating fluid retention. The absence of data supporting therapy and the potential for adverse reactions underscores the importance of judicious use. Excessive diuresis should be avoided because hypovolaemia may reduce cardiac output, impair renal function, and cause electrolyte disturbances that precipitate arrhythmias, exacerbate neurohormonal activation, and, importantly, adversely impact quality of life by producing weakness, lethargy, and postural symptoms.[63]

As discussed above, there are multiple contributors to the symptom of dyspnoea apart from fluid congestion, and so titrating with diuretics to a symptom target is problematic. The use of flexible diuretic regimens where dosages are titrated in response to fluid retention is more effective. If the patient's fluid decreases the diuretic dose may need to be decreased. Figure 9.6 provides some guidelines for titrating diuretic therapy. In patients

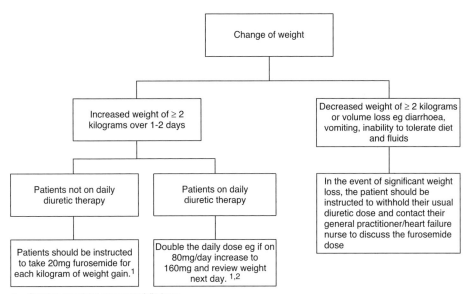

1. Only if no associated symptoms of dizziness.
2. Additional potassium replacement needs to be on an individualised basis with consideration of renal function and concomitant medications.

Fig. 9.6 Guidelines for titrating diuretic therapy.

with HF treated with a loop diuretic, blockade of sodium reabsorption is thought to occur at different sites in the nephron in response to stimulation of proximal and distal tubular sodium reabsorption. Diuretic resistance is defined as a clinical state in which diuretic response is diminished or lost before the therapeutic goal of relief from oedema has been reached. Common causes of diuretic resistance include: renal dysfunction, compensatory mechanisms to restore arterial blood volume, hyponatraemia, and altered diuretic pharmacokinetics. Strategies to overcome diuretic resistance include: sodium and fluid restriction, ensuring optimal pharmacotherapy (in particular ACE inhibitors), and alteration in route and timing, and combination of diuretic agents. Intravenous diuretic therapy, including infusions, may overcome issues of bioavailability and intestinal oedema.[63] If the daily dose of frusemide exceeds 160 mg, the addition of another diuretic at another site of action of the nephron may be useful. The addition of hydrochlorthiazide (25 mg), metolazone (2.5 mg), or acetazolamide (250 mg) may be effective in reducing oedematous symptoms.

Resistance to oral therapy results in interstitial salt and water accumulation. This can occur in the gastrointestinal system impairing absorption. Intravenous administration of a loop diuretic may overcome problems of intestinal absorption. A continuous intravenous infusion of frusemide appears to achieve greater diuresis and natriuresis than intermittent intravenous doses. Continuous infusion prevents a rebound in post-diuretic sodium reabsorption, thereby maximizing diuretic efficacy. Further, frusemide administered as an infusion causes fewer ototoxic effects than bolus injections. It is important to consider that the route of administration needs to be accommodated to the person's choice for place of care and available resources. Diuretics can be administered by subcutaneous and intramuscular routes as well, although there is very little reported evidence for subcutaneous use.[64,65] As doses escalate the potential for electrolyte depletion, especially of potassium, magnesium, as well as thiamine, increases and so monitoring these parameters may be useful. A general principle is to regularly appraise fluid status and diuretic dose and to aim for the lowest possible dose. High doses can exacerbate the sensation of fatigue and dyspnoea.[66] An important strategy in minimizing the use of diuretics is ensuring that the patient monitors fluid and sodium intake.

Novel and contentious HF therapies to improve symptom management

The burden of HF has fuelled research resulting in a range of therapeutic advances, in acute, decompensated, and chronic HF. Many of these advances focus on decreasing symptomatic burden, in particular dyspnoea. In recent times the introduction of agents such as natriuretic peptide infusions (neseritide), ventricular assist devices (VADs), automated implantable cardiac defibrillators (AICDs), cardiac resynchronisation therapy (CRT) ultrafiltration, and novel inotropic agents such as levosimendan have increased the range of treatment options available and potentially the confusion and conflict for many clinicians who strive to do not only the *best* they can but *all* they can for the patient. Findings from many of the clinical trials, with the exception of AICDs and CRT, remain controversial because of conflicting findings and questions remaining regarding dosing and duration of therapy. Treatment allocation of novel therapies should be assessed according to the needs of the patient and potential risks and benefits. Interdisciplinary care, a defining feature of a supportive approach to HF management, can assist individual clinicians in making rational, ethical, and accountable decisions regarding therapy. Further, the range of skills derived from an interdisciplinary approach including physicians, nurses, pharmacists, physiotherapists, occupational therapists, social workers, and pastoral care can increase the range of symptom management options available.

Deterioration in HF leads many clinicians to consider inotropic therapy. To date, most trials of inotropic therapy, with the exception of digoxin and more recently levosimendan, have shown an increase in mortality, albeit in spite of improvements in symptoms. Many of the issues surrounding the use of many of these therapies relate to methodological uses such as choice of endpoints, dosing, and patient selection.[67,68] The discussion of these issues is beyond the scope of this chapter, yet it does underscore the complexity of HF therapy and the importance of assessing the goals and preferences for treatment. However, it is important to note that patients and their families should be informed of the increased risk with many of these treatments.

Anxiety–dyspnoea cycle

Anxiety and sympathetic activation is closely related to the sensation of dyspnoea. Benzodiazepines may be used to relieve the anxiety associated with dyspnoea[3] and are often even more effective with a concomitant behavioural strategy. As with many other conditions, unless the cause is treated the symptom persists. Often having access to someone over the phone and/or systems such as 'vital call' can increase the sense of control for the patients in the home setting. When panic attacks occur it is often difficult to differentiate in the community setting between intense anxiety and potential myocardial ischaemia. Management and treatment of panic attacks is critical not just for the patient's psychological benefit but to also decrease the deleterious increases in myocardial oxygen demand. Cognitive behavioural approaches may be useful in minimizing the anxiety-dyspnoea cycle. Benzodiazepines can also be used to manage panic attacks arising from the anxiety associated with dyspnoea.[3] Lorazepam is often useful as it can be administered sublingually in distressed patients, acts quickly, and is less sedating than other agents such as diazepam.[56]

Opioids

Opioids are an integral part of the management of dyspnoea, in people who are breathless at rest, particularly in the advanced stages and those resistant to other treatment strategies. Opioids have been shown to be useful in increasing patients' exercise tolerance, resulting in a decrease in respiratory effort and a lesser sensation of dyspnoea. Williams et al.[69] conducted a trial of a bolus dose (1–2 mg) of intravenous diamorphine in 16 stable HF patients and produced an improvement in exercise capacity. Another small trial of 10 patients in NYHA Class III/IV using 2.5–5 mg of oral morphine demonstrated an improvement in the sensation of breathlessness.[70] Therapeutic dosages of opioids act by reducing preload, reducing the responsiveness of the dominant respiratory control centre, and decreasing anxiety.[71] The optimum route and dose regime remain unclear but it appears that opioids do improve dyspnoea. Well designed and sufficiently powered randomized controlled trials are required to explore optimal dosing, timing, and tolerability of opioid therapy.

Opioids are able to be administered orally, transdermally, rectally, intravenously, intramuscularly, and subcutaneously. Therefore a range of therapeutic regimens is available. Frequent bolus doses may be more effective than slow-release formulations or continuous infusions.[72] Sadly, many clinicians withhold opioids for fear of causing respiratory depression and excessive drowsiness, denying patients potential benefits. Opioids should be titrated to the level of symptoms and can be used without causing respiratory depression or excessive drowsiness.[73] The therapeutic benefits of opioids can be achieved at doses that do not cause respiratory depression. When introducing any form of pharmacotherapy the risks and benefits have to be carefully weighed up, and in this respect opioids are not different. Clinicians are well aware of the need for the judicious introduction of ACE inhibitors and β-blockers. A similar approach of 'starting low and going slow' is important, as is warning patients and their families about possible deleterious effects. As in most clinical scenarios, confidence comes in the use of the medication and as cardiology clinicians start to use these agents it may be appropriate to consult their palliative care colleagues and pharmacists to assist them in these therapies. Nebulized opioids can also be administered, but in a recent systematic review their efficacy has been questioned and as a result they are not recommended.[74,75] It is important to anticipate potential adverse effects such as constipation and nausea associated with these therapies and to implement prophylactic strategies, such as added dietary fibre or aperients, to minimize patient distress.[73,76] It is useful to know that effects such as increased sedation often pass over time with dose adjustment and increased tolerability. Clinicians should be mindful that some opioids can induce bronchospasm through a mechanism of histamine release, although this is not common.[56] It is also important for the clinician to appreciate that there are a range of opioid agents and preparations, and as in other drug therapies, changing the agent, dose, timing of dosage, and medication route may improve tolerability.

Non-invasive ventilation

CPAP may relieve dyspnoea through decreasing the neuromechanical dissociation of the respiratory drive and counterbalancing the inspiratory load on respiratory muscles and haemodynamic benefits on ventricular remodelling.[6,77] CPAP also decreases left-ventricular afterload by increasing intrathoracic pressure, increasing stroke volume, and reducing cardiac sympathetic activity. CPAP decreases preload by impeding venous return and reducing right- and left-ventricular end-diastolic pressure. The unloading of the inspiratory muscles is possibly the result of increased lung compliance due to redistribution of fluid in the extrathoracic cavity. The Canadian Continuous Positive Airway Pressure for Patients with Central Sleep Apnea and Heart Failure trial randomized 258 patients to either CPAP or no CPAP and followed this group for 2 years. Although this trial has no impact on survival, hospitalization rates, and quality of life improvements were shown in nocturnal oxygenation, ejection fraction, norepinephrine levels, and 6-min walk distances.[78] The use of CPAP has to be weighed against the potential benefit and level of burden for the patient and their family. It is important to consider issues related to treatment adherence in HF and to ensure that masks are appropriately fitted and air flow settings adapted to maximize comfort and tolerance.

Environmental factors

The sensation of dyspnoea can be exacerbated by extremes of temperature, both hot and cold as well as environmental pollution. The humidity associated with peak summer periods can be troublesome to some patients. Of particular concern is pollution of environments by cigarette smoking. Families of people with dyspnoea should be encouraged to provide smoke-free environments.

Positioning and comfort measures

A key strategy to promote comfort and management of dyspnoea is in the positioning of the patient. Sitting the patient up can relieve dyspnoea by increasing vital capacity and reducing abdominal splinting. The inability of the HF patient to lie in the supine position without experiencing dyspnoea is known as orthopnoea. Using extra pillows to sit themselves up whilst asleep often relieves the symptom. Involvement of the patient's family in activities to promote comfort can increase their sense of involvement and promote intimacy with their loved one. Advice on posture, relaxation techniques, and having a flow of air across the face (e.g. from a fan or an open window) may also provide relief of symptoms. The relief provided by such a flow of air is thought to be mediated by activation of inhibitory fibres from facial receptors.[79]

Exercise and promotion of activity

Exercise and physical activity are recommended therapies across the HF trajectory from diagnosis to palliative care. Asthenia and generalized weakness are key characteristics of people with HF. Exercise capacity is limited in HF due to abnormalities in skeletal and respiratory muscle metabolism.[80,81] Cachexia can also be a feature of end-stage HF.[82,83] Impairment of nutritional metabolism can exacerbate muscle dysfunction (cachexia is discussed in detail in Chapter13). Even in the later stages of disease strength training can be effective and decrease symptom burden. Selective respiratory muscle training has been shown to improve the endurance and strength of respiratory muscles, enhancing submaximal and maximal exercise capacity in patients with HF.[84] Strategies to promote exercise reconditioning and improve nutritional status can improve the patient's sense of well-being and also their sense of control. Promotion of optimal nutrition can assist in aiding optimal muscle function and modify the severity of anaemia which affects exercise capacity. Where possible, formal cardiac rehabilitation programmes can be accessed; however, home-based programmes can also be useful for patients (see Chapter 11 for further details).

Fluid and sodium restriction

A range of adverse effects occur from oedematous symptoms in the advanced stages of HF. As well as dyspnoea associated with pulmonary congestion, pedal, sacral, and scrotal oedema associated with fluid overload may cause significant distress and make the patient more vulnerable to pressure sores. Avoiding fluid overload and retention requires careful attention to the fluid balance status. Where possible patients should be weighed daily to monitor fluid status. This may become difficult as the patient becomes more frail and debilitated, although weigh chairs and other technological solutions are becoming more readily available. Where weighing the patient becomes difficult it is then necessary to observe the patient closely for increasing oedema, particularly in dependent areas such as the sacrum.

An important part of the disease management approach to HF management is monitoring fluid balance. Patients and their families often need assistance in the management of fluid restrictions. Evidence-based guidelines recommend restricting total fluid intake to1.5 L day^{-1} and 1 L in severe cases of HF. Patients and their families require tangible examples of volume amounts and need to be informed of hidden sources of sodium, such as in processed foods, and to count fluid volumes in soups, fruits, and desserts. It is also important to make people aware that salt substitutes may substitute potassium for sodium and this may cause hyperkalaemia, particularly within the context of renal impairment.

Complementary and alternative therapies

The use of complementary and alternative treatments, such as massage to decrease anxiety, is increasing, despite the sparse evidence base for such approaches. Emotional responses such as anxiety and anger can precipitate and aggravate dyspnoea and therefore addressing these factors is critical.[85] Although some studies have been undertaken to assess these therapies the widespread recommendation is limited due methodological factors such as small sample sizes. Relaxation and biofeedback techniques have demonstrated some efficacy in breathlessness in COPD and in HF patients. A critical strategy is to address anxiety before it escalates into a situation of panic. Precarious and fragile haemodynamics mean that it is important to address activation of the sympathetic nervous system. Distraction is a useful technique, and the playing of music and getting the patient to watch a movie can be useful. Breathing exercises and meditation strategies such as Buteyko and Pranyama that use diaphragmatic breathing can relieve the sensation of dyspnoea and promote a sense of control.[86,87] Bernardi and colleagues[88] demonstrated in a small study that training using the Ave Maria (in Latin) or a yoga mantra induced favourable psychological responses and in baroreflex sensitivity. It is generally useful to introduce these strategies early in the HF trajectory so that they become part of the self-management technique. As HF progresses and the clinical condition worsens it is difficult to teach these skills as concentration diminishes. Cognitive impairment becomes increasingly evident in HF as the physical condition deteriorates and cardiac output falls. One feature of this cognitive decline is a diminished capacity to learn new tasks. Many patients may choose to try alternative therapies when they feel they have exhausted conventional approaches. Some studies have suggested the benefit of acupuncture.[89,90] Strategies that promote a sense of control are likely to improve the patient's sense of well-being and minimize feelings of hopelessness. It is important that patients and their families feel comfortable in discussing alternative approaches and in disclosing the treatments that they are undertaking. It is also important for clinicians to weigh particular risks and benefits of these naturopathic agents. The potential for deleterious drug interactions with herbs and vitamins increases as metabolic derangements occur in the advanced stages of disease at the end of life.

An important strategy in the management of symptomatic HF is the introduction of energy conservation techniques. As symptoms worsen activities of daily living become increasingly difficult. Taking a shower can be very tiring so implementation of a range of strategies such as sitting in a shower chair and using a towelling robe instead of hand drying with a towel can reduce energy expenditure.[91]

Dyspnoea in advanced HF

A key issue limiting effective symptom management for people with HF requiring supportive care is the failure to appreciate what is meant by the integration of a palliative approach within care planning. For some clinicians, a palliative approach means giving up hope and abandoning usual care. However, a palliative approach refers to care delivered to provide symptom relief, comfort, and support for patients and their families. These key premises are encapsulated in a supportive approach to HF care. For people with HF, pharmacological and non-pharmacological strategies are not automatically discontinued.[92] In contrast the capacity of individual therapies to provide symptom relief needs to be appraised. When the patient deteriorates to a stage where the focus should be exclusively on a palliative approach to dyspnoea management it is important that the goals of therapy be clearly defined and an advance care plan formulated in accordance with institutional and legal regulatory frameworks.[93]

The conversations necessary to formulate these plans, although challenging and difficult, when performed proficiently can occur within a context of hope.[94] This hope is based not upon a cure but the hope for satisfying and fulfilling moments, promotion of control and autonomy over events, and reassurance that amidst uncertainty and upheaval that there will be people there to help and support them.[94]

Perhaps before discussing the treatment and management strategies it is important to consider the relationship between the treating team and the patient and their family. It is easy for clinicians to underestimate the great source and comfort patients derive from contact and recognition, particularly with their cardiologists. As many people with HF have been under the care of the same cardiologist and general practitioner for many years, they respect and value these doctors. To abruptly cease this relationship and hand over to specialist palliative care services can be devastating to patients and their families in the midst of uncertainty and upheaval. Therefore a supportive approach to HF management and the use of a multidisciplinary approach can interface readily with palliative care strategies and minimize distress and role conflict.[4] Our work to date has demonstrated that patients fear abandonment by their clinicians.[95] As in advance care planning it is the words and communication skills that are most effective and powerful in structuring these relationships. Dialogue such as 'the palliative care team are going to work with us to ensure that you are kept the most comfortable; I will still be part of the team and will play an active role in your care and I am available if you want to talk with me' makes the patient feel in control and promotes a sense of acceptance and continuity as they make the transition into a palliative care setting if necessary. The majority of HF patients can be managed at the end of life by cardiology and primary-care clinicians with access to consultancy models where appropriate. Although case conferencing and care planning can appear labour intensive, this investment of time in the communication and clarification of goals often prevents crisis situations, discontent, conflict, and inappropriate and unnecessary interventions.[96]

Conclusions

Beyond the core treatment for HF management, effective management of dyspnoea is limited. Key symptom management strategies are summarized in Table 9.3. As the burden of HF continues to escalate there is a need for large randomized controlled clinical trials to determine optimal management strategies. The absence of evidence for dyspnoea management related to HF is not an excuse to allow patients and their families to suffer unnecessarily. The use of a supportive approach to HF management allows the integration of physical, social, psychological, and spiritual considerations in the care of the patient and their family not just in the later stages of illness but across the entire illness trajectory.

In spite of the sparse evidence in relation to pharmacological strategies to inform practice, clinicians can be comforted by the fact that many of the needs identified by

Table 9.3 Summary of symptomatic strategies to improve symptom management

Symptom	Pharmacological	Non-pharmacological
Dyspnoea	Diuretics, opioid, oxygen	Positioning, airflow
Oedema	Diuretics	Skin care, compression, support
Fatigue	Psychostimulants	Energy conservation, exercise
Anaemia	Erythropoietin plus iron. Transfusion	Dietary modifications
Pain	WHO guidelines. Nitrates for ischaemia	Positioning, heat packs, massage
Anorexia, constipation	Appetite stimulants. Aperients	Dietary modification
Anxiety	Benzodiazepines	Relaxation, action plan
Depression	Selective serotonin reuptake inhibitors	Psychological support

patients and their families relate to effective communication and coordination of care. These barriers to satisfaction with care can be readily addressed within an integrated, supportive care approach to HF management. The success of this approach is largely dependent on the clinician's capacity for accurate assessment of a patient's needs and their capacity to create a professional and meaningful bond with the patient and their family. The management of dyspnoea is a critical HF management strategy from diagnosis to death. As underscored in many of the other chapters in this book relating to symptom management, as the patient advances along the illness trajectory there needs to be a tapering in the introduction of pharmacological and non-pharmacological strategies to achieve symptom management. Although dyspnoea remains a challenging and distressing symptom, a range of strategies are available to the clinician to decrease symptom burden.

References

1. Goodlin SJ (2005). Palliative care for end-stage heart failure. *Curr Heart Fail Rep* **2**: 155–60.
2. Voduc N, Webb K, O'Donnell DE (2005). Pulmonary rehabilitation. In: *Dyspnoea in Advanced Disease. A Guide to Clinical Management* (ed. S Booth, D Dudgeon), pp. 137–55. Oxford: Oxford University Press.
3. Dutka D, Johnson MJ (2005). Breathlessness in heart failure. In: *Dyspnoea in Advanced Disease. A Guide to Clinical Management* (ed. S Booth, D Dudgeon), Oxford: Oxford University Press.
4. Goodlin SJ, Hauptman PJ, Arnold R, Grady K, Hershberger RE, Kutner J *et al.* (2004). Consensus statement: palliative and supportive care in advanced heart failure. *J Cardiac Fail* **10**: 200–9.
5. Killian K (2005). History of dyspnea. In: *Dyspnea. Mechanisms, Measurement, and Management*, 2nd edn (ed. DE O'Donnell). Boca Raton, FL: Taylor & Francis.
6. Friedman MM (1997). Older adults' symptoms and their duration before hospitalization for heart failure. *Heart Lung* **26**: 169–76.
7. American Thoracic Society (1999). Dyspnea. Mechanisms, assessment, and management: a consensus statement. *Am J Respir Crit Care Med* **159**: 321–40.
8. Eriksson H, Caidahl K, Larsson B, Ohlson LO, Welin L, Wilhelmsen L *et al.* (1987). Cardiac and pulmonary causes of dyspnoea–validation of a scoring test for clinical-epidemiological use: the Study of Men Born in 1913. *Eur Heart J* **8**: 1007–14.
9. Wasserman K (1982). Dyspnea on exertion. Is it the heart or the lungs? *J Am Med Assoc* **248**: 2039–43.
10. Caroci Ade S, Lareau SC (2004). Descriptors of dyspnea by patients with chronic obstructive pulmonary disease versus congestive heart failure. *Heart Lung* **33**: 102–10.
11. McKee PA, Castelli WP, McNamara PM, Kannel WB (1971). The natural history of congestive heart failure: the Framingham study. *New Engl J Med* **285**: 1441–6.
12. Mandak JS, McConnell TR (1998). Pulmonary manifestations of chronic heart failure. *J Cardiopul Rehab* **18**: 89–93.
13. Manning HL, Schwartzstein RM (1995). Pathophysiology of dyspnea. *New Engl J Med* **333**: 1547–53.
14. Goodlin SJ (2005). Heart failure in the elderly. *Exp Rev Cardiovasc Ther* **3**: 99–106.
15. Eriksson H, Svardsudd K, Larsson B, Ohlson LO, Welin L, Tibblin G *et al.* (1987). Dyspnoea in a cross-sectional and a longitudinal study of middle-aged men: the study of men born in 1913 and 1923. *Eur Heart J* **8**: 1015–23.
16. Mahler DA (1987). Dyspnea: diagnosis and management. *Clin Chest Med* **8**: 215–30.

17. Rogers RL, Feller ED, Gottlieb SS (2006). Acute congestive heart failure in the emergency department. *Cardiol Clin* **24**: 115–23.

18. Spector N, Klein D (2001). Chronic critically ill dyspneic patients: mechanisms and clinical measurement. *AACN Clin Issues: Adv Pract Acute Crit Care* **12**: 220–33.

19. Scano, G., Stendardi, L., and Grazzini, M. Understanding dyspnoea by its language. *Eur Respir J*, (2005) **25**(2): 380–85.

20. Simon PM, Schwartzstein RM, Weiss JW, Fencl V, Teghtsoonian M, Weinberger SE (1990). Distinguishable types of dyspnea in patients with shortness of breath. *Am Rev Respir Dis* **142**: 1009–14.

21. Beach D, Schwartzstein RM (2005). The genesis of breathlessness. What do we understand? In: *Dyspnoea in Advanced Disease. A Guide to Clinical Management* (ed. S Booth, D Dudgeon), pp. 1–18. Oxford: Oxford University Press.

22. McConnell TR, Mandak JS, Sykes JS, Fesniak H, Dasgupta H (2003). Exercise training for heart failure patients improves respiratory muscle endurance, exercise tolerance, breathlessness, and quality of life. *J Cardiopul Rehab* **23**: 10–16.

23. Laoutaris I, Dritsas A, Brown MD, Manginas A, Alivizatos PA, Cokkinos DV (2004). Inspiratory muscle training using an incremental endurance test alleviates dyspnea and improves functional status in patients with chronic heart failure. *Eur J Cardiovasc Prevent Rehab* **11**: 489–96.

24. Mahler DA (ed.) (1990). *Dyspnea*. New York: Futura Publishing Company.

25. Mandak JS, McConnell TR (1998). Pulmonary manifestations of chronic heart failure. J *Cardiopul Rehab* **18**: 89–93.

26. Nordgren L, Sorensen S (2003). Symptoms experienced in the last six months of life in patients with end-stage heart failure. *Eur J Cardiovas Nurs* **2**: 213–17.

27. Grady KL, Dracup K, Kennedy G, Moser DK, Piano M, Warner Stevenson L *et al.* (2000). Team management of patients with heart failure. A statement for healthcare professional from the Cardiovascular Nursing Council of the American Heart Association. *Circulation* **102**: 2443–56.

28. Felker GM, Adams KF, Jr, Gattis WA, O'Connor CM (2004). Anemia as a risk factor and therapeutic target in heart failure. *J Am Coll Cardiol* **44**: 959–66.

29. Johnson JL (2000). Pleural effusions in cardiovascular disease. Pearls for correlating the evidence with the cause. *Postgrad Med* **107**: 95–101.

30. Anderson WF (1976). The clinical assessment of ageing and problems of diagnosis in the elderly. *S Afr Med J* **50**: 1257–9.

31. Rich MW (2001). Heart failure in the 21st century: a cardiogeriatric syndrome. *J Gerontol Ser A: Biol Sci Med Sci* **56**: M88–M96.

32. Bradley TD, Floras JS (2003). Sleep apnea and heart failure: Part I: obstructive sleep apnea. *Circulation* **107**: 1671–8.

33. Bradley TD, Floras JS (1996). Pathophysiologic and therapeutic implications of sleep apnea in congestive heart failure. *J Card Fail* 1996. p. 223–40.

34. Ingbir M, Freimark D, Motro M, Adler Y (2002). The incidence, pathophysiology, treatment and prognosis of Cheyne-Stokes breathing disorder in patients with congestive heart failure. *Herz* **27**: 107–12.

35. Pepin JL, Chouri-Pontarollo N, Tamisier R, Levy P (2006). Cheyne-Stokes respiration with central sleep apnoea in chronic heart failure: proposals for a diagnostic and therapeutic strategy. *Sleep Med Rev* **10**: 33–47.

36. Sin DD, Fitzgerald F, Parker JD, Newton G, Floras JS, Bradley TD (1999). Risk factors for central and obstructive sleep apnea in 450 men and women with congestive heart failure. *Am J Respir Crit Care Med* **160**: 1101–6.

37. Staniforth AD, Kinnear WJ, Cowley AJ (2001). Cognitive impairment in heart failure with Cheyne-Stokes respiration. *Heart* **85**: 18–22.

38. Swedberg K, Cleland J, Dargie H, Drexler H, Follath F, Komajda M *et al.* (2005). Guidelines for the diagnosis and treatment of chronic heart failure: executive summary (update 2005): The Task Force for the Diagnosis and Treatment of Chronic Heart Failure of the European Society of Cardiology.[see comment]. *Eur Heart J* **26**: 1115–40.

39. Hunt SA, Baker DW, Chin MH, Cinquegrani MP, Feldmanmd AM, Francis GS *et al.* (2001). ACC/AHA Guidelines for the evaluation and management of chronic heart failure in the adult: Executive summary a report of the American College of Cardiology/American Heart Association Task Force on Practice Guidelines (Committee to revise the 1995 Guidelines for the evaluation and management of heart failure). *Circulation* **104**: 2996–3007.

40. Krum H, National Heart Foundation of Australia, Cardiac Society of Australia & New Zealand, and Chronic Heart Failure Clinical Practice Guidelines Writing Panel (2001). Guidelines for management of patients with chronic heart failure in Australia. *Med J Aust* **174**: 459–66.

41. Hunt SA, Abraham WT, Chin MH, Feldman AM, Francis GS, Ganiats TG *et al.* (2005). ACC/AHA 2005 Guideline update for the diagnosis management of chronic heart failure in the adult: a report of the American College of Cardiology/American Heart Association Task Force on Practice Guidelines (Writing Committee to Update the 2001 Guidelines for the Evaluation and Management of Heart Failure). *Circulation* **112**: 154–235.

42. Mills R, Al-Mallah M. (2006). Heart failure secondary to coronary artery disease. In: *Congestive Heart Failure*, 3rd edn (ed. B. Greenberg), pp. 285–304. Philadelphia: Lippincott Williams & Wilkins.

43. Barkham TM, Martin FC, Eykyn SJ (1996). Delay in the diagnosis of bacteraemic urinary tract infection in elderly patients. *Age Ageing* **25**: 130–2.

44. Richards M, Nicholls MG, Espiner EA, Lainchbury JG, Troughton RW, Elliott J *et al.* for the Christchurch Cardioendocrine Research Group, and Australia-New Zealand Heart Failure Group (2006). Comparison of B-type natriuretic peptides for assessment of cardiac function and prognosis in stable ischemic heart disease. *J Am Coll Cardiol* **47**: 52–60.

45. Mehta RL, Pascual MT, Soroko S, Chertow GM, Group PS (2002). Diuretics, mortality, and nonrecovery of renal function in acute renal failure. *J Am Med Assoc* **288**: 2547–53.

46. Nohria A, Mielniczuk LM, Stevenson LW (2005). Evaluation and monitoring of patients with acute heart failure syndromes. *Am J Cardiol* **96**: 32G–40G.

47. Mattison LE, Coppage L, Alderman DF, Herlong JO, Sahn SA (1997). Pleural effusions in the medical ICU: prevalence, causes, and clinical implications. *Chest* **111**: 1018–23.

48. Carrieri-Kohlman V, Stulbarg MS (2003). Dyspnea. In: *Pathological Phenomena in Nursing* (ed. C. West), p. 175–209. Saunders.

49. McCord M, Cronin-Stubbs, D (1992). Operationalizing dyspnea: focus on measurement. *Heart Lung* **21**: 167–79.

50. Mahler DA (2005). Measurement of dyspnea: clinical ratings. In: *Dyspnea. Mechanisms, Measurement, and Management*, 2nd edn (ed. DE O'Donnell), pp. 147–65. Boca Raton, FL: Taylor & Francis.

51. Gift AG (1989). Validation of a vertical visual analogue scale as a measure of clinical dyspnea. *Rehab Nurs* **14**: 323–5.

52. Heart Failure Society of America (2006). HFSA 2006 Comprehensive heart failure practice guideline. *J Card Fail* **12**: e1–e122.

53. Smart N, Marwick TH (2004). Exercise training for patients with heart failure: a systematic review of factors that improve mortality and morbidity.[Review: see comment]. *Am J Med* **116**: 693–706.

54. McAlister FA, Stewart S, Ferrua S, McMurray JJV (2004). Multidisciplinary strategies for the management of heart failure patients at high risk for admission: a systematic review of randomized trials. *J Am Coll Cardiol* **44**: 810–19.

55. Abernethy AP, Currow DC, Frith P, Fazekas B (2005). Prescribing palliative oxygen: a clinician survey of expected benefit and patterns of use. *Palliat Med* **19**: 168–70.

56. Prodigy Guidance. *Palliative care dyspnoea* (available at http://www.prodigy.nhs.uk/palliative_care_dyspnoea/extended_information/management_issues, Accessed 26 September, 2006)

57. Booth S, Anderson H, Swannick M, Wade R, Kite S, Johnson M (2004). The use of oxygen in the palliation of breathlessness. A report of the expert working group of the scientific committee of the association of palliative medicine. *Respir Med* **98**: 66–77.

58. Carrieri-Kohlman V, Douglas MK, Gormley JM, Stulbarg MS (1993). Desensitization and guided mastery: treatment approaches for the management of dyspnea. *Heart Lung* **22**: 226–34.

59. Tomaka J, Thompson S, Palacios R (2006). The relation of social isolation, loneliness, and social support to disease outcomes among the elderly. *J Aging Health* **18**: 359–84.

60. Flather MD, Yusuf S, Kober L, Pfeffer M, Hall A, Murray G *et al.* (2000). Long-term ACE-inhibitor therapy in patients with heart failure or left-ventricular dysfunction: a systematic overview of data from individual patients. ACE-Inhibitor Myocardial Infarction Collaborative Group. *Lancet* **355**: 1575–81.

61. Packer M, Bristow MR, Cohn JN, Colucci WS, Fowler MB, Gilbert EM *et al.* (1996). The effect of carvedilol on morbidity and mortality in patients with chronic heart failure. U.S. Carvedilol Heart Failure Study Group. *New Engl J Med* **334**: 1349–55.

62. The CAPRICORN Investigators (2001). Effect of carvedilol on outcome after myocardial infarction in patients with left-ventricular dysfunction: the CAPRICORN randomised trial. *Lancet* **357**: 1385–90.

63. Davidson P, Macdonald P, Paull G, Rees D, Howes L, Cockburn J *et al.* (2003). Diuretic therapy in chronic heart failure: implications for heart failure nurse specialists. *Aust Crit Care* **16**: 59–69.

64. Verma AK, da Silva JH, Kuhl DR (2004). Diuretic effects of subcutaneous furosemide in human volunteers: a randomized pilot study. *Ann Pharmacother* **38**: 544–9.

65. Fonzo-Christe C, Vukasovic C, Wasilewski-Rasca AF, Bonnabry P (2005). Subcutaneous administration of drugs in the elderly: survey of practice and systematic literature review. *Palliat Med* **19**: 208–19.

66. Ellison DH (1991). The physiologic basis of diuretic synergism: its role in treating diuretic resistance. *Ann Intern Med* **114**: 886–94.

67. Thackray S, Easthaugh J, Freemantle N, Cleland JG (2002). The effectiveness and relative effectiveness of intravenous inotropic drugs acting through the adrenergic pathway in patients with heart failure-a meta-regression analysis. *EurJ Heart Fail* **4**: 515–29.

68. Cleland JG, McGowan J (2002). Levosimendan: a new era for inodilator therapy for heart failure? *Curr Opin Cardiol* **17**: 257–65.

69. Williams SG, Wright DJ, Marshall P, Reese A, Tzeng BH, Coats AJ *et al.* (2003). Safety and potential benefits of low dose diamorphine during exercise in patients with chronic heart failure. *Heart* **89**: 1085–6.

70. Johnson MJ, McDonagh TA, Harkness A, McKay SE, Dargie HJ (2002). Morphine for the relief of breathlessness in patients with chronic heart failure–a pilot study. *Eur J Heart Fail* **4**: 753–6.

71. Gutstein H, Akil H (2001). Opioid analgesics. In: *Goodman & Gilman's the Pharmacological Basis of Therapeutics*, 10th edn (ed. J Hardman, L Limbird, A Gilman), pp. 569–619. New York: McGraw-Hill.

72. Enck R (1999). The role of nebulized morphine in managing dyspnea. *Am J Hospice Palliat Care* **16**(1): p. 373–374.

73. Abernethy AP, Currow DC, Frith P, Fazekas BS, McHugh A, Bui C (2003). Randomised, double blind, placebo controlled crossover trial of sustained release morphine for the management of refractory dyspnoea. *Br Med J* **327**: 523–8.

74. Davis C (1995). The role of nebulised drugs in palliating respiratory symptoms of malignant disease. *Eur J Palliat Care* **2**: 9–15.

75. Jennings AL, Davies AN, Higgins JP, Gibbs JS, Broadley KE (2002). A systematic review of the use of opioids in the management of dyspnoea. *Thorax* **57**: 939–44.

76. Twycross R, Wilcock A, Charlesworth S, Dickman A (2006). *Palliative care formulary* (available at http://www.palliativedrugs.com/, accessed 26 September 2006).

77. Yan AT, Bradley TD, Liu PP (2001). The role of continuous positive airway pressure in the treatment of congestive heart failure. *Chest* **120**: 1675–85.

78. Bradley TD, Logan AG, Kimoff RJ, Series F, Morrison D, Ferguson K *et al.* (2005). Continuous positive airway pressure for central sleep apnea and heart failure. *New Engl J Med* **353**: 2025–33.

79. Manning HL, Schwartzstein RM (1995). Pathophysiology of dyspnea. *N Engl J Med* **333**:1547–53.

80. Drexler H, Riede U, Munzel T, Konig H, Funke E, Just H (1992). Alterations of skeletal muscle in chronic heart failure. *Circulation* **85**: 1751–9.

81. Mancini D, Henson D, LaManca J, Levine S (1992). Respiratory muscle function and dyspnea in patients with chronic congestive heart failure. *Circulation* **86**: 909–18.

82. Anker SD (2002). Imbalance of catabolic and anabolic pathways in chronic heart failure. *Scand J Nutr* **46**: 3–10.

83. Anker SD, Sharma R (2002). The syndrome of cardiac cachexia. *Int J Cardiol* **85**: 51–66.

84. Mancini DM, Henson D, LaManca J, Levine S (1992). Respiratory muscle function and dyspnea in patients with chronic congestive heart failure. *Circulation* **86**: 909–18.

85. Smoller JW, Pollack MH, Otto MW, Rosenbaum JF, Kradin RL (1996). Panic anxiety, dyspnea, and respiratory disease. Theoretical and clinical considerations. *Am J Respir Crit Care Med* **154**: 6–17.

86. Cooper S, Oborne J, Newton S, Harrison V, Thompson Coon J, Lewis S *et al.* (2003). Effect of two breathing exercises (Buteyko and pranayama) in asthma: a randomised controlled trial. *Thorax* **58**: 674–9.

87. Bowler SD, Green A, Mitchell CA (1998). Buteyko breathing techniques in asthma: a blinded randomised controlled trial. *Med J Aust* **169**: 575–8.

88. Bernardi L, Sleight P, Bandinelli G, Cencetti S, Fattorini L, Wdowczyc-Szulc J *et al.* (2001). Effect of rosary prayer and yoga mantras on autonomic cardiovascular rhythms: comparative study. *Br Med J* **323**: 1446–9.

89. Filshie J, Penn K, Ashley S, Davis CL (1996). Acupuncture for the relief of cancer-related breathlessness. *Palliat Med* **10**: 145–50.

90. Jobst K, Mcpherson K, Brown V, Fletcher H, Mole P, Hua Chen J *et al.* (1986). Controlled trial of acupuncture for disabling breathlessness. *Lancet* **328**: 1416–19.

91. Schaefer KM, Potylycki MJS (1993). Fatigue associated with congestive heart failure: use of Levine's conservation model. *J Adv Nurs* **18**: 260–8.

92. Pantilat SZ, Steimle AE (2004). Palliative care for patients with heart failure. *J Am Med Assoc* **291**: 2476–82.

93. NSW Health. *Using advanced care directives* (available at http://www.health.nsw.gov.au/pubs/2004/pdf/adcare_directive.pdf, accessed 26 September, 2006).

94. Davidson P, Dracup K, Phillips J, Padilla G, Daly J (2007). Preparing for the worst while hoping for the best: the relevance of hope in the heart failure illness trajectory. *J Cardiovasc Nurs* **22**: 159–65

95. Davidson P, Paull G, Rees D, Daly J, Cockburn J (2005). Narrative analysis of documentation: authentication of the home-based heart failure nurse specialist role and function. *Am J Crit Care* **14**: 1–8.

96. Mitchell G, Cherry M, Kennedy R, Weeden K, Burridge L, Clavarino A *et al.* (2005). General practitioner, specialist providers case conferences in palliative care–lessons learned from 56 case conferences. *Aust Fam Physician* **34**: 389–92.

Chapter 10

Sleep-disordered breathing in heart failure

Lip Bun Tan, Thomas Köhnlein, Mark W. Elliot

The association between heart failure (HF) and sleep disturbance can be divided into two major categories:

1. The symptoms of HF which result in direct disruption of sleep and insomnia.

2. Sleep apnoea syndromes:

    (i) central sleep apnoea syndrome, which is usually a consequence of worsening HF;

    (ii) obstructive sleep apnoea syndrome, which may be a precursor of cardiac diseases leading to the development of chronic HF.

Sleep-related HF symptoms

One of the most troublesome symptoms in patients with severe HF is dyspnoea, especially during sleep. If patients suffer from exertional dyspnoea, a natural reaction is to avoid any exertion that will precipitate breathlessness. Similarly, dyspnoea precipitated by splinting the diaphragm by bending forward or over-eating can also be consciously avoided. Orthopnoea can to some extent also be volitionally avoided by patients sleeping propped up, for example by using multiple pillows or special cushions, or even by sleeping in a chair. However, sleep-related dyspnoea is even more distressing, because there is no volitional manoeuvre that patients can undertake to avoid such symptoms. Affected patients feel utterly helpless.

The symptoms and burden of chronic HF can seriously impair the physiological sleep architecture. Frequent awakening might impede progression into deep and refreshing sleep stages. Sleep deprivation with lack of sufficient amounts of slow wave sleep (SWS) and rapid eye movement (REM) sleep, which are understood as the physiological states for bodily and mental recuperation, may result not only in physical but also, and more importantly, mental or psychological fatigue. This state can be described as insomnia associated with chronic HF. The more severe the extent of the HF, the worse the distressing symptom becomes. During the hyperpnoeic phases, HF patients may have to drive the respiratory muscles so hard as to induce lactic acidosis so that they feel unbearably exhausted. From the patient's perspective, since they are somnolent during the apnoeic phases, what they are most disturbed by is waking up to an awareness of troublesome breathlessness during the hyperpnoeic phases. It is not surprising that when patients reach these stages, they may entertain suicidal thoughts or even request euthanasia.

What is even more frustrating for them is that the standard therapies for managing HF or sleep disturbance often paradoxically worsen the condition. Sedative pharmacological agents, such as benzodiazepines, benzodiazepine receptor activators, antidepressants, neuroleptics, antihistamines, and others can exacerbate sleep apnoea (see below). Treatment of HF which often produces dramatic improvements in patients admitted for acute left ventricular (LV) failure, namely the use of loop diuretics and diamorphine, can also paradoxically exacerbate sleep-related breathing disorders in patients with chronic severe HF because of reductions in cardiac output through excessive lowering of the requisite LV filling pressures. Similarly, aggressive introduction and up-titration of the drugs proven to be of prognostic benefit to HF patients, such as β-adrenergic receptor blockers, can also reduce cardiac output to such an extent as to tip them over the threshold into the vicious cycle of worsening dyspnoea.

It is clear therefore that for carers and physicians aiming to look after patients with severe HF, a lack of awareness of the complex pathophysiological mechanisms responsible for precipitating such distressing symptoms and ignorance about what therapies to avoid and which to institute are not acceptable options.

Sleep apnoea syndromes

The term 'sleep apnoea' encompasses a number of different clinical problems. In *obstructive sleep apnoea syndrome* (OSAS), the most common form of sleep apnoea, episodes of apnoea occur during sleep as a result of airway obstruction at the level of the pharynx. *Central sleep apnoea syndrome* (CSAS) describes nocturnal disturbances in the central control of breathing. In pure central sleep apnoea, no anatomical abnormality can be found. Many patients with CSAS can also have obstructive events, so-called *mixed sleep apnoea syndrome*.

Central sleep apnoea syndrome (CSAS)

Advanced chronic congestive HF is one of the most frequent reasons for CSAS.[1,2] The typical pattern of periodic breathing (PB) during wakefulness, and during sleep, was first described in the first half of the 19th century by Cheyne[3] and Stokes,[4] and is therefore referred to as Cheyne–Stokes respiration (CSR).

CSR or PB is characterized by a regular, crescendo–decrescendo oscillation of tidal volume (Fig. 10.1). This results in slow oscillations between central hypopnoea or central apnoea, and hyperventilation.[5,6] The typical length of one period is 30–120 seconds, but longer periods have been observed. In the majority of patients, PB begins during light sleep in stages 1 and 2, and rarely during REM sleep. Variations of PB can be found during a single night, and studies over successive nights have shown different expressions of PB in the same individual.[7] The amount of PB varies widely between different patients with the same extent of HF.

During prolonged hypopnoea or apnoea the oxygen saturation decreases, combined with a slow rise in the partial pressure of carbon dioxide ($PaCO_2$) and a decline in blood

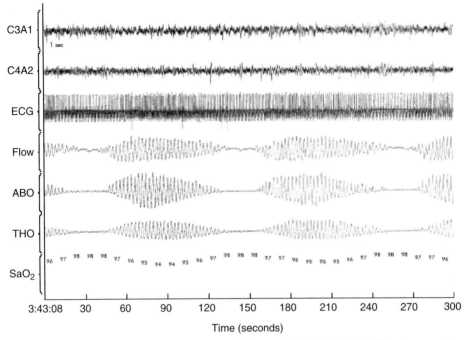

Fig. 10.1 Five-minute section of a polysomnographic record of EEG (C3A1, C4A2), electrocardiogram (ECG), oronasal air flow (Flow), abdominal ventilatory effort (ABD), thoracic ventilatory effort (THO), and oxygen saturation measured at the finger tip of the left hand (SaO$_2$) in a 57-year-old man with moderate ischaemic HF (NYHA Class II–III). This is a typical breathing pattern with Cheyne–Stokes respiration with hyperpnoeic and apnoeic sequences in sleep stage 2. There are fluctuations in oxygen saturation in response to PB, with delay of the transit time from the lungs to the finger tip of the left hand.

and tissue pH. Central nervous system activity may be unaffected until late apnoea, which means that sleep is maintained during an apnoeic episode.[8] The resumption of ventilation is associated with EEG arousals, which are markers of central nervous system activation.[9] At that moment, sleep is seriously disturbed, and the patient is forced to change to a more superficial level of sleep.

Prevalence of CSAS

The highest prevalence of PB is found in patients with severe, chronic LV insufficiency. Recent reports estimate the prevalence of PB in patients with underlying ischaemic heart disease or idiopathic dilated cardiomyopathy, LV ejection fraction of ≤ 40%, and optimized medical therapy at 30–40%.[10] The majority of these patients are male.[11]

Prognosis of CSAS

The presence of PB during sleep in patients with congestive HF has significant implications. The prognosis of a patient with any degree of HF is worse if CSAS is present.[12] The cumulative survival and transplant-free rate was found to be significantly

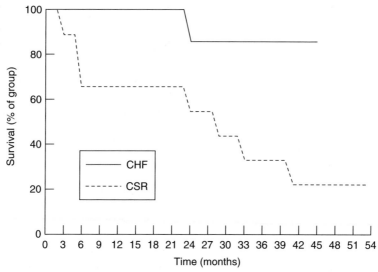

Fig. 10.2 Cumulative survival of patients in chronic HF (CHF) with or without central sleep apnoea and PB (CSR). Adapted from Hanly and Zuberi-Khokhar.[13]

worse for patients with PB (100% versus 66% after 1 year, 86% versus 56% after 2 years, respectively; Fig. 10.2).[13]

The severity of PB, assessed by the apnoea–hypopnoea index (AHI) (see below) has been shown to be an independent predictor of poor prognosis.[14] Andreas and co-workers[6] found an increased likelihood of dying within a few months in patients with congestive HF and PB during sleep and wakefulness.

The prognosis of HF patients with CSAS has not been shown to be significantly improved by long-term continuous positive airways pressure (CPAP) therapy. A Canadian multi-centre study[15] included 258 patients with a mean observational period of 24 months. Overall, long-term CPAP treatment improved some worthwhile clinical features of HF patients, such as attenuated central sleep apnoea, improved nocturnal oxygenation, improved daytime alertness and wellbeing, increased the distance walked in 6 min, and increased LV ejection fraction. The study was underpowered due to recruitment problems and terminated earlier than expected due to initially higher mortality rates in the CPAP group, but the mortality rates reversed later in the study. Subgroup analyses are awaited to get further insights into the therapeutic value of CPAP in CSAS. A key take-home message is that in selected patients who can tolerate using it, CPAP can be empirically used to improve their quality of life but there is no mandate to use it as a means to improve HF prognosis.

Clinical presentation of CSAS

The typical symptoms of all forms of sleep apnoea are daytime hypersomnolence and fatigue. Many patients are likely to fall asleep in quiet or monotonous situations or whenever they are not busy during the day. Despite apparently sleeping for many hours during the night, patients with CSAS (and with OSAS, see below) may not feel fully refreshed. These symptoms impair patients' quality of life and may contribute to their more sedentary lifestyle.[16] They also overlap with and exacerbate the typical symptoms of congestive HF, such as lethargy, impaired exercise capacity, and paroxysmal nocturnal dyspnoea.[17] Fatigue can also be a side-effect of cardiac medication (e.g. β-blockers), but hypersomnolence and excessive lethargy should alert the clinician to the possibility of sleep apnoea.

Patients with congestive HF and PB are more limited in their physical performance and develop dyspnoea at lower workloads compared with patients with disease of similar severity but without PB.[18] The prevalence of cardiac arrhythmia is significantly higher compared with patients with the same degree of HF but without PB.[19,20]

Pathophysiology

In healthy subjects, the tidal volume and frequency of breathing (minute ventilation) is principally controlled by the arterial partial pressure of carbon dioxide ($PaCO_2$), blood pH, and the partial pressure of oxygen (PaO_2).[21] These parameters are sensed in the arterial blood by peripheral chemoreceptors located in the carotid bodies and the aortic arch. These peripheral chemoreceptors are thought to react rapidly to short-term changes in blood gas.[22] Central chemoreceptors are located at the ventral surface of the medulla oblongata, behind the blood–brain barrier, which may delay responses to changes in arterial blood gases. Information from all chemoreceptors is transferred to, and processed in, the respiratory centres in the brainstem, adjacent to centres which control the cardiovascular system.[23] Further inputs into the respiratory centres come from receptors in the lungs (stretch and pressure receptors), and from proprioceptors in the respiratory muscles. Output from the respiratory centre is conducted by efferent nerves to the respiratory muscles.[24,25]

The control of breathing maintains blood gases within a tight range, according to the metabolic demands of the body. PB reflects uncompensated instability of the feedback control of ventilation. This can occur if information transfer to the controller is delayed or the controller gain is altered.[26,27]

Increased controller gain seems to be important in the pathogenesis of PB.[28] Various hormones and drugs can alter the sensitivity of human chemoreceptors, including the endogenous catecholamines noradrenaline and adrenaline.[29] Levels of both hormones are increased in the blood and urine of patients with HF, probably as compensation for cardiac pump failure.[30] Increased circulating concentrations of these catecholamines might increase the responsiveness of the respiratory controller to CO_2, leading to hyperventilation.[31,32] Latent hyperventilation during wakefulness is a common finding in patients with chronic HF, and a relationship between an abnormally increased ventilatory response to CO_2 during the day and PB during sleep has been observed.[33]

A single deep breath is a common finding at the onset of a sequence with PB during sleep. $PaCO_2$ may fall below the apnoeic threshold, causing the first apnoea of the sequence.[34] As mentioned above, arousals are frequently observed in association with respiratory events. Arousals may trigger the release of endogenous catecholamines. The responsiveness to CO_2 may be increased if arousals are frequent, which further destabilizes the respiratory control system.[35] This induces an accelerating ventilatory drive producing tidal volumes and frequencies that overshoot what was required to normalize blood gases after a hypopnoea or apnoea phase. The net effect is a reduction in $PaCO_2$ below the apnoeic threshold, thereby precipitating a new apnoeic/hypopnoeic phase, thus perpetuating the cyclic PB.[36] Therefore CSAS can be understood as a phenomenon of hyperventilation during sleep with subsequent compensatory phases of apnoea or hypopnoea, rather than a sleep disorder resulting from apnoea, like obstructive sleep apnoea syndrome, as discussed below.

Chemoreceptor gain can be diminished pharmacologically by benzodiazepines, dopamine, codeine, morphine, and alcohol.[37,38] Dihydrocodeine has been shown in small clinical studies to reduce the amount of PB in patients with HF, but none of these substances can be applied clinically for CSAS.[39]

In the majority of patients, PB episodes are transient phenomena during some phases of the night and sometimes during the day, whereas impaired cardiac function, delayed circulation time, and increased chemoreceptor susceptibility are present chronically. This observation lends further support to the hypothesis that factors other than low cardiac output contribute to the fluctuations of ventilation.[40]

Consequences of PB

Repetitive arousals during sleep may cause sleep fragmentation with a reduction in the amount of SWS and REM sleep, which are the most recuperative sleep stages.[41,42] The clinical signs of non-refreshing sleep are frequently observed (see above).

The most critical situation in PB is during late apnoea when arousal occurs. At this time the heart is supplied with the smallest amount of oxygen, and sympathetic activation with rapid release of catecholamines exposes the circulation to high workloads. In patients with severe PB, several hundred of these episodes may occur during a single night. This has given rise to speculation that these repetitive increases in cardiac stress might be the decisive reason for the poorer prognosis of patients with PB.[43]

Large amounts of endogenous catecholamines seem to promote the progression of structural damage to the heart.[44] Recent studies have demonstrated that catecholamines induce a direct toxic effect on cardiac myocytes *in vivo* and subsequent myocardial fibrosis,[45] and accelerated cardiac myocyte hypertrophy, possibly promoting the progression of structural heart diseases.[46]

Obstructive sleep apnoea syndrome

Prevalence

The obstructive sleep apnoea syndrome (OSAS) is one of the largest health-care problems in the Western world. It is estimated that in western European countries, up to 9% of the middle-aged population fulfil at least one definition of OSAS (apnoea/hypopnea index of ≥5 plus a complaint of daytime sleepiness).[47,48]

Pathophysiology

The site of pathophysiological processes in OSAS is the pharynx, which is abnormal in size and/or collapsibility. On the one hand, the pharynx must be flexible and deformable to allow speech and deglutition, but as a conduit for airflow it must resist collapse. These functions are provided by active tone of the muscles of the lower pharynx that protect the pharynx from collapsing. The collapsibility of the pharynx during sleep might be due to altered tonic input for the muscles, and due to diminished reflex activity. Sleep is associated with pharyngeal narrowing and a substantial increase in air flow resistance even in normal individuals. An abnormal pharynx can be kept open in wakefulness by compensatory increase in dilator muscle activity, but during sleep this compensation fails and the airway may collapse.[49] Upper airway obstruction may occur anywhere from the nose to the glottis, with the most frequent site of primary obstruction being the nasopharynx, at the level of the soft palate (Fig. 10.3). Partial collapse or vibrations of the velum results in snoring, hypopnoea, and, in some cases, prolonged obstructive hypoventilation. Complete obstruction results in apnoea.[50]

Hypopnoea and apnoea reduce the airflow to and from the site of gas exchange in the lung. Oxygenation and the pH of the blood and tissues slowly fall, while the $PaCO_2$ rises. The changes in blood gases are thought to be one stimulus for a central change of state, an arousal (for details see 'Pathophysiology of PB' above). Another powerful stimulus for arousal is the effect of the Mueller manoeuvre, which is performed involuntarily by patients during an obstructive apnoea, producing major negative swings of the intrathoracic pressure.[51]

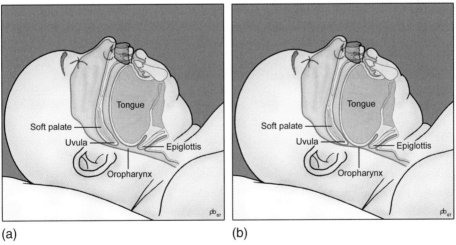

(a)   (b)

Fig. 10.3 Sleep is associated with pharyngeal narrowing and a substantial increase in air flow resistance even in normal individuals (a). Partial collapse or vibrations of the velum result in snoring, hypopnoea, and, in some cases, prolonged obstructive hypoventilation. Complete obstruction results in an apnoea (b).

Arousals are associated with increased muscle tone in the pharynx and a subsequent reopening of the obstructed upper airways to restore normal air flow. As described above, arousals can seriously disturb the continuum of physiological sleep stages. A rate of 10 arousals or more per hour of sleep is associated with clinically relevant sleep fragmentation and impairment of the recuperative sleep stages of SWS and REM sleep. It seems evident that sleep fragmentation from repetitive arousals is the primary cause of daytime hypersomnolence.[52]

Clinical presentation

Witnessed snoring and nocturnal apnoeas, combined with choking during sleep are important indicators for OSAS. Severe sleepiness during the day and the tendency to fall asleep, even in inappropriate situations, are further suggestive of sleep apnoea. However, the affected individual might not be aware of his or her snoring and hypersomnolence. Patients may develop daytime sleepiness over years, so that they do not realize how they are losing their physiological alertness. In addition, susceptibility to sleep fragmentation and deprivation varies between individuals.[53] Frequently reported symptoms of OSAS include restless sleep with frequent awakening, dry mouth and sore throat in the morning, morning headaches, personality changes, intellectual impairment, and impotence.

OSAS is associated with a number of other medical problems. The details for OSAS and the disorders described below are under continuous discussion, but there are reasons to claim OSAS as an independent risk factor at least for arterial hypertension,[54,55] ischaemic heart disease,[56] and stroke[57] (see Table 10.1). Obesity and OSAS are frequently associated. Significant sleep apnoea is present in 40% of obese individuals,[58] and more than 70% of OSAS patients are obese.[59] A 10% weight gain seems to be associated with a six-fold

Table 10.1 Spectrum of the acute and chronic effects of OSAS on the heart and circulation

	Prevalence (%)	Level of evidence
Acute effects (during sleep)		
Surges of blood pressure (pulmonary and systemic)	Up to 100	+++
Sinus arrhythmia	Up to 100	+++
Sinus arrest/AV block	5–10	++
Ventricular extra systoles	5–10	+
Atrial fibrillation	5–10	++
Chronic effects (during the day)		
Systemic arterial hypertension	40–60	+++
Pulmonary hypertension	20–30	++
Coronary heart disease	20–30	++
Stroke	5–10	++
Left-heart insufficiency	5–10	++

+/++/+++, level of evidence for causality, assessed by epidemiological, clinical, and experimental studies: low/moderate/high.

increase in the odds ratio of development of sleep apnoea.[60] High-density lipoprotein (HDL) levels are inversely related to the severity of OSAS. In a study of 470 patients with OSA, a higher AHI was associated with lower HDL levels.[61] OSAS is associated with type II diabetes mellitus. In a cross-sectional and longitudinal analysis of 1387 patients with sleep-disordered breathing, patients with an AHI ≥15 were more likely to have diabetes than patients with an AHI <5 (15% versus 3%, respectively).[62] Secondary pulmonary hypertension may be due to OSAS, although the magnitude of the risk is uncertain.[63] Patients with OSAS frequently develop pro-coagulatory changes like an increased aggregation of platelets and higher average serum concentrations of fibrinogen.

Repetitive oxygen desaturation and reoxygenation produces intravascular pro-inflammatory cytokines and highly reactive oxygen species. These disturbances in the microvessel milieu may result in endothelial dysfunction. Impairment of endothelial-dependent vasodilatation is an established precursor for the development of arterial hypertension and arteriosclerosis.[64,65] Nocturnal arrhythmia is frequently detected in OSAS patients. Obstructive apnoeas and the resulting Mueller manoeuvres are strong triggers for parasympathetic activation, whereas arousals are associated with activation of the sympathetic system. The resulting pattern of nocturnal bradycardia and tachycardia should not be misinterpreted as tachy–brady syndrome.

Atrial fibrillation is common in OSAS patients. OSAS may trigger phases of atrial fibrillation during sleep.[66] More than 50% of unselected patients with atrial fibrillation have OSAS.[67] Ventricular extrasystolic beats might appear when the nocturnal oxygen saturation drops below 60% (not uncommon in OSAS). A higher risk of sudden cardiac death in OSAS patients was suggested by Gami and co-workers,[68] but this is still speculative and unproven.

Patients with OSAS perform worse than control subjects on driving simulators and have a higher automobile crash rate than other drivers. Studies using data from car insurers reveal that sleepy drivers have a hugely elevated risk for severe automobile accidents (odds ratio 64.38; CI 45–91) compared with well-matched healthy drivers.[69] However, this increased risk can be normalized with effective treatment of sleep apnoea.[70]

Prognosis

Similar to CSAS, frequent obstructions of the upper airways during sleep may seriously impair the prognosis of the patient. OSAS is associated with a number of diseases, which in themselves are reasons for morbidity and premature death. There are no clear-cut data on the prognosis of OSAS in different stages of the disease, but it has been speculated that survival of OSAS may be similarly reduced as in CSAS when associated with advanced cardiac insufficiency.[71]

Diagnosis of sleep apnoea syndromes

Full polysomnography is regarded as the 'gold' standard method for the diagnosis of nocturnal breathing disorders (of central or obstructive origin). The typical ventilatory pattern of OSAS or PB is identified visually, according to the guidelines of the American

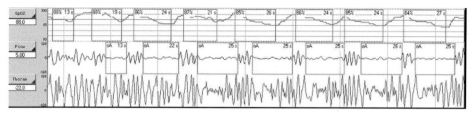

Fig. 10.4 Five-minute section of a patient with repetitive obstructive apnoea. The airflow in front of the mouth and nose (Flow channel) shows regular complete cessation of ventilation (oA), while the Thorax channel shows uninterrupted ventilatory efforts. Regular drops of the oxygen saturation (SaO$_2$) can be seen as a response to the apnoeas. As a result of the oxygen saturation being measured at the finger tip, the oxygen measurement is delayed by the blood travelling time to the site of measurement.

Thoracic Society[1] (see Figs 10.1 and 10.4). Obstructive apnoeas are sometimes followed by reflex central apnoeas, superficially mimicking primary central apnoea.[72]

Several indices describing the severity of the disorder have been established, such as the AHI, indicating the average number of respiratory events during an hour of sleep. Up to 15 apnoeic or hypopnoeic episodes per hour of sleep (irrespective of their central or obstructive origin) can be considered as normal or mild, above this and up to 30 reflects moderate, and an AHI of >30 reflects severe sleep apnoea.[73]

Moreover, important information on the severity of the problem and the possible impact on the quality of sleep are given by the arousal index (AI), which is pathological if above 15 arousals per hour of sleep. PB can be quantified as a proportion of the total sleep time. The average oxygen saturation during the night, and the time spent below an oxygen saturation of 90%, give further insights into the severity of the syndrome.

Sleep studies with full polysomnography are expensive and may be difficult to organize. There are screening systems on the market which can be handled by the patient at home, but which record only a limited number of sleep parameters.

Treatment of sleep apnoea syndromes

Specific drug treatment for sleep apnoea has been studied in recent years.[74–81] Substances such as theophylline, morphine derivatives, and supplementation of inhaled air with 3% CO$_2$ have been applied under experimental conditions in small studies.[82–84] None of these treatments can be recommended for routine practice. The prescription of sedatives for patients with any form of sleep-disordered breathing should be discouraged. Sedatives may further reduce the refreshing sleep stages of SWS and REM sleep. Sedatives worsen a patient's sleep quality and daytime performance.[85]

Well-established treatments for OSAS includes continuous positive airway pressure (CPAP) via nasal mask, oral protrusion appliances, and in rare cases nocturnal non-invasive ventilation (see below). Before considering patients for specific treatment for CSAS, medical therapy of the underlying heart disease must be optimized,[86,87] since improvement of cardiac output has been shown to reduce PB.[27,88] (See also Chapter 3 on optimal pharmacological therapy.)

Treatment options

Continuous positive airway pressure (CPAP)

CPAP has been used for the treatment of patients with obstructive or central sleep apnoea since the late 1980s. In OSAS it has been hypothesized that continuous positive pressure in the airways (6 mbar or above) prevents collapse of the soft tissue in the pharynx. This has been described as 'pneumatic splinting' of the upper airways. CPAP stabilizes the patient's ventilation, and reduces the frequency of apnoeic/hypopnoeic episodes, arousals, and the number of oxygen desaturations during sleep.[89] Advanced CPAP devices adjust the CPAP pressure automatically during the night (Auto-CPAP), depending on the body position or other parameters which necessitate higher or lower treatment pressures.

Although the mechanism of action of CPAP in CSAS is not fully understood, CPAP has been shown to be an effective method of treatment.[90] It can be difficult to introduce CPAP in some patients[91] but a relatively low pressure level of 5 mbar has been shown to be effective in adults with a normal body mass index.[92] The mean oxygen saturation increases and the transcutaneous CO_2 increases back into the normal range.[83] Studies of sympathetic nervous system activation during treatment with CPAP have shown a significant reduction in noradrenaline, but not adrenaline excretion, in overnight urine collections.[75]

CPAP also has direct haemodynamic effects, increasing the intrathoracic pressure thereby reducing cardiac afterload and preload, by reducing venous return to the right atrium. This results in lower diastolic filling pressures and more effective pump function.[93,94] CPAP recruits atelectatic lung areas improving oxygen transfer in the lungs, and the higher intrapulmonary oxygen content might prevent recurrent rises of right-ventricular afterload and subsequent pulmonary hypertension.[95] However, a recently published randomized study investigating chronic HF patients with and without PB, revealed an improvement in LV ejection fraction and mortality in patients with PB only, suggesting that any beneficial effect from CPAP is a consequence of an improvement in PB.[96] As described above with the Canadian multi-centre study, the beneficial effects of CPAP on the long-term prognosis are uncertain.[15]

Non-invasive ventilation

Patients with both forms of sleep apnoea have been treated with non-invasive pressure support ventilation (PSV). In OSAS this seems to have advantages over CPAP in very severely affected patients who would need high levels of CPAP (≥ 15 mbar). Patients' tolerance to the procedure might be improved with two pressure levels for inspiration and expiration. In CSAS, PSV has been tested in one prospective controlled randomized study.[97] PSV was not found to be superior to CPAP.

In recent years new forms of 'intelligent' ventilation have been developed for patients with CSAS. As an example, 'Adaptive Servo Ventilation' is designed for patients with PB to prevent hyperventilation and to support the patient's own breathing if necessary. Adaptations of the ventilatory pressure are possible for each single breath.[98] The outcome for patients has been studied in some smaller studies only, but all available reports found better treatment success than CPAP. Nothing is known as yet about hard endpoints such as progression of the underlying heart disease or mortality.

Oxygen

In patients with obstructive sleep apnoea, application of oxygen may only slightly improve oxygenation during sleep, and therefore oxygen is irrelevant in the treatment of OSAS.

In CSAS, the application of 4 L min^{-1} of oxygen via nasal cannulae has been shown to improve nocturnal PB. Some investigators have demonstrated an almost complete abolition of PB and an improved mean overnight oxygen saturation,[89] whereas others observed only a partial (approximately 50%) reduction in the number of hypopnoeas and apnoeas.[87,99] Andreas et al.[79] demonstrated a significant increase in exercise tolerance (peak oxygen consumption) in a cohort of 22 HF patients with PB during sleep after 1 week of nocturnal oxygen therapy. The same study revealed a significant correlation between the increase in peak oxygen consumption during ergospirometry and a decrease in PB, in arousals, and in the amount of time spent in bed with an oxygen saturation of <90%. Staniforth and colleagues[100] conducted a study with oxygen versus room air in a randomized, double-blind crossover study design. Four weeks of nocturnal oxygen treatment reduced the number of apnoeic and PB episodes during sleep, as well as the nocturnal urinary noradrenaline excretion in a cohort of 11 patients with stable HF. No significant changes in sleep quality, patient symptoms, or cognitive function could be demonstrated. It has been postulated that the effect of high oxygen concentrations is due to enhanced cellular metabolism in the peripheral chemoreceptors and a subsequent alteration of their setting.[101]

Pacemakers

One recent randomized trial by Garrigue et al.[102] demonstrated that in patients without HF, overdrive pacing of the heart by 15 beats min^{-1} above its average rate during sleep reduces the frequency of central and obstructive apnoeas and hypopnoeas by 50%. The mechanisms responsible for that observation are not clear, and nothing was reported about the frequency of arousals, sleep quality, or tolerance by patients.

Three further trials[103–105] studied atrial overdrive pacing in patients with moderate to severe sleep apnoea but without HF. All investigators found no significant effect on the severity of any form of sleep apnoea syndrome. Possible adverse effects of long-term pacing in patients are not known but a potential harm in pacing-induced HF[106] should not be ignored, therefore pacemaker implantation is not a treatment option for sleep apnoea.

Conclusions

CSAS with PB is frequent, but often unrecognized, in patients with advanced congestive HF. In many patients, daytime fatigue and impaired physical performance is not just a symptom of the heart disease or a side-effect of treatment, but an indicator of sleep-disordered breathing. The prognosis of patients with chronic HF seems to be significantly worse if CSAS is present. The causal relationship between chronic HF and CSAS is not fully understood, but delayed circulation time, increased chemoreceptor sensitivity to CO_2, and input into the respiratory centres from other brain centres and from peripheral receptors might have pathophysiological importance. Treatment options include CPAP and supplemental oxygen. CPAP is the most widespread therapy, but because of relatively poor patient acceptance in some studies more sophisticated ventilatory support strategies need to be developed. Adequately powered prospective randomized controlled trials with survival and health status as endpoints are needed to establish whether the correction of sleep-related abnormalities of breathing in patients with HF really does improve outcome.

Appendix: glossary

AHI (apnoea–hypopnoea index): the apnea–hypopnea index is defined as the total number of episodes of apnoea and hypopnoea per hour of sleep. A value of ≥5 is abnormal.

AI (arousal index): the number of arousals related to the total sleep time. It is useful for quantifying sleep fragmentation.

CSA (central sleep apnoea): a pattern of fluctuating breathing which can be classified into hypocapnic or hypercapnic forms. The former is seen mainly in patients with congestive HF. The latter is seen mainly in patients with central nervous system disorders that have caused loss of normal breathing control, e.g. in patients with encephalitis, neuromuscular disease, or kyphoscoliosis.

CSR (Cheyne–Stokes respiration): characterized by a regular, crescendo–decrescendo oscillation of tidal volume; also known as periodic breathing (see Fig. 10.1).

Orthopnoea: breathlessness precipitated by lying flat horizontally, most commonly due to pulmonary oedema secondary to left-ventricular failure, but may be caused by pleural effusions, diaphragmatic hernia, or phrenic nerve palsy.

OSA (obstructive sleep apnoea): apnoeic episodes occurring during sleep as a result of airway obstruction at the level of the pharynx.

PB (periodic breathing): characterized by a regular, crescendo–decrescendo oscillation of tidal volume; also known as Cheyne–Stokes respiration (Fig. 10.1).

PND (paroxysmal nocturnal dyspnoea): intermittent attacks of breathlessness waking the patient from sleep. Traditionally, students have been taught that this is because the patient slips into the horizontal torso position during sleep thereby precipitating orthopnoea, and to gain relief they usually have to sit up and dangle their feet over the edge of the bed. CSA, CSR, or OSA may also be responsible for PND. Alternatively, paroxysmal or intermittent arrhythmia (e.g. AF, SVT, VT) may be responsible.

REM (rapid eye movement) sleep: the stage of sleep characterized by rapid movements of the eyes, during which, the activity of the brain neurons is quite similar to that during waking hours and vivid dreams occur.

References

1. American Thoracic Society (1989). Indications and standards for cardiopulmonary sleep studies. *Am Rev Respir Dis* **139**:559–68.

2. Mortara A, Sleight P, Pinna GD *et al.* (1999). Association between hemodynamic impairment and Cheyne-Stokes respiration and periodic breathing in chronic stable congestive heart failure secondary to ischemic or idiopathic dilated cardiomyopathy. *Am J Cardiol* **84**: 900–4.

3. Cheyne J (1818). A case of apoplexy in which the fleshy part of the heart is turned to fat. *Dublin Hospital Rep* **2**: 216–23.

4. Stokes W (1854). *The Disease of the Heart and the Aorta*. Dublin: Hodges and Smith, pp. 323–6.

5. Hanly PJ, Millar TW, Steljes DG *et al.* (1989). Respiration and abnormal sleep in patients with congestive heart failure. *Chest* **96**: 480–8.

6. Andreas S, Hagenah G, Möller C (1996). Cheyne-Stokes respiration and prognosis in congestive heart failure. *Am J Cardiol* **78**: 1260–4.

7. Guilleminault C, Robinson A (1996). Central sleep apnoea. *Neurol Clin* **14**: 611–28.

8. Davies RJO, Bennet LS, Barbour C *et al.* (1999). Second by second patterns in cortical electroencephalography and systolic blood pressure during Cheyne-Stokes respiration. *Eur Resp J* **14**: 940–5.

9. Bonnet M, Carley D, Carskadon M *et al.* (1992). EEG arousals: scoring rules and examples. A preliminary report from the Sleep Disorders Atlas Task Force of the American Sleep Disorders Association. *Sleep* **15**: 173–84.

10. Javaheri S (2006). Sleep disorders in systolic heart failure: a prospective study of 100 male patients. The final report. *Int J Cardiol* **106**: 21–8.

11. Sin DD, Fitzgerald F, Parker JD *et al.* (1999). Risk factors for central and obstructive sleep apnoea in 450 men and women with congestive heart failure. *Am J Resp Crit Care Med* **160**: 1101–6.

12. Wilcox I, McNamara SG, Wessendorf T *et al.* (1998). Prognosis and sleep disordered breathing in heart failure. *Thorax* **53**: S33–S36.

13. Hanly PJ, Zuberi-Khokhar NS (1996). Increased mortality associated with Cheyne-Stokes respiration in patients with congestive heart failure. *Am J Respir Crit Care Med* **153**: 272–6.

14. Lanfrachi PA, Braghiroli A, Bosimini E *et al.* (1999). Prognostic value of nocturnal Cheyne-Stokes respiration in chronic heart failure. *Circulation* **99**: 1435–40.

15. Bradley TD, Logan AG, Kimoff RJ *et al.*; the CANPAP investigators (2005). Continuous positive airway pressure for central sleep apnea and heart failure. *New Engl J Med* **353**: 2025–33.

16. Tandon PK, Stander H, Schwarz RP, Jr (1989). Analysis of quality of life data from a randomized, placebo-controlled heart-failure trial. *J Clin Epidemiol* **42**: 955–62.

17. Struthers AD (2000). The diagnosis of heart failure. *Heart* **84**: 334–8.

18. Corra U, Pistono M, Mezzani A *et al.* (2006). Sleep and exertional periodic breathing in chronic heart failure: prognostic importance and interdependence. *Circulation* **113**: 44–50.

19. Leung RS, Bowman ME, Diep TM, Lorenzi-Filho G, Floras JS, Bradley TD (2005). Influence of Cheyne-Stokes respiration on ventricular response to atrial fibrillation in heart failure. *J Appl Physiol* **99**: 1689–96.

20. Leung RS, Diep TM, Bowman ME, Lorenzi-Filho G, Bradley TD (2004). Provocation of ventricular ectopy by Cheyne-Stokes respiration in patients with heart failure. *Sleep* **27**: 1337–43.

21. Campbell JMH, Douglas CG, Haldane JS *et al.* (1913). The response of the respiratory centre to carbonic acid, oxygen and hydrogen ion concentration. *J Physiol* **46**: 301–18.

22. Chua TP, Coats AJS (1995). The reproducibility and comparability of tests of the peripheral chemoreflex: comparing the transient hypoxic ventilatory drive test and the single-breath carbon dioxide response test in healthy subjects. *Eur J Clin Invest* **25**: 887–92.

23. Millhorn DE, Eldrodge FL (1986). Role of ventrolateral medulla in regulation of respiratory and cardiovascular systems. *J Appl Physiol* **61**: 1249–63.

24. Paintal AS (1969). Mechanism of stimulation of type J pulmonary receptors. *J Physiol* **203**: 511–32.

25. Roberts AM, Bhattacharya J, Schulz HD *et al.* (1986). Stimulation of pulmonary vagal afferent C-fibers by lung edema in dogs. *Circ Res* **58**: 512–22.

26. Cherniack NS (1999). Apnoea and periodic breathing during sleep. *New Engl J Med* **341**: 985–7.

27. Khoo MCK, Gottschalk A, Pack A (1991). Sleep induced periodic breathing and apnoea: a theoretical study. *J Appl Physiol* **70**: 2014–24.

28. Chua TP, Clark AL, Amadi AA *et al.* (1996). Relation between chemosensitivity and the ventilatory response to exercise in chronic heart failure. *J Am Coll Cardiol* **27**: 650–7.

29. Cunningham DJC, Hey EN, Patrick JM *et al.* (1963). The effect of noradrenaline infusion on the relation between pulmonary ventilation and the alveolar pO_2 and pCO_2 in man. *Ann NY Acad Sci* **109**: 756–71.

30. Swedberg K, Eneroth P, Kjekshus J (1990). Hormones regulating cardiovascular function in patients with severe congestive heart failure and their relation to mortality. *Circulation* **82**: 1730–6.

31. Chua TP, Ponikowski P, Harrington D *et al.* (1997). Clinical correlates and prognostic significance of the ventilatory response to exercise in chronic heart failure. *J Am Coll Cardiol* **29**: 1585–90.

32. Cunningham DJC, Hey EN, Patrick JM *et al.* (1963). The respiratory effect of infused noradrenaline at raised partial pressures of oxygen in man. *J Physiol* **165**: 45–6.

33. Andreas S, v. Breska B, Kopp E *et al.* (1993). Periodic respiration in patients with heart failure. *Clin Invest* **71**: 281–5.

34. Naughton M, Benard D, Tam A *et al.* (1993). Role of hyperventilation in the pathogenesis of central sleep apnoeas in patients with congestive heart failure. *Am Rev Respir Dis* **148**: 330–8.

35. Phillipson EA, Bowes G (1986). Control of breathing during sleep. In: *Handbook of Physiology: Respiration* (ed. NS Cherniack *et al.*), pp. 649–90. Bethesda, MD: American Physiological Society.

36. Naughton MT, Bradley TD (1998). Sleep apnoea in congestive heart failure. *Clin Chest Med* **19**: 99–113.

37. Schoene RB (1992). Regulation of ventilation. In: *Foundations of Respiratory Care* (ed. DJ Pierson, RM Kacmarek), pp. 129–34. New York: Churchill Livingstone.

38. van de Borne P, Oren R, Somers VK (1998). Dopamine depresses minute ventilation in patients with Heart Failure. *Circulation* **98**: 126–31.

39. Ponikowski P, Anker SD, Chua TP *et al.* (1999). Oscillatory breathing patterns during wakefulness in patients with chronic heart failure. Clinical implications and role of augmented peripheral chemosensitivity. *Circulation* **100**: 2418–24.

40. Skatrud JB, Dempsey JA (1983). Interaction of sleep state and chemical stimuli in sustaining rhythmic ventilation. *J Appl Physiol* **55**: 813–22.

41. Hanly PJ, Zuberi-Khokhar N (1995). Daytime sleepiness in patients with congestive heart failure and Cheyne-Stokes respiration. *Chest* **107**: 952–8.

42. Levine B, Roehrs T, Stepanski E *et al.* (1987). Fragmenting sleep diminishes its recuperative value. *Sleep* **10**: 590–9.

43. Kaye DM, Lefkovits J, Jennings GL *et al.* (1995). Adverse consequences of high sympathetic nervous activity in the failing human heart. *J Am Coll Cardiol* **26**: 1257–63.

44. Cohn JN, Levine TB, Olivari MT *et al.* (1984). Plasma norepinephrine as a guide to prognosis in patients with congestive heart failure. *New Engl J Med* **311**: 819–23.

45. Goldspink DF, Burniston JG, Clark WA, Tan LB (2004). Catecholamine-induced apoptosis and necrosis in cardiac and skeletal myocytes of the rat *in vivo*: the same or separate death pathways? *Exp Physiol* **89**: 407–16.

46. Mann DL, Kent RL, Parson B *et al.* (1992). Adrenergic effects on the biology of the adult mammalian cardiocyte. *Circulation* **85**: 790–804.

47. Young T, Palta M, Dempsey J *et al.* (1993). The occurrence of sleep-disordered breathing among middle-aged adults. *New Engl J Med* **328**: 1230.

48. Tishler PV, Larkin EK, Schluchter MD, Redline S (2003). Incidence of sleep disordered breathing in an urban adult population: the relative importance of risk factors in the development of sleep-disordered breathing. *J Am Med Assoc* **289**: 2230–7.

49. Mezzanotte WS, Tangel DJ, White DP (1992). Waking genioglossal EMG in sleep apnoea patients versus normal controls (a neuromuscular compensatory mechanism). *J Clin Invest* **89**: 1571.

50. Gould GA, Whyte KF, Rhind GB *et al.* (1988). The sleep hypopnea syndrome. *Am Rev Respir Dis* **137**: 895–8.

51. Rees K, Kingshott RN, Wraith PK, Douglas NJ (2000). Frequency and significance of increased upper airway resistance during sleep. *Am J Respir Crit Care Med* **162**: 1210–14.

52. Engleman HM, Douglas NJ (2004). Sleep. 4: Sleepiness, cognitive function, and quality of life in obstructive sleep apnoea/hypopnoea syndrome. *Thorax* **59**: 618–22.

53. Van Dongen HP, Vitellaro KM, Dinges DF (2005). Individual differences in adult human sleep and wakefulness: leitmotif for a research agenda. *Sleep* **28**: 479.

54. Nieto FJ, Young TB, Lind BK *et al.* (2000). Association of sleep-disordered breathing, sleep apnoea, and hypertension in a large community-based study: Sleep Heart Health Study. *J Am Med Assoc* **283**: 1829–36.

55. Peppard PE, Young T, Palta M, Skatrud J (2000). Prospective study of the association between sleep-disordered breathing and hypertension. *New Engl J Med* **342**: 1378–84.

56. Peker Y, Hedner J, Norum J, Kraiczi H, Carlson J (2002). Increased incidence of cardiovascular disease in middle-aged men with obstructive sleep apnoea: a 7-year follow-up. *Am J Respir Crit Care Med* **166**: 159–65.

57. Yaggi H, Mohsenin V (2004). Obstructive sleep apnoea and stroke. *Lancet Neurol* **3**: 333–42.

58. Young T, Peppard PE, Gottlieb DJ (2002). Epidemiology of obstructive sleep apnoea: a population health perspective. *Am J Respir Crit Care Med* **165**: 1217–39.

59. Vgontzas AN, Tan TL, Bixler EO, Martin LF, Shubert D, Kales A (1994). Sleep apnoea and sleep disruption in obese patients. *Arch Intern Med* **154**: 1705–11.

60. Peppard PE, Young T, Palta M, Dempsey J, Skatrud J (2000). Longitudinal study of moderate weight change and sleep-disordered breathing. *J Am Med Assoc* **284**: 3015–21.

61. Borgel J, Sanner BM, Bittlinsky A *et al.* (2006). Obstructive sleep apnoea and its therapy influence high-density lipoprotein cholesterol serum levels. *Eur Respir J* **27**: 121.

62. Reichmuth KJ, Austin D, Skatrud JB, Young T (2005). Association of sleep apnoea and type 2 diabetes: a population-based study. *Am J Respir Crit Care Med* **172**: 1590.

63. Marrone O, Bonsignore MR (2002). Pulmonary haemodynamics in obstructive sleep apnoea. *Sleep Med Rev* **6**: 175–93.

64. Ip MS, Tse HF, Lam B, Tsang KW, Lam WK (2004). Endothelial function in obstructive sleep apnea and response to treatment. *Am J Respir Crit Care Med* **169**: 348–53.

65. Nieto FJ, Herrington DM, Redline S, Benjamin EJ, Robbins JA (2004). Sleep apnea and markers of vascular endothelial function in a large community sample of older adults. *Am J Respir Crit Care Med* **169**: 354–60.

66. Schulz R, Eisele HJ, Seeger W (2005). Nocturnal atrial fibrillation in a patient with obstructive sleep apnoea. *Thorax* **60**: 174.

67. Gami AS, Pressman G, Caples SM *et al.* (2004). Association of atrial fibrillation and obstructive sleep apnea. *Circulation* **110**: 364–7.

68. Gami AS, Howard DE, Olson EJ, Somers VK (2005). Day–night pattern of sudden death in obstructive sleep apnea. *New Engl J Med* **352**: 1206–14.

69. Lardelli-Claret P, Luna-Del-Castillo J de D, Jimenez-Moleon JJ *et al.* (2003). Association of main driver-dependent risk factors with the risk of causing a vehicle collision in Spain, 1990–1999. *Ann Epidemiol* **13**: 509–17.

70. George CF (2001). Reduction in motor vehicle collisions following treatment of sleep apnoea with nasal CPAP. *Thorax* **56**: 508–12.

71. Campos-Rodriguez F, Pena-Grinan N, Reyes-Nunez N *et al.* (2005). Mortality in obstructive sleep apnea-hypopnea patients treated with positive airway pressure. *Chest* **128**: 624–33.

72. Arand DL, Bonnet MH (1997). Sleep-disordered breathing. In: *Respiratory Care* (ed. GG Burton *et al.*), pp. 295–308. Philadelphia: Lippincott.

73. Gottlieb DJ, Whitney CW, Bonekat WH *et al.* (1999). Relation of sleepiness to respiratory disturbance index: the Sleep Heart Health Study. *Am J Respir Crit Care Med* **159**: 502–7.

74. Naughton MT, Benard DC, Rutherford R *et al.* (1994). Effect of continuous positive airway pressure on central sleep apnoea and nocturnal pCO$_2$ in heart failure. *Am J Respir Crit Care Med* **150**: 1598–604.

75. Naughton MT, Liu PP, Benard DC *et al.* (1995). Treatment of congestive heart failure and Cheyne-Stokes Respiration during sleep by continuous positive airway pressure. *Am J Respir Crit Care Med* **151**: 92–7.

76. Javaheri S (2000). Effects of continuous positive airway pressure on sleep apnoea and ventricular irritability in patients with heart failure. *Circulation* **101**: 392–7.

77. Wilson GN, Wilcox I, Piper AJ *et al.* (1998). Treatment of central sleep apnoea in congestive heart failure with nasal ventilation. *Thorax* **53**: S41–S46.

78. Hanly PJ, Millar TW, Steljes DG *et al.* (1989). The effect of oxygen on respiration and sleep in patients with congestive heart failure. *Ann Intern Med* **111**: 777–82.

79. Andreas S, Clemens C, Sandholzer H *et al.* (1996). Improvement of exercise capacity with treatment of Cheyne-Stokes respiration in patients with congestive heart failure. *J Am Coll Cardiol* **27**: 1486–90.

80. Franklin KA, Eriksson P, Sahlin C *et al.* (1997). Reversal of central sleep apnoea with oxygen. *Chest* **111**: 163–9.

81. Xie A, Rankin F, Rutherford R *et al.* (1997). Effects of inhaled CO$_2$ and added dead space on idiopathic central sleep apnoea. *J Appl Physiol* **82**: 918–26.

82. Pesek CA, Cooley R, Narkiewicz K *et al.* (1999). Theophylline therapy for near-fatal Cheyne-Stokes respiration. A case report. *Ann Intern Med* **130**: 427–30.

83. Lorenzi-Filho G, Rankin F, Bies J *et al.* (1999). Effects of inhaled carbon dioxide and oxygen on Cheyne-Stokes Respiration in patients with heart failure. *Am J Respir Crit Care Med* **159**: 1490–8.

84. Steens RD, Millar TW, Su X *et al.* (1994). Effect of inhaled 3% CO$_2$ on Cheyne-Stokes respiration in congestive heart failure. *Sleep* **17**: 61–8.

85. Bonnet MH, Dexter JR, Arand DL (1990). The effect of triazolam on arousal and respiration in central sleep apnoea patients. *Sleep* **13**: 31–41.

86. The Task Force of the Working Group on Heart Failure of the European Society of Cardiology (1997). The treatment of heart failure. *Eur Heart J* **18**: 736–53.

87. Tan LB, Mills J, Wright DJ (1999). Management of heart failure. *J R Coll Physicians Lond* **33**: 25–30.

88. Yasuma F, Hayashi H, Noda S *et al.* (1995). A case of mitral regurgitation whose nocturnal periodic breathing was improved after mitral valve replacement. *Japan Heart J* **36**: 267–72.

89. Loredo JS, Ancoli-Israel S, Kim EJ, Lim WJ, Dimsdale JE (2006). Effect of continuous positive airway pressure versus supplemental oxygen on sleep quality in obstructive sleep apnea: a placebo-CPAP-controlled study. *Sleep* **29**: 564–71.

90. Krachman SL, D'Alonzo GE, Berger TJ *et al.* (1999). Comparison of oxygen therapy with nasal continuous positive airway pressure on Cheyne-Stokes respiration during sleep in congestive heart failure. *Chest* **116**: 1550–7.

91. Buckle P, Millar T, Kryger MH (1992). The effect of short-term nasal CPAP on Cheyne-Stokes respiration in congestive heart failure. *Chest* **102**: 31–5.

92. Bradley TD, Holloway RM, McLaughlin PR *et al.* (1992). Cardiac output response to continuous positive airway pressure in congestive heart failure. *Am Rev Resp Dis* **145**: 377–82.

93. Naughton MT, Rahman MA, Hara K *et al.* (1995). Effect of continuous positive airway pressure on intrathoracic and left ventricular transmural pressure in patients with congestive heart failure. *Circulation* **91**: 1725–31.

94. Metha S, Liu PP, Fitzgerald FS *et al.* (2000). Effects of continuous positive airway pressure on cardiac volumes in patients with ischemic and dilated cardiomyopathy. *Am J Respir Crit Care Med* **161**: 128–34.

95. Welte T (2000). Noninvasive ventilation in acute respiratory insufficiency. *Pneumologie* **54**: 5–9.

96. Sin SS, Logan AG, Fitzgerald FS *et al.* (2000). Effects of continuous positive airway pressure on cardiovascular outcomes in heart failure patients with and without Cheyne-Stokes respiration. *Circulation* **102**: 61–6.

97. Köhnlein T, Welte T, Tan LB, Elliott MW (2002). Assisted ventilation for heart failure patients with Cheyne-Stokes respiration. *Eur Respir J* **20**: 934–41.

98. Teschler H, Dohring J, Wang YM, Berthon-Jones M (2001). Adaptive pressure support servo-ventilation: a novel treatment for Cheyne-Stokes respiration in heart failure. *Am J Respir Crit Care Med* **164**: 614–19.

99. Köhnlein T, Golpon H, Hoffmann B *et al.* (1998). Ventilation in patients with Cheyne-Stokes respiration. *Pneumologie* **52**: 648.

100. Staniforth AD, Kinnear WJ, Starling R *et al.* (1998). Effect of oxygen on sleep quality, cognitive function and sympathetic activity in patients with chronic heart failure and Cheyne-Stokes respiration. *Eur Heart J* **19**: 922–8.

101. Cherniack NS, Longobardo GS (1986). Abnormalities in respiratory rhythm. In: *Handbook of Physiology* (ed. NS Cherniack, JG Widdicombe), pp. 729–49. Bethesda, MD: American Physiological Society.

102. Garrigue S, Bordier P, Jais P *et al.* (2002). Benefit of atrial pacing in sleep apnoea syndrome. *New Engl J Med* **346**: 404–12.

103. Luthje L, Unterberg-Buchwald C, Dajani D, Vollmann D, Hasenfuss G, Andreas S (2005). Atrial overdrive pacing in patients with sleep apnoea with implanted pacemaker. *Am J Respir Crit Care Med* **172**: 118–22.

104. Pepin JL, Defaye P, Garrigue S, Poezevara Y, Levy P (2005). Overdrive atrial pacing does not improve obstructive sleep apnoea syndrome. *Eur Respir J* **25**: 343–7.

105. Unterberg C, Luthje L, Szych J, Vollmann D, Hasenfuss G, Andreas S (2005). Atrial overdrive pacing compared to CPAP in patients with obstructive sleep apnoea syndrome. *Eur Heart J.*

106. Moe GW, Armstrong P (1999). Pacing-induced heart failure: a model to study the mechanism of disease progression and novel therapy in heart failure. *Cardiovasc Res* **42**: 591–9.

Chapter 11

Fatigue and exercise intolerance

Rebecca Boxer and Ileana Piña

Introduction

Fatigue is a prominent symptom in patients with heart failure (HF) and has a profound effect on quality of life. Fatigue limits a person's daily activity, their ability to perform activities of daily living (ADLs), and initiates a cycle of physical decline in the chronically ill.[1,2] Fatigue may be one of the only symptoms recognized by the patient with HF, especially in older adults. Older patients may simply curb their activities rather than challenging their fatigue and/or bringing it to medical attention (see also Chapter 17). Fatigue is also difficult to study due its subjective nature. Fatigue can be described as an ongoing chronic tiredness throughout the day or exercise intolerance. A poor ability to tolerate exercise can set up a cycle of advancing fatigue and deconditioning resulting in physical disability. The contributors to fatigue are multifactorial and the interaction between multiple physiological and psychosocial factors is not well understood. Physiological contributors include decreased cardiac output, skeletal muscle abnormalities, endothelial dysfunction, neurohormonal derangements, and inflammation. In addition, many non-cardiovascular abnormalities common in patients with HF contribute to fatigue and include: anemia, pulmonary disease, sleep apnea, deconditioning, poor nutrition, depression, diabetes, and medications. Although many of these co-morbidities have been studied to some extent, only very infrequently have they been definitively linked to fatigue. In this chapter we will review fatigue and exercise intolerance as well as management strategies for the patient with HF.

Heart failure

Poorly compensated or inadequately treated HF is an important contributor to fatigue and exercise intolerance in patients and should spearhead investigation. Increased fluid volume in the lungs and other body tissues will greatly impact a patient's daily physical function, appetite, and cardiopulmonary reserve (see also Chapter 3). However, overly zealous diuresis may also lead to fatigue and poor physical function due to activation of the renin–angiotensin–aldosterone system (RAAS), volume and electrolyte depletion, and worsening of renal dysfunction. Utilization of medication to treat and stabilize HF according to published guidelines should be initiated and maximized as tolerated.[3,4] These include angiotensin-converting enzyme inhibitors (ACE-I) and/or angiotensin II receptor blockers (ARBs) for those who are ACE-I intolerant. Blockade of the RAAS with medication has been linked to a reduction in fatigue[5] and improvement in submaximal exercise capacity.[6] A comprehensive review of ACE-I demonstrates that they may have a beneficial effect on body composition and physical performance and highlights the influence that RAAS blockade can have on muscle.[7] β-Blockers (BBs) are also a critical part of this regimen. Initial fatigue from BBs is often mild and transitory and will often dissipate. Should BB-induced fatigue be a concern, dosing could be administered at bedtime to minimize symptoms. Recovery of cardiac function and reverse remodeling are the intended goals of these therapies and can improve function and quality of life[3,4] in addition to decreasing mortality and hospitalizations. Upward titration to guideline doses of medication should be sought, even in those who are predominantly receiving palliation and end-of-life care in that the medications can markedly reduce symptoms and increase patient comfort (see also Chapter 4).

Pathogenesis

There has been great effort to identify causal relationship between physiologic changes in the HF syndrome and fatigue. It has become clear that fatigue in HF patients is due to a network of physiological changes in multiple body systems (Table 11.1). These changes are not uniform and do not take place in all patients.

Cardiac output

Decreased cardiac output is a hallmark of HF and is evident in the poorly perfused patient who is vasoconstricted and cool to the touch in the extremities. Cardiac output responds to increased demand of tissues with physical exercise by increasing heart rate and stroke volume. As exercise intensifies increased cardiac output is accomplished mostly by increased heart rate. Patients with HF are unable to augment cardiac output in

Table 11.1 Factors which contribute to fatigue in HF

Inadequate control of volume/pressures
Decreased cardiac output with poor response to activity
Metabolic and structural skeletal muscle changes
Decreased skeletal muscle blood flow
Endothelial dysfunction
Inflammation/cytokine release
Ischemia
Chronic renal disease/uremia
Anemia
Dehydration (from over-diuresis)
Sleep apnea (central and/or obstructive)
Malnutrition/protein wasting
Medication side-effects
Depression
Deconditioning
Other conditions: diabetes, thyroid disease, peripheral vascular disease

response to exercise due to an already maximized stroke volume, although in the well-compensated patient this may only become obvious when nearing peak exercise. In the era of BBs, increase of heart rate with exercise may also be blunted. Decreased cardiac output and inability to augment cardiac output with exercise has traditionally been thought to be the largest contributor to fatigue, breathlessness, and exercise intolerance. However, there is no convincing correlation between cardiac function at rest and cardiac function with exercise.[8,9] Reported symptoms of fatigue and dyspnea with exercise do not necessarily correlate with hemodynamic parameters.[10] Skeletal muscle perfusion is an important part of exercise intolerance, but some of those with abnormal cardiac output do not have impaired skeletal blood flow.[11] In addition, clinical trials that aimed to increase cardiac output and improve function with inotropes have shown an increase in arrhythmias and mortality.[12,13] In fact, left ventricular (LV) end-diastolic pressures (filling pressures) are better correlated with survival than cardiac output.[14]

Skeletal muscle

Skeletal muscle plays an important role in fatigue and exercise intolerance in patients with HF. Muscle strength has been found to be predictive of adverse outcome.[15] Changes occur in skeletal muscle structure, metabolism, and perfusion although the relationship to fatigue and exercise intolerance is still not well understood. Structurally, type I muscle fibers (slow fibers) utilized in low-endurance exercise and more resistant to fatigue are decreased while type II fibers utilized for short bursts of activity (fast fibers) and more easily fatigued are increased.[16–19] Resistance to fatigue with exercise correlates with measures of fiber size.[19] Myosin heavy chain type I fibers have been correlated with peak oxygen uptake (VO_2)[20] and apoptosis in skeletal muscle has also been correlated with exercise capacity.[21] Skeletal muscle metabolism represented by reduced glycogen content has been linked to exertional fatigue in both normals and HF patients.[22–24] Oxidative enzymes such as citrate synthase have also been shown to be reduced[25] and inversely related to blood lactate accumulation (Table 11.2).[26]

Blood flow to exercising muscle has also been studied, but no definitive link has been made to fatigue.[11] Decreased blood flow to exercising muscle is due to a variety of reasons including abnormalities in the vascular endothelium. Endothelial release of nitric oxide (a vasodilator) can be attenuated in HF but some reversal can take place with exercise.[27] Stimulation of the renin–angiotensin system and sympathetic nervous system as well as elevated endothelin all contribute to an increase in vasoconstriction and diminished blood flow. Decreased perfusion to exercising skeletal muscle results in anaerobic metabolism and a build-up of lactic acid. For any given workload, the HF patient will develop muscle fatigue and anaerobic metabolism faster then healthy subjects. Poorly perfused skeletal muscle can ultimately result in muscle wasting and decreased oxygen extraction and muscle fatigue. Muscle recovery from exercise may also be prolonged. However, a percentage of patients with poor exercise tolerance will have abnormalities in lactate despite normal muscle blood flow perfusion, suggesting intrinsic muscle abnormalities to be a cause.[11]

Table 11.2 Skeletal muscle changes in HF

Changes in structure	Changes in metabolism
Loss of Type I (slow twitch) fibers (endurance fibers)	Reduced glycogen content
Increase in Type II (fast twitch) fibers (easily fatigued)	Decreased citrate synthase (mitochondrial oxidative enzyme)
Decreased fiber size (cross- sectional area)	Increase in reactive oxygen species
Decreased capillary density	Decreased pH
Decreased mitochondrial size and number	Ergoreflex overactivity
Apoptosis	

Respiratory muscles may also be affected and can impact upon exercise tolerance, resulting in a patient easily becoming dyspneic with exertion and losing ventilatory reserve.[28] Training of these muscles may improve function and decrease dyspnea.[29,30]

The muscle hypothesis (Fig 11.1) of HF describes the relationship between multiple systems which contribute to physiological decline in the patient with HF.[32] Aberrant signals from the skeletal muscle system via ergoreflex play an important role in the cycle of neurohormonal response and may play an important role in exercise intolerance. Ergoreceptors in exercising muscle respond to the accumulation of metabolic by-products.

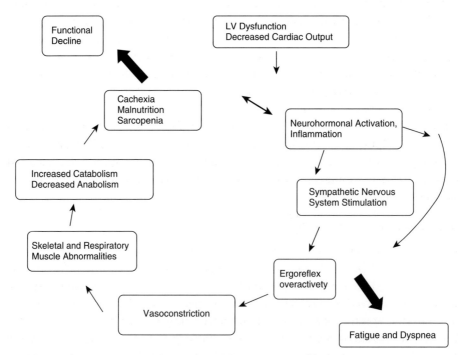

Fig. 11.1 The muscle hypothesis of HF. Adapted from Coats et al.[31] (adapted and reproduced with permission from the BMJ Publishing Group).

Initially the response of ergoreceptors is to compensate for exercising skeletal muscle and improve delivery of nutrients by increasing sympathetic activity, vasoconstriction in non-exercising muscle, and ventilation. Over-stimulation of the sympathetic nervous system, decreased vagal tone, and hyperventilation contribute to dyspnea and exercise intolerance.[32] This can result in an increase in peripheral resistance and ultimately perfusion of exercising muscles Decreased peripheral muscle mass may also occur due to increased ergoreflex activity.[33] Exercise training probably attenuates these responses to ergoreflex overactivity.[34]

Neuroendocrine changes and cachexia

Neuroendocrine disturbance in patients with the HF syndrome affect skeletal muscle wasting and fatigue. There has been increased interest in the endocrinology of HF and the development of cachexia. An association of decreased anabolic hormones such as testosterone, dehydroepiandrosterone (DHEA), and insulin-growth factor-I has been identified. Repletion of anabolic hormones has been unimpressive but has shown some benefit in physical function.[35,36] Increased markers of catabolism, such as cortisol and cytokines, have been theorized to contribute to the development of muscle loss.[37,38] Inflammatory mediators such as tumor necrosis factor-α (TNFα), interleukin-1 (IL-1), and IL-6 affect muscle catabolism and fatigue in HF as in other diseases but the mechanism for this is unknown.[39] However, trials that have studied antagonism of inflammatory markers have failed to show improvements in outcome.[40] Excess sympathetic stimulation, resulting in elevations of epinephrine and norepinephrine often seen in HF, may affect skeletal muscle resulting in local vasoconstriction, poor perfusion, ischemia, and radical formation.[41]

Development of cardiac cachexia is a well-known phenomenon in end-stage HF. Approximately 20% of HF patients are cachectic.[42] Often cachexia is defined by weight loss alone with loss in all body compartments: fat, muscle, and bone.[43,44] It has become clear that the syndrome is more far-reaching and includes changes in hormonal balance,[37,45] increased inflammation,[46] and insulin resistance.[48] An increase in resting metabolic rate may occur in some patients.[48] Decreased nutrition due to poor intake and/or poor absorption due to bowel edema may also play a role. Cachectic patients are markedly fatigued and have poor exercise tolerance. Although not yet adequately studied, exercise may have an important role in reversing the cachectic state in HF patients (see also Chapter 13).

Inactivity and deconditioning

HF is associated with physical decline that includes difficulty performing ADLs, development of frailty, falls, disability, and increased utilization of health services.[49–51] Currently, the physiological mechanisms underlying the development of physical decline are poorly understood. Inactivity due to the symptoms of poorly controlled HF including breathlessness and fatigue rapidly result in deconditioning, especially in the older adult. Co-morbidities such as coronary artery disease with angina, arthritis, diabetic neuropathy, and peripheral vascular disease will also contribute to inactivity. Individuals continue to lose muscle strength and stamina which enhances their decline. Repeat hospitalizations are an important part of this downward spiral of functioning in the chronically ill.[52,53] Older patients who are frequently hospitalized rapidly lose strength and become dependent in basic daily activities. The cycle of deconditioning leads to further fatigue and it becomes difficult to different between symptoms of HF, co-morbidities, and/or deterioration due to inactivity. Breaking this cycle takes increasing activity through regular daily activity and exercise and pain control if needed. Utilizing physical therapy and rehabilitation can help in this process.

Post-exercise fatigue

Fatigue during exercise is a prominent symptom in patients with HF. The ability to perform ADLs has been shown to be reduced in HF patients and may be more relevant to the patient's quality of life than peak aerobic capacity.[54] ADLs involve a slow, low level of work and may be equated with a 'slow' treadmill exercise protocol. This may be more likely to provoke fatigue that a 'fast' protocol, which is more likely to provoke dyspnea.[55] Patients often report fatigue that can last beyond the performance of activity and complain of post-exercise fatigue that appears to be out of proportion to an exercise bout.[1,18,56] Often the symptom of fatigue can persist for up to 24 h after an exercise test. Post-exercise fatigue may also be a disincentive to attending cardiac rehabilitation sessions. Currently, the mechanism responsible for this post-exercise fatigue is unknown but is probably as complex as the fatigue symptoms experienced during activity.[11,16,57–59] The sensation of post-exercise fatigue may have an impact on the quality of life in these patients and may be a deterrent to the performance of regular physical activity. Subsequently, HF patients may avoid activities that could evoke symptoms of post-activity fatigue[54,60] thus perpetuating a cycle of decreased exercise tolerance and deconditioning.

Exercise and cardiac rehabilitation

Evidence indicates that exercise training can improve exercise tolerance and quality of life for the patient with HF.[61] There are a variety of small studies which have looked at the effects of exercise in the patient with HF. Belardinelli et al.[62] conducted the one study that retrospectively evaluated morbidity and mortality and showed that cardiac-related mortality and HF-related hospitalizations were decreased as well. A Cochrane Review of 29 studies found that exercise training increased exercise duration, work capacity, and maximal oxygen consumption (VO_2 max). In those studies that measured quality of life, the majority found an improvement with exercise, although different instruments were used.[63] It is unclear if exercise training will impact upon a patient's generalized fatigue. Submaximal exercise (exercise which does not reach the anaerobic threshold) may be more representative of day to day activity. Therefore improvement in submaximal exercise capacity may be more important for the fatigue-limited patient. Studies that have demonstrated improvement in submaximal exercise capacity have utilized both aerobic and endurance training.[64–66] There is also some evidence that something as simple as a home walking program may provide benefit as well.[67,68]

Heart failure with preserved systolic function

Fatigue and exercise intolerance are commonly seen in patients with preserved systolic function (PSF), also called HF with normal ejection fraction (HFNEF). Although these patients have a better prognosis than those with depressed systolic function, symptoms of breathlessness and fatigue can be prominent. More common in older adults and women,[69] the relationship with the development of fatigue and deconditioning is not completely understood. In comparison with those with systolic failure, those with PSF have equally reduced peak and submaximal exercise performance as well as measures of quality of life.[70,71] Post-hospitalization, those with PSF maintain or decline in physical function similarly to those with isolated systolic failure.[52,72]

Co-morbidities and fatigue

There are multiple co-morbidities that are commonly seen in the HF patient which can contribute to fatigue and exercise intolerance. This section will review these disorders.

Anemia

Anemia contributes to both fatigue and dyspnea by reducing the oxygen-carrying capacity of the blood. This is complicated by the decreased physiologic reserve and the HF patients' inability to compensate to the anemic state. These patients are at increased risk for muscle tissue hypoxia and anerobic metabolism. The prevalence of anemia in HF patients varies widely due to study differences in the laboratory definition of anemia and differences in populations studied. In a recent systematic review of the literature the prevalence ranged from 9–69.7% but increases with increasing HF severity[73] and tends to be more common in those with higher New York Heart Association (NYHA) class. Those HF patients with anemia tended to have a lower quality of life, decreased oxygen utilization at maximal exercise (VO_2max), decreased exercise duration as well as shorter 6-min walk distance.[74] Studies which have addressed functional capacity with administration of erythropoietin and correction of anemia in HF patients have seen improvement in NYHA class,[75] and one small study showed improvement in exercise capacity.[76] Adverse effects of this treatment have also been demonstrated, and include thrombogenic effects and hypertension. At present there are no established recommendations for treatment of anemia in the HF Practice Guidelines 2006.[3,4] Evaluation and treatment of underlying causes of anemia such as iron or vitamin B_{12} deficiency should be treated. In the very fatigued patient the clinician may choose to treat anemia with erythropoietin for symptomatic relief. A randomized controlled trial using darbepoetin has been initiated.

Dehydration and electrolytes

Chronic dehydration and over-diuresis should be considered when evaluating a patient for fatigue. Usually uremic toxins need to become quite elevated before a patient will experience the lethargy of renal failure. Losses of electrolytes such as magnesium, potassium, and calcium, common with the use of loop diuretics, can lead to muscle fatigue and generalized weakness. Vitamin D deficiency may be associated with low magnesium and calcium levels and vitamin D should be repleted in these patients. Patients on diuretics should have electrolytes followed and routinely replaced.

Minimizing diuretics by utilizing other HF-stabilizing medications such as angiotensin converting enzyme inhibitors (ACE-I), angiotensin receptor blockers (ARBs), and β-blockers (BBs) is an important part of HF management as well as preserving renal function. Use of these other medications may actually preclude the use of diuretics. In addition medications, that block RAAS may have a direct effect on exercise tolerance and fatigue (see Chapter 4).

Medical therapy

β-blockers, which are a cornerstone of HF management are known to cause fatigue, although, the frequency of this side effect may be overestimated.[77] The value of BB therapy will outweigh the adverse effects for most patients. Strategies to decrease BB-related fatigue are important and include once a day dosing; particularly dosing at bedtime. Many patients will find that BB-related fatigue abates with time.

Physiological changes in HF such as decreased hepatic and renal perfusion, gut congestion, hypoalbuminemia, and chronic kidney disease contribute to changes in drug absorption and metabolism. Changes in body composition may result in alterations in the volume of distribution of many medications. This can result in higher serum concentrations of various drugs as well as a prolonged half-life. This is of particular concern with sedating medication in HF patients. These medications should be used cautiously and at the lowest effective dose. Patients with HF often complain of poor sleep, and careful investigation of causative factors should be initiated. This includes evaluation for paroxysmal nocturnal dyspnea, orthopnea, angina, and sleep apnea. Sleep medications may actually compound the problem in terms of daytime fatigue and sleepiness. Treatment of the underlying disorder is often more effective. Careful review of over-the-counter medications and herbal remedies is an important part of the fatigue assessment in HF patients. Classes of medications that tend to be the most fatigue provoking are antidepressants, antipsychotics, antihistamines, benzodiazepines, muscle relaxants, opiates, and other sleep aids. Over-the-counter medications usually contain antihistamines, often diphenhydramine. This medication can last in a patient's system into the following day resulting in daytime fatigue and somnolence as well as being a frequent cause of confusion in the older adult.

Depression

Depression is a well-known co-morbidity with cardiovascular disease and is common in HF. In the outpatient setting close to 50% of patients are depressed,[78] although a wide range has been noted at 9–60%.[79] Depression has been linked to decreased adherence to the medication regimen[82] which is a well known cause of readmission.[81] Fatigue is often a common symptom of depression, although it may be subjective and not proven with objective physiological testing.[81] Depression also may be linked to functional decline over time in these patients.[83] Patients with HF should be evaluated for depression and treated aggressively. There are multiple screening tools which can easily be used in the office setting: two examples are the Geriatric Depression Scale[84] for older patients or the Beck Depression Inventory[85] (see also Chapter 15).

Sleep disorders

Lack of adequate, restful sleep can be a chronic problem for the patient with HF and a major contributor to fatigue. A careful sleep history can illuminate the source of difficulty. Those who have prominent night-time symptoms, such as paroxysmal nocturnal dyspnea and orthopnea, which disrupt sleep may benefit from the addition of nitrates at bedtime. If nocturia is the major source of disruption, diuretics can be administered later in the day and prior to bedtime. Volume is thus removed before sleep and may decrease the need for frequent urination at night. Anxiety and depression can also be disruptive to sleep and should be addressed as mentioned. A review of sleep hygiene can be helpful and advice to the patient should include:

- Sleep only when sleepy.
- If you can't fall asleep within 20 min, get up and do something relaxing and quiet such as reading.
- Avoid daytime naps so you will be tired at bedtime.
- Get up and go to bed the same time every day.
- Regular exercise may improve sleep, but not before bedtime.
- Listen to relaxing music, read something soothing for 15 min, have a cup of caffeine-free tea, do relaxation exercises.
- Avoid watching TV before bedtime.
- Avoid caffeine, nicotine, and alcohol for at least 4–6 h before bedtime.
- Have a light snack before bedtime so your stomach is not too empty.
- Make sure your bed and bedroom are quiet and comfortable: a cooler room is often ideal.
- Use sunlight to set your biological clock and get out into the sun during the day.

Sleep apnea is also common in patients with HF, with up to 50% of patients with the disorder, including central, obstructive, and mixed types. Sleep apnea can be a major source of fatigue and daytime somnolence. It tends to be more common in men than women. HF patients suspected of having sleep apnea should be evaluated. Sleep apnea will not only disrupt sleep but can also increase systemic and pulmonary pressures resulting in worsening HF (see also Chapter 10).

Malnutrition

The role that malnutrition plays in fatigue in the HF patient is unclear. Malnutrition is a well-known part of the HF syndrome and includes caloric deficiency, micronutrient deficiencies, as well as protein malnutrition. Loss of appetite in chronic HF is well known and is probably due to circulating cytokines and gut edema. Edema of the bowel is also

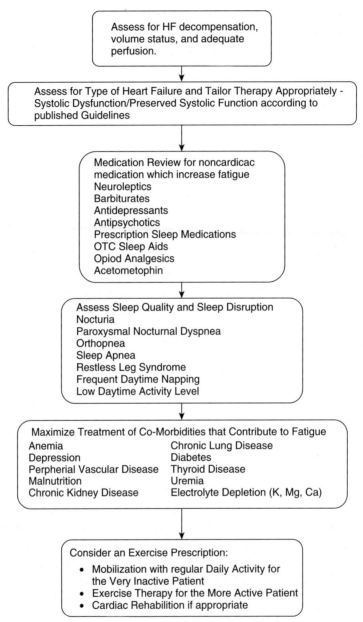

Fig. 11.2 Algorithm for assessing fatigue in the HF Patient.

likely to affect the ability to absorb nutrients.[86,87] In addition, the edematous bowel is cited as an important factor in inflammation due to bacterial translocation and endotoxins entering the circulation.[86] In addition the chronic use of loop diuretics can result in chronic losses of micronutrients such as potassium, calcium, magnesium, and zinc.

There has been little study on the effect of the replacement of nutrients in this patient population. There is increasing evidence that vitamin D deficiency is common in HF patients and this theoretically could affect physical function, as seen in other populations (Boxer, unpublished data).[88–90] Low levels of co-enzyme Q (an antioxidant and a factor in mitochondrial synthesis of ATP) has also been cited as deficient in HF patients with repletion improving exercise tolerance.[91] Witte *et al.*[87] reported improvement in quality of life scores, mostly due to improvement in fatigue and breathlessness with a high-dose micronutrient supplement in HF patients.

Associated conditions

Many conditions are commonly seen in those with HF and can affect exercise performance and fatigue.

- Peripheral vascular disease and claudication will perpetuate physical decline and exercise intolerance. This can add to the cycle of deconditioning in these patients.
- Diabetes with poorly controlled glucose can result in chronic fatigue and muscle weakness. This in addition to peripheral neuropathy can have an additive effect in the chronic deconditioning seen in the HF patient.
- Thyroid disease is also an important contributor to fatigue as well as the cause of HF in some circumstances. Correction of thyroid disorders is necessary in these patients.

Quantifying fatigue and exercise intolerance

A variety of methods can be used to try and quantify a patient's fatigue and exercise intolerance. Health status questionnaires such as the Minnesota Living with Heart Failure,[92] Kansas City Cardiomyopathy Questionnaire,[93] and the Medical Outcomes Study 36-Item Short-Form General Health Survey (SF36) will all give information on fatigue as well as vitality and physical function. A specific scale for fatigue can be used as well. The Yale Dyspnea-Fatigue Index is a validated tool used in HF patients to determine the magnitude and pace of a task that produces either dyspnea or fatigue and the level of functional impairment. The index has three components graded from 0–4. The aggregate score is then 0–12 with 0 for the worst symptoms and 12 for no symptoms.[94]

Exercise tests including the 6-min walk test and graded exercise tests give insight into a patient's fatigue, dyspnea, and exercise intolerance. These tests help correlate a subject's sense of fatigue and dyspnea with their actual exercise capacity. Cardiopulmonary testing (CPX) is the gold standard to assess a patient's physical ability and provides information not only on cardiac and pulmonary function but also skeletal muscle function and deconditioning. The respiratory exchange ratio ($RER = VCO_2/VO_2$) measured during CPX testing is a good measure of patient effort during the test. A patient's perceived effort can also be measured by the Borg scale.[95] The Borg scale requires that the patient understands the measure as 'total body effort'. Tolerance for submaximal exercise can also be measured and may be the closest correlate with regular daily activity.

Exercise recommendations

Guidelines in exercise training in HF patients are not yet available and are an area of active research. The following recommendations are adapted from Piña *et al.*[61] An exercise prescription for the stable HF patient should be initiated to maintain function and muscle strength. Prescriptions should be tailored to the individual patient and in the very debilitated patient may be as simple as performing their own ADLs. Cardiopulmonary exercise testing at the outset of an exercise program is an objective assessment of functional capacity and can help guide an appropriate exercise prescription. Basing exercise intensity on heart rate (HR) alone may not be possible for patients on BBs. Exercise intensity can be based on 70–80% of peak VO_2 in the stronger more stable patient and 60% of peak VO_2 in the more functionally impaired patient. In patients taking BBs, the percentage of HR reserve can also be used to guide intensity. HR reserve is the difference between the resting HR and the peak HR on an exercise test, added to the baseline HR. A level of 60–70% of HR reserve is a reasonable intensity recommendation. Patients who cannot tolerate CPX testing should be stabilized before an exercise regimen is initiated. Exercise should be symptom driven and interval training with periods of rest may be better tolerated. Initiation of an exercise program is best done in a supervised setting and then transitioned to home.

Patients should be instructed on an appropriate warm-up period prior to exercise and a cool down post-exercise. Warm-up should be at least 15 min prior to an exercise period of 20–30 min at a variable intensity depending on the patient. Patients may need to have a day of rest between days with exercise, although if they are able they should be encouraged to walk on days without more strenuous exercise.

The recommendations, benefits, and safety of resistance training in the patient with HF have not yet been established. Strengthening of specific muscle groups is encouraged, including the upper and lower extremities.

Whether exercise in HF patients improves outcomes is the focus of a large multicenter randomized US National Institutes of Health trial, HF ACTION, which will be completed in 2008. The trial is testing the hypothesis that aerobic training in addition to excellent evidenced-based medical therapy will improve the combined endpoint of all-cause hospitalizations and mortality when compared with medical therapy alone. The results of this trial are eagerly awaited.

Summary

Fatigue and dyspnea are common symptoms in the patient with HF and often worsen with advancing HF. Fatigue probably results from derangements in multiple physiological systems. Guideline recommended medical management of HF and treatment of underlying disorders is important in controlling symptoms. Attention to nutrition and exercise is important when developing a treatment plan.

References

1. Cohen-Solal A, Laperche T, Morvan D, Geneves M, Caviezel B, Gourgon R (1995). Prolonged kinetics of recovery of oxygen consumption after maximal graded exercise in patients with chronic heart failure. Analysis with gas exchange measurements and NMR spectroscopy. *Circulation* **91**: 2924–32.
2. Oka RK, Stotts NA, Dae MW, Haskell WL, Gortner SR (1993). Daily physical activity levels in congestive heart failure. *Am J Cardiol* **71**: 921–5.

3. Hunt SA, Abraham WT, Chin MH *et al.* (2005). ACC/AHA 2005 guideline update for the diagnosis and management of chronic heart failure in the adult. *J Am Coll Cardiol* **46**: 1116–43.

4. HFSA 2006 comprehensive heart failure practice guideline. *J Card Fail* **12**: e1–e122.

5. Riegger GA, Bouzo H, Petr P *et al.* (1999). Improvement in exercise tolerance and symptoms of congestive heart failure during treatment with candesartan cilexetil. Symptom, Tolerability, Response to Exercise Trial of Candesartan Cilexetil in Heart Failure (STRETCH) investigators. *Circulation* **100**: 2224–30.

6. Blanchet M, Sheppard R, Racine N *et al.* (2005). Effects of angiotensin-converting enzyme inhibitor plus irbesartan on maximal and submaximal exercise capacity and neurohumoral activation in patients with congestive heart failure. *Am Heart J* **149**: 938.

7. Carter CS, Onder G, Kritchevsky SB, Pahor MR (2005). Angiotensin-converting enzyme inhibition intervention in elderly persons: effects on body composition and physical performance. *J Gerontol A: Biol Sci Med Sci* **60**: 1437–46.

8. Franciosa JA, Park M, Levine TB (1981). Lack of correlation between exercise capacity and indexes of resting left ventricular performance in heart failure. *Am J Cardiol.* **47**: 33–9.

9. Myers J, Froelicher VF (1991). Hemodynamic determinants of exercise capacity in chronic heart failure. *Ann Intern Med* **115**: 377–86.

10. Wilson JR, Rayos G, Yeoh TK, Gothard P, Bak K (1995). Dissociation between exertional symptoms and circulatory function in patients with heart failure. *Circulation* **92**: 47–53.

11. Wilson JR, Mancini DM, Dunkman WB (1993). Exertional fatigue due to skeletal muscle dysfunction in patients with heart failure. *Circulation* **87**: 470–5.

12. Packer M, Carver JR, Rodeheffer RJ, Ivanhoe RJ *et al.* (1991). Effect of oral milrinone on mortality in severe chronic heart failure. The PROMISE Study Research Group. *New Engl J Med* **325**: 1468–75.

13. Cuffe MS, Califf RM, Adams KF, Jr *et al.* for Outcomes of a Prospective Trial of Intravenous Milrinone for Exacerbations of Chronic Heart Failure (OPTIME-CHF) investigators (2002). Short-term intravenous milrinone for acute exacerbation of chronic heart failure: a randomized controlled trial. *J Am Med Assoc* **287**: 1541–7.

14. Stevenson LW, Tillisch JH, Hamilton M *et al.* (1990). Importance of hemodynamic response to therapy in predicting survival with ejection fraction less than or equal to 20% secondary to ischemic or nonischemic dilated cardiomyopathy. *Am J Cardiol* **66**: 1348–54.

15. Hulsmann M, Quittan M, Berger R *et al.* (2004). Muscle strength as a predictor of long-term survival in severe congestive heart failure. *Eur J Heart Fail* **6**: 101–7.

16. Sullivan MJ, Green HJ, Cobb FR (1990). Skeletal muscle biochemistry and histology in ambulatory patients with long-term heart failure. *Circulation* **81**: 518–27.

17. Lipkin DP, Jones DA, Round JM, Poole-Wilson PA (1988). Abnormalities of skeletal muscle in patients with chronic heart failure. *Int J Cardiol* **18**: 187–95.

18. Drexler H, Riede U, Munzel T, Konig H, Funke E, Just H (1992). Alterations of skeletal muscle in chronic heart failure. *Circulation* **85**: 1751–9.

19. Massie BM, Simonini A, Sahgal P, Wells L, Dudley GA (1996). Relation of systemic and local muscle exercise capacity to skeletal muscle characteristics in men with congestive heart failure. *J Am Coll Cardiol* **27**: 140–5.

20. Sullivan MJ, Duscha BD, Klitgaard H, Kraus WE, Cobb FR, Saltin B (1997). Altered expression of myosin heavy chain in human skeletal muscle in chronic heart failure. *Med Sci Sports Exerc* **29**: 860.

21. Vescovo G, Volterrani M, Zennaro R *et al.* (2000). Apoptosis in the skeletal muscle of patients with heart failure: investigation of clinical and biochemical changes. *Heart* **84**: 431–7.

22. Mancini D, Benaminovitz A, Cordisco ME, Karmally W, Weinberg A (1999). Slowed glycogen utilization enhances exercise endurance in patients with heart failure. *J Am Coll Cardiol* **34**: 1807–12.

23. Coyle EF, Coggan AR, Hemmert MK, Ivy JL (1986). Muscle glycogen utilization during prolonged strenuous exercise when fed carbohydrate. *J Appl Physiol* **61**: 165–72.

24. Musch TI, Ghaul MR, Tranchitella V, Zelis R (1990). Skeletal muscle glycogen depletion during submaximal exercise in rats with chronic heart failure. *Basic Res Cardiol* **85**: 606–18.

25. Schaufelberger M, Eriksson BO, Held P, Swedberg K (1996). Skeletal muscle metabolism during exercise in patients with chronic heart failure. *Heart* **76**: 29–34.

26. Sullivan MJ, Green HJ, Cobb FR (1991). Altered skeletal muscle metabolic response to exercise in chronic heart failure. Relation to skeletal muscle aerobic enzyme activity. *Circulation* **84**: 1597–607.

27. Hambrecht R, Fiehn E, Weigl C *et al.* (1998). Regular physical exercise corrects endothelial dysfunction and improves exercise capacity in patients with chronic heart failure. *Circulation* **98**: 2709–15.

28. Mancini DM, Henson D, LaManca J, Levine S (1994). Evidence of reduced respiratory muscle endurance in patients with heart failure. *J Am Coll Cardiol* **24**: 972–81.

29. Laoutaris I, Dritsas A, Brown MD, Manginas A, Alivizatos PA, Cokkinos DV (2004). Inspiratory muscle training using an incremental endurance test alleviates dyspnea and improves functional status in patients with chronic heart failure. *Eur J Cardiovasc Prev Rehabil* **11**: 489–96.

30. McConnell TR, Mandak JS, Sykes JS, Fesniak H, Dasgupta H (2003). Exercise training for heart failure patients improves respiratory muscle endurance, exercise tolerance, breathlessness, and quality of life. *J Cardiopulmon Rehabil* **23**: 10–16.

31. Coats AJ, Clark AL, Piepoli M, Volterrani M, Poole-Wilson PA (1994). Symptoms and quality of life in heart failure: the muscle hypothesis. *Br Heart J* **72**(Suppl.): S36–S39.

32. Ponikowski PP, Chua TP, Francis DP, Capucci A, Coats AJ, Piepoli MF (2001). Muscle ergoreceptor overactivity reflects deterioration in clinical status and cardiorespiratory reflex control in chronic heart failure. *Circulation* **104**: 2324–30.

33. Piepoli MF, Kaczmarek A, Francis DP *et al.* (2006). Reduced peripheral skeletal muscle mass and abnormal reflex physiology in chronic heart failure. *Circulation* **114**: 126–34.

34. Piepoli M, Clark AL, Volterrani M, Adamopoulos S, Sleight P, Coats AJ (1996). Contribution of muscle afferents to the hemodynamic, autonomic, and ventilatory responses to exercise in patients with chronic heart failure: effects of physical training. *Circulation* **93**: 940–52.

35. Niebauer J, Pflaum CD, Clark AL *et al.* (1998). Deficient insulin-like growth factor I in chronic heart failure predicts altered body composition, anabolic deficiency, cytokine and neurohormonal activation. *J Am Coll Cardiol* **32**: 393–7.

36. Malkin CJ, Pugh PJ, West JN, van Beek EJ, Jones TH, Channer KS (2006). Testosterone therapy in men with moderate severity heart failure: a double-blind randomized placebo controlled trial. *Eur Heart J* **27**: 57–64.

37. Anker SD, Chua TP, Ponikowski P *et al.* (1997). Hormonal changes and catabolic/anabolic imbalance in chronic heart failure and their importance for cardiac cachexia. *Circulation* **96**: 526–34.

38. Kontoleon PE, Anastasiou-Nana,MI, Papapetrou PD *et al.* (2003). Hormonal profile in patients with congestive heart failure. *Int J Cardiol* **87**: 179–83.

39. Kotler DP (2000). Cachexia. *Ann Intern Med* **133**: 622–34.

40. Mann DL, McMurray JJ, Packer M *et al.* (2004). Targeted anticytokine therapy in patients with chronic heart failure: results of the Randomized Etanercept Worldwide Evaluation (RENEWAL). *Circulation* **109**: 1594–602.

41. Mann DL, Reid MB (2003). Exercise training and skeletal muscle inflammation in chronic heart failure: feeling better about fatigue. *J Am Coll Cardiol* **42**: 869–72.

42. Anker SD, Rauchhaus MR (1999). Insights into the pathogenesis of chronic heart failure: immune activation and cachexia. *Curr Opin Cardiol* **14**: 211–16.

43. Anker SD, Clark AL, Teixeira MM, Hellewell PG, Coats AJ (1999). Loss of bone mineral in patients with cachexia due to chronic heart failure. *Am J Cardiol* **83**: 612–15, A10.

44. Kenny AM, Boxer R, Walsh S, Hager WD, Raisz LG (2006). Femoral bone mineral density in patients with heart failure. *Osteoporosis Int* **17**: 1420–7.

45. Clark AL (2006). Origin of symptoms in chronic heart failure. *Heart* **92**: 12–16.

46. Levine B, Kalman J, Mayer L, Fillit HM, Packer M (1990). Elevated circulating levels of tumor necrosis factor in severe chronic heart failure. *New Engl J Med* **323**: 236–41.

47. Swan JW, Anker SD, Walton C *et al.* (1997). Insulin resistance in chronic heart failure: relation to severity and etiology of heart failure. *J Am Coll Cardiol* **30**: 527–32.

48. Poehlman ET, Scheffers J, Gottlieb SS, Fisher ML, Vaitekevicius P (1994). Increased resting metabolic rate in patients with congestive heart failure. *Ann Intern Med* **121**: 860–2.

49. Newman AB, Gottdiener JS, McBurnie MA *et al.* (2001). Associations of subclinical cardiovascular disease with frailty. *J Gerontol A: Biol Sci Med Sci* **56**: M158–M166.

50. Aronow WS (1997). Treatment of congestive heart failure in older persons. *J Am Geriatr Soc* **45**: 1252–7.

51. Bickenbach JE (2003). Functional status and health information in Canada: proposals and prospects. *Health Care Finance Rev* **24**: 89–102.

52. Smith GL, Masoudi FA, Vaccarino V, Radford MJ, Krumholz HM (2003). Outcomes in heart failure patients with preserved ejection fraction: mortality, readmission, and functional decline. *J Am Coll Cardiol* **41**: 1510–18.

53. Landefeld CS, Palmer RM, Kresevic DM, Fortinsky RH, Kowal J (1995). A randomized trial of care in a hospital medical unit especially designed to improve the functional outcomes of acutely ill older patients. *New Engl J Med* **332**: 1338–44.

54. Belardinelli R, Georgiou D, Cianci G, Purcaro A (1999). Randomized, controlled trial of long-term moderate exercise training in chronic heart failure: effects on functional capacity, quality of life, and clinical outcome. *Circulation* **99**: 1173–82.

55. Lipkin DP, Canepa-Anson R, Stephens MR, Poole-Wilson PA (1986). Factors determining symptoms in heart failure: comparison of fast and slow exercise tests. *Br Heart J* **55**: 439–45.

56. Belardinelli R, Barstow TJ, Nguyen P, Wasserman K (1997). Skeletal muscle oxygenation and oxygen uptake kinetics following constant work rate exercise in chronic congestive heart failure. *Am J Cardiol* **80**: 1319–24.

57. Tanabe Y, Takahashi M, Hosaka Y, Ito M, Ito E, Suzuki K (2000). Prolonged recovery of cardiac output after maximal exercise in patients with chronic heart failure. *J Am Coll Cardiol* **35**: 1228–36.

58. Wilson JR, Mancini DM (1993). Factors contributing to the exercise limitation of heart failure. *J Am Coll Cardiol* **22**(Suppl. A): 93A–98A.

59. Sullivan MJ, Knight JD, Higginbotham MB, Cobb FR (1989). Relation between central and peripheral hemodynamics during exercise in patients with chronic heart failure. Muscle blood flow is reduced with maintenance of arterial perfusion pressure. *Circulation* **80**: 769–81.

60. Picozzi NM, Clark AL, Lindsay KA, McCann GP, Hillis WS (1999). Responses to constant work exercise in patients with chronic heart failure. *Heart* **82**: 482–5.

61. Pina IL, Apstein CS, Balady GJ *et al.* (2003). Exercise and heart failure: a statement from the American Heart Association Committee on exercise, rehabilitation, and prevention. *Circulation* **107**: 1210–25.

62. Belardinelli R, Georgiou D, Scocco V, Barstow TJ, Purcaro A (1995). Low intensity exercise training in patients with chronic heart failure. *J Am Coll Cardiol* **26**: 975–82.

63. Rees K, Taylor RS, Singh S, Coats AJ, Ebrahim S (2004). Exercise based rehabilitation for heart failure. *Cochrane Database Syst Rev* 2004(3) CD003331.

64. Meyer K, Schwaibold M, Westbrook S *et al.* (1997). Effects of exercise training and activity restriction on 6-minute walking test performance in patients with chronic heart failure. *Am Heart J* **133**: 447–53.

65. Tyni-Lenne R, Gordon A, Jansson E, Bermann G, Sylven C (1997). Skeletal muscle endurance training improves peripheral oxidative capacity, exercise tolerance, and health-related quality of life in women

with chronic congestive heart failure secondary to either ischemic cardiomyopathy or idiopathic dilated cardiomyopathy. *Am J Cardiol* **80**: 1025–9.

66. Sullivan MJ, Higginbotham MB, Cobb F (1989). Exercise training in patients with chronic heart failure delays ventilatory anaerobic threshold and improves submaximal exercise performance. *Circulation* **79**: 324–9.

67. Corvera-Tindel T, Doering LV, Woo MA, Khan S, Dracup K (2004). Effects of a home walking exercise program on functional status and symptoms in heart failure. *Am Heart J* **147**: 339–46.

68. Oka RK, De Marco T, Haskell WL *et al.* (2000). Impact of a home-based walking and resistance training program on quality of life in patients with heart failure. *Am J Cardiol* **85**: 365–9.

69. Vasan RS, Benjamin EJ, Levy D (1995). Prevalence, clinical features and prognosis of diastolic heart failure: an epidemiologic perspective. *J Am Coll Cardiol* **26**: 1565–74.

70. Kitzman DW, Little WC, Brubaker PH *et al.* (2002). Pathophysiological characterization of isolated diastolic heart failure in comparison to systolic heart failure. *J Am Med Assoc* **288**: 2144–50.

71. Rao A, Asadi-Lari M, Walsh J, Wilcox R, Gray D (2006). Quality of life in patients with signs and symptoms of heart failure–does systolic function matter? *J Card Fail* **12**: 677–83.

72. Lindenfeld J (2005). Prevalence of anemia and effects on mortality in patients with heart failure. *Am Heart J* **149**: 391–401.

73. Silverberg DS, Wexler D, Blum M *et al.* (2000). The use of subcutaneous erythropoietin and intravenous iron for the treatment of the anemia of severe, resistant congestive heart failure improves cardiac and renal function and functional cardiac class, and markedly reduces hospitalizations. *J Am Coll Cardiol.* **35**: 1737–44.

74. Silverberg DS, Wexler D, Sheps D *et al.* (2001). The effect of correction of mild anemia in severe, resistant congestive heart failure using subcutaneous erythropoietin and intravenous iron: a randomized controlled study. *J Am Coll Cardiol* **37**: 1775–80.

75. Mancini DM, Katz SD, Lang CC, LaManca J, Hudaihed A, Androne AS (2003). Effect of erythropoietin on exercise capacity in patients with moderate to severe chronic heart failure. *Circulation* **107**: 294–9.

76. Ko DT, Hebert, PR, Coffey CS, Sedrakyan A, Curtis JP, Krumholz HM (2002). B-blocker therapy and symptoms of depression, fatigue, and sexual dysfunction. *J Am Med Assoc* **288**: 351–7.

77. Gottlieb SS, Khatta M, Friedmann E *et al.* (2004). The influence of age, gender, and race on the prevalence of depression in heart failure patients. *J Am Coll Cardiol* **43**: 1542–9.

78. Rutledge T, Reis VA, Linke SE, Greenberg BH, Mills PJ (2006). Depression in heart failure a meta-analytic review of prevalence, intervention effects, and associations with clinical outcomes. *J Am Coll Cardiol* **48**: 1527–37.

79. Gehi A Haas D, Pipkin S, Whooley MA (2005). Depression and medication adherence in outpatients with coronary heart disease: findings from the Heart and Soul Study. *Arch Intern Med* **165**: 2508–13.

80. Vinson JM, Rich MW, Sperry JC, Shah AS, McNamara T (1990). Early readmission of elderly patients with congestive heart failure. *J Am Geriatr Soc* **38**: 1290–5.

81. Skotzko CE, Krichten C, Zietowski G *et al.* (2000). Depression is common and precludes accurate assessment of functional status in elderly patients with congestive heart failure. *J Card Fail* **6**: 300–5.

82. Rumsfeld JS, Havranek E, Masoudi FA *et al.* (2003). Depressive symptoms are the strongest predictors of short-term declines in health status in patients with heart failure. *J Am Coll Cardiol* **42**: 1811–17.

83. Yesavage JA, Brink TL, Rose TL *et al.* (1982). Development and validation of a geriatric depression screening scale: a preliminary report. *J Psychiatr Res* **17**: 37–49.

84. Beck AT (1978). *Depression Inventory*. Philadelphia: Center for Cognitive Therapy.

85. Krack A, Sharma R, Figulla HR, Anker SD (2005). The importance of the gastrointestinal system in the pathogenesis of heart failure. *Eur Heart J* **26**: 2368–74.

86. Witte KK, Clark AL (2006). Micronutrients and their supplementation in chronic cardiac failure. An update beyond theoretical perspectives. *Heart Fail Rev* **11**: 65–74.

87. Zittermann A, Schleithoff SS, Tenderich G *et al.* (2003). Low vitamin D status: a contributing factor in the pathogenesis of congestive HF? *J Am Coll Cardiol* **41**: 105–12.

88. Visser M, Deeg DJ, Lips P *et al.* (2003). Low vitamin D and high parathyroid hormone levels as determinants of loss of muscle strength and muscle mass. *J Clin Endocrinol Metab* **88**: 5766–72.

89. Verhaar HJ, Samson MM, Jansen PA *et al.* (2000). Muscle strength, functional mobility and vitamin D in older women. *Aging (Milano)* **12**: 455–60.

90. Witte KK, Clark AL, Cleland JG (2001). Chronic heart failure and micronutrients. *J Am Coll Cardiol.* **37**: 1765–74.

91. Rector T, Kubo S, Cohn J (1987). Patient self-assessment of their heart failure 2: Content, reliability and validity of a new measure, the Minnesota Living with Heart Failure questionnaire. *Heart Fail* 198–209.

92. Green CP, Porter CB, Bresnahan DR, Spertus JA (2000). Development and evaluation of the Kansas City Cardiomyopathy Questionnaire: a new health status measure for heart failure. *J Am Coll Cardiol* **35**: 1245–55.

93. Feinstein AR, Fisher MB, Pigeon JG (1989). Changes in dyspnea-fatigue ratings as indicators of quality of life in the treatment of congestive heart failure. *Am J Cardiol* **64**: 50–5.

94. Borg G (1998). *Borg's Perceived Exertion and Pain Scale.* Champaign, IL: Human Kinetics.

Chapter 12

Pain in heart failure patients

Sue Wingate and Mary S. Wheeler

Introduction

Pain is a common co-existing problem in persons with heart failure (HF), yet there are scant data available to guide the management of pain in these persons. The assessment and treatment of pain in this population is complex because of: (1) the inability to use non-steroidal anti-inflammatory medications (NSAIDs) and corticosteroids because of their adverse effects, (2) the multiple medications that are used to treat HF, (3) the many co-morbidities and associated interventions used in this population, and (4) the high prevalence of elderly people in this population.[1]

Anecdotally, HF clinicians note a high frequency of pain as a patient complaint during a HF consultation, and several studies have noted that pain and/or physical discomfort is reported in 30–80% of patients with advanced HF.[2–7]

The purpose of this chapter is to examine the complex issues of pain and pain management in persons with HF. Limited literature provides evidence for practice in this area; thus, content presented in this chapter also includes appropriate general pain management principles, pharmacology, and clinical experience. A general review of pain concepts will first be presented. We will then outline the evidence for the existence of pain in persons with HF and discuss the assessment and treatment of pain, with a focus on persons with HF. Finally, we will suggest areas for future research.

General pain concepts

Pain is a personal event that most, if not all, of those reading this chapter will have experienced. There are times when the pain is easy to describe and the reasons for the pain are easily identified. At other times, words to describe the sensation are elusive or do not seem to quite capture what is being felt. The word 'pain' describes a concept used to focus and label a group of sensations, thoughts, emotions, and behaviors.[8]

Current pain nomenclature differentiates between acute and chronic pain. Acute pain follows an injury to the body and generally disappears as the injury heals. It is usually associated with objective physical signs that include elevations of heart rate, blood pressure, and respiratory rate.[9] Acute pain generally lasts for less than 6 months, and responds well to pharmacologic and non-pharmacologic interventions.[10] Acute pain should be treated aggressively, including treatment during the time frame during which a diagnosis is being made.[9] Current pain terminology also includes references to *physiological pain* and *inflammatory pain*, which share many of the elements of the definition of acute pain. Physiological pain is an essential early warning device that alerts us to the presence in the environment of damaging stimuli. This type of pain is activated by specialized sensory nociceptor fibers located in the peripheral tissues and activated only by noxious stimuli. Inflammatory pain is also initiated by tissue damage, and results in hypersensitivity at the site of injury. Once activated in the periphery, the sensory input travels to the spinal cord and the brain.[11]

Chronic pain occurs as a result of unresolved pain, and reflects changes in the nervous system. Terminology used in chronic pain states includes hyperalgesia (referring to a heightened pain perception to noxious stimuli) and allodynia (referring to pain evoked from non-noxious stimuli). These changes may develop due to low thresholds in primary afferent nociceptors or changes in the central mechanisms in the spinal cord or fore-brain.[12] Chronic pain exists longer than the expected time for healing, does not serve any purpose to the body, becomes very resistant to therapy, and may exist in the absence of any physical reason that supports the subjective report of pain.[1] Chronic pain results in an increased utilization of health-care services[10] and a decrease in function and quality of life. The terms 'chronic' and 'persistent' pain are often used interchangeably in the medical literature. The term 'chronic pain' may be associated with negative stereotypes; the term 'persistent pain' may foster a more positive attitude by both patients and professionals to the many treatment options that are available to alleviate suffering.[13]

Chronic pain may be associated with an increased risk of hypertension. Research suggests that the blood pressure/pain regulatory relationship may be altered in the chronic pain condition. It appears that chronic pain may be associated with dysfunction in overlapping systems that modulate both the pain response and the blood pressure response. It is postulated that chronic pain contributes to the development of hypertension through its effects on sympathetic arousal and the failure of normal homeostatic pain regulatory mechanisms. Therefore, early aggressive assessment and management of chronic pain may have an impact on cardiovascular disease risk.[14]

When the pain is a result of a primary lesion or dysfunction in the nervous system, neuropathic pain is diagnosed. In the periphery, it may result from diseases (such as diabetes, herpes zoster, or HIV), neuroma formation, or nerve compression (tumors, crush, entrapment). When the damage occurs in the brain or spinal cord it is labeled a central pain syndrome. Following the nerve injury, the peripheral and central systems undergo changes that result in a combination of factors that result in neuropathic pain.[15]

Surveys from several Western countries indicate that chronic and recurring pain is a significant problem for a substantial proportion of the population.[8] Over half of adults in the United States (US) experience chronic or recurrent pain, and a significant number have to make lifestyle changes to accommodate the pain.[16] Further, almost half of the adults in the US report inadequate pain relief and that chronic pain adversely affects their quality of life—both in terms of their day-to-day activities and their emotional well-being.[16] Nearly two-thirds of adults in a large population-based sample noted pain of greater than 3 months duration; indeed, many of these respondents were 'silent sufferers' as they had not informed their health-care provider of their pain. Nearly three-quarters of these silent sufferers had moderate to severe pain, and half had pain for more than 8 days per month.[17]

Regarding the elderly, one in five older Americans takes analgesic medications several times a week or more and over half of these persons have taken pain medication for more than 6 months.[13] Previous studies have noted that 25–50% of community-dwelling older people have chronic or recurrent pain[18-20] and that 45–80% of nursing home residents have substantial pain that is under-treated.[21,22] In addition, both community-dwelling patients and nursing home patients have been found to have several sources of pain. The consequences of pain in the elderly include depression, anxiety, decreased socialization, sleep disturbances, impaired ambulation, and increased health-care utilization and costs.[13] Further, other conditions may worsen with the presence of pain, such as gait disturbances, rehabilitation, and adverse effects from multiple drug prescriptions.[23]

Evidence for pain in persons with HF

Several studies document pain in persons with HF (Table 12.1). This literature summary highlights deficiencies in our knowledge of pain in HF patients. Studies have included only patients with advanced HF, indeed, several have included patients considered terminally ill, and thus we have no data on pain in those HF patients whose disease is in an earlier stage. Importantly, a few of the studies just noted a 'cardiac' diagnosis, and this may or may not have included patients with HF (although HF is usually the common pathway for end-stage cardiac illness). Several studies did not differentiate the responses of cardiac patients from those of others with advanced illnesses. Only cross-sectional and retrospective studies have been reported, no longitudinal trials have been done on this topic. No information on pain location or etiology has been reported, except for the study which noted pain as anginal pain.[6] No data on interventions for pain have been collected. Studies have not noted the effect of pain on the patient's quality of life. Studies do suggest that persons with advanced HF have a similar prevalence of pain as do persons with cancer.[4,5,24]

Although, as mentioned, there is no evidence to guide what pain treatments should be used in HF patients, we do have evidence about what *not* to use for treatment. HF patients should avoid the use of NSAIDs, common medications used in treating pain, especially inflammatory pain such as arthritis pain. NSAIDs inhibit the enzymes cyclooxygenase 1 and 2 (COX-1 and -2) which leads to impairment of prostaglandin synthesis and a subsequent decrease in inflammation and pain. Inhibition of prostaglandin synthesis can also cause sodium and water retention and a decrease in renal blood flow and glomerular filtration rate.[1] Use of NSAIDs has been associated with a two-fold increased risk for hospitalization for new HF in older persons taking diuretics[26] and with a 10-fold adjusted relative risk for a HF relapse in patients with pre-existing HF.[27,28] The odds of a first hospital admission with HF have been directly related to the NSAID dose and to those NSAIDs with a longer (rather than shorter) half-life.[27] Published guidelines for care of the patient with chronic HF clearly state to avoid the use of NSAIDs, including COX-2 inhibitors, in this population.[29,30] Corticosteroids should also be used sparingly in HF patients because of the potential for hypertension and edema due to sodium and fluid retention.

Table 12.1 Literature summary

Author	Design	Setting/Subjects	Methods	Outcomes	Comments
Kutner et al.[2]	Cross-sectional survey	Providers in 16 hospices rated 347 patients (14% with CHF or other cardiac diagnosis); median age 78 years	Providers completed the Memorial Symptom Assessment Scale	76% of patients reported pain	(1) 76% may be conservative estimate as symptoms assessed by proxy not by the patient. (2) No separate report of pain in CHF patients
Levensen et al.[3]	Retrospective	Subgroup of SUPPORT cohort of patients post-hospitalization for exacerbation of CHF at 5 tertiary care academic medical centers; surrogate decision-makers of 539 patients who died from chronic HF	Surrogate decision-maker interviews	41% of surrogates reported patient in severe pain in the 3 days before death	Rate of pain in non-cancer illnesses in SUPPORT similar to rate of pain in cancer illnesses[25]
Walke et al.[4]	Cross-sectional	226 community-dwelling persons >60 years old with CHF (66 patients with mean age 75 years), advanced COPD, or cancer	In-home interviews using Edmonton Symptom Assessment System	(1) Physical discomfort reported by 38% overall. (2) Of CHF patients, 27% reported physical discomfort, 20% reported pain	No difference in the proportion of patients having pain among the 3 groups of patients
Weiss et al.[5]	Cross-sectional	988 terminally ill patients (predicted to live <6 months; 18% with cardiac etiology) from 6 geographically diverse sites; 59% of total subjects >65 years	Patient interview with 135-question survey form; degree of pain assessed with questions adapted from Wisconsin BPI	(1) 50% of total sample noted moderate to severe pain. (2) 47% of cardiac patients noted moderate to severe pain	(1) Degree of pain was similar between patients with and without a cancer diagnosis. (2) Specific cardiac diagnoses not known

Anderson et al.[6]	Cross-sectional survey	Palliative care (213 patients) and end-stage CHF (66 patients with median age 67 years, 49% classified as NYHA Class III or IV)	(1) Listing of troublesome symptoms. (2) Symptom checklist	(1) 32% noted pain as 2nd most troublesome symptom. (2) 41% of CHF patients checked pain on checklist	Pain was defined as 'angina' for troublesome symptoms; unknown how pain was defined on checklist
Rabow and Dibble[7]	Cross-sectional	90 outpatients with advanced CHF (31), COPD or cancer with prognosis of 1–5 years; overall sample with mean age of 68.6 years	BPI at entry, 6 months, and 12 months	Report of 'any pain' 84% at baseline, 86% at 6 months, 79% at 12 months	Patients of color reported more pain than whites
Zambroski et al.[26]	Retrospective	90 CHF patients in hospice; mean age 81 years	Chart review	At hospice admission, 3% had chest pain, 20% had other pain, 75% had no pain	Relative lack of pain may have been due to patients' moribund condition at time of admission or use of morphine for managing symptoms

CHF congestive heart failure COPD, chronic obstructive pulmonary disease; NYHA, New York Heart Association; BPI, Brief Pain Inventory.

Assessment

Pain is more than a physical sensation. Traditionally, providers focus on the physical and biological domain and pay little, if any, attention to the spiritual, social, psychological, emotional, and cultural domains. Considering the patient's past pain experiences, current emotional state, and the personal and cultural meaning of pain leads to an effective treatment plan. Viewing pain within a context of a mind–body experience highlights the importance of a comprehensive assessment that seeks information on all domains.[31]

Pain is always subjective. No neurophysiological or laboratory test can measure pain. Clinicians must accept the patient's report of pain.[9] Since pain is so prevalent, every encounter with a health-care provider should include a screen for pain. The screening for

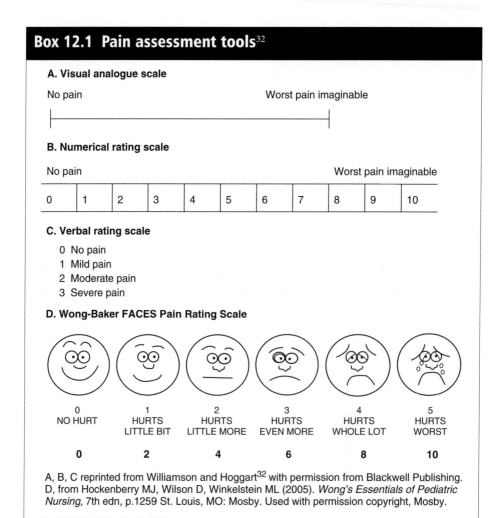

Box 12.1 Pain assessment tools[32]

A. Visual analogue scale

No pain   Worst pain imaginable

B. Numerical rating scale

No pain   Worst pain imaginable

0	1	2	3	4	5	6	7	8	9	10

C. Verbal rating scale

0 No pain
1 Mild pain
2 Moderate pain
3 Severe pain

D. Wong-Baker FACES Pain Rating Scale

0 NO HURT	1 HURTS LITTLE BIT	2 HURTS LITTLE MORE	3 HURTS EVEN MORE	4 HURTS WHOLE LOT	5 HURTS WORST
0	2	4	6	8	10

A, B, C reprinted from Williamson and Hoggart[32] with permission from Blackwell Publishing. D, from Hockenberry MJ, Wilson D, Winkelstein ML (2005). *Wong's Essentials of Pediatric Nursing*, 7th edn, p.1259 St. Louis, MO: Mosby. Used with permission copyright, Mosby.

pain can be accomplished by the patient independently completing a screening or assessment tool, by non-professional staff offering the tool and recording the results, or by professional staff. There are numerous tools that have been shown to be valid and reliable for clinical use to determine pain severity and four are highlighted in Box 12.1.[10,13,32] Having more than one tool available in the clinical area is recommended, so that patients may use the tool that makes the most sense to them. Once chosen, the health-care team should consistently offer that tool to the patient to provide consistency in the measurement and the scores recorded.

If the screen for pain is positive, then a comprehensive assessment should be completed. Since 2000, the Joint Commission on Accreditation of Healthcare Organizations (JCAHO) has made pain assessment part of the scoring criteria for an accreditation visit. The format for the assessment is not mandated, but the required assessment standards are defined.[10] In addition to regulatory requirements, a pain assessment provides a presumptive diagnosis upon which further diagnostics and a treatment strategy can be based.[33] Many tools exist to guide the clinician in obtaining the data, including the Brief Pain Inventory and the Initial Pain Assessment Tool.[34] Include the patient in the assessment phase by asking them to keep a 'pain diary' that documents such elements as date and time of pain experienced, severity rating, pain triggers, and the effectiveness of pain relief measures.[35] No matter what tool is used, a comprehensive assessment includes the items listed in Box 12.2.

Patients may present with both acute pain and chronic pain—a very confusing picture. These patients may have a difficult time rating their pain and identifying all the places that are painful, and may report severe pain but appear comfortable to the interviewer.[36] To get a sense of the chronicity of the pain, the clinician might ask, 'How many days in the past six months have you been unable to do what you like to do because of pain?'.[37]

Box 12.2 Components of comprehensive pain assessment

Location of pain

Intensity

Quality of pain—helps to determine whether somatic, visceral, and/or neuropathic structures are involved

Onset, duration, rhythms, variations

What causes/increases the pain

What decreases/relieves the pain

Effects of pain—on sleep, appetite, activity, emotions, relationships

Quality of life

Goals for pain relief

Patients with chronic pain may or may not have presenting symptoms reflecting sympathetic arousal. They may be frustrated with telling their story multiple times and not obtaining satisfactory relief. They may report the same pain rating information despite multiple interventions, leading to frustration for the clinician. Individuals with chronic pain may also present with vague and multifocal complaints.[36]

It is important to ask a patient in pain about the quality of their sleep. The relationship between sleep and pain continues to be investigated.[38] It is postulated that there are shared mechanisms underlying both pain and sleep disturbances. A recent study demonstrated that even moderate sleep deprivation in HF patients negatively influenced quality of life, with body pain being one of the largest areas of impairment.[39]

Assessment of pain in the elderly is complicated by a high prevalence of dementia, sensory impairment, and disability. Not only are the elderly reluctant to report pain, but many older people expect pain with aging and do not think their pain can be alleviated. In addition, they may fear the need for diagnostic tests or medications that have side-effects. Although many will deny the presence of 'pain', many older adults will acknowledge the terms 'discomfort', 'hurting', or 'aching'; thus it is helpful to use a variety of terms synonymous with pain when screening older patients.[13]

Patients with HF should undergo the same screening for pain as other patients. Attention should be paid to the location of the pain, as patients with advanced HF may have pain from a variety of sources—angina, pericarditis, device implants, or edematous limbs.[40] Assessing pain in the patient with advanced HF may be confounded by the use of opioids to treat symptoms other than pain (i.e. dyspnea).[25]

Chest pain presents a diagnostic challenge for the clinician, and more so in the HF patient. Is the chest pain due to cardiac causes, or is it musculoskeletal, gastrointestinal, psychosocial, pulmonary, or nonspecific?[41] Multiple tests can be ordered to identify or rule out the cause of the pain. In supportive care, if the test result will not change the treatment plan, then obtaining the test may be more of a burden than a benefit to the patient and serious consideration should be given to not ordering the test.

After the interview, a physical exam would include inspection and palpation of the painful area(s), observing for swelling, tender points, strength, range of motion, gait changes, and temperature changes.[36] A more thorough exam would include reflexes, cranial nerve function, dermatome evaluation, skin changes, and joint evaluations.[42]

Treatment

General issues

Goal setting for a patient in pain is important both to guide therapy and as a patient education tool. Relief from chronic pain remains elusive and total relief is rare. Currently available medications do not eliminate pain, but we can hope to reduce pain.[8] Discussing what the patient has tried in the past, both successfully and unsuccessfully, will help to establish trust and set realistic expectations of the pain management plan. The goals may be stated in terms of function, return to work, and ability to engage in social activities.

Listening to the patient's goals gives the clinician an end-point for therapy, and allows one to give a sense of the realistic ability to meet the stated goals.

Education of the patient and family (if available and the patient wants their involvement) should be part of the treatment plan. They need to know how to use medications for maintenance therapy and acute exacerbations. Preparing them for the physical and mental changes that represent patient declines is a priority intervention. Discussion about discontinuing medications, or alternative dosing routes/schedules/amounts should occur in a proactive mode, not as crisis intervention.

There are many options for treating pain, with pharmacological approaches being the mainstay for both acute and chronic pain. The American Pain Society has published recommendations for the pharmacologic treatment of acute pain (Box 12.3); no such list exists for the treatment of chronic pain. One common reference used to guide pharmacologic choices for pain management is the World Health Organization (WHO) Analgesic Ladder which has been in use since the early 1980s and which was originally developed to treat cancer pain (Fig. 12.1). The ladder has been modified for use in other disease states; most recently the drug choices for each step of the ladder have been adapted for those patients with renal insufficiency.[43]

In the WHO ladder, the choice of drug class is based on a pain rating of mild, moderate, or severe. In general, mild pain is treated with non-opioids [e.g. acetaminophen and NSAIDs (although NSAIDs are *not* to be used in HF)], moderate pain is treated with the

Box 12.3 American Pain Society recommendations for the treatment of acute pain and cancer pain[9]

1. Individualize the route, dosage, and schedule
2. Administer analgesics on a regular schedule if pain is present most of the day
3. Know the dose and time course of several opioid analgesic preparations
4. Give infants and children adequate doses of opioids
5. Follow patients closely
6. Use care when changing to a new opioid or route of administration
7. Recognize and treat side-effects
8. Do not use meperidine and beware of potential hazards of mixed agonist–antagonists, especially pentazocine
9. Do not use placebos to assess the nature of pain
10. Monitor for the development of tolerance and treat appropriately
11. Expect physical dependence and prevent withdrawal
12. Do not diagnose patients with an opioid addiction based only on the presence of opioid dependence
13. Be alert to the psychological state of the patient

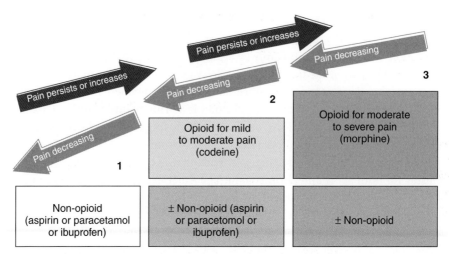

Fig. 12.1 World Health Organization Pain Ladder. Reprinted with permission from: WHO (2003). *Palliative Care: Symptom Management and End-of-life Care. Integrated Management of Adult and Adolescent Illness* (http://whqlibdoc.who.int/hq/2004/WHO_CDS_IMAI_2004.4.pdf).

'weak' opioids (e.g. combination opioid/non-opioid preparations), and severe pain is treated with 'strong' opioids (e.g. morphine, oxycodone, fentanyl, methadone). Adjuvants and non-pharmacologic therapies can be used at any level of the ladder (previous versions of the WHO ladder have listed adjuvants on the ladder steps).[1]

When starting an oral opioid medication on an opioid-naïve patient with constant pain, use an immediate-release preparation and administer a dose every 4 h. This is based on the 4 h half-life of the opioids. This strategy provides stable blood levels in five half-lives (approximately 24 h) of the drug. If the patient has a good response to the immediate-release preparation, consider converting the patient to a long-acting preparation. This provides a more convenient dosing schedule and uninterrupted sleep.[35]

Effective treatment of pain includes prescription of analgesics, prescription of physical therapy and modalities, use of assistive devices and alternative therapies, as well as an explanation of the nature of the pain, discussion of lifestyle modifications, modification of the pathological process, and modification of the pain perception.[44] Non-pharmacologic interventions are important tools in pain management and may be used alone or in combination with pharmacologic strategies. Table 12.2 lists several non-pharmacologic interventions that may be utilized. There are no known studies that have targeted these interventions for pain in HF patients, but it is possible that persons with HF may benefit from these therapies.[1]

Transcutaneous electrical nerve stimulation (TENS) is a non-pharmacologic intervention often used in pain management. Caution is required when using this modality in patients with pacemakers or internal cardioverter defibrillators (ICDs). A case study has been reported regarding the successful use of TENS in a patient with a pacemaker.[45] Use of TENS in patients with ICDs may be associated with an increased risk of inappropriate shocks due to device interactions.[46] Crevenna *et al.*[47] described electromagnetic interference

Table 12.2 Non-pharmacologic Interventions (from Wheeler and Wingate[13])

Intervention	Explanation
Physical Activity Program	Reduces pain improves psychologic health, lessens the clinical impact of age-related biologic changes Include exercises that improve joint range of motion, increase muscle strength and power, enhance postural and gait stability, and restore cardiovascular fitness Individualize to meet the needs and preferences of each patient; individuals may require referral to a specialized therapist or trainer
Patient Education	Include information about self-help techniques (relaxation, distraction), known cause of pain, goals of treatment, treatment options, expectations of pain management, analgesic drug use Encourage patients to educate themselves by using local available resources Include families and caregivers Reinforce content and self-help efforts at each visit Provide focused education prior to special treatment or procedures
Cognitive-Behavioral Therapies	Cognitive therapies are designed to modify factors such as helplessness, low self-efficacy, and catastrophizing Cognitive therapies include distraction methods to divert attention from pain, mindfulness methods to enhance acceptance of pain, methods for altering self-defeating thought patterns, Behavioral strategies help patients control pain by pacing activities, increasing involvement in pleasurable activities, and using relaxation methods, Cognitive and behavioral strategies are usually combined Can be conducted individually or in group and may include involvement of spouse or other partners Usually requires 6-10 sessions with a trained therapist
Spiritual Involvement	Rising interest in religion and spirituality as a means to reduce suffering Important part of treating pain holistically

that occurred in three of eight ICD patients receiving TENS therapy and recommended individualized assessments for patients with ICDs who are considering TENS therapy.[47]

The elderly

The majority of patients with HF are elderly and this adds to the complexity of managing pain in this population. Most older people have been excluded from trials of analgesics.[48] Older persons are also more likely to experience side-effects of analgesic medications and they may be more sensitive to analgesic properties, especially those of opioid analgesics.[49] However, the American Geriatric Society has noted in its guidelines that the chronic use of opioids for persistent pain may have fewer life-threatening risks than does the long-term daily use of high-dose NSAIDs.[13] If opioids are used in the elderly, it is recommended to start with low doses and titrate up slowly.

Heart failure

Acute pain

Common causes of acute pain in persons with HF are gout, migraines, musculoskeletal pain, or post-operative pain. Ascertain the level of the patient's pain and consider pharmacotherapy choices for that step of the WHO ladder, avoiding the use of NSAIDs. For mild pain, acetaminophen (maximal daily dose of 4000 mg daily) is a first-line choice. An acetaminophen dose of 650 mg is approximately equal to 30 mg of codeine. Acetaminophen can also be combined with an opioid for additive effects and to potentially minimize the opioid dose. Many patients can be managed with an acetaminophen–codeine combination.[1]

Episodes of acute gout are common in HF patients on high-dose diuretic therapy. Most patients seek treatment for acute gout via their primary-care provider or an urgent care provider—both situations where these providers may unknowingly prescribe an NSAID for the patient. This emphasizes the importance of pro-actively educating persons with HF about the untoward effects of NSAIDs and the need for them to advocate for themselves to avoid these drugs either in an over-the-counter situation or when prescribed by another provider. For acute gout, colchicine as tolerated (usually 1.2 mg initially followed by 0.6 mg b.i.d.) can be used, with an opioid or acetaminophen–opioid combination added if needed. Patients prone to gout should be taught to avoid triggers such as trauma to affected joints, binge alcohol ingestion, fasting, and a very low carbohydrate diet.[50]

Patients with migraine pain should try prophylactic migraine relief therapy. HF patients may note a decrease in their migraine pain after they have been started on a β-blocker for their HF treatment. Drugs in the triptan class should be used with caution in HF patients because of possible untoward side-effects such as palpitations, syncope, arrhythmias, and precipitation of angina in those patients with ischemic heart disease.[1]

A unique cause of acute pain in patients with HF is the potential discomfort associated with firing of an ICD. These devices are placed to treat life-threatening ventricular arrhythmias. The shock sensation from this device has been rated as a '6' on a 0–10 pain scale.[51,52] Although the physical discomfort of this shock may be short-lived, possible psychological ramifications remain. Some patients experience multiple, repeated shocks over a brief time interval (an 'ICD' storm defined as two or more shocks in a 24-h period); others may experience occasional, or no, shocks. For frequent shocks, the device needs to be checked for malfunction, and electrolytes need to be checked and corrected if abnormal. An anti-arrhythmic drug may be prescribed to decrease the occurrence of the arrhythmia.[29] Some patients, especially those in the advanced stage of HF, may decide to deactivate the ICD. If the ICD is not deactivated, a plan needs to be established related to the physical and psychological issues that may arise if the device fires as the patient is dying.

Atrial defibrillators are also being implanted now to treat recurrent atrial fibrillation, and the discomfort from these shocks is also an issue. A difference with atrial defibrillators, however, is that shocks from these devices are 'planned' shocks initiated by the patient or health-care provider when the offending rhythm is detected, as opposed to the sudden, unplanned shocks from an ICD. Thus, trials are under way to determine the most effective sedation to use when a cardioversion is done with an atrial defibrillator.[53]

Chronic pain

Common causes of chronic, or persistent, pain in persons with HF are musculoskeletal problems (especially arthritis), neuropathy, and refractory anginal pain. For musculoskeletal pain, again following the WHO ladder and avoiding NSAIDs, acetaminophen is a good first choice for mild pain. Opioids can be added if needed. Topical capsaicin cream, which works by depleting substance P, may be helpful for some patients; however, it takes several weeks to achieve full effects and requires dosing two to three times daily.

Many patients with arthritis pain take glucosamine and chondroitin supplements. Small studies on the efficacy of these agents noted mixed results. A recent multicenter randomized trial investigating the use of glucosamine, chondroitin, combined glucosamine and chondroitin, celecoxib, and placebo in patients with knee pain from osteoarthritis found that glucosamine and chondroitin alone or in combination did not effectively reduce pain (defined as a 24% decrease in pain from baseline to week 24). Adverse effects were mild, infrequent, and evenly distributed among the groups.[54] If patients do use these supplements, note that diuretics may decrease the effectiveness of glucosamine and that close monitoring of glucose levels is needed in patients with diabetes as glucosamine may increase insulin resistance.[55]

Neuropathic pain is common especially in those HF patients with diabetes or cancer. Adjuvant medications (Box 12.4), especially the tricyclic antidepressants (TCAs) and anticonvulsants, are used to treat this pain as these drugs alter, attenuate, or otherwise modulate pain perception.[56] They may be used alone or in combination with other pharmacologic agents. The use of certain adjuvants raises important issues in HF patients. The anticholinergic side-effects of TCAs (orthostatic hypotension, dizziness, dry mouth) may be intolerable for some patients, especially elders. Desipiramine may be the best choice in this category as it has fewer of the anticholinergic side-effects and also less cardiotoxicity potential.[56] Of the anticonvulsants, gabapentin is the most commonly used due to its low side-effect profile; however, it can cause fluid retention in some patients and thus requires close evaluation in the HF patient. Local anesthetics are second-line choices for those who have not received relief from TCAs or anticonvulsants. Mexilitine, an oral local anesthetic, has multiple cardiac side-effects and should not be used to manage pain in persons with HF.[57]

Box 12.4 Adjuvant medications

Tricyclic antidepressants

Anticonvulsants

Alpha 2-adrenergic agonists

Antihistamines

Oral local anesthetics

Topical analgesics

Psychostimulants

Methadone is being used more frequently in chronic pain management, especially for neuropathic pain and to slow the development of opioid tolerance.[13] Ventricular arrhythmias, especially torsade de pointes, have been reported in patients treated with high doses of methadone.[58–60] There are no data regarding the use of this drug in HF patients. If methadone is used as part of the pain management plan, it should be prescribed and titrated by pain management specialists or clinicians familiar with this drug's unique properties.[1]

Chronic angina should be treated with conventional medical and surgical therapies, as appropriate and desired by the patient and family. If conventional therapy fails, and angina becomes intractable, treatment options become more limited. Intractable angina pain has been successfully treated with an implanted spinal cord stimulator.[61,62] In one case, the placement of the temporary spinal cord stimulator was successfully accomplished at the bedside, with placement confirmed post-procedure with a bedside chest X-ray.[62]

Enhanced external counterpulsation (EECP) is another treatment option for angina. During this procedure the patient's legs are wrapped in pairs of pneumatic cuffs around the upper thighs, lower thighs and calves. The cuffs are sequentially inflated and deflated to increase diastolic pressure and decrease systolic pressure, similar to the hemodynamic effects of the intra-aortic balloon pump. This treatment has been shown to significantly reduce anginal symptoms and extend time to exercise-induced ischemia[63] and has been approved by the US Food and Drug Administration (FDA) as a non-surgical out-patient treatment for angina. Most patients tolerate the procedure, but it does require commitment and the ability to attend treatments in an out-patient center for several hours a week for approximately 4 to 7 weeks. The use of EECP has been specifically studied in patients with refractory angina and left-ventricular dysfunction and was found to decrease angina and improve quality of life, with these outcomes maintained at a 2-year follow-up.[64] Trials focusing on the use of EECP to treat persistent symptoms (not angina) in HF patients are ongoing. At this time, the US FDA has not approved the use of EECP for the treatment of HF symptoms.

Pain at the end of life

End-stage disease is characterized by a series of acute exacerbations of symptoms that may or may not improve with medical interventions. It is difficult to determine when the patient moves from the chronic to the end-stage of the HF disease trajectory. Symptoms noted for HF patients during the last 7 days of life in a hospice included shortness of breath, edema, incontinence, confusion, poor appetite, and pain.[25] Further, the SUPPORT study noted family perceptions that 41% of HF patients were in severe pain in the 3 days before death.[3] Knowing that the change from end-stage illness to actively dying is difficult to identify, treating pain appropriately whenever reported should be the standard of care for persons with HF.

Barriers to pain management

At one time, opioids were withheld from cancer patients because of the fear of addiction and side-effects.[35] Now, opioids are the mainstay treatment for cancer pain, with a large body of research supporting their use, along with non-opioids and non-pharmacologic approaches.[9] We know that untreated cancer pain leads to changes in the peripheral and central nervous system, resulting in exaggerated pain sensitivity or hypersensitivity. Studies of this nature for the HF patient are lacking, leaving the clinician in a position to extrapolate best practice guidelines from other disease states.

The relief of pain from life-threatening illness needs to expand beyond the cancer patient to other disease states.[35] If your patient does not get relief from non-opioids and disease-specific treatment, then a trial of opioids is in order.[35] However, the long-term use of opioids in pain other than cancer pain remains controversial. It raises questions about tolerance, tolerability, drug diversion, side-effects, polypharmacy, drug interactions, and the risk/benefit ratio.[8,65] When clinicians become more aware of the correct definitions of addiction, tolerance, and dependence (Box 12.5), they will be less likely to confuse requests for pain relief with addiction. Medical use of opioids is generally not associated with addiction; however, in some cases, there may be cause for caution. Potential warnings against the use of opioid therapy include patients with extreme emotional distress, poor perception of effective coping, use of multiple pain descriptors or pain sites, poor social support, poor employment history and long term reliance on the health care system.[65]

Evaluation of pain management therapy

The goal of therapy should be appropriate and adequate doses to reduce pain and improve quality of life. Quality of life will be defined by the patient and family, and will be unique to the individuals involved. The evaluation should include multiple factors, such as physical activity, return to work, decrease in pain severity, reduction in use of

Box 12.5 Definitions related to the use of opioids for the treatment of pain[8]

1. **Addiction**—a primary, chronic, neurobiological disease, with genetic, psychosocial, and environmental factors influencing its development and manifestations. It is characterized by behaviors that include one or more of the following: impaired control over drug use, compulsive use, continued use despite harm, and craving

2. **Physical dependence**—a state of adaptation that is manifested by a class-specific drug withdrawal syndrome that can be produced by abrupt cessation, rapid dose reduction, decreasing blood levels of the drug, and/or administration of an antagonist

3. **Tolerance**—a state of adaptation in which exposure to a drug induces changes that result in a diminution of one or more of the drug's effects over time

4. **Pseudoaddiction**—a term that describes patient behaviors that may occur when pain is undertreated. Pseudoaddiction can be distinguished from true addiction in that the behaviors resolve when pain is effectively treated

rescue doses of medication, and sleep. This is a complex area, and no single measure can capture all relevant areas.[65] It is recommended not to use a reduction in pain medication as an outcome and recognize that the relationship between pain reports and function is modest.[8]

Ongoing discussion about treatment goals and progress toward the goals should be documented. The treatment plan should be adjusted as goals are met or changed. As the patient's functional condition changes, changes in caregiving needs should be anticipated and planned for. As nutritional and hydration conditions change, and as liver and kidney function change, medications may need to be adjusted for dosing amounts or intervals, or may need to be stopped altogether.

Future research

Multiple unanswered questions remain regarding pain and treatment of pain in persons with HF. Introductory work is critically needed to establish the actual incidence, location, and etiology of pain in this population. Inflammatory markers and neurohormonal activation need to be examined to determine if there are common pathways and/or mediators between the pain response and the neurohormonal milieu in HF. Intervention studies are needed on the efficacy and safety of various pain treatments and whether these treatments also affect HF outcomes such as mortality, hospitalizations, and quality of life. Importantly, studies are needed that are longitudinal in design and assess HF patients at all stages of the disease trajectory.

A new trial under way will help to answer some of the important introductory questions about this topic. Pain Assessment Incidence and Nature in Heart Failure (PAIN-HF) is a multi-site, nationwide study that will enroll approximately 400 advanced HF patients from out-patient clinics and home hospice settings. PAIN-HF is designed to: (1) identify the prevalence of pain, its location and possible causes; (2) identify the severity of pain, its interference with activities and its impact on quality of life; (3) understand the correlates of other symptoms and issues in patients' lives on their perception of pain, and (4) identify current treatments for pain and their effectiveness in relieving pain.

References

1. Wheeler M, Wingate S (2004). Managing noncardiac pain in heart failure patients. *J Cardiovas Nurs* **19**(6, Suppl.): S75–S83.
2. Kutner JS, Kassner CT, Nowels DE (2001). Symptom burden at the end of life: Hospice providers' perceptions. *J Pain Symptom Manage* **21**: 473–80.
3. Levenson JW, McCarthy EP, Lynn J, Davis RB, Phillips RS (2000). The last six months of life for patients with congestive heart failure. *J Am Geriatr Soc* **48**(5, Suppl.): S101–S109.
4. Walke LM, Gallo WT, Tinetti ME, Fried TR (2004). The burden of symptoms among community-dwelling older persons with advanced chronic disease. *Arch Intern Med* **164**: 2321–4.
5. Weiss SC, Emanuel LL, Fairclough DL, Emanuel EJ (2001). Understanding the experience of pain in terminally ill patients. *Lancet* **357**: 1311–15.
6. Anderson H, Ward C, Eardley A *et al*. (2001). The concerns of patients under palliative care and a heart failure clinic are not being met. *Palliat Med* **15**: 279–86.

7. Rabow MW, Dibble SL (2005). Ethnic differences in pain among outpatients with terminal and end-stage chronic illness. *Pain Med* **6**: 235–41.

8. Turk DC (2002). Clinical effectiveness and cost-effectiveness of treatments for patients with chronic pain. *Clin J Pain* **18**: 355–65.

9. American Pain Society (2003). *Principles of Analgesic Use in the Treatment of Acute Pain and Cancer Pain*, 5th edn. Glenview, IL: American Pain Society.

10. Joint Commission on Accreditation of Healthcare Organizations (2003). *Improving the Quality of Pain Management Through Measurement and Action*. Oakbrook Terrace, IL: Joint Commission on Accreditation of Healthcare Organizations.

11. Woolf C, Salter M (2000). Neuronal plasticity: increasing the gain in pain. *Science* **288**: 1765–8.

12. Bolay H, Moskowitz M (2002). Mechanisms of pain modulation in chronic syndromes. *Neurology* **59**(Suppl. 2): S2–S7.

13. AGS Panel on Persistent Pain in Older Persons (2002). The management of persistent pain in older persons. *J Am Geriatr Soc* **50**: S205–S224.

14. Bruehl S, Ok YC, Jirjis JN, Biridepalli S (2005). Prevalence of clinical hypertension in patients with chronic pain compared to nonpain general medical patients. *Clin J Pain* **21**: 147–53.

15. Suzuki R, Dickenson AH (2000). Neuropathic pain: nerves bursting with excitement. *NeuroReport* **11**: R17–R21.

16. American Pain Foundation http://www.painfoundation.org/page.asp?file=Library/PainSurveys.htm

17. Watkins E, Wollan PC, Melton LJ, Yawn BP (2006). Silent pain sufferers. *Mayo Clin Proc* **81**: 167–71.

18. Helme RD, Gibson SJ (1999). Pain in older people. In: *Epidemiology of Pain* (ed. IK Crombie, PR Croft, SJ Linton, L LeResche, M Von Korff), pp. 103–112. Seattle: IASP Press.

19. Blythe FM, March LM, Brnabic AJ *et al.* (2001). Chronic pain in Australia: a prevalence study. *Pain* **89**: 127–34.

20. Mantyselka P, Kumpusalo E, Ahonen R *et al.* (2001). Pain as a reason to visit the doctor: a study in Finnish primary health care. *Pain* **89**: 175–80.

21. Ferrell BA (1995). Pain evaluation and management in the nursing home. *Ann Intern Med* **123**: 681–7.

22. Bernabei R, Gambassi G, Lapane K *et al.* (1998). Management of pain in elderly patients with cancer. SAGE Study Group. Systematic Assessment of Geriatric Drug use via Epidemiology. *J Am Med Assoc* **279**(23): 1877–82.

23. AGS Panel on Chronic Pain in Older Persons (1998). The management of chronic pain in older persons. *J Am Geriatr Soc* **46**: 635–51.

24. Lynn J, Teno JM, Phillips RS, Wu AW *et al.* (1997). Perceptions by family members of the dying experience of older and seriously ill patients. *Ann Intern Med* **126**: 97–106.

25. Zambroski CH, Moser DK, Roser LP, Heo S, Chung ML (2005). Patients with heart failure who die in hospice. *Am Heart J* **149**: 558–64.

26. Heerdink ER, Leufkenslt G, Herings RM *et al.* (1998). NSAIDs associated with increased risk of congestive heart failure in elderly patients taking diuretics. *Arch Intern Med* **158**: 1108–12.

27. Page J, Henry D (2000). Consumption of NSAIDs and the development of congestive heart failure in elderly patients: an underrecognized public health problem. *Arch Intern Med* **160**: 777–84.

28. Feenstra J, Heerdink ER, Grobbee DE *et al.* (2002). Association of nonsteroidal anti-inflammatory drugs with first occurrence of heart failure and with relapsing heart failure: the Rotterdam Study. *Arch Intern Med* **162**: 265–70.

29. Hunt SA, Abraham WT, Chin MH *et al.* (2005). AHA/ACC 2005 guideline update for the diagnosis and management of chronic heart failure in the adult: a report of the American College of Cardiology/American Heart Association Task Force on Practice Guidelines (Writing Committee to Update the 2001 Guidelines for the Evaluation and Management of Heart Failure). *Circulation* **112**: 154–235.

30. Adams KF, Lindenfeld J, Arnold JMO *et al.* (2006). Executive Summary: HFSA 2006 Comprehensive Heart Failure Practice Guideline. *J Card Fail* **12**: 10–38.

31. McCaffery, M (1999). Pain management. In: *Pain: Clinical Manual*, 2nd edn (ed. M McCaffery, C Pasero). St Louis, MO: Mosby.

32. Williamson A, Hoggart B (2005). Pain: a review of three commonly used pain rating scales. *J Clin Nurs* **14**: 798–804.

33. Pacl D (2001). Managing the pain of advanced chronic disease. *Texas Med* **97**: 38–41.

34. Pasero C, McCaffery M (2005). No self-report means no pain-intensity rating. *Am J Nurs* **105**: 50–3.

35. Brookoff D (2000). Chronic pain: 2. The case for opioids. *Hosp Prac* **35**: 69–72, 75–6, 81–4.

36. D'Arcy Y (2005). Field guide to pain. *Nurse Practitioner* **30**: 46–8.

37. Herr K (2002). Chronic pain: Challenges and assessment strategies. *J Gerontol Nurs* **28**: 20–7.

38. Parker KP, Kimble LP, Dunbar SB, Clark PC (2005). Symptom interactions as mechanisms underlying symptom pairs and clusters. *J Nurs Scholar* **37**: 209–15.

39. Skobel E, Norra C, Sinha A, Breuer C, Hanrath P, Stelbrink C (2005). Impact of sleep-related breathing disorders on health-related quality of life in patients with chronic heart failure. *Eur J Heart Fail* **7**: 505–11.

40. Horne G, Taylor S (2005). Palliative care in advanced heart disease. In: *Handbook of Palliative Care* (ed. C Faull, Y Carr), pp. 331–44. Oxford: Blackwell Publishing.

41. Cayley WE (2005). Diagnosing the cause of chest pain. *Am Fam Physician* **272**: 2012–21.

42. Simons SM (2000). Physical examination of the patient in pain. In: *Practical Management of Pain*, 3rd edn (ed. PP Raj). St Louis, MO: Mosby.

43. Launay-Vacher V, Karie S, Fau JB, Izzedine H, Deray G (2005). Treatment of pain in patients with renal insufficiency: the World Health Organization three-step ladder adapted. *J Pain* **6**: 137–48.

44. Bennett M, Forbes K, Faull C (2005). The principles of pain management. In: *Handbook of Palliative Care* (ed. C Faull, Y Carr), pp. 116–47. Oxford: Blackwell Publishing.

45. Shade SK (1985). Use of transcutaneous electrical nerve stimulation for a patient with a cardiac pacemaker. *Phys Ther* **65**: 206–7.

46. Pyatt JR, Trenbath D, Chester M, Connelly DT (2003). The simultaneous use of a biventricular implantable cardioverter defibrillator (ICD) and transcutaneous electrical nerve stimulation (TENS) unit: implications for device interaction. *Eurospace* **5**: 91–3.

47. Crevenna R, Stix G, Pleiner J *et al.* (2003). Electromagnetic interference by transcutaneous neuro-muscular electrical stimulation in patients with bipolar sensing implantable cardioverter defibrillators: a pilot study. *Pacing Clin Electrophysiol* **26**: 626–9.

48. Rochon PA, Fortin PR, Dear KB *et al.* (1993). Reporting of age data in clinical trials of arthritis. Deficiencies and solutions. *Arch Intern Med* **153**: 243–8.

49. Kaiko RF, Wallenstein SL, Rogers AG *et al.* (1982). Narcotics in the elderly. *Med Clin North Am* **66**: 1079–89.

50. (1995). Management of gout. In: *Primary Care Medicine: Office Evaluation and Management of the Adult Patient*, 3rd edn (ed. AH Goroll, LA May, AG Mulley Jr), pp. 795–8. Philadelphia, PA: Lippincott.

51. Pelletier D, Gallagher R, Mitten-Lewis S, McKinely S, Squire J (2002). Australian implantable cardiac defibrillator recipients: quality-of-life issues. *Int J Nursing Pract* **8**: 68–74.

52. Ahmad M, Bloomstein L, Roelke M, Bernstein AD, Parsonnet V (2000). Patients' attitudes toward implanted defibrillator shocks. *Pacing Clin Electrophysiol* **23**: 934–8.

53. Mitchell AR, Spurrell PA, Gerritse BE, Sulke N (2004). Improving the acceptability of the atrial defibrillator for the treatment of persistent atrial fibrillation: the atrial defibrillator sedation assessment study (ADSAS). *Int J Cardiol* **96**: 141–5.

54. Clegg DO, Reda DJ, Harris CL *et al.* (2006). Glucosamine, chondroitin sulfate, and the two in combination for painful knee osteoarthritis. *New Engl J Med* **354**: 795–808.

55. (2001). *Nursing Herbal Medicine Handbook*. Springhouse, PA: Springhouse.

56. World Health Organization (1996). *Cancer Pain Relief: With a Guide to Opioid Availability*, 2nd edn. Geneva: World Health Organization.

57. Coyle N, Layman-Goldstein M (2001). Pain assessment and management in palliative care. In: *Palliative Care Nursing: Quality Care at the End of Life* (ed. ML Matzo, DW Sherman), pp. 362–486. New York: Springer.

58. Walker PW, Klein D, Kasza L (2003). High dose methadone and ventricular arrhythmias: a report of three cases. *Pain* **103**: 321–4.

59. Kornick CA, Kilborn MJ, Santiago-Palma J *et al.* (2003). QTc interval prolongation associated with intravenous methadone. *Pain* **105**: 499–506.

60. Krantz MJ, Lewkowiez L, Hays H, Woodroffe MA, Robertson AD, Mehler PS (2002). Torsade de pointes associated with very-high-dose methadone. *Ann Intern Med* **137**: 501–4.

61. Lanza GA, Sestito A, Sgueglia GA *et al.* (2005). Effects of spinal cord stimulation on spontaneous and stress-induced angina and 'ischemia-like' ST-segment depression in patients with cardiac syndrome X. *Eur Heart J* **26**: 983–9.

62. Janfaza DR, Michna E, Pisini JV, Ross EL (1998). Bedside implantation of a trial spinal cord stimulator for intractable anginal pain. *Anesth Analg* **87**: 1242–4.

63. Arora RR, Chou TM, Jain D *et al.* (1999). The multicenter study of enhanced external counterpulsation (MUST-EECP): effect of EECP on exercise-induced myocardial ischemia and anginal episodes. *J Am Coll Cardiol* **33**: 1833–40.

64. Soran O, Kennard Ed, Kfoury AG, Delsey SF for the IEPR Investigators (2006). Two-year clinical outcomes after enhanced external counterpulsation (EECP) therapy in patients with refractory angina pectoris and left ventricular dysfunction (report from The International EECP Patient Registry). *Am J Cardiol* **97**: 17–20.

65. Bloodworth D (2005). Issues in opioid management. *Am J Phys Med Rehab* **84**: S42–S55.

Chapter 13

Cardiac cachexia

Mitja Lainscak, Anja Sandek, and Stefan D. Anker

Introduction

The lifespan of an adult is usually associated with a slow but constant weight gain until the age of 60 years when it levels off, whereas at the age of 70 years an almost imperceptible weight loss of 0.1–0.2 kg year^{-1} commences.[1] Chronic disease, on the other hand, frequently causes significant weight loss due to body wasting, with resultant loss of muscle, fat, or both.[2,3] Ultimately, the serious complication of cachexia (from the Greek *kakós* 'bad' and *hexis* 'condition') may ensue, and those affected usually die over a short period.[4]

Cachexia has been recognized as an ominous sign of chronic heart failure (HF) for many centuries. Indeed, the earliest report originates from the Hippocratic school of medicine (about 460–370 BC) on the Greek island of Kos. Hippocrates offered his observation in an elegant and detailed description, namely 'the flesh is consumed and becomes water, . . . the abdomen fills with water, the feet and legs swell, the shoulders, clavicles, chest, and thighs melt away . . . the illness is fatal'.[5] This description is still applicable in modern medicine. Thereafter it took more than 1700 years before Withering described another patient, while the term 'cardiac cachexia' was introduced by the French physician Mauriac in 1860. From the historical point of view, another important example of cachexia deserves comment. The former United States president Franklin D. Roosevelt suffered from chronic HF with cardiac cachexia, which certainly affected his judgment at the Yalta meeting and may have impacted upon world history over the following decades.[6]

Cardiac cachexia is usually a feature of end-stage chronic HF and is almost inevitably associated with an adverse outcome. Nonetheless, this clinical feature has only recently attracted the attention of investigators.[7] This chapter will mainly focus on the pathophysiology of cardiac cachexia, describe the possible clinical implications, and outline the potential future development of therapeutic strategies.

Definition

Although several groups have made extensive studies of the scientific aspects of body wasting associated with a variety of chronic diseases, there is no widely accepted definition of cachexia. Growing research interest culminated in the organization in 2000 of the 1st Cachexia Conference. At the 3rd Cachexia Conference in 2005, the definition of cachexia was one of the principal topics, yet no definitive statement has been adopted.

For cardiac cachexia, several proposals have been offered. Some historical definitions focused on body fat and classified patients as malnourished when body fat content was <15% in men and <22% in women or if weight was <90% of ideal weight.[8] Cachexia was also defined as body fat content <27% for men and <29% for women[9] or as a reduction to <85% or even 80% of ideal weight.[10,11] Loss of body weight was highlighted in 1994, when Freeman suggested a definition based on a loss of ≥10% of lean tissue.[12] Due to the unavailability of dual-energy X-ray absorptiometry (DEXA) in everyday clinical practice, further assessments have remained more clinically oriented. In the clinical setting it is important to document only non-oedematous weight loss and to exclude other conditions associated with body wasting and cachexia such as cancer and thyroid disease. Initially, a weight loss of >7.5% of the previous weight over a period of 6 months and body mass index <24 were found to predict a 50% mortality at 18 months.[13] Later, a detailed analysis of the Studies of Left Ventricular Dysfunction (SOLVD) trial database established a weight loss of ≥6% as the optimal cut-off to define cachexia for clinical use[4].

Epidemiology and aetiology

Congestive HF affects about 1% of population at the age of 50 years but the prevalence increases to >10% at the age of 80 years[14]. However, an ever increasing prevalence in the population is anticipated, probably due to greater life expectancy, longer survival of patients with ischaemic heart disease, more awareness of the condition, better diagnosis and management and the use of evidence-based therapy in patients with established chronic HF[15].

Based on several comprehensive large-scale epidemiological analyses, data on the frequency and degree of body wasting in chronic HF are available. In the first prospective study 171 consecutive patients with chronic HF were studied and 28 (16%) were identified as being cachectic.[13] The observed weight loss ranged from 9% to 36% (corresponding to 6–30 kg) over a range of 6 months to 13 years. The mortality of cachectic patients reached 50% at 18 months, significantly worse than that for non-cachectic patients (Fig. 13.1), and worse than the prognosis for most cancers.[16] In a reanalysis of the SOLVD treatment database, 549 of 1929 patients (28%) were identified with new oedema-free weight loss of more than 7.5% and as many as 702 patients (36%) experienced weight loss of >6% over 3 years,[4] with the cross-sectional prevalence ranging from 12% to 14%. A cut-off for weight loss of >6% was identified as the strongest prognostic indicator amongst cut-offs ranging from 5% to 15%, hence the proposal of this parameter as the marker of choice for the identification of cardiac cachexia in clinical practice.

Why patients with chronic HF develop cardiac cachexia is still not fully understood. The development of cardiac cachexia may be associated with three different mechanisms: (1) malabsorption and metabolic dysfunction, (2) dietary deficiency, and (3) loss of nutrients via the urinary or digestive tracts.[2] The first extensive analysis of the pathogenesis of cardiac cachexia was performed by Pittman and Cohen in 1964.[17] Catabolic/anabolic imbalance due to protein loss and cellular hypoxia was proposed as the principal pathogenic

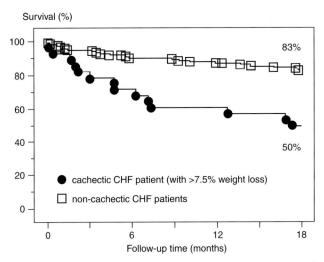

Fig. 13.1 Kaplan–Meier survival curves for 18-month survival of 171 patients with chronic HF subgrouped as cachectic and non-cachectic patients. Data from Anker et al.[13]

factor in a less efficient intermediary metabolism. Moreover, hypoxia was cited as a possible factor in anorexia and in an increased basal metabolic rate.

Anorexia may be related to symptoms (e.g. fatigue and dyspnoea), intestinal oedema with nausea and/or a protein-losing gastroenteropathy, or even as a side-effect of drug therapy [e.g. digoxin, angiotensin-converting enzyme (ACE) inhibitors], and sodium-restricted diets. Indeed, Buchanan found marked anorexia to be the most common cause of the cachectic state in 11 cachectic patients [New York Heart Association (NYHA) Class IV] with mitral valve disease. This investigation found no evidence for malabsorption or cellular hypoxia.[18] Another study offered conflicting results in a report suggesting fat malabsorption in elderly ambulatory patients with cardiac cachexia.[19] Simple starvation and anorexia are often considered to be the main cause of cardiac cachexia, but they would predominantly lead to a loss of fat tissue and reduced plasma albumin levels. Yet neither albumin nor liver enzyme levels are decreased in cachectic patients.[20] Overall, this would argue against a major contribution of starvation, anorexia, gastrointestinal malabsorption, or liver synthetic dysfunction in cachectic patients with chronic HF.

Another important aspect is higher metabolic rate, which has been repeatedly demonstrated in patients with HF.[21–23] In 1994, Poehlman et al.[21] demonstrated increased resting metabolic rates in stable patients with chronic HF compared with controls. Although Obisesan et al.[23] showed a positive correlation between the resting metabolic rate and severity of disease, Poehlman and colleagues[24] failed to confirm the difference when comparing cachectic with non-cachectic patients and healthy control subjects.

Lack of physical activity and deconditioning with subsequent muscle atrophy have also been observed in a substantial proportion of patients with HF.[25] However, histological evidence suggests that the muscle atrophy in chronic HF differs from the atrophy seen in other conditions resulting in reduced activity.[26]

Alterations of body composition

Cachectic chronic HF patients suffer from a general wasting process affecting muscle,[25] fat, and bone tissue stores.[27] Moreover, in a recent study we were also able to demonstrate wasting of the left ventricle itself in cachectic patients.[28] The muscle hypothesis argues that changes in skeletal muscle are key elements in the deterioration of patients with HF.[29] Indeed, a loss of lean body mass is readily demonstrable in patients with cardiac cachexia.[25] A complex interplay of metabolic, neurohormonal, and immune abnormalities affects metabolism, proliferation, differentiation, and apoptosis in skeletal muscle. Finally, muscle wasting ensues and patients develop symptomatic exercise intolerance.[30] We found muscle weakness and early fatigue in chronic HF to be experienced mainly by patients in NYHA Class III and IV,[31] and cachectic patients.[27] Whilst it is known that a loss of lean body mass predicts poor prognosis in cancer and AIDS,[32] this has not been reported for the patients with HF. Cachectic chronic HF patients also present with a 16% reduction of strength per unit muscle (both legs: 39% lower strength) compared with non-cachectic patients.[31] Eventually, combined with the impaired peripheral blood flow commonly seen in chronic HF patients,[33] this may lead to decreased oxidative capacity and impaired effort tolerance.

As well as loss of lean tissue, it has been shown that cachectic chronic HF patients have a significant reduction in fat tissue mass and decreased bone mineral density when compared to non-cachectic patients and healthy controls.[31]

Pathogenesis of cardiac cachexia

The aetiology of catabolic/anabolic imbalance, wasting, and changes in body composition leading to cardiac cachexia in patients with chronic HF is not entirely clear. It appears that this is due to the complex interplay of multiple mechanisms as outlined in Fig. 13.2.

Neuroendocrine abnormalities

The neurohormonal hypothesis, proposed in 1992,[34] suggested that overactivation of the neuroendocrine system is a major contributor to the progression of chronic HF. Initially, or in the acute setting, activation of the sympathetic nervous system, the renin–angiotensin–aldosterone axis, and the natriuretic peptide system seems beneficial, whilst chronic overactivation observed in chronic HF contributes to deleterious effects seen as increased vascular resistance and afterload, ventricular enlargement and adverse remodelling (see also Chapter 3).[35]

Chronic sympathetic overactivation is probably reflected in increased plasma norepinephrine levels[36] where both norepinephrine and epinephrine can cause a metabolic shift towards catabolic processes.[20] Catecholamines promote body wasting through different mechanisms, including an increase in resting energy expenditure in patients with HF.[23] A graded increase in resting metabolic rate corresponds to NYHA class, which supports the hypothesis that the clinical severity of the illness relates to the degree of increase in resting energy demands.[23] Additionally, studies have reported an association between neurohormonal activation and mortality.[37] It is therefore not surprising that catecholamine levels were found to be markedly elevated in cachectic patients with chronic

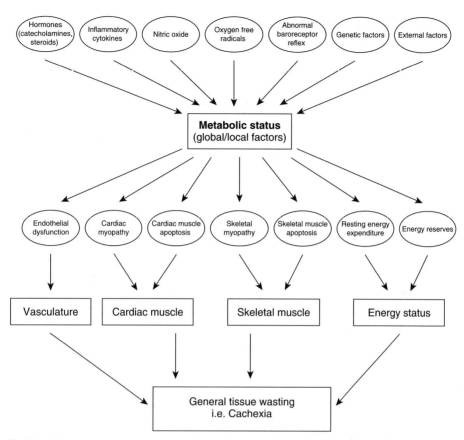

Fig. 13.2 The development of cachexia. Catabolic /anabolic imbalance and complex interaction of different body systems. Data from Anker et al.[27]

HF but remained near normal in those without cachexia.[20] Additionally, plasma aldosterone levels and plasma renin activity were increased in patients with cardiac cachexia, although the duration of chronic HF and pharmacological treatment, including ACE inhibitors and diuretic use were similar.[20] This implies a specific association between cachexia and sympathetic activation in chronic HF where renin, as a potent stimulator of the production of stress hormones (angiotensin II and norepinephrine), may be of particular importance.[38] In addition, angiotensin II can induce apoptosis in cardiac myocytes,[39] fibrosis in smooth muscle cells, and has been shown to reduce circulating levels of insulin-like growth factor 1 (IGF-1) in animal models, thus leading to anorexia with wasting.[40] Finally, a putative role of catecholamines in lipid mobilization has been suggested, which may also be triggered by up-regulation of atrial natriuretic peptide in HF.[51]

General stress is also characterized by elevated cortisol levels, and this is also found in cachectic chronic HF patients.[20] As far back as 1989, Anand et al.[42] demonstrated a 2.5-fold increase in cortisol in untreated chronic HF patients with severe disease. We confirmed these findings only for cachectic patients while cortisol levels in other patient sub-groups remained near normal.[20]

Inflammatory system activation

Inflammatory pathways are involved in all forms of cachexia. Evidence for this first appeared in 1990 when Levine *et al.*[10] reported increased levels of tumour necrosis factor α (TNFα) in patients with cardiac cachexia. This was confirmed in subsequent reports[11] and TNFα was shown to be the strongest predictor of the degree of previous weight loss in patients with HF. As well as TNFα, other cytokines including interleukin-1 (IL-1), IL-6, interferon-γ, and transforming growth factor-β, produced by monocytes/macrophages, endothelial cells, and myocardium, are also important in the development of catabolism. Therefore, the immune system is likely to be one of the key target areas for the future management of cachexia.

At present, three hypotheses for the activation of the immune system seem plausible. Firstly, hypoxia may induce the production of pro-inflammatory cytokines.[43] Secondly, the failing heart itself is capable of producing TNFα, and may be the single most important source of TNFα.[44] Thirdly, the endotoxin hypothesis of endotoxin release and immune activation due to bacterial translocation through an oedematous bowel wall has been postulated.[45] Importantly, bacterial endotoxins are known to be the strongest natural inflammatory stimulus.[46] Supporting this are the demonstrations of elevated endotoxin concentrations in patients during an acute oedematous exacerbation[47] and increased levels of procalcitonin in patients with cardiogenic shock and pyrexia but with negative bacterial cultures.[48] Furthermore, microcirculatory problems and acute venous congestion seem to alter gut permeability for bacteria and endotoxin, which stimulates inflammatory cytokine activation when present in the circulation.[49] This hypothesis, therefore, provides a rationale for important therapeutic strategies directed against bowel bacteria, endotoxin itself, and binding of the endotoxin to the cells of immune system. Lipids may be of particular importance in patients with chronic HF by binding to and detoxifying the effects of endotoxins.[50] Indeed, high lipoprotein levels were found to be inversely related to low levels of TNFα and other cytokines,[51] and low total serum cholesterol was independently associated with a worse prognosis in patients with HF.[52]

Additionally, a recent review suggests a close relation between autonomic imbalance and immune activation.[53] Functional and structural changes in the central nervous system, triggered by autonomic afferent signals from the damaged heart, can reduce central parasympathetic tone with subsequent activation of inflammatory and immune responses. While this hypothesis is interesting, most of the limited evidence is experimental and needs confirmation in a prospective clinical assessment of temporal changes throughout the course of chronic HF.

Along with immune activation, chronic HF is also characterized by elevation of other inflammatory markers such as the erythrocyte sedimentation rate[54] and uric acid.[55] Inflammatory cytokines and catabolic hormone levels are known to be associated with the reduction of muscle, fat, and bone tissue content in cachectic chronic HF patients.[56] Growth hormone resistance may be present as elevated levels of growth hormone, and inappropriately normal or low levels of IGF-1 were also found in cachectic chronic

HF patients.[20] Recently, impaired insulin sensitivity has been shown to be an independent predictor of mortality in patients with stable chronic HF,[57] and a clear relationship between impaired insulin sensitivity and increased pro-inflammatory cytokine load was previously demonstrated.[10]

Therapeutic options

Cachexia is frequent and associated with a poor prognosis in a variety of chronic diseases, including HF. Nonetheless, at present, no unifying mechanism has emerged offering a basis for therapy for this ominous syndrome. Recently, several exciting options have been postulated, and they are predominantly based on the available physiological and pathophysiological evidence.[58]

Pharmacological treatment

Current optimal therapy for patients with chronic HF includes ACE inhibitors, angiotensin receptor blockers (ARBs), β-blockers, and aldosterone antagonists (see Chapter 4).[59] Although not investigated in properly conducted trials in cachectic patients, available data suggest potential benefits in the use of neurohormonal antagonists.

ACE inhibitors reduce morbidity and mortality and improve symptoms in patients with chronic HF. Beneficial effects on neurohormones and endothelial function have also been demonstrated in cardiac cachexia.[27] Indeed, treatment with enalapril reduces the risk of weight loss in patients with chronic HF,[4] which is likely to be associated with prevention of muscle wasting. Angiotensin II induces cachexia secondary to increased muscle proteolysis,[60] thus treatment with ARBs may be useful in wasting conditions through activation of skeletal muscle IGF-1.

β-Blockers now have a widely accepted role in the treatment of HF.[61] Additionally, the beneficial effects of β-blockers on the maintenance of body weight has long been established for a variety of diseases.[62] For patients with chronic HF, preliminary analyses of the COPERNICUS[63] and CIBIS II[64] databases have reported that patients on carvedilol or bisoprolol, respectively, gained on average about 1.0 kg of body weight in 12 months compared with those on placebo. Furthermore, long-acting metoprolol and carvedilol resulted in significantly greater weight gain in cachectic chronic HF patients compared with those without cachexia (5.2 kg vs 0.8 kg, $P < 0.03$).[65] This is consistent with the inhibition of lipolysis and total body fat gain as shown in another study.[66]

Anticytokine treatment seems logical in the setting of chronic HF; however, a large-scale trial with etanercept and a smaller trial with infliximab were stopped prematurely due to a lack of benefit from etanercept[67] and increased mortality in the subgroup receiving the highest dose of infliximab.[68] However, these apparently negative results have to be put into context before anticytokine treatment is dismissed in patients with chronic HF.[69] Importantly, this specific treatment may be effective only in patients with a pronounced inflammatory response or in patients with advanced HF. Further evaluation of the cytokine hypothesis in appropriate patients treated at the correct doses is warranted. This hypothesis is being further investigated in the ACCLAIM trial.[70]

Pentoxifylline, a phosphodiesterase inhibitor, was also investigated as an anti-TNFα agent in patients with HF. Initial results were promising but were not fully confirmed in a subsequent trial on top of ACE inhibitors and β-blockers.[71]

Anabolic steroids, widely adopted by athletes, represent another putative candidate for the treatment of cachexia. Although no data exist for cachectic patients, Malkin *et al.*[72] recently reported that testosterone had improved functional capacity and symptoms in non-cachectic chronic HF patients. However, wide clinical application seems doubtful due to a number of serious side-effects including renal dysfunction and cardiotoxicity.[73] A more suitable option for the treatment of cachexia related to chronic HF may be a specific androgen receptor agonist without mineralocorticoid effects. Another anabolic agent, recombinant human growth hormone, has attracted considerable attention for the treatment of HF patients.[74] Although evidence of clinical effectiveness in general chronic HF patients is lacking,[75] benefits are demonstrable in those with cachexia[76] and with adequate dosing.[77] It seems that growth hormone resistance in cardiac cachexia might require the use of high doses of growth hormone or a combination of growth hormone with IGF-1.[78]

The recently discovered appetite-stimulating peptide hormone ghrelin, an endogenous ligand for the growth hormone secretagogues receptor, is currently the focus of research interest. Ghrelin acts both through growth hormone-dependent and -independent mechanisms, ultimately resulting in a positive energy balance. Initial reports demonstrated improvement in body composition, muscle wasting, functional capacity, and sympathetic augmentation in cachectic patients with chronic HF or chronic obstructive pulmonary disease.[79] However, existing studies included only a limited number of patients, were open-labelled, and not placebo controlled. Although therapy with ghrelin remains attractive, wide clinical application may be limited by cost and the requirement for parenteral administration.

Nutritional support

Nutritional abnormalities are known to contribute to the cachexia of chronic illness.[80] Importantly, healthy elderly people already have a high incidence of inadequate nutrition and hence a higher risk of developing cachexia of chronic disease. Additionally, protein–energy malnutrition is common in chronic illnesses.[81] In a recent trial, micronutrient supplementation improved left-ventricular ejection fraction and quality of life in elderly patients with HF.[82] Another study found that enteral nutritional support of 600 kcal day^{-1} over a 6-week period increased body mass (63.4 kg to 66.0 kg), total body fat mass (15.5 kg to 17.2 kg), 6-min walk test (366 m to 433 m), and decreased TNFα concentration (12.7 pg ml^{-1} to 2.4 pg ml^{-1}) in patients with cardiac cachexia.[83]

Physical training

Although exercise intolerance is the hallmark of chronic HF, systematic assessment of skeletal muscle function in chronic HF is lacking.[30] It has been shown that physical training improves the muscular metabolic abnormalities and atrophy as well as impaired blood flow and neurohormonal abnormalities.[84] Importantly, physical training was reported to reduce local muscle inflammation, increase anti-apoptotic and anabolic factors such as IGF-1, and improve the oxidative capacity of skeletal muscle.[85] A recent meta-analysis of randomized controlled trials indicated that physical training has a prognostic role in patients with HF.[86] As chronic HF, and in particular cardiac cachexia, are inherently linked with exercise intolerance, largely preventing some patients from undertaking any physical activity, an alternative approach with electrical muscle stimulation seems a reasonable option. Indeed, a comparable benefit of home-based electrical stimulation with respect to bicycle training[87] and a reversal of the deleterious effects on skeletal muscle have been reported in patients with advanced HF.[88] A systematic cardiac rehabilitation programme has never been fully studied in cachectic chronic HF patients, thus randomized controlled trials to evaluate the effects of physical training in this clinical cohort would be valuable.

What the future holds

The burden of chronic disease and consequently cachexia, including cardiac cachexia, will increase in years to come. Excessive mortality and lack of proven therapeutic strategies set the stage for properly designed and conducted interventional clinical trials with novel (e.g.. ghrelin) and also established medications (e.g.. β-blockers, ACE inhibitors), whose effectiveness in this therapeutic role may have been overlooked for many years. Additionally, nutritional strategies and physical training are also worthy of further review and clinical trials of these interventions are already in progress.[58]

Conclusions

The current definition of non-oedematous weight loss of 6% over 6 months readily identifies patients with cardiac cachexia and mediates a poor prognosis. Despite recent advances in therapy for chronic HF, this definition still applies to about 15% of patients with congestive HF. Abnormalities in the neuroendocrine and immune systems cause catabolic/anabolic imbalance, body wasting, and cardiac cachexia. With improved knowledge of the underlying pathophysiology, a number of emerging treatment strategies for prevention and treatment are being developed and tested. Although no specific treatment is currently available, several approaches with the use of neurohormonal drugs, nutritional support, ghrelin, and physical training appear to show potential benefits and the results of ongoing clinical trials in cardiac cachexia are awaited.

References

1. Wallace JI, Schwartz RS (2002). Epidemiology of weight loss in humans with special reference to wasting in the elderly. *Int J Cardiol* **85**: 15–21.
2. Anker SD, Sharma R (2002). The syndrome of cardiac cachexia. *Int J Cardiol* **85**: 51–66.
3. Schols AM (2002). Pulmonary cachexia. *Int J Cardiol* **85**: 101–10.
4. Anker SD, Negassa A, Coats AJ *et al.* (2003). Prognostic importance of weight loss in chronic heart failure and the effect of treatment with angiotensin-converting-enzyme inhibitors: an observational study. *Lancet* **361**: 1077–83.

5. Katz AM, Katz PB (1962). Diseases of the heart in the works of Hippocrates. *Br Heart J* **24**: 257–64.

6. Doehner W, Anker SD (2002). Cardiac cachexia in early literature: a review of research prior to Medline. *Int J Cardiol* **85**: 7–14.

7. Anker SD, Steinborn W, Strassburg S (2004). Cardiac cachexia. *Ann Med* **36**: 518–29.

8. Carr JG, Stevenson LW, Walden JA, Heber D (1989). Prevalence and haemodynamic correlates of malnutrition in severe congestive heart failure secondary to ishaemic or idiopathic dilated cardiomyopathy. *Am J Cardiol* **63**: 709–13.

9. McMurray J, Abdullah I, Dargie HJ, Shapiro D (1991). Increased concentrations of tumor necrosis factor in 'cachectic' patients with severe chronic heart failure. *Br Heart J* **66**: 356–8.

10. Levine B, Kalman J, Mayer L, Fillith H, Packer M (1990). Elevated circulating levels of tumor necrosis factor in severe chronic heart failure. *New Engl J Med* **323**: 236–41.

11. Otaki M (1994). Surgical treatment of patients with cardiac cachexia. An analysis of factors affecting operative mortality. *Chest* **105**: 1347–51.

12. Freeman LM, Roubenoff R (1994). The nutritional implications of cardiac cachexia. *Nutr Rev* **52**: 340–7.

13. Anker SD, Ponikowski P, Varney S *et al.* (1997). Wasting as independent risk factor for mortality in chronic heart failure. *Lancet* **349**: 1050–3.

14. Cowie MR, Mosterd A, Wood DA *et al.* (1997). The epidemiology of heart failure. *Eur Heart J* **18**: 208–25.

15. Cleland JGF, Khand A, Clark AC (2001). The heart failure epidemic: exactly how big is it? *Eur Heart J* **22**: 623–6.

16. Stewart S, MacIntyre K, Hole DJ, Capewell S, McMurray JJ (2001). More 'malignant' than cancer? Five-year survival following a first admission for heart failure. *Eur J Heart Fail* **3**: 315–22.

17. Pittman JG, Cohen P (1964). The pathogenesis of cardiac cachexia. *New Engl J Med* **271**: 403–9.

18. Buchanan N, Keen RD, Kingsley R, Eyberg CD (1977). Gastrointestinal absorption studies in cardiac cachexia. *Intens Care Med* **3**: 89–91.

19. King D, Smith ML, Chapman TJ, Stockdale HR, Lye M (1996). Fat malabsorption in elderly patients with cardiac cachexia. *Age Ageing* **25**: 144–9.

20. Anker SD, Chua TP, Ponikowski P *et al.* (1997). Hormonal changes and catabolic/anabolic imbalance in chronic heart failure and their importance for cardiac cachexia. *Circulation* **96**: 526–34.

21. Poehlman ET, Scheffers J, Gottlieb SS, Fisher ML, Vaitekevicius P (1994). Increased resting metabolic rate in patients with congestive heart failure. *Ann Intern Med* **121**: 860–2.

22. Podbregar M, Voga G (2002). Effect of selective and nonselective β-blockers on resting energy production rate and total body substrate utilization in chronic heart failure. *J Card Fail* **8**: 369–77.

23. Obisesan TO, Toth MJ, Kendall D (1996). Energy expenditure and symptom severity in men with heart failure. *Am J Cardiol* **77**: 1250–2.

24. Toth MJ, Gottlieb SS, Goran MI, Fisher ML, Poehlman ET (1997). Daily energy expenditure in free-living heart failure patients. *Am J Physiol* **272**: E469–E475.

25. Mancini DM, Walter G, Reichek N *et al.* (1992). Contribution of skeletal muscle atrophy to exercise intolerance and altered muscle metabolism in heart failure. *Circulation* **85**: 1364–73.

26. Vescovo G, Serafini F, Facchin L *et al.* (1996). Specific changes in skeletal muscle myosin heavy chains composition in cardiac failure: differences compared with disuse atrophy as assessed on microbiopsies by high resolution electrophoresis. *Heart* **76**: 337–43.

27. Anker SD, Swan JW, Volterrani M *et al.* (1997). The influence of muscle mass, strength, fatigability and blood flow on exercise capacity in cachectic and non-cachectic patients with chronic heart failure. *Eur Heart J* **18**: 259–69.

28. Florea VG, Moon J, Pennell DJ, Doehner W, Coats AJ, Anker SD (2004). Wasting of the left ventricle in patients with cardiac cachexia: a cardiovascular magnetic resonance study. *Int J Cardiol* **97**: 15–20.

29. Coats AJS, Clark AL, Piepoli M *et al.* (1994). Symptoms and quality of life in heart failure; the muscle hypothesis. *Br Heart J* **72**: S6–S39.

30. Strassburg S, Springer J, Anker SD (2005). Muscle wasting in cardiac cachexia. *Int J Biochem Cell Biol* **37**: 1938–47.

31. Harrington D, Anker SD, Chua TP *et al.* (1997). Skeletal muscle function and its relation to exercise tolerance in chronic heart failure. *J Am Coll Cardiol* **30**: 1758–64.

32. Kotler DP, Tierney AR, Wang J, Pierson RN (1989). Magnitude of body-cell-mass depletion and the timing of death from wasting in AIDS. *Am J Clin Nutr* **50**: 444–7.

33. Volterrani M, Clark AL, Ludman PF *et al.* (1994). Predictors of exercise capacity in chronic heart failure. *Eur Heart J* **15**: 801–9.

34. Packer M (1992). The neurohormonal hypothesis: a theory to explain the mechanism of disease progression in heart failure. *J Am Coll Cardiol* **20**: 248–54.

35. Francis GS (1985). Neurohormonal mechanisms involved in congestive heart failure. *Am J Cardiol* **55**(Suppl.): 15A–21A.

36. Goldstein DS (1981). Plasma norepinephrine as an indicator of sympathetic neural activity in clinical cardiology. *Am J Cardiol* **48**: 1147–54.

37. Cohn JN, Levine B, Olivari MT *et al.* (1984). Plasma norepinephrine as a guide to prognosis in patients with chronic congestive heart failure. *New Engl J Med* **311**: 819–23.

38. Staroukine M, Devriendt J, Decoodt P, Verniory A (1984). Relationships between plasma epinephrine, norepinephrine, dopamine and angiotensin II concentrations, renin activity, hemodynamic state and prognosis in acute heart failure. *Acta Cardiol* **39**: 131–8.

39. Kajstura J, Cigola E, Malhotra A *et al.* (1997). Angiotensin II induces apoptosis of adult ventricular myocytes *in vitro*. *J Mol Cell Cardiol* **29**: 859–70.

40. Brink M, Wellen J, Delafontaine P (1996). Angiotensin II causes weight loss and decreases circulating insulin-like growth factor I in rats through a pressor-independent mechanism. *J Clin Invest* **97**: 2509–16.

41. Lafontan M, Moro C, Sengenes C *et al.* (2005). An unsuspected metabolic role for atrial natriuretic peptides: the control of lipolysis, lipid mobilization, and systemic nonesterified fatty acids levels in humans. *Arterioscler Thromb Vasc Biol* **25**: 2032–42.

42. Anand IS, Ferrari R, Kalra GS, Wahi PL, Poole-Wilson PA, Harris PC (1989). Edema of cardiac origin. Studies of body water and sodium, renal function, hemodynamic indexes, and plasma hormones in untreated congestive cardiac failure. *Circulation* **80**: 299–305.

43. Hasper D, Hummel M, Kleber FX, Reindl I, Volk HD (1998). Systemic inflammation in patients with heart failure. *Eur Heart J* **19**: 761–5.

44. Torre-Amione G, Kapadia S, Lee J *et al.* Tumor necrosis factor-alpha and tumor necrosis factor receptors in the failing human heart. *Circulation* **93**: 704–11.

45. Anker SD, Egerer KR, Volk HD, Kox WJ, Poole-Wilson PA, Coats AJ (1997). Elevated soluble CD14 receptors and altered cytokines in chronic heart failure. *Am J Cardiol* **79**: 1426–30.

46. Von Haehling, Genth-Zontz S, Anker SD, Volk HD (2002). Cachexia: a therapeutic approach beyond cytokine antagonism. *Int J Cardiol* **85**: 173–85.

47. Niebauer J, Volk HD, Kemp M *et al.* (1999). Endotoxin and immune activation in chronic heart failure: a prospective cohort study. *Lancet* **353**: 1838–42.

48. Brunkhorst F, Clark A, Forycki Z, Anker S (1999). Pyrexia, procalcitonin, immune activation and survival in cardiogenic shock: the potential importance of bacterial translocation. *Int J Cardiol* **72**: 3–10.

49. Krack A, Sharma R, Figulla HR, Anker SD (2005). The importance of the gastrointestinal system in the pathogenesis of heart failure. *Eur Heart J* **26**: 2368–74.

50. Rauchhaus M, Coats AJ, Anker SD (2000). The endotoxin-lipoprotein hypothesis. *Lancet* **356**: 930–3.

51. Rauchhaus M, Koloczek V, Volk H *et al.* (2000). Inflammatory cytokines and the possible immuno-logical role for lipoproteins in chronic heart failure. *Int J Cardiol* **76**: 125–33.

52. Rauchhaus M, Clark AL, Doehner W *et al.* (2003). The relationship between cholesterol and survival in patients with chronic heart failure. *J Am Coll Cardiol* **42**: 1933–40.

53. Jankowska EA, Ponikowski P, Piepoli MF, Anker SD, Poole-Wilson PA (2006). Autonomic imbalance and immune activation in chronic heart failure – pathophysiological links. *Cardiovasc Res* **70**:434–45.

54. Sharma R, Rauchhaus M, Ponikowski PP et al (2000). The relationship of the erythrocyte sedimentation rate to inflammatory cytokines and survival in patients with chronic heart failure treated with angiotensin-converting enzyme inhibitors. *J Am Coll Cardiol* **36**: 523–8.

55. Anker SD, Doehner W, Rauchhaus M *et al.* (2003). Uric acid and survival in chronic heart failure; validation and application in metabolic, functional, and hemodynamic staging. *Circulation* **107**: 1991–7.

56. Anker SD, Ponikowski PP, Clark AL *et al.* (1999). Cytokines and neurohormones relating to body composition alterations in the wasting syndrome of chronic heart failure. *Eur Heart J* **20**: 683–93.

57. Doehner W, Rauchhaus M, Ponikowski P *et al.* (2005). Impaired insulin sensitivity as an independent risk factor for mortality in patients with stable chronic heart failure. *J Am Coll Cardiol* **46**: 1019–26.

58. Springer J, Filippatos G, Akashi YJ, Anker SD (2006). Prognosis and therapy approaches of cardiac cachexia. *Curr Opin Cardiol* **21**: 229–33.

59. Swedberg K, Cleland J, Dargie H *et al.* (2005). Guidelines for the diagnosis and treatment of chronic heart failure: full text (update 2005). *Eur Heart J* **26**: 1115–40.

60. Song Yao-Hua, Li Y, Du J *et al.* (2005). Muscle-specific expression of IGF-1 blocks angiotensin-induced skeletal muscle wasting. *J Clin Invest* **115**: 451–8.

61. Shibata MC, Flather MD, Wang D (2001). Systematic review of the impact of beta blockers on mortality and hospital admissions in heart failure. *Eur J Heart Fail* **3**: 351–9.

62. Sharma AM, Pischon T, Hardt S, Kunz I, Luft FC (2001). Beta-adrenergic receptor blockers and weight gain: a systematic analysis. *Hypertension* **37**: 250–4.

63. Anker SD, Coats AJS, Roecker EB, Scherhag A, Packer M (2002). Does Carvedilol prevent and reverse cardiac cachexia in patients with severe heart failure? Results of the COPERNICUS study.[abstract] *Eur Heart J* **23**(Suppl. S): 394

64. Anker SD, Lechat P, Dargie HJ (2003). Prevention of cachexia in patients with chronic heart failure by bisoprolol: results from the CIBIS-II study.[abstract] *J Am Coll Cardiol* **41**(Suppl.): 156A–157A.

65. Hyrniewicz K, Androne AS, Hudaihed A, Katz SD (2003). Partial reversal of cachexia by beta-adrenergic receptor blocker therapy in patients with chronic heart failure. *J Card Fail* **9**: 464–8.

66. Lainscak M, Keber I, Anker SD (2006). Body composition changes in patients with systolic heart failure treated with beta blockers: a pilot study. *Int J Cardiol* **106**: 319–22.

67. Mann DL, McMurray JJ, Packer M *et al.* (2004). Targeted anticytokine therapy in patients with chronic heart failure: results of the Randomized Etanercept Worldwide Evaluation (RENEWAL). *Circulation* **109**: 1594–602.

68. Chung ES, Packer M, Lo KH, Fasanmade AA, Willerson JT. Anti-TNF Therapy Against Congestive Heart Failure Investigators (2003). Randomized, double-blind, placebo-controlled, pilot trial of infliximab, a chimeric monoclonal antibody to tumor necrosis factor-alpha, in patients with moderate to severe heart failure: results of the anti-TNF Therapy Against Congestive Heart Failure (ATTACH) trial. *Circulation* **107**: 3133–40.

69. Anker SD, Coats AJS (2002). How to RECOVER from RENAISSANCE? The significance of the results of RECOVER, RENAISSANCE, RENEWAL, and ATTACH. *Int J Cardiol* **86**: 123–30.

70. Von Haehling S, Anker SD (2005). Future prospects of anticytokine therapy in chronic heart failure. *Expert Opin Investig Drugs* **14**: 163–76.

71. Batchelder K, Mayosi BM (2005). Pentoxyfilline for heart failure: a systematic review. *S Afr Med J* **95**: 171–5.

72. Malkin CJ, Pugh PJ, West JN, van Beek EJ, Jones TH, Channer KS (2006). Testosterone therapy in men with moderate severity heart failure: a double-blind randomized placebo controlled trial. *Eur Heart J* **27**: 57–64.

73. Rauchhaus M, Doehner W, Anker SD (2006). Heart failure therapy: testosterone replacement and its implications. *Eur Heart J* **27**: 10–12.

74. Fazio S, Sabatini D, Capaldo B *et al.* (1996). A preliminary study of growth hormone in the treatment of dilated cardiomyopathy. *New Engl J Med* **334**: 809–14.

75. Osterziel KJ, Strohm O, Schuler J *et al.* (1998). Randomised, double-blind, placebo controlled trial of human recombinant growth hormone in patients with chronic heart failure due to dilated cardiomyopathy. *Lancet* **351**: 1233–7.

76. O'Driscoll JG, Green DJ, Ireland M *et al.* (1997). Treatment of end-stage cardiac failure with growth hormone. *Lancet* **349**: 1068.

77. Bocchi E, Moura L, Guimaraes G *et al.* (2005). Beneficial effects of high doses of growth hormone in the introduction and optimization of medical treatment in decompensated congestive heart failure. *Int J Cardiol* **110**: 313–17.

78. Cicoria M, Kalra PR, Anker SD (2003). Growth hormone resistance in chronic heart failure and its therapeutic implications. *J Card Fail* **9**: 219–26.

79. Nagaya N, Kojima M, Kangawa K (2006). Ghrelin, a novel growth hormone-releasing peptide, in the treatment of cardiopulmonary-associated cachexia. *Intern Med* **45**: 127–34.

80. Witte KK, Clark AL (2002). Nutritional abnormalities contributing to cachexia in chronic illness. *Int J Cardiol* **85**: 23–31.

81. Moriwaki H, Tajika M, Miwa Y *et al.* (2000). Nutritional pharmacotherapy of chronic liver disease: from support of liver failure to prevention of liver cancer. *J Gastroenterol* **35**(Suppl. 12): 13–17.

82. Witte KK, Nikitin NP, Parker AC *et al.* (2005). The effect of micronutrient supplementation on quality-of-life and left ventricular function in elderly patients with heart failure. *Eur Heart J* **26**: 2238–44.

83. Rozentryt P, Michalak A, Nowak JU, Brachowska A, Polonski L, Anker SD (2005). The effects of enteral supplementation in patients with cardiac cachexia – a prospective, randomised, double-blind, placebo controlled trial. In: *3rd Cachexia Conference, Final Program and Abstract Book*, p. 82 (available at: http://www.lms-events.com/18/Cachexia_2005_Final_Abstract.pdf).

84. Coats AJ, Adamopoulos S, Meyer TE *et al.* (1990). Effects of physical training in chronic heart failure. *Lancet* **335**: 63–6.

85. Gielen S, Adams V, Linke A *et al.* (2005). Exercise training in chronic heart failure: correlation between reduced local inflammation and improved oxidative capacity in skeletal muscle. *Eur J Cardiovasc Prev Rehabil* **12**: 393–400.

86. Piepoli MF, Davos C, Francis DP, Coats AJ; ExTraMATCH Collaborative (2004). Exercise training meta-analysis of trials in patients with chronic heart failure (ExTraMATCH). *Br Med J* **328**: 189–95.

87. Harris S, LeMaitre JP, Mackenzie G, Fox KA, Denvir MA (2003). A randomised study of home-based electrical simulation of the legs and conventional bicycle exercise training for patients with chronic heart failure. *Eur Heart J* **24**: 871–8.

88. Nuhr MJ, Pette D, Berger R *et al.* (2004). Beneficial effects of chronic low-frequency stimulation of thigh muscles in patients with advanced chronic heart failure. *Eur Heart J* **25**: 136–43.

Chapter 14

Cognitive impairment

Giuseppe Zuccalà, Alice Laudisio, and Roberto
Bernabei

Historical perspective

The first concept of a neuropsychological disorder characterized by 'lack of concentration and memory impairment' due to several physically disabling conditions might be identified in the description of 'nervous exhaustion' or 'neurasthenia' by G. M. Beard in 1869.[1]

However, it was only in 1977 that an editorial in *The Lancet*, dealing with the effects of bradycardia on cerebral electrical activity and performance among older subjects, coined the term 'cardiogenic dementia'.[2] Noticeably, the author indicated elderly patients as a particularly vulnerable population, suggesting that, considering the high sensitivity to anoxia of the aged brain, bradycardia might easily impair cerebral blood flow in older subjects thus causing or aggravating cognitive abnormalities. A few years later, a study found multiple cognitive deficits, including 'significant' memory impairment, in 70% of patients undergoing cardiac rehabilitation.[3] The authors proposed the term 'circulatory dementia' to describe this form of cognitive impairment, of which the aetiology, however, was considered 'unknown'.

In the late 1990s, the issue of 'cardiogenic' or 'circulatory' dementia was revived by repeated reports on the effect of pacemaker implantation and cardiac transplantation on cognitive function in patients with end-stage heart failure (HF) or extreme bradycardia.[4–6] According to these studies, cognitive impairment associated with low cardiac output states seemed to represent quite a rare condition, limited to selected populations of patients with severe cardiac dysfunction. However, subsequent studies also demonstrated an excess prevalence of cognitive impairment (ranging from 35% to 58%) in older populations with only mild to moderate HF.[7–10]

Most recently, studies performed in large older populations with HF, such as the 'Gruppo Italiano di Farmacoepidemiologia nell'Anziano' (Italian Pharmacoepidemiology in the Elderly Study Group) demonstrated that among older patients with HF cognitive dysfunction, even when mild, is associated with a fivefold increase in the risk of mortality and a six-fold increase in the probability of dependence in the activities of daily living.[10,11] These figures are important from the perspective of clinicians as well as national health systems, because, despite recent advances in pharmacological treatment, HF in older populations is still associated with astonishingly high rates of mortality and disability. In fact, it has been found that, following hospital discharge, over 20% of patients aged over 75 with a diagnosis of HF die within 1 month, and less than 50% are still alive at 1 year.[12] Also, a recent study compared period-specific 5-year survival among incident HF cases in 1970 to 1974, and 1990 to 1994 in an older population. In this study, analysis of 38,800 and 127,419 person-years for 1970 to 1974 and 1990 to 1994, respectively, indicated that the spread of state-of-the-art treatment for HF in clinical practice has yielded only minimal changes in the survival of male patients, and no variations in the survival rates of women.[13] Such observations cast doubts on our knowledge of the determinants of survival in older patients with HF, as well as on the efficacy and safety of 'acknowledged' drug treatment for HF in older populations.[14] This concern was fuelled by the demonstration of an inverse association between systolic blood pressure and cognitive performance among older patients with HF who were treated with vasodilating agents.[15] This finding, that was in keeping with repeated epidemiological observations of an increased risk of developing cognitive impairment in older subjects with lower baseline blood pressure levels, raised the issue of possible deleterious effects of treatment with vasodilating agents on cerebral perfusion.[16,17] However, a subsequent study indicated that, among the hospitalized elderly with HF, starting treatment with angiotensin-converting enzyme (ACE) inhibitors was associated with an increased probability of improving cognitive performance, independently of baseline or discharge blood pressure levels.[18] Such results also confirmed the potential reversibility of cognitive impairment associated with HF; this issue is crucial from the clinical and economic perspective, as cognitive impairment is a major determinant of the loss of functional ability among older patients with HF.[11] Disability, in turn, is a major determinant of the increased resource consumption associated with HF that currently represents the most costly medical illness in the United States.[19–22] Accordingly, it has been calculated that even moderate gains in cognitive functioning among these patients might allow substantial reductions in mortality rates and resource consumption (See also Chapter 19).[22,23]

The adverse effects of cardiovascular diseases on cognitive function in the aged are only beginning to be recognized. At present 'cardiogenic dementia' is generally considered a major component of 'vascular' dementias.[23] The growing body of evidence on the prevalence and clinical implications of 'cardiogenic dementia', particularly in view of the increasing incidence and prevalence rates of HF in older populations, is conferring increasing relevance to the detection and treatment of cognitive deficits in patients with left ventricular dysfunction. In the 2003 annual congress of the Heart Failure Society of America a symposium was dedicated to cognitive impairment in HF.[24] Subsequently, a position statement of the society highlighted the opportunity for including the variations in cognitive functioning among the outcomes of trials on ventricular assist devices;[25] this aim is being increasingly pursued by researchers.[26] In addition, assessment and monitoring of cognitive performance has been suggested as a primary endpoint of any pharmacological trial in HF,[27] and is being introduced into clinical guidelines.[28] Research on the determinants and potential treatment of 'cardiogenic dementia' was included among the most relevant studies in the field of HF in 2005.[29]

Epidemiology

Currently available epidemiological data indicate that vascular cognitive impairment is the second most common form of dementia after Alzheimer's disease; in fact, this form of cognitive dysfunction might represent 15–20% of all dementias.[23] However, this figure is thought to underestimate the true prevalence of this form of cognitive impairment, which should probably be considered the most common cause of dementia in Western countries, at least among subjects older than 85.[30] Indeed, some studies performed in Eastern populations seem to indicate that this form of dementia is far more common than Alzheimer's disease; these differences in incidence rates have not yet been explained, even though genetic factors might play a role.[31] Independently of current prevalence rates, it is generally agreed that, due to progressive aging of the world's population, both the incidence and prevalence of vascular dementias will increase in the next decades.[23] Also, the prevalence rates of HF are increasing, chiefly among the older age strata of populations. In fact, in the United States, the rates of hospital admission for HF increased by 25% between 1985 and 1995 among patients older than 85; due to progressive aging of populations, the number of patients with HF will double within the next 40 years.[32] Accordingly, HF represents by far the most common diagnosis in hospitalized elderly patients; a recent study of incident cases has found that patients older than 60 years represent 88% of patients admitted with HF as first diagnosis; of these, 49% are older than 80, so that HF has been defined as a 'cardiogeriatric syndrome'.[33] In addition, these data and projections are likely to underestimate the true epidemiological reality, as it has been demonstrated that more than 50% of older subjects with left ventricular systolic dysfunction have never been diagnosed with HF(See also Chapter 2).[34]

As already mentioned, the reported prevalence of cognitive dysfunction in older populations with HF varies across studies, according to diagnostic criteria as well as to the criteria adopted to rule out primary neurodegenerative disorders and cerebrovascular disease. In a large study of ambulatory, unselected older subjects with reported diagnosis of HF, cognitive impairment has been detected in nearly 60% of participants.[7] In the GIFA database, after the exclusion of patients with any ICD-9 CM codes of Alzheimer's or cerebrovascular disease, cognitive impairment, as diagnosed by a short screening method (the Hodkinson Abbreviated Mental Test) was found in 35% (647 of 1,860) of participants with verified diagnosis of HF, but only in 28% (4,229 of 15,053) of subjects without such a diagnosis.[10] In another population of older patients with HF, after excluding subjects who met the NINCDS/ADRDA criteria for Alzheimer's disease and those with a Hachinski ischaemic score suggestive of possible cerebrovascular disease, use of a thorough mental deterioration battery identified cognitive dysfunction in 53% of cases.[8]

Even when considering the most conservative estimate (26%) of prevalence rates, it has been calculated that, in the United States only, over 1 million subjects might be affected by undiagnosed cognitive dysfunction associated with HF.[23] Hence, a relevant quota of 'cardiogenic dementia' cases, and thus a relevant source of functional disability and reduced survival, is currently being missed in clinical practice. In fact, a study of co-morbid conditions reported in 122,630 Medicare beneficiaries with HF found a diagnosis of any form of dementia (thus including Alzheimer's disease and post-stroke cases along with cardiogenic dementia) in only 9% of patients.[35]

Aetiology

Cerebral embolism was initially considered to be the major culprit for the development of cognitive impairment among patients with HF.[16] However, an excess prevalence of cognitive dysfunction has also been demonstrated among elderly people with HF after the exclusion of cases with cerebrovascular disease;[8,10] in addition, in these patients atrial fibrillation, either chronic or paroxysmal, is not associated with increased probability of cognitive impairment.[11] Indeed, the incidence of cerebral embolism among patients with HF is too low to account for most cases of cognitive dysfunction in these subjects.[36] On the other hand, cognitive dysfunction among older patients with HF has been associated with left ventricular dysfunction (i.e. left ventricular ejection fraction below 30%),[8] and with systolic blood pressure levels lower than 130 mmHg.[15] Cohort studies have generally shown that hypertension is a risk factor for the development of cognitive impairment or dementia[37,38] and that antihypertensive treatment can prevent cognitive dysfunction.[39] However, in several cohort studies blood pressure has been found to decrease well before the onset of dementia.[40,41] Recently, worsening cognitive function has been documented in cohort studies among subjects with baseline systolic blood pressure below 130 mmHg.[42,43] Among older subjects, both HF and systolic hypotension have been associated with the presence of white matter lesions; such lesions, in turn, have been associated with increased prevalence of dementia.[44] Subcortical alterations have also been associated with conditions of chronic hypoperfusion in neuropathological studies.[45] The pattern of cognitive dysfunction in older subjects with HF and reduced left ventricular function further supports the involvement of subcortical areas.[8] Noticeably, cerebral blood flow is heavily dependent upon systolic blood pressure in patients with HF,[46] as well as in general older populations,[47] due to impaired autoregulation of cerebral circulation. The impairment of cognitive functioning in patients with HF is thought to be associated with specific damage in the white subcortical matter of selected cerebral areas that seem to be more sensitive to hypoperfusional damage. These areas include the periventricular white matter, the basal ganglia and the hippocampus. The damage of subcortical white matter causes disarrangement of intra- and interhemispherical connections; this has relevant consequences, due to the ensuing interruption of neuronal circuits that link prefrontal areas to the basal ganglia, thalamocortical junctions, and the limbic lobe. Such pathways are crucial for memory, attention, executive functions, and continence.[48] Most recently, the volume of periventricular white matter hyperintensities has been shown to be associated with declining mental processing speed in a prospective study of older subjects without baseline dementia.[49]

The bulk of these observations definitely support the role of cerebral hypoperfusion as the major determinant of cognitive impairment in patients with HF.[16,17,23] This issue does not represent a mere academic matter. In fact, while cerebral embolism would result in permanent damage to cognitive processes, the hypoperfusive mechanism implies potential reversibility of cognitive deficits, at least before the development of structural cerebral alterations.[16,18,23] However, other mechanisms might underlie the development of cognitive dysfunction in subjects with HF, together with reduced cerebral perfusion. In fact, the rapid changes in cognitive performance produced by both ACE-inhibitors and angiotensin-I receptor blockers in patients with hypertension or HF suggest that activation of the renin–angiotensin system might play a role in the pathogenesis of vascular dementia.[18] Indeed, cerebral AT-1 receptors are thought to be involved in the development of neurological deficits, as well neuronal injury, apoptosis, and inflammatory responses (probably via the expression of c-Fos and c-Jun proteins) after cerebral ischaemia.[50,51]

The bulk of co-morbid conditions generally associated with HF in older populations might also account for some cases of cognitive impairment in these subjects. For instance, diabetes has been associated with executive dysfunction in older patients.[52] Noticeably, in the GIFA study about 20% of older patients with HF had diabetes mellitus.

Eventually, inflammation represents another potential cause of, or factor contributing to, cognitive impairment in patients with HF. In fact, increased secretion of pro-inflammatory cytokines is a hallmark of HF;[53] however, increased serum and cerebral pro-inflammatory cytokine levels have been associated with both Alzheimer's disease and multi-infarct dementia.[54]

Clinical features

From the clinical point of view, vascular dementia (that is currently thought to include 'cardiogenic dementia') is characterized by early loss of executive control functions (Table 14.1).[55] It is generally acknowledged that impairment of executive control functions mediates the development of disability (i.e. dependence for the activities of daily living, such as walking, dressing, bathing, using the toilet, or eating) in subjects with mild cognitive impairment.[56] This might explain the observed development of disability among the elderly with HF with even mild cognitive impairment.[11] Impairment in calculation, memory, and language functions seem to occur only later, and the severity of such deficits has no relation, at least initially, with the degree of subcortical damage.

Table 14.1 Characteristics of cognitive impairment associated with HF

Onset	Sudden or gradual
Progression	Usually slow, with stepwise fluctuations
Objective findings	Focal deficits
Executive control functions	Early and severely impaired
Dementia type	Subcortical
Neuroimaging	White matter lesions, possibly infarcts
Gait	Often early compromised
Continence	Often early compromised
Functional ability	Early impaired
Left ventricular systolic function	Often severely impaired

Impairment of executive functions results in psychomotor slackening, postural disturbances, disorganization of sequential tasks, and difficulty in managing personal effects. Patients cannot start any kind of activity by themselves, have reduced mental flexibility, and are unable to pay attention to relevant aspects of their actions. They have a low capacity of discrimination and abstraction. In fact, deterioration of the executive functions causes a dissociation between will and action. For instance, patients do not lose the ability to get dressed, but are unable to start the action or choose the appropriate clothes. When considering these features, it is not difficult to explain why cognitive impairment has been associated in older patients with HF with a six-fold increase in the probability of dependence for the activities of daily living.[11]

As already mentioned, disability is a major determinant of the excess expenditure associated with HF.[22] However, cognitive dysfunction is also independently associated with a fivefold increase in mortality rates among subjects with diagnosis of HF, even 1 year after hospital discharge.[10] It could easily be hypothesized that, among elderly subjects with HF, the prognostic role of cognitive impairment might simply reflect the severity of left ventricular dysfunction or, as most recently suggested, of other factors such as anaemia, electrolyte imbalance, or renal failure.[57] Nevertheless, a study conducted in patients with severe HF has proven that reduced perfusion-associated cerebral metabolism, as detected by proton magnetic resonance spectroscopy, is a powerful and independent determinant of decreased survival.[58] Therefore, cerebral metabolic abnormalities could represent a determinant, rather than a marker, of early mortality among patients with left ventricular dysfunction. It is unclear how brain dysfunction might influence the survival of patients with HF; however, impaired autonomic control of cardiac rhythm could represent the link between brain dysfunction and cardiovascular mortality in these subjects. In fact, increased QT dispersion and decreased heart rate variability have been observed in patients with Alzheimer's disease or mild cognitive impairment; in these subjects, the degree of derangement in both electrocardiographic parameters paralleled the severity of cognitive impairment.[59] Noticeably, several reports indicate that both increased QT dispersion and decreased heart rate variability are associated with decreased survival of patients with HF.[60]

At present, there are no acknowledged tests to detect and quantify cognitive impairment among patients with HF. Indeed, the use of complex mental deterioration batteries that have been applied in some studies would be excessively time-consuming for routine ambulatory practice; in addition, the administration and interpretation of such sets of diagnostic tools require specific expertise. Thus, most studies conducted in older populations with HF explored cognitive performance using simple screening tools, such as the Mini Mental State Examination Test or the Hodkinson Abbreviated Mental Test. These tests generally allowed the detection of impairment in complex reasoning (calculation and visual-spatial intelligence).[8,15] However, such screening tests do not allow the detection of dysexecutive syndrome that probably represents, as already discussed, the first sign of cognitive impairment in patients with HF. Indeed, there is no consensus about the best methods for assessing disturbances of executive control functions in clinical practice. The Trail Making B, for instance, is among the most commonly used tests in this setting;

however, this test is quite time-consuming and is strongly dependent upon education. [61] Probably, use of the clock drawing test might represent the best compromise between efficacy and ease of administration in clinical practice. This test, in which patients are asked to draw a clock showing a certain hour (most commonly 11:10), has been proven to detect executive dysfunction in subjects who do not exhibit difficulty in performing visuospatial tasks, such as the copying of polygons in the Mini Mental State test.[62] This test has been proven to be independent of education, and has been proposed for the assessment of older patients in outpatient practices.[62] Thus, a combination of a general baseline neuropsychological assessment tool with a variety of clock drawing test might be adopted for the screening and, possibly, follow-up of cognitive dysfunction among patients with HF in routine clinical practice.

Treatment

As described above, neuroanatomical and neuropathological studies indicate that patients with HF eventually develop structural cerebral alterations that lead to permanent cognitive dysfunction.[44,45] Also, it must be emphasized that even though some descriptive studies have shown that cognitive impairment associated with HF might be improved by cardiac transplantation, pacemaker implantation, or pharmacological treatment,[4–6,18] no intervention has so far been proven to reverse this form of vascular dementia in a randomized trial.

Therefore, the prevention of cerebral vascular damage, based upon the most accurate and early control of vascular risk factors, currently represents the key intervention.[23]

Older patients, and even physicians, are often uncertain about the benefits of preventive interventions in older age. Nevertheless, even though the relative risk associated with single cardiovascular risk factors decreases with advancing age, the absolute risk increases steeply. Thus, the 'number needed to treat' for preventive interventions is markedly reduced in older subjects, so rendering the cost-effectiveness ratio of both primary and secondary prevention more favourable among older subjects.[63]

The relevance of healthy lifestyle habits, including smoking cessation, moderate alcohol consumption, and regular physical activity, should be stressed to any patients with HF. Also, strict control of diabetes and dyslipidaemia is essential for preventing structural and functional cerebral damage. Noticeably, it has been suggested that statins might improve cognition in general, as well as in demented older populations.[64,65] Most recently, analyses performed in 1,511 hospitalized elderly people with a diagnosis of HF enrolled in the GIFA study demonstrated that, among the elderly, the presence of hyperglycaemia was associated with a 33% increased probability of cognitive impairment, after adjusting for potential confounders.[57] On the other hand, restoration of normal serum glucose levels was associated with improved cognitive performance at discharge. The same study found that abnormal sodium and potassium serum levels were independently associated with detection of cognitive dysfunction, and that normalization of serum potassium was associated with improving cognition through hospital stay.

Increased serum creatinine and reduced albumin and haemoglobin levels were other potentially reversible predictors of cognitive impairment among patients with HF in the GIFA database; again, normalization of haemoglobin levels was independently associated with improving cognitive performance at discharge.[57] Renal dysfunction is increasingly being found to be a relevant marker of decreased survival and functional status among patients with HF. The issue of anaemia deserves particular attention. In fact, neurological symptoms are commonly reported in elderly patients with anaemia.[66] Although data on specific neurological effects of anaemia are limited, the presence of anaemia (and consequent hypoxia) appears to contribute to impaired cognitive function in patients with chronic renal failure, who frequently suffer from confusion, inability to concentrate, decreased mental alertness, and impaired memory.[66,67] Correction of anaemia with erythropoietin treatment may reverse brain dysfunction not directly attributable to uraemia. In fact, it improves both cognitive function and brain electrophysiology by raising levels of sustained attention, thereby increasing the speed and efficiency of scanning and perceptual motor function, and enhancing learning and memory.[67] The association between anaemia and cognitive function is also suggested by the increasing evidence indicating a relationship between erythropoietin and nervous system function.[68] Treatment of anaemia also yields relevant haemodynamic and metabolic effects. In fact, treatment of anaemia by erythropoietin in patients with HF has been proven to increase peripheral oxygen delivery and, in older patients undergoing haemodialysis, to increase cerebral blood flow, oxygen extraction, and metabolic rate for oxygen.[69,70] In addition, normalization of haemoglobin levels in anaemic patients with HF has been found to improve left ventricular ejection fraction, stroke volume, and cardiac output, which, in turn, might improve cerebral perfusion.[71] This issue is of particular interest in the view of a potential negative effect of ACE-inhibitors on haemoglobin levels.[72] Therefore, treatment of anaemia might become a mainstay in the prevention, and possibly treatment, of cognitive dysfunction associated with HF.

The issue of the effects of blood pressure control on cognitive functioning of patients with HF is more complex. In fact, systolic blood pressure below 130 mmHg has been associated with increased probability of cognitive impairment among hospitalized patients with HF, including those who received vasodilating agents.[15] Indeed, systolic blood pressure below 130 mmHg has been associated with increased risk of cognitive decline also in general older populations.[42,43] These findings, along with other reports on reduced cerebrovascular reactivity in HF patients, raised concern about the potential detrimental effects of agents yielding vasodilating effects on cerebral perfusion of subjects with left ventricular dysfunction.[16,17] Nevertheless, a study of 1,220 older inpatients with diagnosis of HF who did not take ACE-inhibitors before hospital admission recently indicated that starting treatment with ACE-inhibitors was independently associated with increased probability of improving cognitive performance during hospital stay.[18] In this study, the probability of improving cognitive performance was higher for dosages above the median values, as compared with lower doses, and increased with the duration of treatment. Most importantly, such effects of ACE-inhibitors on cognitive functioning were independent of baseline as well as achieved blood pressure levels.

Noticeably, ACE-inhibitors and angiotensin-I receptor blockers (ARBs) have been proven to prevent cognitive decline, or even to reverse cognitive deficits, in hypertensive populations.[73,74] In addition, enalapril has been found to increase cerebral blood flow in patients with HF.[75] As a whole, these data indicate that either ACE-inhibitors or ARBs should be administered to subjects with HF also with the aim of improving cognitive performance, independently of blood pressure. Also, adequate up-titration of these agents might be required to yield the greatest benefit.[18] Noticeably, ACE-inhibitors are characterized by poor diffusibility through the blood–brain barrier; ARBs, on the contrary, yield high intracerebral concentrations.[76,77] In addition, selective blockade of cerebral angiotensin-I receptors by ARBs has been shown to blunt neurological deficits and to reduce neuronal apoptosis following experimental ischaemia.[50,51] Also, treatment with ARBs should allow angiotensin II to interact with angiotensin II receptors, that yield non-haemodynamic neuroprotective effects and modulate glutamatergic and GABAergic synaptic transmission.[78,79] Accordingly, several clinical studies found that ARBs, but not ACE-inhibitors, yield neuroprotective effects in subjects with cerebral ischaemia.[78,80] However, whether ARBs might be superior to ACE-inhibitors in improving the cognitive performance of patients with HF has to be ascertained by randomized trials.

Conclusions

A multitude of data currently indicate that 'cardiogenic dementia' is a major, potentially reversible cause of functional disability and reduced survival in patients with HF. However, research on the determinants and potential treatment of 'cardiogenic dementia' is only just beginning. In fact, there still needs to be a consensus on the methods to adopt for the routine assessment of cognitive functioning in patients with HF; also, the effects of treatment for HF on cognitive performance have yet be ascertained in randomized trials. Overall, all the available evidence regarding cognitive impairment associated with HF clearly indicates that mortality and readmission rates cannot be considered any longer the only outcome variables in the management of patients with HF. As stated by several authors, research in the field of HF should broaden to a comprehensive view of health outcomes, so yielding evidence that might support clinical decision-making, improve clinical practice, and guide health policy. Focusing on health status outcomes would also be in keeping with the Institute of Medicine's promotion of patient-centred care, among the six strategies designated to improve the quality of care in the United States. The course of research on the multidimensional assessment of older patients with HF, that begun nearly 20 years ago,[81] is still far from its end.

References

1. Beard GM (1869). Neurasthenia or nervous exhaustion. *Boston Med Surg J* **3**: 217–21.
2. Editorial (1977). Cardiogenic dementia. *Lancet* **1**: 27–8.
3. Barclay LL, Weiss EM, Mattis S *et al.* (1988). Unrecognized cognitive impairment in cardiac rehabilitation patients. *J Am Geriatr Soc* **36**: 22–8.

4. Koide H, Kobayashi S, Kitani M *et al.* (1994). Improvement of cerebral blood flow and cognitive function following pacemaker implantation in patients with bradycardia. *Gerontology* **40**: 79–85.

5. Bornstein RA, Starling RC, Myerowitz P, Haas GJ (1995). Neuropsychological function in patients with end-stage heart failure before and after cardiac transplantation. *Acta Neurol Scand* **91**: 260–5.

6. Grimm M, Yeganehfar W, Laufer G *et al.* (1996). Cyclosporine may affect improvement of cognitive brain function after successful cardiac transplantation. *Circulation* **94**: 1339–45.

7. Cacciatore F, Abete P, Ferrara N *et al.* (1998). Congestive heart failure and cognitive impairment in an older population. *J Am Geriatr Soc* **46**: 1343–8.

8. Zuccalà G, Cattel C, Gravina-Manes E *et al.* (1997). Left ventricular dysfunction: a clue to cognitive impairment in older patients with heart failure. *J Neurol Neurosurg Psychiat* **63**: 509–12.

9. Almeida OP, Flicker L (2001). The mind of a failing heart: a systematic review of the association between congestive heart failure and cognitive functioning. *Intern Med J* **31**: 290–5.

10. Zuccalà G, Pedone C, Cesari M *et al.* (2003). The effects of cognitive impairment on mortality among hospitalized patients with heart failure. *Am J Med* **115**: 97–103.

11. Zuccalà G, Onder G, Pedone C *et al.* (2001). Cognitive dysfunction as a major determinant of disability in patients with heart failure: results from a multicentre survey. *J Neurol Neurosurg Psychiat* **70**: 109–12.

12. MacIntyre K, Capewell S, Stewart S *et al.* (2000). Evidence of improving prognosis in heart failure: trends in case fatality in 66 547 patients hospitalized between 1986 and 1995. *Circulation* **102**: 1126–31.

13. Barker WH, Mullooly JP, Getchell W (2006). Changing incidence and survival for heart failure in a well-defined older population, 1970–1974 and 1990–1994. *Circulation* **113**: 799–805.

14. Konstam MA (2000). Progress in heart failure management? Lessons from the real world. *Circulation* **102**: 1076–8.

15. Zuccalà G, Onder G, Pedone C *et al.* (2001). Hypotension and cognitive impairment: selective association in patients with heart failure. *Neurology* **59**: 1986–92.

16. Pullicino PM, Hart J (2001). Cognitive impairment in congestive heart failure? Embolism vs hypoperfusion. *Neurology* **57**: 1945–6.

17. Mathias CJ (2000). Cerebral hypoperfusion and impaired cerebral function in cardiac failure. *Eur Heart J* **21**: 346.

18. Zuccalà G, Onder G, Marzetti E *et al.* (2005). Use of angiotensin-converting enzyme inhibitors and variations in cognitive performance among patients with heart failure. *Eur Heart J* **26**: 226–33.

19. Konstam V, Salem D, Pouleur H *et al.* (1996). Baseline quality of life as a predictor of mortality and hospitalization in 5,025 patients with congestive heart failure. SOLVD Investigations. Studies of Left Ventricular Dysfunction Investigators. *Am J Cardiol* **78**: 890–5.

20. Wolinsky FD, Smith DM, Stump TE *et al.* (1997). The sequelae of hospitalization for congestive heart failure among older adults. *J Am Geriatr Soc* **45**: 558–63.

21. Haldeman GA, Croft JB, Giles WH *et al.* (1999). Hospitalization of patients with heart failure: National Hospital Discharge Survey, 1985 to 1995. *Am Heart J* **137**: 352–60.

22. Rich MW, Nease RF (1999). Cost-effectiveness analysis in clinical practice. The case of heart failure. *Arch Intern Med* **159**: 1690–700.

23. Roman GC (2004). Brain hypoperfusion: a critical factor in vascular dementia. *Neurol Res* **26**: 454–8.

24. Normand SL, Rector TS, Neaton DJ *et al.* (2005). Clinical considerations in the study of health status in device trials for heart failure. *J Card Fail* **11**: 396–403.

25. Konstam MA, Lindenfeld J, Pina IL *et al.* (2004). Key issues in trial design for ventricular assist devices: a position statement of the Heart Failure Society of America. *J Card Fail* **10**: 91–100.

26. Zimpfer D, Wieselthaler G, Czerny M *et al.* (2006). Neurocognitive function in patients with ventricular assist devices. A comparison of pulsatile and continuous blood flow devices. *ASAIO J* **52**: 24–7.

27. Lang CC, Mancini DM (2007). Noncardiac comorbidities in heart failure. *Heart* **93**: 665–71.

28. Arnold JMO, Demers C, Dorian P *et al.* (2006). Canadian cardiovascular society consensus conference recommendations on heart failure 2006: diagnosis and management. *Can J Cardiol* **22**: 23–45.

29. Tang WHW, Francis GS (2005). The year in heart failure. *J Am Coll Cardiol* **46**: 2125–33.

30. Neuropathology Group of the Medical Research Council Cognitive Function and Ageing Study (2001). Pathological correlates of late-onset dementia in a multicentre, community-based population in England and Wales. *Lancet* **357**: 169–75.

31. Slooters AJC, Tang M-X, van Duijn CM *et al.* (1997). Apolipoprotein E epsilon 4 and the risk of dementia with stroke. A population-based investigation. *J Am Med Assoc* **277**: 818–21.

32. McCullough PA, Philbin EF, Spertus JA *et al.* (2002). Confirmation of a heart failure epidemic: findings from the Resource Utilization Among Congestive Heart Failure (REACH) study. *J Am Coll Cardiol* **39**: 60–9.

33. Rich MW (2001). Heart failure in the 21st century: a cardiogeriatric syndrome. *J Gerontol A Biol Sci Med Sci* **56**: M88–M96.

34. Mosterd A, Hoes AW, de Bruyne MC *et al.* (1999). Prevalence of heart failure and left ventricular dysfunction in the general population: the Rotterdam Study. *Eur Heart J* **20**: 447–55.

35. Braunstein JB, Anderson GF, Gerstenblith G *et al.* (2003). Noncardiac comorbidity increases preventable hospitalizations and mortality among Medicare beneficiaries with chronic heart failure. *J Am Coll Cardiol* **42**: 1226–33.

36. Katz SD, Marantz PR, Biasucci L *et al.* (1993). Low incidence of stroke in ambulatory patients with heart failure: a prospective study. *Am Heart J* **126**: 141–6.

37. Kilander L, Nyman H, Boberg M *et al.* (1998). Hypertension is related to cognitive impairment. *Hypertension* **31**: 780–6.

38. Whitmer RA, Sidney S, Selby J *et al.* (2005). Midlife cardiovascular risk factors and risk of dementia in late life. *Neurology* **64**: 277–81.

39. Tzourio C, Anderson C, Chapman N *et al.* (2003). Effects of blood pressure lowering with perindopril and indapamide therapy on dementia and cognitive decline in patients with cerebrovascular disease. Arch Intern Med 2003;163:1069–75.

40. Launer LJ, Masaki R, Petrovich H *et al.* (1995). Association between midlife blood pressure levels and late-life cognitive function. *J Am Med Assoc* **274**: 1846–51.

41. Skoog I, Lernfelt B, Landahal S *et al.* (1996). A 15 year longitudinal study on blood pressure and dementia. *Lancet* **347**: 1141–5.

42. Glynn RJ, Beckett LA, Herbert LE *et al.* (1999). Current and remote blood pressure and cognitive decline. *J Am Med Assoc* **281**: 438–45.

43. Verghese J, Lipton RB, Hall CB *et al.* (2003). Low blood pressure and the risk of dementia in very old individuals. *Neurology* **61**: 1667–72.

44. Tarvonen S, Roytta M, Raiha I *et al.* (1996). Clinical features of leukoaraiosis. *J Neurol Neurosurg Psychiat* **60**: 431–6.

45. Cummings JL (1994). Vascular subcortical dementias: clinical aspects. *Dementia* **5**: 177–80.

46. Georgiadis D, Sievert M, Cencetti S *et al.* (2000). Cerebrovascular reactivity is impaired in patients with cardiac failure. *Eur Heart J* **21**: 407–13.

47. Melamed E, Lavy S, Bentin S *et al.* (1980). Reduction in regional cerebral blood flow during normal aging in man. *Stroke* **11**: 31–5.

48. Breteler MM, Van Swieten JC, Bots ML *et al.* (1994). Cerebral white matter lesions, vascular risk factors, and cognitive function in a population-based study: the Rotterdam study. *Neurology* **44**: 1246–52.

49. Van den Heuvel DM, ten Dam VH, de Craen AJ *et al.* (2006). Increase in periventricular white matter hyperintensities parallels decline in mental processing speed in a non-demented elderly population. *J Neurol Neurosurg Psychiat* **77**: 149–53.

50. Lou M, Blume A, Zhao Y *et al.* (2004). Sustained blockade of brain AT1 receptors before and after focal cerebral ischemia alleviates neurological deficits and reduces neuronal injury, apoptosis, and inflammatory responses in the rat. *J Cereb Blood Flow Metab* **24**: 536–47.

51. Dai WL, Funk A, Herdegen T *et al.* (1999). Blockade of central angiotensin AT1 receptors improves neurological outcome and reduces expression of AP-1 transcription factors after focal brain ischemia in rats. *Stroke* **30**: 2391–9.

52. Qiu WQ, Price LL, Hibberd P *et al.* (2006). Executive dysfunction in homebound older people with diabetes mellitus. *J Am Geriatr Soc* **54**: 496–501.

53. Deswal A, Petersen NJ, Feldman AM *et al.* (2001). Cytokines and cytokine receptors in advanced heart failure: an analysis of the cytokine database from the VESnarinone Trial (VEST). *Circulation* **103**: 2055–9.

54. Yaffe K, Kanaya A, Lindquist K *et al.* (2004). The metabolic syndrome, inflammation, and risk of cognitive decline. *J Am Med Assoc* **292**: 2237–42.

55. Buffon F, Porcher R, Hernandez K *et al.* (2006). Cognitive profile in CADASIL. *J Neurol Neurosurg Psychiat* **77**: 175–80.

56. Royall DR, Palmer R, Chiodo LK *et al.* (2005). Executive control mediates memory's association with change in instrumental activities of daily living: the Freedom House Study. *J Am Geriatr Soc* **53**: 11–17.

57. Zuccalà G, Marzetti E, Cesari M *et al.* (2005). Correlates of cognitive impairment among patients with heart failure: results of a multicenter survey. *Am J Med* **118**: 496–502.

58. Lee CW, Lee JH, Lim T *et al.* (2001). Prognostic significance of cerebral metabolic abnormalities in patients with congestive heart failure. *Circulation* **103**: 2784–7.

59. Zulli R, Nicosia F, Borroni B *et al.* (2005). QT dispersion and heart rate variability abnormalities in Alzheimer's disease and in mild cognitive impairment. *J Am Geriatr Soc* **53**: 2135–9.

60. Adamson PB, Smith AL, Abraham WT *et al.* (2004). Continuous autonomic assessment in patients with symptomatic heart failure: prognostic value of heart rate variability measured by an implanted cardiac resynchronization device. *Circulation* **110**: 2389–94.

61. Barnes DE, Tager IB, Satariano WA *et al.* (2004). The relationship between literacy and cognition in well-educated elders. *J Gerontol A Biol Sci Med Sci* **59**: 390–5.

62. Royall DR, Cordes JA, Polk M (1998). CLOX: an executive clock drawing task. *J Neurol Neurosurg Psychiat* **64**: 588–94.

63. Carbonin PU, Zuccalà G, Marzetti E *et al.* (2003). Coronary risk factors in the elderly: their interactions and treatment. *Curr Pharm Design* **9**: 2465–78.

64. Sparks DL, Sabbagh MN, Connor DJ *et al.* (2005). Atorvastatin for the treatment of mild to moderate Alzheimer disease: preliminary results. *Arch Neurol* **62**: 753–7.

65. Zamrini E, McGwin G, Roseman JM (2004). Association between statin use and Alzheimer's disease. *Neuroepidemiology* **23**: 94–8.

66. Lipschitz D (2003). Medical and functional consequences of anemia in the elderly. *J Am Geriatr Soc* **51**: S10–S13.

67. Nissenson AR (1999). Epoetin and cognitive function. *Am J Kidney Dis* **20**: 21–4.

68. Lipton SA (2004). Erythropoietin for neurologic protection and diabetic neuropathy. *New Engl J Med* **350**: 2516–17.

69. Silveberg DS, Wexler D, Sheps D *et al.* (2001). The effect of correction of mild anemia in severe, resistant congestive heart failure using subcutaneous erythropoietin and intravenous iron: a randomized controlled study. *J Am Coll Cardiol* **37**: 1775–80.

70. Metry G, Wickstrom B, Valind S *et al.* (1999). Effect of normalization of hematocrit on brain circulation and metabolism in hemodialysis patients. *J Am Soc Nephrol* **10**: 854–63.

71. Nissenson AR, Goodnough LT, Dubois RW (2003). Anemia—not just an innocent bystander? *Arch Intern Med* **163**: 1400–4.

72. Ishani A, Weinhandl E, Zhao Z *et al.* (2005). Angiotensin-converting enzyme inhibitor as a risk factor for the development of anemia, and the impact of incident anemia on mortality in patients with left ventricular dysfunction. *J Am Coll Cardiol* **45**: 391–9.

73. Tzourio C, Anderson C, Chapman N *et al.* (2003). Effects of blood pressure lowering with perindo-pril and indapamide on dementia and cognitive decline in patients with cerebrovascular disease. *Arch Intern Med* **163**: 1069–75.

74. Fogari R, Mugellini A, Zoppi A *et al.* (2003). Influence of losartan and atenolol on memory function in very elderly hypertensive patients. *J Hum Hypertens* **17**: 781–5.

75. Kamishirado H, Inoue T, Fujito T *et al.* (1997). Effect of enalapril maleate on cerebral blood flow in patients with chronic heart failure. *Angiology* **48**: 707–13.

76. Fabris B, Chen BZ, Pupic V *et al.* (1990). Inhibition of angiotensin-converting enzyme (ACE) in plasma and tissue. *J Cardiovasc Pharmacol* **15**(Suppl. 2): S6–S13.

77. Hu K, Bahner U, Gaudron P *et al.* (2001). Chronic effects of ACE-inhibiiton (quinapril) and angiotensin-II type-1 receptor blockade (losartan) on atrial natriuretic peptide in brain nuclei of rats with experimental myocardial infarction. *Basic Res Cardiol* **96**: 258–66.

78. Li J, Culman J, Hortnagl H *et al.* (2005). Angiotensin AT2 receptor protects against cerebral ischemia-induced neuronal injury. *FASEB J* **19**: 617–19.

79. Pan HL (2004). Brain angiotensin II and synaptic transmission. *Neuroscientist* **10**: 422–31.

80. Fournier A, Messerli FH, Achard JM *et al.* (2004). Cerebroprotection mediated by angiotensin II – a hypothesis supported by recent randomized clinical trials. *J Am Coll Cardiol* **43**: 1343–7.

81. Rubenstein LZ, Wieland GD, Josephson KR *et al.* (1988). Improved survival for frail elderly inpatients on a geriatric evaluation unit (GEU): who benefits? *J Clin Epidemiol* **41**: 441–9.

Chapter 15

Depression and anxiety in patients with chronic heart failure

David Bekelman and Mark D. Sullivan

Because psychological distress, particularly depression, is strongly associated with health status, morbidity, and mortality in patients with heart failure (HF), the management of depression and anxiety plays an important role in the supportive care of patients with HF. This chapter reviews research concerning the assessment, epidemiology, and management of depression and anxiety in patients with chronic HF. While the majority of research in depression in cardiovascular disease has been in patients with coronary artery disease and myocardial infarction, a growing literature exists for patients with HF. Anxiety has been under-researched in patients with heart disease even though it may play a significant role in quality of life.[1,2] For the purposes of this chapter, the word 'depression' refers to clinically significant depressive symptoms, while 'depressive disorder' means a mood disorder as classified by the Diagnostic and Statistical Manual of Mental Disorders (DSM-IV). We use the term 'sadness' or 'demoralization' to refer to mood states short of a DSM-IV mood disorder that occur in patients with HF. We use the term 'anxiety' to refer to clinically significant symptoms of anxiety, and specific anxiety disorders will be labeled as such (e.g. panic disorder, generalized anxiety disorder).

We first discuss the measurement, assessment, and diagnosis of depression and anxiety through structured diagnostic interviews and self-report measures. Specifically, we discuss the challenges in diagnosis of depression given that some symptoms of depression may be due to symptoms from HF (such as sleep disturbance, appetite, and weight changes). We make recommendations about how to screen for depression in HF. Second, we describe the epidemiology of depression and anxiety in HF, including incidence and prevalence. Third, we discuss risk factors for depression and anxiety in HF as well as complications and outcomes. We introduce a conceptual model of risk factors and outcomes that describes the relationship between depression/anxiety and HF health status and the mediators of this relationship. Finally, we describe the management of depression and anxiety in HF using psychological and pharmacological modalities.

Measurement/assessment/diagnosis

The underdiagnosis and undertreatment of depression in the medically ill is a serious problem.[3] The likelihood of psychiatric disorder increases with increasing severity of medical illness but the recognition and treatment of psychiatric disorders decreases.

Indeed, clinicians often consider patients who have serious medical illnesses such as HF to have 'good reasons' to be depressed and are therefore reluctant to make the diagnosis.[4] At other times, clinicians fear that a psychiatric diagnosis 'blames' their patients for their distress and labels them as 'failures' in coping with their medical illness. While temporary sadness may be a normal aspect of coping with a new diagnosis or declining function (see Chapter 20), depressive or anxiety disorders are not normal responses to medical illness. In fact, the majority of patients with HF or even terminal cancer do not have depressive or anxiety disorders.[5,6] Thus, explaining away clinically significant depression or anxiety as 'understandable' is not only empirically incorrect but also risks denying patients beneficial treatment. Even patients with severe medical illness can respond to standard psychiatric treatments for depressive disorders. In medically ill patients with depressive disorders, psychiatric treatment may be the most effective strategy for improving the patient's quality of life.

Similar difficulties exist in the diagnosis and treatment of anxiety in the medically ill and similar arguments can be made to advocate for case-finding and treatment. However, there is a paucity of research in anxiety and HF. Few studies have measured anxiety separately from overall psychological distress in patients with HF and even fewer have distinguished anxiety symptoms from anxiety disorders. The majority of clinical recommendations made in this chapter concerning anxiety management are based on studies in other populations (medically ill and healthy).

Measuring depression

Depression and anxiety are challenging to diagnose and research because symptoms occur on a spectrum that ranges from sadness or nervousness to depressive and anxiety disorders. These challenges are more difficult in people with medical disorders such as HF, since many of the symptoms of HF or its treatment are also symptoms of depression and anxiety (sleep disturbance, loss of appetite, lack of energy). However, when symptoms such as fatigue, chest pain, or dyspnea have been studied carefully in HF[7] or in other chronic illnesses such as diabetes[8] or multiple sclerosis,[9] the severity of these symptoms is more strongly related to the severity of depression and anxiety than to the severity of the medical disease.

There are four ways to approach the problem of measuring depression and diagnosing depressive disorders in the medically ill.[4] First, one can include all symptoms of depression and diagnose depression in the medically ill in the same way as in healthy persons. This is called the *inclusive* approach, where sensitivity is high, specificity is low, and etiology is ignored. A second, *etiologic* approach, focuses on determining the cause of each depression symptom and excludes those symptoms that are related to the medical illness (such as fatigue from HF). While more specific, it is often difficult to determine whether the symptom is indeed caused by the medical illness. The third approach is known as the *exclusive* approach. Here, symptoms of depression that may be related to medical illness are excluded (such as fatigue, sleep disturbance, anorexia), and diagnosis of a depressive disorder relies on the remaining symptoms. This approach improves specificity but loses sensitivity and may overlook cases. Finally, the *substitutive* approach replaces physical symptoms of depression with alternative criteria that are cognitive (e.g. thoughts like 'I'm a failure' or decreases in cognitive functioning) or mood-related (e.g. irritability, brooding).

Different measurement/diagnostic approaches yield different rates of depression. Kathol et al.[10] operationalized and compared the four sets of criteria and found that diagnosis of major depressive disorder in 152 cancer patients differed by as much as 13%. Koenig et al.[11] conducted a similar study in medical inpatients aged 60 years and older and found prevalence differences of 11%. A study of patients with chronic pain using three sets of criteria found prevalence rates of depressive disorder to differ by as much as 16%.[12] Thus, choice of approach leads to different case-finding of depression.

The choice of approach should depend on the context and purpose of the depression assessment.[4] *For research purposes, the exclusive approach is the best* because it maximizes specificity. It decreases variability in the depressed group and minimizes the likelihood of confounding variables. For example, to research the risk of mortality associated with depression the exclusive approach may be superior.[13] While the exclusive approach is most specific and preferentially detects the most severe depression, the inclusive approach is the most sensitive.[11] *For clinical purposes, an inclusive or substitutive approach is preferred* because of the risk of missing potential cases and the generally low burden of treatment. In addition, the inclusive approach offers a diagnostic strategy that balances the tendency to underdiagnose depression in the medically ill.[12] Finally, a sensitive depression diagnostic strategy is also preferred in clinical practice because depressive symptoms that are not associated with a full-blown depressive disorder are associated with poor outcomes and may benefit from treatment.[14]

Measuring anxiety

Anxiety and depression commonly coexist. Patients with depressive disorders often manifest symptoms of anxiety, and patients with anxiety disorders may develop sleep disturbance, depressed mood, anorexia, and other symptoms of depression. When patients with anxiety or depressive disorders are followed long-term, they tend to show symptoms of both types of disorder over time.[15]

Specialists often see anxiety and depression as manifestations of a broader notion of psychological distress, sometimes termed 'negative affectivity'.[16,17] Specialists seeking to distinguish depression and anxiety often do so in terms of positive and negative affect. There is good evidence that these two aspects of emotion are not simply the opposites of each other, but can vary independently. Both anxiety and depression are characterized by high levels of negative affect, with depression also characterized by low levels of positive affect.[18,19]

Symptoms of anxiety can be divided into two domains: cognitive and physical. Cognitive symptoms include nervousness, worry, feeling keyed up or on edge, difficulty concentrating, irritability, fear of losing control or going crazy, fear of dying, and derealization (feelings of unreality) or depersonalization (being detached from oneself). Physical symptoms of anxiety include trembling, twitching, feeling shaky, muscle tension/aches/soreness, restlessness, easy fatigability, palpitations/accelerated heart rate, sweating, sensations of shortness of breath or smothering, feelings of choking, chest pain/discomfort, dry mouth, dizziness/light-headedness, nausea/diarrhea/abdominal distress, hot flushes, chills, numbness/tingling, frequent urination, trouble swallowing or lump in the throat.

Assessment and differential diagnosis of depression and anxiety

An assessment of depression or anxiety in a patient with HF should include a thorough history and sometimes a physical examination and laboratory testing or imaging. The history should focus on elucidating when symptoms developed, what role environmental stressors, illness, or treatments have played, and what symptoms of depression or anxiety are present. It is often important to understand the relationship of the psychological symptom to HF exacerbations (e.g. breathlessness) or to treatments (e.g. implantable cardioverter-defibrillator (ICD) firings). Screening instruments are often useful for documenting symptoms. A broader psychosocial assessment is very useful for placing these symptoms in context. This includes consideration of current relationships, educational level, family structure, financial status, and illness experience, among other items. The past psychiatric history, including previous episodes of depression or anxiety and response to treatment, as well as history of suicidality, is valuable. Asking about suicidality is critical. It is not true that asking about suicidal thoughts increases risk or suicide or suicidal ideation. Evaluation of mental status and cognitive screening is important. A medication and substance use history is important in differential diagnosis. Finally, obtaining a medical history is valuable because certain medical illnesses may cause depression and/or anxiety.

Considering a differential diagnosis of depression and anxiety will help determine any further evaluation, appropriate treatment, and follow up. First, clinicians should look for the effects of substance intoxication or withdrawal (e.g. alcohol or caffeine). Second, an underlying medical basis should be considered. For example, a patient with anxiety and tachycardia may have a new pulmonary embolus or an exacerbation of chronic pulmonary disease. A depressed patient may have hypothyroidism. Third, depression or anxiety may be due to a psychological response to HF. In evaluating this distress response, it in important to assess the severity and duration of the current episode and the presence of any past episodes. The epidemiology of mood disorders in older, medically ill adults suggests that most of those meeting criteria for major or minor depression have had depressive episodes prior to the onset of their medical illness.[20,21]

Finally, there may be an underlying psychiatric disorder. Besides the depressive and anxiety disorders described in the next section, other psychiatric disorders may cause depressive or anxious symptoms, including personality disorders, somatoform disorders, schizophrenia, delirium, and dementia. These are reasons why the evaluation of mental status and cognitive screening is important, especially in the elderly and severely ill patient with HF (see also Chapter 17). The reader is referred to more comprehensive reviews of the differential diagnosis of depression and anxiety for further detail.[22]

Diagnosis of depressive and anxiety disorders in patients with HF

As mentioned previously, depressive and anxiety symptoms occur on a spectrum from normal/mild to disabling/severe. Criterion-based diagnostic systems, such as the DSM-IV, define a threshold at which a set of depressive or anxiety symptoms become a depressive or anxiety disorder.[23] These disorders are generally based on number, severity, frequency, and duration of symptoms, as well as association with impairment in function. The diagnosis of DSM-IV major depressive disorder requires either depressed mood or anhedonia (a marked loss of interest or pleasure in most or all activities) plus four other core symptoms most of the day nearly every day for at least 2 weeks. Minor depressive disorder is characterized by the presence of two to four total depressive symptoms instead of five or more for major depressive disorder. While major and minor depressive disorders are generally episodic conditions, dysthymia is a chronic depressive disorder in which low-grade depressive symptoms are present for the majority of at least 2 years. It is important to note that depressed mood (i.e. sadness, dysphoria) is neither necessary nor sufficient to diagnose a depressive disorder. Thus, determining whether a patient's sadness is a 'normal' reaction to HF is not relevant to diagnosis of a depressive disorder.[4]

There are few studies of specific anxiety disorders in patients with HF. Some specific anxiety disorders that may be seen include panic disorder, agoraphobia, post-traumatic stress disorder, obsessive–compulsive disorder, and generalized anxiety disorder. Anxiety appears to be a significant problem in many patients with ICDs which are now becoming the standard of care for many patients with HF due to their demonstrated benefit in reducing mortality.[24] The relative importance of a past history of anxiety disorder vs. past experience of defibrillator shocks is as yet undetermined.[25]

Clinical interviews

The 'gold standard' for the diagnosis of depressive and anxiety disorder in patients with HF varies by context. In the clinical setting, a diagnostic clinical interview by a mental health professional is the gold standard. These interviews, of course, may vary in their content and structure. In the research setting, structured interviews provide a more reliable criterion standard for the diagnosis of these disorders. Several structured interview approaches exist, included the Diagnostic Interview Scale (DIS), the Structured Clinical Interview for the DSM (SCID), the Schedule of Affective Disorders and Schizophrenia (SADS), and the World Health Organization's Composite International Diagnostic Interview (CIDI). These will not be described in further detail here, although it should be noted that they use different approaches to deal with the problem that symptoms of depression and physical illness overlap (see 'Measurement' section).

Screening instruments for depression and anxiety

While self-report instruments are not generally designed to diagnose depressive disorders, the different measurement/diagnostic approaches previously described are reflected in these instruments. The Beck Depression Inventory (BDI), for example, has been used commonly in studies of depression in patients with cardiovascular disease and HF. It was not specifically designed for medically ill patients and uses an *inclusive* approach, including many physical symptoms of depression. Thus, case-finding rates for depression using the BDI are often higher compared with case-finding using other screening instruments. The Geriatric Depression Scale (GDS), for example, *excludes* many physical symptoms and *substitutes* cognitive symptoms, such as views of oneself and the future.

We recommend considering several instruments for screening of depression and anxiety in patients with HF. For interested readers, reviews of mood disorder screening instruments can be found elsewhere.[26] The Patient Health Questionnaire-9 (PHQ-9, reprinted with permission as an appendix to this chapter) and the Generalized Anxiety Disorder-7 (GAD-7) are used to screen for depression and anxiety, respectively. Both were developed in large samples of primary-care patients. The PHQ-9 is a nine-item self-report instrument that has strong psychometric properties and is useful for diagnosing depressive disorder as well as to track depression symptoms over time.[27] The PHQ-9 has also been validated for phone use.[28] The PHQ-2 is the first two items from the nine-item scale of the PHQ-9. A score of 3 or more on the Patient Health Questionnaire-2 (PHQ-2) has a sensitivity of 87% and specificity of 78% for major depressive disorder in medical outpatients using the SCID as the gold standard.[27] The GAD-7 is a seven-item self-report instrument that also has strong psychometric properties and is a valid tool for screening for generalized anxiety disorder and assessing its severity.[29]

The Hospital Anxiety and Depression Scale (HADS) is a 14-item self-report instrument that has been in use longer than the PHQ-9.[30] The main benefit of the HADS is that one can track both symptoms of anxiety and depression in one instrument. The HADS is less good as a screening tool for the diagnosis of depressive disorder and there are fewer data regarding responsiveness to change over time compared with the PHQ-9.

Epidemiology of depression and anxiety

In this section, we describe findings on the prevalence, incidence, risk factors, complications, and outcomes of depression and anxiety in patients with HF. Studies vary in their findings depending on the population of patients enrolled (inpatients, outpatients) and the manner in which HF and mood disturbances are diagnosed.

Prevalence

Clinically significant depression is present in 21.5% of HF patients according to a recent meta-analysis.[31] Prevalence varies most by whether questionnaires are used (33.6% prevalence of clinically significant depression) versus diagnostic interviews (19.3% prevalence). Readers are referred to a recent meta-analysis for a comprehensive review of prevalence studies of depression in HF.[31]

Inpatients

Using diagnostic psychiatric interviews, rates of major depressive disorder in hospitalized HF patients range from 13.9% to 36.5%.[32-34] Using structured diagnostic interviews, Freedland *et al.*[32] evaluated 682 patients aged 40 years or older at one hospital and found that 20% met DSM-IV criteria for a current major depressive episode,16% for a current minor depressive episode, and the remainder (64%) were not currently depressed. Ninety per cent of the enrolled patients completed the Beck Depression Inventory and 51% ($n = 140$) scored 10 or more, the usual cut-off for clinically significant depression. Forty-five per cent of these 140 patients were classified as not being depressed according to the structured diagnostic interview. This illustrates the difficulties in using certain screening instruments which we discussed earlier in the chapter. Koenig[34] studied 542 patients age 60 or older at one hospital using structured psychiatric interviews and found that 36.5% had a current major depressive episode and 17% had a current minor depressive episode. Inpatient prevalence rates will show more variability due to varying severity of medical illness and method of assessment. Depressive disorder prevalence in HF inpatients appears to be at least as high as the 15–20% reported for patients post-myocardial infarction.

Outpatients

Both depressive disorder and clinically significant depressive symptoms are common in outpatients with HF, although prevalence rates are lower than in inpatients. This is typical of other medically ill populations and is probably related to the strong association between health status and depression.[35–37] What qualifies as clinically significant depressive symptoms has varied from study to study, but a prevalence figure of 20% is a reasonable consensus estimate.

Incidence

Several studies have determined the incidence of depression in outpatients with HF. In a multicenter prospective cohort study of 245 outpatients with HF and ejection fraction <0.40, 52 (21.2%) developed clinically significant depressive symptoms at 1 year according to the Medical Outcomes Study-Depression (MOS-D) questionnaire.[38] In another study, 203 inpatients were followed for 24 weeks after discharge with the GDS and the SCID-NP.[39] Of the 130 subjects who initially screened negative for depression according to the GDS, at 4 weeks 12% had a positive screen and at 24 weeks 6% had a positive screen. These findings are limited in this study, however, by unclear methods of accounting for missing data.

Risk factors and outcomes

Depression, anxiety, and HF: conceptual model

The conceptual model in Fig. 15.1 displays relationships between depression and anxiety and HF. Central to the model is the notion that depression and anxiety (see the boxes 'Depression and anxiety disorders' and 'Subsyndromal depression and anxiety' in Fig. 15.1) are risks for poor HF health status and outcomes (box 'Heart failure health status') and that these in turn are risks for depression/anxiety. In between these two boxes in the conceptual model are the mediators thought to be responsible for these relationships.

This section reviews some of the evidence to support this conceptual model. Later in the chapter, the conceptual model is used to show how interventions can reduce the risk of depression or anxiety, decrease depression or anxiety severity, and reduce the adverse outcomes from depression and anxiety.

Risk factors for depression and anxiety in HF patients

Studies have evaluated both clinical and biomarker risk factors for depression and HF. Most of these studies have been cross-sectional and thus show association rather than true longitudinal predictive risk.

Clinical risk factors

One study evaluated longitudinal predictors of depressive symptoms in patients with HF.[38] In multivariate analysis, living alone, alcohol abuse, perception of medical care as being a substantial economic burden, and health status (measured by the Kansas City Cardiomyopathy Questionnaire) were independent predictors of developing depressive symptoms. There was a graded relationship between the number of risk factors present and the risk of developing clinically significant depression as measured by the MOS-D.

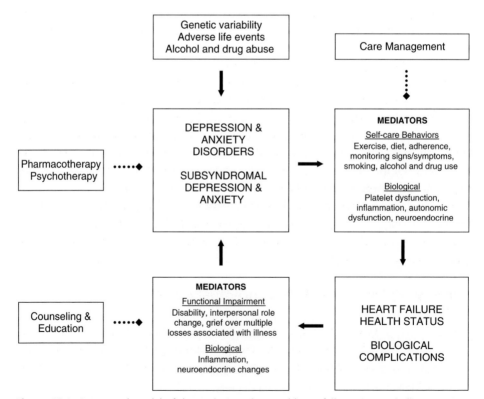

Figure. 15.1 Conceptual model of depression, anxiety, and heart failure. Arrows indicate hypothesized causal pathways, and dotted lines indicate targets for intervention.

For patients who had none of these risk factors, 7.9% developed depression at 1 year, and when three were present, the risk of depression was 69.2% at 1 year. No other sociode-mographic factors were predictive of the onset of depression. In addition, neither ejection fraction, New York Heart Association (NYHA) functional class, performance on a 6-min walk test, nor brain natriuretic peptide were predictive. Risk associated with a past history of depression was not included in this study.

Other factors associated with depression have been found in cross-sectional studies of patients with HF. These have included gender, age, income, past history of major depression, NYHA class, activities of daily living (ADL) or instrumental ADL (IADL) dependence, co-morbid medical or psychiatric illnesses, physical symptoms (e.g. short-ness of breath, fatigue), inability to work because of disability, a distressed personality type, and spiritual well-being.[34, 35, 38, 40–42] Cross-sectional studies are inconsistent in finding relationships between these factors and depression. In addition, it is not possible to determine from these cross-sectional studies if these associations are causes or conse-quences of depression.

Biomarker risk factors

Much of the research on biological risks for depression in medically ill patients is in patients with cancer. This research suggests that both inflammation and neuroendocrine changes may mediate the relationship between medical illness and depression.[43–46] Thus, the biological risks for depression in patients with HF are simply hypothesized in the conceptual model.

Based on these data and other research, risk factors for depression and anxiety are grouped into two boxes in the conceptual model.[47] In one box are genetic vulnerability, adverse life events, and alcohol and drug abuse. These are risk factors for depression and anxiety regardless of HF. Individuals with these risk factors may have had depression and anxiety prior to developing HF. The box that includes HF health status/biological complications is the second group of risk factors. The relationship between HF health status/biological complications and depression/anxiety is mediated by functional impairment and hypothesized biological mechanisms. Functional impairment as a medi-ator between HF health status and depression/anxiety is particularly important as a management target. Through supportive counseling and education techniques described later in the chapter, clinicians who care for HF patients can help patients cope with their functional impairment and potentially prevent or reduce depression and/or anxiety.

Complications/outcomes from depression and anxiety in HF patients

Depression is related to worse short-term health status, declines in functioning, increased rehospitalization and mortality, and increased health service utilization and cost. In this section, we review studies that demonstrate these outcomes and then discuss mediators of these outcomes.

Depressed patients were at significantly higher risk for worsening of HF symptoms, physical and social function, and quality of life in a national sample of 460 outpatients with HF.[36] Depression was also the strongest predictor of these outcomes in this study compared with multiple demographic, cardiac, non-cardiac, and treatment variables. Depression has been more strongly associated with poor health-related quality of life and health status in patients with HF than NYHA class or HF disease severity indicators.[7,48–52]

Depression has also been independently related to increased rehospitalization[53–54] and mortality[53,55] in patients with HF. In multivariate analyses, depression was associated with 2.18 [95% confidence interval (CI) 0.97, 4.92] times the risk of mortality at 1 year and 2.62 (95% CI 1.19, 5.79) times the risk of hospitalization at 1 year.[53] Vaccarino et al.[56] found depression to independently predict a combined end-point of decreased ADLs and mortality after 6 months. Sullivan et al.[54] found that patients with HF followed for a mean of 3 years were more likely to progress to the combined endpoint of transplant or death if they were depressed (hazard ratio 2.54, 95% CI 1.16, 5.55). Finally, depression was found to be an independent predictor of all-cause mortality and cardiovascular death or hospitalization after acute myocardial infarction complicated by HF.[57]

Depression may also lead to more health service utilization, controlling for severity of illness, including medical visits and rehospitalization days,[58] although another study suggested that severity of illness accounted for a significant percentage of higher health service use.[34] A retrospective cohort study found that annualized health-care costs were 26% higher in patients with HF who were receiving antidepressants and 29% higher in patients who had a depression diagnosis and were receiving antidepressants when compared with HF patients with no evidence of depression.[59] The analysis was adjusted for age, gender, medical co-morbidity, and length of stay at index hospitalization (as a proxy for HF severity).

Many patients with HF have ICDs, and the role of depression in the morbidity and mortality of patients with life-threatening arrhythmias or with ICDs is significant. Depression is strongly associated with the risk of out-of-hospital sudden cardiac death.[60] Higher levels of anxiety and depression independently predict subsequent arrhythmia events in patients with ICDs.[61] Depression, anxiety, fears about ICD firing, and fears of death are the most common psychological problems after implantation of an ICD.[62] Stress, difficulty adjusting, sexual dysfunction, and loss of control are also described.[63] However, it is unclear how much of the psychological distress is related to ICD implantation versus having HF, being predisposed towards depression or anxiety, or other factors.[63] Several studies have demonstrated that the experience of ICD shocks is associated with clinically significant anxiety disorders and decrements in health status (see also Chapter 5).[64,65] However, psychological variables are much stronger predictors of health status outcomes in these patients than the occurrence of ICD shocks.[51]

Anxiety is understudied in patients with HF, although it is a significant contributor to poor heath status in other populations.[1,66] One study measured symptoms of anxiety in HF patients and found that while anxiety symptoms were highly correlated with depression symptoms, they did not predict 1-year mortality while depression symptoms did.[67]

However, in another study in patients with ischemic heart disease, anxiety symptoms were found to predict cardiac events and increased health-care consumption.[68]

In summary, these studies provide strong evidence that depression and possibly anxiety are associated with multiple adverse outcomes in HF patients as well as increased health-care utilization and cost. Many factors may mediate these outcomes in HF patients. The mechanisms linking depression with HF health status and adverse outcomes are not certain, but evidence supports both biological and behavioral mechanisms.[69]

Potential biological mediators of the relationship between depression and health status and outcomes in HF patients include platelet dysfunction, inflammation, autonomic dysfunction, and neuroendocrine abnormalities (see Fig. 15.1). A variety of platelet abnormalities, including increased platelet reactivity, occur in patients with depression that could be associated with an increased likelihood of thrombosis.[70] Elevations in pro-inflammatory cytokines are found in depressed patients[71] and are implicated in the pathogenesis and progression of HF.[72] Autonomic dysfunction in patients with depression, such as low heart rate variability, may lead to arrhythmias in HF patients.[73] Higher levels of anxiety and depression predict subsequent arrhythmia events in patients with ICDs even after controlling for left-ventricular ejection fraction, arrhythmia history, and medication use.[74] Finally, depression is associated with hyperactivity of the hypothalamic–pituitary–adrenal axis, manifested by hypercortisolemia, sympathetic hyperactivity, including elevated plasma norepinephrine levels, and other abnormalities; these abnormalities represent another possible mediator of depression on HF outcomes.[75,76]

Behavioral mediators of the relationship between depression and health status and outcomes in HF patients include self-care behaviors such as exercise, diet, adherence, monitoring of signs/symptoms, smoking, and alcohol and drug use (see Fig. 15.1).[77–82] In addition, multiple intervention studies have targeted self-care behaviors and demonstrate improved HF patient health status and other outcomes.[83]

Management of depression in patients with HF

Both pharmacotherapy and certain forms of psychotherapy have been shown to be effective for the treatment of depression in patients with ischemic heart disease and patients with other medical illnesses, including cancer. We are not aware of any published randomized trials evaluating the effectiveness of treatments for depression specifically in patients with HF, although the ongoing SADHART-HF trial was designed to evaluate the safety and effectiveness of pharmacological treatment for depression in HF.[84] Two major randomized trials have evaluated treatments for depression in cardiac patients, SADHART and ENRICHD.

SADHART was a double-blind, placebo-controlled, randomized trial that evaluated the efficacy and safety of 24 weeks of sertraline for the treatment of major depression in 369 patients within 30 days of an acute coronary syndrome.[85] Sertraline had no effect on ejection fraction, heart rate, blood pressure, electrocardiographic measures, or 24-h heart rate variability. Sertraline was more effective than placebo for the treatment of depression in patients with a prior history of depression, but not in patients without a prior history of depression. There was no effect on cardiac outcomes, although the trial was not powered to identify a change in cardiac outcomes.

The ENRICHD trial tested the effect of 6-months of cognitive-behavioral psychotherapy (with sertraline at 5 weeks if needed) compared with usual care in 2481 patients who had a recent myocardial infarction and either low social support and/or major or minor depression.[86] The intervention did not differ from placebo on the primary endpoint of combined all-cause mortality and non-fatal, recurrent myocardial infarction. There was a modest effect of the intervention on depressive symptoms and social support. A secondary observational analysis of ENRICHED data comparing depressed patients who did and did not receive selective serotonin reuptake inhibitor (SSRI) therapy suggested that SSRI treatment of depressed patients who experience an acute myocardial infarction might reduce subsequent cardiovascular morbidity and mortality.[87]

Pharmacotherapy

Antidepressants have a well-documented record of efficacy for the treatment of depression, even in the presence of severe chronic medical illness.[88] In the absence of contraindications, we recommend using the starting dose (Table 15.1) in the elderly or patients with more serious medical illness for 3–7 days (use more rapid dose escalation in hospitalized patients or more severe depressive illness). Younger patients with less severe medical illness often tolerate starting with the lowest therapeutic dose. Continue dose increases every 3–7 days to achieve the therapeutic dose. Initial therapeutic benefit may be seen as quickly as 1–3 weeks, although benefits may take as long as 4–8 weeks to appear. If improvement is not seen within 4–6 weeks, we recommend switching to an alternative antidepressant. When improvement is seen, additional medication benefit may occur over 3–6 months. Medications generally have similar efficacy and should be chosen based on safety in cardiac patients and on side-effect profile.

SSRIs

SSRIs are the first-line treatment for major depressive disorder and for dysthymia in patients with HF. The SSRIs all have a favorable cardiac safety profile. They are much safer in regular use and in overdose than the older tricyclic antidepressants. The tricyclic antidepressants should generally be avoided in patients with HF because of their potential for arrhythmias, hypotension, and anticholinergic side-effects.[89] We recommend starting with either citalopram or sertraline because these medications have documented cardiac safety and the lowest risk of drug interactions.[85,90] All SSRIs can cause nausea, headache, sexual dysfunction, insomnia or sedation, and diarrhea or constipation. Other common side-effects include dry mouth, nervousness, tremor, and sweating. Except for sexual dysfunction, these side-effects tend to resolve with time. Rare but potentially serious side-effects include the syndrome of inappropriate antidiuretic hormone secretion and platelet dysfunction that may be associated with increased bleeding time.

Table.15.1 Recommended medications for treatment of depression in HF patients

Name	Starting dose in elderly patients	Therapeutic dose	Dosing schedule	Common side-effects	Drug interactions
SSRIs					
Sertraline	12.5–25 mg	50–200 mg	Once daily	Diarrhea, nausea, agitation, sexual dysfunction	β-blockers, flecainide, warfarin
Citalopram	5–10 mg	20–40 mg	Once daily	Nausea, dry mouth, somnolence	β-blockers, flecainide, warfarin
SNRIs					
Venlafaxine	37.5–75 mg	75–300 mg	Once daily (immediate release); twice daily (extended release)	Nausea, headache, somnolence	Ranolazine, warfarin
Duloxetine	20–30 mg	60–120mg	Once or twice daily	Nausea, dry mouth, constipation	Amiodarone, β-blockers
Other antidepressants					
Bupropion	37.5–75 mg	150–400 mg	Once daily (immediate release); twice daily (extended release)	Insomnia, dry mouth, headache, agitation	β-blockers, flecainide, warfarin
Mirtazapine	7.5–15 mg	15–45 mg	Once daily	Sedation, weight gain	Quinadine
Stimulants					
Methylphenidate	2.5–5 mg	5–20 mg	8 a.m. and noon	Agitation, insomnia	Clonidine, warfarin

Other medications

Venlafaxine and duloxetine are serotonin–norepinephrine reuptake inhibitors (SNRIs) with side-effects that are similar to SSRIs. Since they also inhibit norepinephrine reuptake, they may also produce shaking or sweating early in therapy. They may be associated with elevations in blood pressure, especially in doses greater than the recommended range. These medications have relatively few drug interactions, though they both interact with warfarin, commonly used in HF patients. Both these medications have documented efficacy in neuropathic pain.[91]

Bupropion is a norepinephrine and dopamine modulator. Bupropion has major benefits over SSRIs in that it is not sedating, does not cause sexual dysfunction, and has little cardiovascular toxicity.[92] It may be particularly useful in patients with fatigue. Agitation, insomnia, and rarely seizures may be seen at higher doses. We generally avoid using bupropion in patients with seizures or brain tumors. Since bupropion is approved by the US Food and Drug Administration for use in smoking cessation, there is an established safety record in coronary disease patients.[93] Bupropion has mild positive inotropic effects in animal models, though these may be reversed in the presence of β-blockade.[94] It has very few drug interactions. In our clinical experience, many patients with HF and depression find the activating properties of bupropion to be helpful.

Mirtazapine increases norepinephrine and serotonin concentrations by blocking inhibitory receptors. Several advantages in side-effect profile are that mirtazapine is generally not associated with nausea, anxiety, insomnia, or sexual dysfunction. It may be useful for treating nausea because of its blockade of serotonin-3 receptors. It is quite sedating and may produce significant weight gain due to appetite stimulation.[95] Mirtazapine may thus be useful in certain patients with insomnia or cardiac cachexia. It has few drug interactions.[96]

Methylphenidate

Methylphenidate is effective for treatment of depression in a variety of medical conditions.[97,98] It is generally well tolerated and can rapidly elevate mood, increase appetite, and diminish fatigue. In addition it may be effective as an adjuvant analgesic, improve attention and concentration, and reduce sedation caused by opiates or other medicines. Many would consider psychostimulants such as methylphenidate to be first-line antidepressants in the palliative care population.[99] Side-effects are typically mild and dose-related and may include anxiety, agitation, nausea, and insomnia. Rarely, psychotic symptoms or tachycardia and hypertension may occur.[100] Some cardiologists are concerned about using stimulants in HF patients at high risk for tachyarrhythmias.[101]

Electroconvulsive therapy (ECT)

ECT is another treatment modality for major depressive disorder. It should be considered early for patients who have depression with psychotic symptoms, severe suicidal ideation, or worsening nutritional status.

Supportive communication and psychotherapeutic approaches for depression and anxiety

The relationship between the HF patient and the primary-care provider or cardiologist is an important therapeutic tool (see Fig. 15.1 box 'Counseling and education'). Communication between the provider and patient has a significant role in diagnostic accuracy, therapeutic adherence, and patient satisfaction.[102–107] While treatment with medications or more formal counseling or psychotherapy may be needed, supportive communication and attention to the provider–patient relationship is always an essential first step. In fact, the quality of provider–patient communication is also associated with provider satisfaction.[108] Reassuring the patient that you see their emotional reaction as a reasonable and expected response to their medical disease can go a long way to establishing empathy (see also Chapter 22). This reassurance, however, should not exclude the possibility that the patient's emotional reaction requires further evaluation and/or treatment. Rather, the provider should explain that many people experience emotional distress such as depression or anxiety related to their HF. In addition, further evaluation and/or treatment is important and often leads to less distress and improved quality of life and may lead to better HF health status (see Fig. 15.1).

Supportive communication involves a variety of skills such as active listening, non-verbal communication, and empathy. Empathy is particularly important skill and may help in preventing or reducing symptoms of depression and anxiety (see Fig. 15.1 box 'Counseling and education').[109] These skills are regarded as teachable and learnable and should be within the therapeutic armamentarium of providers of HF care.[110,111] A systematic review found improvement in symptoms over 6 months with supportive, non-directive counseling.[112]

Several factors are important in considering a referral for psychotherapy.[3] These include the severity of the patient's distress, the patient's health status and life expectancy, the availability of trained psychotherapists and means to pay for treatment, the available support network, the patient's motivation for psychological therapy, and the patient's ability to learn new coping strategies. The choice of type of psychotherapy will depend on some of these factors as well as the patient's ability to engage in a process that involves introspection and the expression of feelings.

The ENRICHD study (described above) tested a cognitive/behavioral therapy in targeted patients with cardiovascular disease, but other psychotherapeutic techniques have had success in patient populations with general medical illness. Randomized controlled trials support the use of interpersonal psychotherapy in specific medically ill populations, and a large randomized controlled trial has recently been designed to evaluate its use in cardiac patients.[113,114] In addition, two randomized controlled trials have found that problem-solving therapy is effective in reducing symptoms of depression in primary-care patients.[115,116] Finally, several studies have demonstrated the effectiveness of collaborative depression care management in elderly patients with depression who often have medical co-morbidities.[117–120] These collaborative depression care management interventions include medication for depression as well as education, behavioral activation, and/or problem-solving or interpersonal psychotherapy.

Management of anxiety in patients with HF

The first step towards managing anxiety is to help the patient identify what he or she is feeling and why. The underlying cause should be treated if symptoms are due to substance intoxication/withdrawal or a medical problem (see 'Assessment and differential diagnosis of depression and anxiety'). If the symptoms related to anxiety are determined to be due to a psychological response to illness, simply naming a set of symptoms as 'anxiety' often helps to contain the anxiety and the symptoms. For example, patients can be reassured when they learn that the shortness of breath, sweating, shaking, and chest tightness they are experiencing is anxiety and not ischemia, and thus not immediately life-threatening. Identifying the psychological cause for why the patient is anxious can be difficult. However, once patients realize that it is alright to talk about their anxiety with their medical doctor, and if a trusting relationship exists, some patients can readily describe the origins of their anxiety.

Many psychological causes for anxiety have been described in patients with general medical illnesses and specifically in patients with HF (see Table 15.2).[121] Communication about diagnosis, prognosis, or treatment using language that the patient and family can understand can help decrease anxiety. Reassurance is an important tool when used at the right time and in the right dose. However, premature reassurance can actually increase anxiety when patients do not feel adequately understood. Many action-oriented physicians underestimate the value of helping the patient feel understood, empathic communication, and assured regular contact with patients. These non-specific techniques can be quite powerful in reducing anxiety.

Because of the lack of studies of anxiety in patients with HF, definitive treatment recommendations are difficult. Medications such as antidepressants have been studied for the treatment of anxiety disorders (generalized anxiety disorder, panic disorder, post-traumatic stress disorder, obsessive–compulsive disorder) in relatively healthy populations.

Pharmacotherapy

Benzodiazepines

Benzodiazepines are the treatment of choice when a time-limited and situational cause of anxiety is identified.[4] These medications are sometimes useful for patients with

Table 15.2 Psychological causes of anxiety and depression in patients with heart failure and potential responses

Loss of control	Identify areas of the patient's life that are under his/her control. Determine how the patient would like to hear medical information and make medical decisions (greater/lesser input from family, physician)
Fear of dying	Demonstrate willingness to discuss ('Some of my patients are anxious/ concerned about what will happen in their future. If you have any of these concerns, I'm happy to talk with you about them.')
Loss of function, disability	Help patient identify things that still can be done with remaining function, consider OT/PT/cardiac rehab referral
Loss of social support, alienation	Encourage patient's supports to come to a medical visit; reassure patient that you will continue to be involved in care at every stage of illness
Attribution of symptoms to mean impending death/ worsening illness severity	Correct misattributions; educate about what different symptoms may mean; consider educating about the illness course and what the future may hold; reframe hope

primary anxiety disorders (e.g. panic disorder) and for patients with secondary anxiety from a medical cause. Other references provide comprehensive lists of benzodiazepines available. We recommend considering midazolam or lorazepam for hospitalized patients, and lorazepam or clonazepam for outpatients. Midazolam has a very short half-life and is thus useful in hospitalized patients for short-term treatment of anxiety, especially when the level of anxiety is changing quickly over time (such as prior to a procedure or test). It can only be given intravenously or intramuscularly. Lorazepam can be given by mouth, intravenously, or intramuscularly. It is metabolized through conjugation so is less problematic in patients with liver disease than some other benzodiazepines which are metabolized through oxidation.[122] Clonazepam has a longer half-life and is useful for patients with relatively constant or longer-term anxiety. Benzodiazepines should generally be used for a time-limited course to maintain effectiveness, minimize psychological and physical dependence, and minimize side-effects. We generally aim for no more than a month or two of benzodiazepine therapy unless there are no viable alternatives. SSRIs or psychotherapy are almost always better choices for chronic anxiety therapy.

Benzodiazepines have several side-effects and should be used with caution in certain patient populations. In general they are much safer in overdose than barbiturates. They can cause sedation and motor and cognitive disturbances. Because of these side-effects they should be used cautiously in patients with brain injury (e.g. dementia, head trauma, mental retardation). Because of the risk of respiratory suppression, caution should be taken in patients with pulmonary disease who retain carbon dioxide or those with sleep apnea. However, fear of causing respiratory suppression should not hinder adequate control of anxiety. The likelihood of respiratory depression is minimized by using short-acting benzodiazepines (midazolam, lorazepam) and careful monitoring. Benzo-diazepines should be avoided at the beginning or end of pregnancy. A reduced dose may be needed in patients with liver disease, brain dysfunction from any cause, and advanced pulmonary disease. There is little evidence to support dosing recommendations in advanced HF, but a 'start low and go slow' strategy should be considered as in all elderly patients. Finally, use in patients with a substance abuse history should be avoided or made very cautiously.

Antidepressants

SSRIs are the treatment of choice for most anxiety disorders including generalized anxiety disorder, panic disorder, obsessive–compulsive disorder, social anxiety disorder, and post-traumatic stress disorder. In general, similar dosing is used for anxiety disorders and depressive disorders, though this is not always true (e.g. in obsessive–compulsive disorder, higher dosing is often needed). Venlafaxine is approved for treatment of gener-alized anxiety disorder and social anxiety disorder. These medicines may take 2–6 weeks to adequately relieve anxiety. Patients may benefit from initial treatment with benzodi-azepines that can be gradually tapered off after 1–2 months. Treatment of anxiety with antidepressants should continue for 4–9 months prior to trials of tapering and discontinuing the medication.

Other anti-anxiety medications

Antipsychotics are the treatment of choice for anxiety associated with delirium or when anxiety is associated with psychotic symptoms such as delusions or hallucinations.[123] They are also useful when there is a legitimate concern of respiratory compromise, when cognitive dysfunction is present, or when anxious patients are being weaned from the ventilator.

Buspirone is a partial serotonin 1A receptor agonist that is approved for treatment of generalized anxiety disorder. It generally takes 5–10 days at a therapeutic dose and may take up to 4 weeks for therapeutic effect and is thus useful only for chronic anxiety. The starting dose is 5 mg three times daily and the minimum effective dose for many patients respond is 10 mg three times daily. The dose can be increased by 10 mg every 7–10 days to a maximum of 60 mg per day. It has benefits in not causing sedation, respiratory depression, cognitive dysfunction, or euphoria and thus is generally safe in the medically ill and substance abusers. It is usually well-tolerated but clinical experience suggests it is not very potent as an anxiolytic.

Supportive communication and psychotherapeutic approaches

Approaches to supportive communication and psychotherapy are discussed under 'Depression' on pages 289–291.

Conclusion

Patients with HF often experience clinically significant depression and/or anxiety. Depression and anxiety are important to assess, diagnose, and treat because they are associated with poor quality of life and health status as well as cardiovascular morbidity and mortality. Inquiring about depression and anxiety symptoms and how patients experience their HF is a critical first step towards diagnosis and treatment. Screening instruments are also helpful. Supportive communication, education, and brief counseling are appropriate initial approaches that may prevent or reduce these symptoms. Medications and psychotherapy are safe and effective and should be a standard part of supportive care for patients with HF.

Appendix

The Patient Health Questionnaire-9 (PHQ-9). Copyright (c)1999 Pfizer Inc. All rights reserved. Reproduced with permission.

PATIENT HEALTH QUESTIONNAIRE (PHQ-9)

NAME: _____   DATE:_____

Over the *last 2 weeks,* how often have you been bothered by any of the following problems? (use "✓" to indicate your answer)	Not at all	Several days	More than half the days	Nearly every day
1. Little interest or pleasure in doing things	0	1	2	3
2. Feeling down, depressed, or hopeless	0	1	2	3
3. Trouble falling or staying asleep, or sleeping too much	0	1	2	3
4. Feeling tired or having little energy	0	1	2	3
5. Poor appetite or overeating	0	1	2	3
6. Feeling bad about yourself—or that you are a failure or have let yourself or your family down	0	1	2	3
7. Trouble concentrating on things, such as reading the newspaper or watching television	0	1	2	3
8. Moving or speaking so slowly that other people could have noticed. Or the opposite—being so fidgety or restless that you have been moving around a lot more than usual	0	1	2	3
9. Thoughts that you would be better off dead, or of hurting yourself in some way	0	1	2	3

add columns: [____] + [____] + [____]

(Healthcare professional: For interpretation of TOTAL, please refer to accompanying scoring card.) TOTAL: [_____]

10. If you checked off *any* problems, how *difficult* have these problems made it for you to do your work, take care of things at home, or get along with other people?	Not difficult at all _____ Somewhat difficult _____ Very difficult _____ Extremely difficult _____

Fold back this page before administering this questionnaire

INSTRUCTIONS FOR USE

for doctor or healthcare professional use only

PHQ-9 QUICK DEPRESSION ASSESSMENT

For initial diagnosis:

1. Patient completes PHQ-9 Quick Depression Assessment on accompanying tear-off pad.

2. If there are at least 4 ✓s in the blue highlighted section (including Questions #1 and #2), consider a depressive disorder. Add score to determine severity.

3. *Consider Major Depressive Disorder*
—if there are at least 5 ✓s in the blue highlighted section (one of which corresponds to Question #1 or #2)

Consider Other Depressive Disorder
—if there are 2 to 4 ✓s in the blue highlighted section (one of which corresponds to Question #1 or #2)

Note: Since the questionnaire relies on patient self-report, all responses should be verified by the clinician and a definitive diagnosis made on clinical grounds, taking into account how well the patient understood the questionnaire, as well as other relevant information from the patient. Diagnoses of Major Depressive Disorder or Other Depressive Disorder also require impairment of social, occupational, or other important areas of functioning (Question #10) and ruling out normal bereavement, a history of a Manic Episode (Bipolar Disorder), and a physical disorder, medication, or other drug as the biological cause of the depressive symptoms.

To monitor severity over time for newly diagnosed patients or patients in current treatment for depression:

1. Patients may complete questionnaires at baseline and at regular intervals (eg, every 2 weeks) at home and bring them in at their next appointment for scoring or they may complete the questionnaire during each scheduled appointment.

2. Add up ✓s by column. For every ✓: Several days = 1   More than half the days = 2   Nearly every day = 3

3. Add together column scores to get a TOTAL score.

4. Refer to the accompanying PHQ-9 Scoring Card to interpret the TOTAL score.

5. Results may be included in patients' files to assist you in setting up a treatment goal, determining degree of response, as well as guiding treatment intervention.

PHQ-9 SCORING CARD FOR SEVERITY DETERMINATION

for healthcare professional use only

Scoring—add up all checked boxes on PHQ-9

For every ✓: Not at all = 0; Several days = 1;
More than half the days = 2; Nearly every day = 3

Interpretation of Total Score

Total Score	Depression Severity
0-4	None
5-9	Mild depression
10-14	Moderate depression
15-19	Moderately severe depression
20-27	Severe depression

References

1. Smith EM, Gomm SA, Dickens CM (2003). Assessing the independent contribution to quality of life from anxiety and depression in patients with advanced cancer. *Palliat Med* **17**: 509–13.

2. Surtees PG, Wainwright NW, Khaw KT, Day NE (2003). Functional health status, chronic medical conditions and disorders of mood. *Br J Psychiat* **183**: 299–303.

3. Rodin GM, Nolan RP, Katz MR (2005). Depression. In: *Textbook of Psychosomatic Medicine* (ed. JL Levenson), pp. 193–270. Arlington, VA: American Psychiatric Publishing.

4. McDaniel JS, Brown FW, Cole SA (2000). Assessment of depression and grief reactions in the medically ill. In: *Psychiatric Care of the Medical Patient* (ed. A Stoudemire, BS Fogel, DB Greenberg), pp. 149–64. New York: Oxford University Press.

5. Shapiro PA (2005). Heart disease. In: *Textbook of Psychosomatic Medicine* (ed. JL Levenson), pp. 423–44. Arlington, VA: Amcrican Psychiatric Publishing.

6. Chochinov HM (2001). Depression in cancer patients. *Lancet Oncol* **2**: 499–505.

7. Sullivan MD, Newton K, Hecht J, Russo JE, Spertus JA (2004). Depression and health status in elderly patients with heart failure: a 6-month prospective study in primary care. *Am J Geriatr Cardiol* **13**: 252–60.

8. Ludman EJ, Katon W, Russo J et al. (2004). Depression and diabetes symptom burden. *Gen Hosp Psychiat* **26**: 430–6.

9. Chwastiak LA, Gibbons LE, Ehde DM et al. (2005). Fatigue and psychiatric illness in a large community sample of persons with multiple sclerosis. *J Psychosom Res* **59**: 291–8.

10. Kathol RG, Mutgi A, Williams J, Clamon G, Noyes R, Jr (1990). Diagnosis of major depression in cancer patients according to four sets of criteria. *Am J Psychiat* **147**: 1021–4.

11. Koenig HG, George LK, Peterson BL, Pieper CF (1997). Depression in medically ill hospitalized older adults: prevalence, characteristics, and course of symptoms according to six diagnostic schemes. *Am J Psychiat* **154**: 1376–83.

12. Wilson KG, Mikail SF, D'Eon JL, Minns JE (2001). Alternative diagnostic criteria for major depressive disorder in patients with chronic pain. *Pain* **91**: 227–34.

13. von Ammon CS, Furlanetto LM, Creech SD, Powell LH (2001). Medical illness, past depression, and present depression: a predictive triad for in-hospital mortality. *Am J Psychiat* **158**: 43–8.

14. Lyness JM, Heo M, Datto CJ et al. (2006). Outcomes of minor and subsyndromal depression among elderly patients in primary care settings. *Ann Intern Med* **144**: 496–504.

15. Tyrer P, Seivewright H, Johnson T (2004). The Nottingham Study of Neurotic Disorder: predictors of 12-year outcome of dysthymic, panic and generalized anxiety disorder. *Psychol Med* **34**(8): 1385–94.

16. Watson D, Clark LA (1984). Negative affectivity: the disposition to experience aversive emotional states. *Psychol Bull* **96**: 465–90.

17. Kubzansky LD, Cole SR, Kawachi I, Vokonas P, Sparrow D (2006). Shared and unique contributions of anger, anxiety, and depression to coronary heart disease: a prospective study in the normative aging study. *Ann Behav Med* **31**: 21–9.

18. Crawford JR, Henry JD (2004). The positive and negative affect schedule (PANAS): construct validity, measurement properties and normative data in a large non-clinical sample. *Br J Clin Psychol* **43**: 245–65.

19. Voogt E, van der Heide A, van Leeuwen AF et al. (2005). Positive and negative affect after diagnosis of advanced cancer. *Psychooncology* **14**: 262–73.

20. McCusker J, Cole M, Dufouil C et al. (2005). The prevalence and correlates of major and minor depression in older medical inpatients. *J Am Geriatr Soc* **53**: 1344–53.

21. Norton MC, Skoog I, Toone L et al. (2006). Three-year incidence of first-onset depressive syndrome in a population sample of older adults: the Cache County study. *Am J Geriatr Psychiat* **14**: 237–45.

22. Levenson JL (ed.) (2005). *Textbook of Psychosomatic Medicine*. Arlington, VA: American Psychiatric Publishing.

23. American Psychiatric Association Task Force on DSM-IV (1994). *Diagnostic and Statistical Manual of Mental Disorders DSM-IV*, 4th edn. Washington, DC: American Psychiatric Association.

24. Pauli P, Wiedemann G, Dengler W, Blaumann-Benninghoff G, Kuhlkamp V (1999). Anxiety in patients with an automatic implantable cardioverter defibrillator: what differentiates them from panic patients? *Psychosom Med* **61**: 69–76.

25. Pedersen SS, van Domburg RT, Theuns DA, Jordaens L, Erdman RA (2005). Concerns about the implantable cardioverter defibrillator: a determinant of anxiety and depressive symptoms independent of experienced shocks. *Am Heart J* **149**: 664–9.

26. Dew MA, Switzer GE, Myaskovsky L, DiMartini AF, Tovt-Korshynska MI (2006). Rating Scales for Mood Disorders. In: *Textbook of Mood Disorders* (ed. DJ Stein, DJ Kupfer, AF Schatzberg), pp. 69–97. Washington, DC: American Psychiatric Publishing.

27. Lowe B, Unutzer J, Callahan CM, Perkins AJ, Kroenke K (2004). Monitoring depression treatment outcomes with the patient health questionnaire-9. *Med Care* **42**: 1194–201.

28. Pinto-Meza A, Serrano-Blanco A, Penarrubia MT, Blanco E, Haro JM (2005). Assessing depression in primary care with the PHQ-9: can it be carried out over the telephone? *J Gen Intern Med* **20**: 738–42.

29. Spitzer RL, Kroenke K, Williams JB, Lowe B (2006). A brief measure for assessing generalized anxiety disorder: the GAD-7. *Arch Intern Med* **166**: 1092–7.

30. Zigmond AS, Snaith RP (1983). The hospital anxiety and depression scale. *Acta Psychiatr Scand* **67**: 361–70.

31. Rutledge T, Reis VA, Linke SE, Greenberg BH, Mills PJ (2006). Depression in heart failure: a meta-analytic review of prevalence, intervention effects, and associations with clinical outcomes. *J Am Coll Cardiol* **48**: 1527–37.

32. Freedland KE, Rich MW, Skala JA, Carney RM, Davila-Roman VG, Jaffe AS (2003). Prevalence of depression in hospitalized patients with congestive heart failure. *Psychosom Med* **65**: 119–28.

33. Vaccarino V, Kasl SV, Abramson J, Krumholz HM (2001). Depressive symptoms and risk of functional decline and death in patients with heart failure. *J Am Coll Cardiol* **38**: 199–205.

34. Koenig HG (1998). Depression in hospitalized older patients with congestive heart failure. *Gen Hosp Psychiat* **20**: 29–43.

35. Freedland KE, Rich MW, Skala JA, Carney RM, Davila-Roman VG, Jaffe AS (2003). Prevalence of depression in hospitalized patients with congestive heart failure. *Psychosom Med* **65**: 119–28.

36. Rumsfeld JS, Havranek E, Masoudi FA *et al.* (2003). Depressive symptoms are the strongest predictors of short-term declines in health status in patients with heart failure. *J Am Coll Cardiol* **42**: 1811–17.

37. Sullivan MD, Newton K, Hecht J, Russo JE, Spertus JA (2004). Depression and health status in elderly patients with heart failure: a 6-month prospective study in primary care. *Am J Geriatr Cardiol* **13**: 252–60.

38. Havranek EP, Spertus JA, Masoudi FA, Jones PG, Rumsfeld JS (2004). Predictors of the onset of depressive symptoms in patients with heart failure. *J Am Coll Cardiol* **44**: 2333–8.

39. Fulop G, Strain JJ, Stettin G (2003). Congestive heart failure and depression in older adults: clinical course and health services use 6 months after hospitalization. *Psychosomatics* **44**: 367–73.

40. Turvey CL, Schultz K, Arndt S, Wallace RB, Herzog R (2002). Prevalence and correlates of depressive symptoms in a community sample of people suffering from heart failure. *J Am Geriatr Soc* **50**: 2003–8.

41. Bekelman DB, Dy S, Becker D, Wittstein I, Hendricks D, Yamashita T, Gottlieb S (2007). Spiritual well-being and depression in patients with heart failure. *J Gen Intern Med* **22**: 470–7 [erratum in *J Gen Intern Med* **22**: 1066].

42. Schiffer AA, Pedersen SS, Widdershoven JW, Hendriks EH, Winter JB, Denollet J (2005). The distressed (type D) personality is independently associated with impaired health status and increased depressive symptoms in chronic heart failure. *Eur J Cardiovasc Prev Rehabil* **12**: 341–6.

43. Capuron L, Ravaud A, Dantzer R (2000). Early depressive symptoms in cancer patients receiving interleukin 2 and/or interferon alfa-2b therapy. *J Clin Oncol* **18**: 2143–51.

44. Capuron L, Ravaud A, Neveu PJ, Miller AH, Maes M, Dantzer R (2002). Association between decreased serum tryptophan concentrations and depressive symptoms in cancer patients undergoing cytokine therapy. *Mol Psychiat* **7**: 468–73.

45. Musselman DL, Miller AH, Porter MR *et al.* (2001). Higher than normal plasma interleukin-6 concentrations in cancer patients with depression: preliminary findings. *Am J Psychiat* **158**: 1252–7.

46. Pasic J, Levy WC, Sullivan MD (2003). Cytokines in depression and heart failure. *Psychosom Med* **65**: 181–93.

47. Katon WJ (2003). Clinical and health services relationships between major depression, depressive symptoms, and general medical illness. *Biol Psychiat* **54**: 216–26.

48. Lee DT, Yu DS, Woo J, Thompson DR (2005). Health-related quality of life in patients with congestive heart failure. *Eur J Heart Fail* **7**: 419–22.

49. Carels RA (2004). The association between disease severity, functional status, depression and daily quality of life in congestive heart failure patients. *Qual Life Res* **13**(1): 63–72.

50. Godemann F, Butter C, Lampe F, Linden M, Werner S, Behrens S (2004). Determinants of the quality of life (QoL) in patients with an implantable cardioverter/defibrillator (ICD). *Qual Life Res* **13**: 411–16.

51. Sears SF, Lewis TS, Kuhl EA, Conti JB (2005). Predictors of quality of life in patients with implantable cardioverter defibrillators. *Psychosomatics* **46**: 451–7.

52. Sullivan M, Levy WC, Russo JE, Spertus JA (2004). Depression and health status in patients with advanced heart failure: a prospective study in tertiary care. *J Card Fail* **10**: 390–6.

53. Jiang W, Alexander J, Christopher E *et al.* (2001). Relationship of depression to increased risk of mortality and rehospitalization in patients with congestive heart failure. *Arch Intern Med* **161**: 1849–56.

54 Sullivan MD, Levy WC, Crane BA, Russo JE, Spertus JA (2004). Usefulness of depression to predict time to combined end point of transplant or death for outpatients with advanced heart failure. *Am J Cardiol* **94**: 1577–80.

55. Murberg TA, Bru E, Svebak S, Tveteras R, Aarsland T (1999). Depressed mood and subjective health symptoms as predictors of mortality in patients with congestive heart failure: a two-years follow-up study. *Int J Psychiat Med* **29**: 311–26.

56. Vaccarino V, Kasl SV, Abramson J, Krumholz HM (2001). Depressive symptoms and risk of functional decline and death in patients with heart failure. *J Am Coll Cardiol* **38**: 199–205.

57. Rumsfeld JS, Jones PG, Whooley MA *et al.* (2005). Depression predicts mortality and hospitalization in patients with myocardial infarction complicated by heart failure. *Am Heart J* **150**: 961–7.

58. Fulop G, Strain JJ, Stettin G (2003). Congestive heart failure and depression in older adults: clinical course and health services use 6 months after hospitalization. *Psychosomatics* **44**: 367–73.

59. Sullivan M, Simon G, Spertus J, Russo J (2002). Depression-related costs in heart failure care. *Arch Intern Med* **162**: 1860–6.

60. Empana JP, Jouven X, Lemaitre RN *et al.* (2006). Clinical depression and risk of out-of-hospital cardiac arrest. *Arch Intern Med* **166**: 195–200.

61. Dunbar SB, Kimble LP, Jenkins LS *et al.* (1999). Association of mood disturbance and arrhythmia events in patients after cardioverter defibrillator implantation. *Depress Anxiety* **9**: 163–8.

62. Sola CL, Bostwick JM (2005). Implantable cardioverter-defibrillators, induced anxiety, and quality of life. *Mayo Clin Proc* **80**: 232–7.

63. McCready MJ, Exner DV (2003). Quality of life and psychological impact of implantable cardioverter defibrillators: focus on randomized controlled trial data. *Card Electrophysiol Rev* **7**: 63–70.

64. Irvine J, Dorian P, Baker B *et al.* (2002). Quality of life in the Canadian Implantable Defibrillator Study (CIDS). *Am Heart J* **144**: 282–9.

65. Schron EB, Exner DV, Yao Q *et al.* (2002). Quality of life in the antiarrhythmics versus implantable defibrillators trial: impact of therapy and influence of adverse symptoms and defibrillator shocks. *Circulation* **105**: 589–94.

66. Surtees PG, Wainwright NW, Khaw KT, Day NE (2003). Functional health status, chronic medical conditions and disorders of mood. *Br J Psychiat* **183**: 299–303.

67. Jiang W, Kuchibhatla M, Cuffe MS *et al.* (2004). Prognostic value of anxiety and depression in patients with chronic heart failure. *Circulation* **110**: 3452–6.

68. Strik JJ, Denollet J, Lousberg R, Honig A (2003). Comparing symptoms of depression and anxiety as predictors of cardiac events and increased health care consumption after myocardial infarction. *J Am Coll Cardiol* **42**: 1801–7.

69. Rumsfeld JS, Ho PM (2005). Depression and cardiovascular disease: a call for recognition. *Circulation* **111**: 250–3.

70. Nemeroff CB, Musselman DL (2000). Are platelets the link between depression and ischemic heart disease? *Am Heart J* **140**(4 Suppl.): 57–62.

71. Pasic J, Levy WC, Sullivan MD (2003). Cytokines in depression and heart failure. *Psychosom Med* **65**: 181–93.

72. Mann DL (2002). Inflammatory mediators and the failing heart: past, present, and the foreseeable future. *Circ Res* **91**: 988–98.

73. Gorman JM, Sloan RP (2000). Heart rate variability in depressive and anxiety disorders. *Am Heart J* **140**(4 Suppl.): 77–83.

74. Dunbar SB, Kimble LP, Jenkins LS *et al.* (1999). Association of mood disturbance and arrhythmia events in patients after cardioverter defibrillator implantation. *Depress Anxiety* **9**: 163–8.

75. Plotsky PM, Owens MJ, Nemeroff CB (1998). Psychoneuroendocrinology of depression. Hypothalamic-pituitary-adrenal axis. *Psychiatr Clin North Am* **21**: 293–307.

76. Maas JW, Katz MM, Koslow SH *et al.* (1994). Adrenomedullary function in depressed patients. *J Psychiatr Res* **28**: 357–67.

77. Morgan AL, Masoudi FA, Havranek EP *et al.* (2006). Difficulty taking medications, depression, and health status in heart failure patients. *J Card Fail* **12**: 54–60.

78. Rosal MC, Ockene JK, Ma Y *et al.* (2001). Behavioral risk factors among members of a health maintenance organization. *Prev Med* **33**: 586–94.

79. DiMatteo MR, Lepper HS, Croghan TW (2000). Depression is a risk factor for noncompliance with medical treatment: meta-analysis of the effects of anxiety and depression on patient adherence. *Arch Intern Med* **160**: 2101–7.

80. Carney RM, Freedland KE, Eisen SA, Rich MW, Jaffe AS (1995). Major depression and medication adherence in elderly patients with coronary artery disease. *Health Psychol* **14**: 88–90.

81. Blumenthal JA, Williams RS, Wallace AG, Williams RB, Jr, Needles TL (1982). Physiological and psychological variables predict compliance to prescribed exercise therapy in patients recovering from myocardial infarction. *Psychosom Med* **44**: 519–27.

82. Patton GC, Carlin JB, Coffey C, Wolfe R, Hibbert M, Bowes G (1998). Depression, anxiety, and smoking initiation: a prospective study over 3 years. *Am J Public Health* **88**: 1518–22.

83. Phillips CO, Wright SM, Kern DE, Singa RM, Shepperd S, Rubin HR (2004). Comprehensive discharge planning with postdischarge support for older patients with congestive heart failure: a meta-analysis. *J Am Med Assoc* **291**: 1358–67.

84. O'Connor CM, Joynt KE (2004). Depression: are we ignoring an important comorbidity in heart failure? *J Am Coll Cardiol* **43**: 1550–2.

85. Glassman AH, O'Connor CM, Califf RM *et al.* (2002). Sertraline treatment of major depression in patients with acute MI or unstable angina. *J Am Med Assoc* **288**: 701–9.

86. Berkman LF, Blumenthal J, Burg M *et al.* (2003). Effects of treating depression and low perceived social support on clinical events after myocardial infarction: the Enhancing Recovery in Coronary Heart Disease Patients (ENRICHD) Randomized Trial. *J Am Med Assoc* **289**: 3106–16.

87. Taylor CB, Youngblood ME, Catellier D *et al.* (2005). Effects of antidepressant medication on morbidity and mortality in depressed patients after myocardial infarction. *Arch Gen Psychiat* **62**: 792–8.

88. Mann JJ (2005). The medical management of depression. *New Engl J Med* **353**: 1819–34.

89. Jiang W, Davidson JR (2005). Antidepressant therapy in patients with ischemic heart disease. *Am Heart J* **150**: 871–81.

90. Nemeroff CB (2003). Overview of the safety of citalopram. *Psychopharmacol Bull* **37**: 96–121.

91. Stahl SM, Grady MM, Moret C, Briley M (2005). SNRIs: their pharmacology, clinical efficacy, and tolerability in comparison with other classes of antidepressants. *CNS Spectrum* **10**: 732–47.

92. Settle EC, Stahl SM, Batey SR, Johnston JA, Ascher JA (1999). Safety profile of sustained-release bupropion in depression: results of three clinical trials. *Clin Ther* **21**: 454–63.

93. Ludvig J, Miner B, Eisenberg MJ (2005). Smoking cessation in patients with coronary artery disease. *Am Heart J* **149**: 565–72.

94. Cremers B, Schmidt KI, Maack C, Schafers HJ, Bohm M (2003). Catecholamine release in human heart by bupropion. *Eur J Pharmacol* **467**: 169–71.

95. Laimer M, Kramer-Reinstadler K, Rauchenzauner M *et al.* (2006). Effect of mirtazapine treatment on body composition and metabolism. *J Clin Psychiat* **67**: 421–4.

96. De Boer T (1996). The pharmacologic profile of mirtazapine. *J Clin Psychiat* **57**(Suppl. 4): 19–25.

97. Grade C, Redford B, Chrostowski J, Toussaint L, Blackwell B (1998). Methylphenidate in early post-stroke recovery: a double-blind, placebo-controlled study. *Arch Phys Med Rehabil* **79**: 1047–50.

98. Fernandez F, Levy JK, Samley HR *et al.* (1995). Effects of methylphenidate in HIV-related depression: a comparative trial with desipramine. *Int J Psychiat Med* **25**: 53–67.

99. Lander M, Wilson K, Chochinov HM (2000). Depression and the dying older patient. *Clin Geriatr Med* **16**: 335–56.

100. Masand P, Pickett P, Murray GB (1991). Psychostimulants for secondary depression in medical illness. *Psychosomatics* **32**: 203–8.

101. Lucas PB, Gardner DL, Wolkowitz OM, Tucker EE, Cowdry RW (1986). Methylphenidate-induced cardiac arrhythmias. *New Engl J Med* **315**: 1485.

102. Levinson W, Gorawara-Bhat R, Lamb J (2000). A study of patient clues and physician responses in primary care and surgical settings. *J Am Med Assoc* **284**: 1021–7.

103. White J, Levinson W, Roter D (1994). 'Oh, by the way': the closing moments of the medical visit. *J Gen Intern Med* **9**: 24–8.

104. Marvel MK, Epstein RM, Flowers K, Beckman HB (1999). Soliciting the patient's agenda: have we improved? *J Am Med Assoc* **281**: 283–7.

105. Roter DL, Stewart M, Putnam SM, Lipkin M, Jr, Stiles W, Inui TS (1997). Communication patterns of primary care physicians. *J Am Med Assoc* **277**: 350–6.

106. Beckman HB, Frankel RM (1984). The effect of physician behavior on the collection of data. *Ann Intern Med* **101**: 692–6.

107. Nightingale SD, Yarnold PR, Greenberg MS (1991). Sympathy, empathy, and physician resource utilization. *J Gen Intern Med* **6**: 420–3.

108. Suchman AL, Roter D, Green M, Lipkin M, Jr (1993). Physician satisfaction with primary care office visits. Collaborative Study Group of the American Academy on Physician and Patient. *Med Care* **31**: 1083–92.

109. Coulehan JL, Platt FW, Egener B *et al.* (2001). 'Let me see if i have this right': words that help build empathy. *Ann Intern Med* **135**: 221–7.

110. Spiro H (1992). What is empathy and can it be taught? *Ann Intern Med* **116**: 843–6.

111. Platt FW, Keller VF (1994). Empathic communication: a teachable and learnable skill. *J Gen Intern Med* **9**: 222–6.

112. Bower P, Rowland N, Hardy R (2003). The clinical effectiveness of counselling in primary care: a systematic review and meta-analysis. *Psychol Med* **33**: 203–15.

113. Markowitz JC, Kocsis JH, Fishman B *et al.* (1998). Treatment of depressive symptoms in human immunodeficiency virus-positive patients. *Arch Gen Psychiat* **55**: 452–7.

114. Frasure-Smith N, Koszycki D, Swenson JR *et al.* (2006). Design and rationale for a randomized, controlled trial of interpersonal psychotherapy and citalopram for depression in coronary artery disease (CREATE). *Psychosom Med* **68**: 87–93.

115. Mynors-Wallis LM, Gath DH, Day A, Baker F (2000). Randomised controlled trial of problem solving treatment, antidepressant medication, and combined treatment for major depression in primary care. *Br Med J* **320**: 26–30.

116. Barrett JE, Williams JW, Jr, Oxman TE *et al.* (2001). Treatment of dysthymia and minor depression in primary care: a randomized trial in patients aged 18 to 59 years. *J Fam Pract* **50**: 405–12.

117. Gilbody S, Whitty P, Grimshaw J, Thomas R (2003). Educational and organizational interventions to improve the management of depression in primary care: a systematic review. *J Am Med Assoc* **289**: 3145–51.

118. Unutzer J, Katon W, Callahan CM *et al.* (2002). Collaborative care management of late-life depression in the primary care setting: a randomized controlled trial. *J Am Med Assoc* **288**: 2836–45.

119. Bruce ML, Ten Have TR, Reynolds CF, 3rd *et al.* (2004). Reducing suicidal ideation and depressive symptoms in depressed older primary care patients: a randomized controlled trial. *J Am Med Assoc* **291**: 1081–91.

120. Ciechanowski P, Wagner E, Schmaling K *et al.* (2004). Community-integrated home-based depression treatment in older adults: a randomized controlled trial. *J Am Med Assoc* **291**: 1569–77.

121. Epstein SA, Hicks D (2005). Anxiety disorders. In: *Textbook of Psychosomatic Medicine* (ed. JL Levenson), pp. 251–70. Arlington, VA: American Psychiatric Publishing.

122. Stoudemire A (1996). Epidemiology and psychopharmacology of anxiety in medical patients. *J Clin Psychiat* **57**(Suppl. 7): 64–72.

123. Breitbart W, Marotta R, Platt MM *et al.* (1996). A double-blind trial of haloperidol, chlorpromazine, and lorazepam in the treatment of delirium in hospitalized AIDS patients. *Am J Psychiat* **153**: 231–7.

Chapter 16

Spiritual issues in heart failure

Ronald Gillilan and Christina M. Puchalski

Introduction

'Every day that I see the sun rise is like Christmas to me, Doc.' That was Mr K's response to being wished 'Merry Christmas'. Mr K was 70 years old, and now that he has a prosthetic valve, his mitral regurgitation is gone, his heart failure (HF) is improved and he has managed to get through it all and maintain a positive, optimistic view of life. It was a moment of realization for this health-care provider (RG) to acknowledge that he knew very little about this patient's personal life. Were there spiritual elements in this patient's life that enabled him to cope with his disease in such a positive way and, if so, would these elements have any impact on the course of his disease?

Health-care professionals are, for the most part, engrossed in the medical, surgical, and technical complexities of care of their patients and give little attention to the spiritual needs of those in their care.[1] In the case of HF patients, the focus is on diagnosis and management of the physical disease process, on such matters as left-ventricular ejection fraction, and increasingly on evidence-based measures to reduce risk of morbidity and mortality and to improve symptoms.[2,3]Clinicians may be aware that patients with HF are experiencing changes in their personal lives, but how pertinent are spiritual issues in the day to day medical care of these patients? The purely technical aspects of medical care often seem cold and impersonal to both patients and caregivers, yet there is a scientific basis, as well as financial considerations, that persuade those involved to comply with what are currently accepted guidelines for the management of HF. In the Western world of medical care, with the many specialized services and considerations of cost-effectiveness, caregivers need to be reminded that there is both a science and an art of medicine that calls for treating the whole person, not just the malfunctioning physical parts.

The public reminds us that in our routine medical care we are missing important psychological factors, like depression, that may have an impact on outcomes in patients with heart disease.[4] A national health survey on psychological distress in heart disease showed a three-fold increase in self-reported psychological distress in subjects with HF compared with non-diseased persons and only 35% of those reporting distress had seen a mental health professional in the past year.[5] In recent years, there has been research on the impact of anxiety, depression, social support, and style of coping in patients with HF, but there are no standardized procedures for psychological assessment of such patients (see also Chapter 15).[6] Treatment strategies usually focus on medication and not on more holistic forms of treatment that include exploring hope and optimism.[7–9] Hope is an important spiritual resource for people. In addition, most studies indicate that spiritual and religious beliefs may have a positive impact on people with depression.[10]

Religious and spiritual beliefs may also help people with advanced cardiac disease. Several surveys have found that most of the population in the USA is religious, many people (75–80%) turn to religion to cope with stress, and the majority (63–83%) of those surveyed approve of having their doctors address spirituality in their care (at least under circumstances of serious or life-threatening illnesses or loss of loved ones).[11–14] In spite of increasing evidence in medical publications of an important relationship between spirituality/religiosity and health/disease, caregivers often ignore the spiritual factors, which may influence treatment decisions, compliance with treatment, end-of-life decisions, and even survival.[15,16] Studies indicate that physicians only discuss spiritual issues with 10–20% of their patients, and even among seriously ill patients, many with do-not-resuscitate orders, only 6.5% have documentation of a spiritual history being taken.[17,18]

Why do just a small percentage of physicians address spiritual needs in their patients? This may be due to skepticism on the part of some, doubting that spiritual (e.g. religious affiliation, existential concerns, and sense of meaning and purpose) factors have direct effects on heart disease or that interventions related to these factors can improve medical outcomes.[19,20] Surveys have shown that roughly 85–95% of physicians agree that spiritual factors are important health components, and would discuss such matters with patients, but 45% of the doctors responding to the survey questions thought it was inappropriate for the physician to initiate the inquiry.[21,22] These survey results also suggested that a physician's own religious attitudes may play a role, with doctors who consider themselves to be religious or spiritual being more likely to initiate spiritual inquiry. The most important barriers noted by physicians to doing a spiritual assessment, were lack of time (71–95%), and inadequate training (59–65%).[23,24] The diversity of backgrounds of caregivers and patients may impose cultural, language, and religious barriers to understanding. Comparison of religious identity surveys of 1990 and 2001 (these two surveys sampled, respectively, 113,723 and 50,281 English-speaking households in 48 states) show that diversity is increasing in the USA, with fewer households identifying their religion as Christian (86% vs. 77%) or Jewish (1.8% vs. 1.3%) and more as Buddhist (0.2% vs. 0.5%), Hindu (0.1% vs. 0.4%), Muslim (0.3% vs. 0.5%) or no religion (0.8% vs. 14%).[25] It is common for physicians of one denomination or culture to be treating a patient from a different cultural or religious background.

The information provided in this chapter will give caregivers a balanced view of the scientific data relating to the spiritual issues encountered in the care of patients with HF. The techniques discussed here will provide the clinician with a means of making a spiritual inquiry that adds only about 2 minutes to the history-taking process.[26] Health-care professionals are reminded to draw upon other professionals, including chaplains, spiritual directors, and pastoral counselors, when inquiry uncovers significant spiritual needs.

Background

Research over the past couple of decades in a growing new field of spirituality and health has begun to give the notion that the time has come for health-care professionals to be aware of the impact of psychosocial and spiritual issues in their patients.[27] The Joint Commission on Accreditation for Health Care Organizations (JCAHO) requires a spiritual assessment of patients.[28,29] The extent to which health-care professionals should give psychosocial and spiritual support is still evolving, but recognition of the issues that may affect the care of patients is an important first step in the process.

The first rule for those who would be health-care professionals of psychosocial and spiritual support is, as Sam Keen put it, to 'get literate', i.e. to become familiar with the literature in this area.[30] The number of published articles in the recent literature on medicine, psychology, philosophy, and religion is sufficiently large (for spirituality and medicine, nearly 1200 such studies prior to 2000 were reviewed and the number is increasing each year) to offer a challenge to those who wish to step sensitively and ethically into the area of spirituality of their patients.[31] It is the goal of this chapter to increase awareness of psychosocial and spiritual issues in health-care settings and to provide a framework upon which caregivers may further develop knowledge and skills to be supportive of the spiritual needs of patients with chronic HF.

Heart failure

The diagnosis of chronic HF implies a condition of inadequate function of the heart to meet the needs of the tissues of the body and implies the end stage of a number of types of heart disease. HF is a common disease state (accounting for 1 million hospital discharges in the USA in 2001), is the most costly cardiovascular disease (significantly higher in depressed patients with HF), and has devastating effects on the lives of patients and their families.[32,33] Although modern treatments are improving the outlook for patients with HF, recent data suggest that survival in more than 50% of HF patients with preserved left-ventricular systolic function is not improving. The ultimate consequence of this growing public health problem of HF is premature death.[34]

In 2003 the American Heart Association reported that HF was an underlying or contributing cause of death in 286,700 persons in the USA and the overall death rate from HF was 19.7%. There was a 174% increase in the number of patients discharged from hospitals in the USA with the diagnosis of HF from 1979 to 2003.[35] As patients and their families wrestle with the issues of symptoms, treatment options, adverse effects, limitations of and changes in lifestyle, economic consequences, questions of life expectancy, and even end-of-life decisions, psychosocial and spiritual resources are often stretched to the limit; there is great need for supportive and compassionate care from their caregivers.

In the USA, it is safe to assume that patients who suffer from HF often have religious beliefs and engage in spiritual practices.[12,17,36] Koenig found a high prevalence of religious beliefs/attitudes (85%), religious affiliation (98%), practice of daily prayer or scripture reading (70%), and weekly attendance at religious services (48%) in a study of 196 adult patients (age at least 55 years) admitted to Duke University Medical Center with HF or pulmonary disease.[37]

Medical doctors have left the spiritual issues to the chaplains and clergy, although not many physicians have made referrals to chaplains. One study found only 20% of inpatients had visits from chaplains.[38] It may have been considered inappropriate for physicians to address spiritual issues with their patients, as internal medicine and cardiology textbooks address psychosocial issues and give little or no attention to the impact on health of religious or spiritual issues.[39,40] The ACC/AHA 2005 Guideline Update for the Diagnosis and Management of Chronic Heart Failure in the Adult does not deal with the spiritual concerns of patients and their families, other than for a brief section that discusses end-of-life considerations.[3] Published research reports in medical and nursing journals have seldom (varying from less than 1% to no more than 12% in reports from 1994 to 2000) considered spirituality as a variable that may influence outcome.[41–43] Data presented in this chapter make it clear that researchers and clinicians can no longer ignore the spiritual aspects of a patient's life in research and medical care.

Spiritual care: a longstanding tradition

The spiritual area of caregiving is not so new to caregivers. In ancient cultures, and still today in indigenous healing practices, a shaman, a priest, or a medicine man ministers to both the spiritual and health needs of their communities.[44] In the history of Christianity, the first hospitals were established by Christians soon after Constantine closed the temples of Asclepius (335 CE), which had served as refuges for the sick. Since the end of the 17th century, the religious and scientific communities have distanced themselves from one another, but still today roughly 20% of inpatients are in religiously affiliated community hospitals.[45,46]

Over the years, boundaries developed between clinician and priest, separating medical and spiritual care for the sick.[47] While there are professional, social, and ethical boundaries that separate the ministry of the chaplain and the care of the clinician, there should not be barriers that prevent sharing of valuable insights and working together, for the well-being of patients.[48] Most physicians are not comfortable addressing spiritual issues with their patients and often, there is little communication with chaplains or ministers involved with the patient. Clinicians feel 'squeamish' about using the term 'healer' to refer to themselves, for fear of reintroducing the supernatural, pseudoscientific, and religious concepts that held back research and use of the scientific method in past generations.[49,50] Only recently have medical schools introduced the topic of spirituality into curricula; the number of medical schools that offer courses in spirituality had grown from 17 in 1994 to 84 by 2004.[51] Learning objectives for medical students were developed by the Task Force on Spirituality, Cultural Issues, and End of Life Care, and are included in the Association of American Medical Colleges MSOP Report III.[52] In that same task force, the definition of spirituality that was arrived at by consensus as relevant for clinicians is that spirituality is common in all cultures and forms the basis of meaning and purpose in peoples' lives. It may be expressed in religious terms, but meaning may also be found in family, non-theistic beliefs and values, work and humanities, and the arts. It is critical to have a broad based definition for clinical care as patients present with many different expressions of spirituality in the clinical setting. Information provided in this chapter should help both students and practicing caregivers to find appropriate ways to provide spiritual support to patients with HF.

It's a matter of heart

'Yes, Doc, I stopped smoking after my second heart attack. It wasn't so much my doctor telling me I needed to quit, but rather I had to decide here (pointing to his chest), in my heart of hearts, that I was going to quit.' This patient had a 'change in heart' that resulted in his being able to get rid of one of the risk factors for further cardiac events. In his own suffering, he had found the strength to live life in a healthier way. He was not talking about the organ that pumps blood, but he was using the term 'heart' as a metaphor for the seat of the mind, body, or spirit, as a term that has been used since the days of Aristotle.[53]

Sometimes medical treatments are not as potent as the state of mind and spirit that a patient brings to his or her illness.[54] The health-care profession has not been so successful in getting patients to modify their unhealthy behaviors. The average success rate in remaining off smoking at 1 year after various smoking cessation interventions was 5.8% in a meta-analysis of 39 controlled smoking cessation trials.[55] Efforts to promote healthy behaviors may be more successful in preventing habits like smoking than stopping the addictive behavior. Data from a 6-year prospective study of 3968 older persons suggest that religiously involved persons had significantly less smoking, largely because they had never smoked.[56] Interpretation of studies such as these is a challenge, as it may be that religious practices discourage cigarette smoking or that beliefs somehow impact health choices. Spirituality is valued in transforming lifestyles, as shown by an alcoholic participating in Alcoholics Anonymous, who finds spiritual strength for recovery.[57] Perhaps the HF patient can find the strength in his or her spiritual resources to make enormous lifestyle changes. The spiritual process of lifestyle adjustment for 87 patients from HF clinics involved three steps: regret regarding past behaviors and lifestyles; search for meaning in the present HF experience; search for hope for the future and reclaiming of optimism.[58]

There is a higher self, a human spirit that can triumph over the assaults of disease. Perhaps it is, in view of the diversity of cultural and religious beliefs, that the human spirit is indefinable. It is important for professionals to be sensitive to the patient's suffering and to have some understanding of the spiritual dimension and resources of that person's life.[59] Viktor Frankl, who survived a Nazi concentration camp, believed that finding meaning in one's suffering was important to survival.[60] Frankl's idea fits with a hospice definition of spirituality, as a personal and psychological search for [transcendent] meaning.[61] An earlier hospice definition of spirituality was a relationship with God or a Divine Other, but because of the diversity of cultures and beliefs, a broader term was adopted. A distinction is made between spirituality and specific religious beliefs and practices. Whatever definitions are used, it is increasingly clear that spirituality and religiosity are important aspects of life that figure into how patients, family members, and caregivers cope with adversity. A spiritual awakening sometimes helps the victim of serious disease and family members, who also must cope and draw upon their resources, think about what is really important in life and thereby make adjustments in priorities.[62] For Lew Epstein, as his life was being cut short by cancer, the essence of it was 'being loved'. He thanked his family and friends for letting him love them. He also said, 'It isn't the end. It's a new beginning'.[63]

Several patients in a hospital-based outpatient cardiac rehabilitation program passed around a resolution that they had written. The resolution was: 'Many of us, being survivors of serious coronary problems . . . concede that this experience, while somewhat awesome and frightening, has spiritually enriched us and expanded our view of life and its deepest meaning'.[64] These patients had not been cured of their disease, as several of them were left with poor left ventricular function and HF symptoms, but they were healing. Healing involves not only the physical, but encompasses the psychosocial and spiritual parts of our being; healing is about the whole person.

Much like health is more than the absence of disease, the term 'healing' has come to mean something more than recovery from an illness or cure of a disease. In the spiritual sense, healing is a movement from the brokenness of illness and disease toward wholeness.[65] Henri Nouwen applied the term 'Wounded Healer' to suggest that one's own suffering, brokenness, and wounds, if seen to rise 'from the depth of the human condition which all men share', can be the beginning point for compassionate care.[66] Dr Shelia Cassidy, whose own experience of the pain of imprisonment and torture well equipped her to later become medical director of a hospice, states that one who cares for the dying patient must be a 'spiritual companion', to be alongside, to be available, and must 'enter into their darkness, go with them, at least part way, along their lonely and frightening road'.[67] Giving spiritual support and being part of the healing process is a relational experience that requires the caregiver to open himself/herself to the life experience of the patient, the patient's family, and sometimes to other caregivers.

Evidence-based approach: do spiritual factors affect the course of disease?

The pathophysiological mechanisms by which psychosocial stress may adversely affect patients with HF have not been well defined, but there has been work evaluating the responsivity of the sympathetic nervous system, various physiological responses, and endothelial dysfunction to emotional stress in coronary artery disease.[68] Although biological (physiological, neural, endocrine, immune, etc.) responses to personal meditation and repetitive prayer have been reported and modern imaging techniques, such as positron emission tomography (PET), hold promise in defining brain metabolism in conditions like depression, defining pathways by which such interventions may influence the course of disease must await further research.[69–71] There are favorable reports of relaxation techniques for the reduction of mental stress, of meditation reducing sympathetic activation and improving quality of life in patients with HF, and of meditation for various medical conditions (including anxiety), but there are insufficient data to reach a definitive conclusion about effectiveness of the interventions in changing the course of disease.[72–74] Nonetheless, these studies and the anecdotal evidence seen in patients' stories suggest that the area of spiritual interventions in cardiac disease should be a consideration for future research.

Observational studies on spirituality and health

The claim can be made that the preponderance of research publications show a positive relationship of spirituality and good health outcomes.[75] Mueller cites research studies that suggest religiously involved persons: live longer (18 prospective studies), have less cardiovascular disease (12 of 16 studies) and hypertension (9 of 13 studies), do more health-promoting behaviors (better diet, exercise, etc.), have fewer hospitalizations and shorter hospitals stays, have better end-of-life experiences (less anxiety), have less depression (24 of 29 studies), anxiety (70 cross-sectional and prospective studies), and suicide (two large ecological studies and a cross-sectional study), are less likely to abuse alcohol or substances (20 studies), and cope better with illness.[76]

Most large population studies have shown that patients with religious involvement have reduced mortality risk, but there has been controversy about methodology and statistical strength of the association between highly religious persons and better longevity.[19,49,77,78] McCullough et al.[79] conducted a meta-analysis of data from 42 independent studies, totaling roughly 126,000 adults in the USA, and concluded there was a robust inverse association between religious involvement and all-cause mortality. Bagiella et al.[80] analyzed data on 14,456 seniors in the USA and, after controlling for important prognostic moderator factors, concluded that while frequent religious attendance was associated with increased survival over 6 years of follow-up of the entire cohort, the association was not robust.

A review of studies prior to 2000 suggests ways in which religion and spirituality are related to mental health and coping strategies, including: sense of well-being, attitudes of hope and optimism (92 of 120 studies), and finding meaning and purpose in life (15 of 16 studies).[81] Oxman et al.[82] found lack of social participation and absence of strength or comfort from religion were important predictors of mortality during the 6-month period following open-heart surgery in 232 seniors (at least 55 years of age).

There are no large, well-designed, observational studies relating spirituality to outcomes in HF patients. In Koenig's 196 patients (about half the patients had HF) there was an inverse association of religious involvement with measures of the severity of illness and functional disability.[37] Beery et al.[83] conducted a 3-year longitudinal quality of life evaluation in 58 patients with HF and reported a strong relationship between global quality of life and spiritual well-being. Two other studies have considered the role of spirituality in adjustment (87 patients) and spiritual needs (20 patients) of patients with HF and both studies reported that spiritual issues were significant in their patients.[58,84]

Negative influence of religion on health

There are a few studies that have shown some aspects of spirituality to have a negative impact on health outcome. King et al.[85] found stronger spiritual belief to be an independent predictor of a poor outcome in 250 patients with heart disease or gynecological problems admitted to a London teaching hospital. Koenig points to weaknesses in data analysis (e.g. 47 of 197 subjects with religious beliefs were lost to follow-up) as a potential explanation that this study is at variance with others in the literature.[86]

Religious struggle seems to impact upon health in a negative way. A 2-year longitudinal study in 596 elderly (55 years or older) medical inpatients at two hospitals in Durham, NC, showed that ill patients experiencing religious struggle had a significantly greater risk of dying.[87] Two spiritual discontent items ('Wondered whether God had abandoned me' and 'Questioned God's love for me') and one demonic reappraisal item ('Decided the devil made this happen') predicted increased risk of mortality. In a similar study, carried out in 70 congestive HF patients, 71 diabetic outpatients, and 97 oncology inpatients in Chicago, IL, the investigators found religious struggle in 15% of subjects. The investigators reported that emotional distress and depressive symptoms were associated with religious struggle in all three groups of patients, with HF patients having the highest level of struggle. Frequent attendance at religious services correlated with lower levels of religious struggle. The investigators recommend that when religious struggle is detected, referral to a trained professional chaplain or pastoral counselor should be considered.[88]

Another such negative impact of religion on health outcome is religiously motivated medical neglect, as reported in child fatalities in faith-healing sects.[89] One hundred and seventy-two deaths in children of parents who withheld medical care because of reliance on religious rituals with beliefs of medical care avoidance (83% of the deaths were from five religious groups), were examined at the University of California. The investigators deemed that 140 of the fatalities, with appropriate medical care, would have had at least a 90% survival rate.

Randomized clinical trials: prayer research

There are no large, randomized, clinical trials of spiritual interventions in patients with HF, but the randomized prayer research data deserve brief consideration. Before examining the prayer trials, one might ask to what extent prayer is used for spiritual support by patients.

Personal prayer, as a coping mechanism and alternative healing activity, is common in the USA (82% of adults in a Time/CNN survey; 64% of women of 371 upstate New York medical clinic patients; 90% of outpatients with pulmonary disease in Philadelphia).[11,17,90] A survey of 560 adults indicated that 90% turned to religion to cope with the stress of the terrorist attacks of 11 September 2001.[91] Prayer is used by patients with HF and pulmonary disease (41–70% of 254 patients in two studies).[37,83] Some patients (varying from 19% to 48% of 659 patients of family practice physicians in four states) would like their physicians to pray with them.[36,92] Of 476 primary care physicians in three states, only one-third of doctors would initiate prayer, even for a dying patient, but 77% would pray if the dying patient requested prayer.[22] Only 13% of 40 devout physicians had prayed aloud with patients and 67% of the time it had happened only once.[93]

Larry Dossey MD, whose popular book contained a review of the scientific data on healing prayer, also noted that he prayed for his patients.[94] He also indicated that he believed that love or compassion is the power that makes healing possible in prayer. A physician's private and personal prayers for his or her patients or prayers for guidance and wisdom in treating those patients may be an important part of the doctor's self-care, but it is quite a different ethical issue from praying in the presence of and with a patient. To avoid the appearance of 'religious coercion', generally (an exception may be for patients of 'concordant' faith, as well known members of the same denomination or parish), physicians should not initiate prayer with patients, and preferably should have an 'identified religious leader' lead the prayer experience.[1] When requested to pray with the patient, it may be appropriate to ask if the patient would like to offer the prayer and the physician may simply offer an 'Amen' at the conclusion of the patient's prayer or sit silently with the patient as the patient prays.[95,96]

Two randomized trials of distant healing prayer in a total of 1373 patients with heart disease gave results that favored at least some type of positive treatment effect.[97,98] A systematic review of 23 randomized trials of 'distant healing' (including prayer and therapeutic touch), involving 2774 patients with various medical, dental, and psychiatric conditions, showed about 57% of the trials had positive treatment effect.[99] A study of 40 outpatients with rheumatoid arthritis is cited to raise the issue of personal contact or direct prayer, as opposed to distant prayer. In this trial, subjects benefited from six hours of direct contact prayer from intercessors, but had no measurable benefit from the addition of distant intercessory prayer.[100]

Three randomized trials of distant intercessory prayer in a total of 3349 patients with heart disease gave negative results for treatment effect of prayer.[101–103] A pilot study in 150 patients for one of the studies had shown the feasibility of conducting such a trial and had shown a non-significant trend favoring therapeutic benefit with therapy.[104] In one of the trials, patients who knew they were being prayed for (but had to hide that treatment assignment from the bedside staff) had a higher incidence of complications.[103] The study speaks to the need for obtaining informed consent from patients who participate in research, since some such studies in the past have not done so.[98,105] Roberts et al.[106] conducted a systematic search of randomized trials from 1887 to 1999 on the effectiveness of intercessory prayer for health problems and concluded that the data were inconclusive.

Prayer research studies have generated discussion and controversy, not only in the medical profession, but also in the religious community. In the view of some scientists, the issue of construct validity (e.g. prayer inadequately explicated; cannot define or measure adequately the type and dose of prayer and fervor of the intercessors), is but one factor that makes the clinical trial approach to testing the efficacy of prayer difficult or impossible.[78,107] Religious leaders and theologians have expressed diverse understandings of the purpose of prayer—to surrender one's will to an omniscient and sovereign God vs. to request healing from a God who is open to the request of faithful believers.[108,109] The intercessory studies presuppose that the patient's will, i.e. a good clinical outcome, will be met if the prayer 'works'. Theologically however, prayer in most religious traditions is for God's will, not the person's. There is, therefore, an inherent question as to what the function of prayer is and whether the scientific method can even measure prayer's effects! For people of faith, the results of studies such as these do not affect their own spiritual practices since faith does not need science to validate its belief system.

Providing spiritual support

A 70-year-old patient was given adequate time during her visit with her doctor to describe the past several weeks of her life. It was a cough that brought her to the doctor and it turned out to be bad news: cancer. After a day of testing, when her doctor informed her of the diagnosis, he said, 'This hasn't been a very good day for you, has it?' She looked at him with a smile, reached out her hand and patted him on the wrist, saying 'Oh, don't worry about all of that. I've had a good life. I just wanted you to know, this has been the best doctor visit I've ever had. You're the only one who ever listened'.[110]

Compassionate care means taking the time to listen. The late Dr Philip Tumulty said, '. . .effective conversation with a patient is not something a physician stumbles upon. It must be learned and studied and planned and experienced. . .it can't be accomplished in a hurry. Time is its essential ingredient'.[111] What Dr Tumulty said of the effective clinician can also be said of nurses and other compassionate caregivers. Spiritual support requires the investment of time and preparation for the encounter with the patient.

It is important for caregivers to be informed as to the language, beliefs, religious and cultural practices and preferences of the population they serve. Language differences are barriers for communication that often require trained medical interpreters to assist in reliable translations.[112] Understanding religious convictions ('hope for a miracle' or 'belief that suffering can have redemptive value' or 'that every moment of life is a gift from God and is worth preserving at any cost') that explain the demands of patients and families for 'inappropriate' aggressive end-of-life care can be a step in helping all parties arrive at an acceptable solution to such dilemmas.[113] Understanding the patient's faith perspective may require particular effort and often needs to involve an appropriate religious leader, if the caregiver is of a different religious faith.[114] There is diversity in the religious characteristics of physicians and one stratified survey of 2000 US physicians indicated differences in religious beliefs and practices from the general population that influence their practice of medicine.[115] Being attentive to existential and spiritual concerns that underscore the person's need to make sense of his or her suffering and find meaning in life is key to good spiritual support. Listening respectfully is essential to understanding the patient's beliefs and concerns.[116]

One opportunity for the physician to make a spiritual assessment of a patient is during the obtaining of the medical history. A spiritual inquiry must be done in a sensitive way, respecting the patient's privacy and without any implications being given of endorsement of religion as being desirable.[78] An acronym that is a useful spiritual assessment tool is FICA, the details of which are shown in Box 16.1.[26] FICA provides the health-care worker with a framework for spiritual inquiry at an appropriate time, as during the gathering of social information. The FICA questions add only about 2 minutes to the history-taking process, but may open the door to discussion that provides substantial insight into the cultural background and spiritual belief system of the patient. Important understandings that can prevent frustrations, lack of trust, and conflicts due to poor communication can come from learning the cultural and spiritual background, values, and customs of patients.[112]

Box 16.1 The FICA Spiritual Assessment Method: an acronym for obtaining a spiritual history

Faith or belief: what is your faith or belief?

    Do you consider yourself spiritual or religious?

    What things do you believe in that give meaning to your life?

Importance: is it important in your life?

    What influence does it have on how you take care of yourself?

    How have your beliefs influenced your behavior during this illness?

    What role do your beliefs play in regaining your health?

Community: are you part of a spiritual or religious community?

    Is this of support to you and how?

    Is there a person or group of people you really love or who are really important to you?

Address: how would you like me, your health-care provider, to address these issues in your health care?

©cpuchalski, 1996

Open-ended questions are often helpful in an interview. Some examples of such questions are: 'Do you have a way of making sense of the things that happen in your life?' 'What helps you get through tough times?' 'To whom do you turn when you need support?'. These questions may not have been validated as reliable in prospective studies.[76] One such question that was tested in 248 patients with stage IV cancer, severe pulmonary disease, and HF and was, 'Are you at peace?'. The investigators found that peacefulness was strongly associated with emotional and spiritual well-being.[117] A working group on religious and spiritual issues at the end of life, with various medical educators, provided suggestions as to how physicians might help patients think through medical decisions, by clarification with open-ended questions.[116] There are also a number of written questionnaires that have been validated in research projects, but most have not gained acceptance in medical practice. One example of a brief, yet relatively comprehensive, tool is the Duke Religion Index, which is a five-item scale.[118]

There is a growing body of medical literature addressing approaches to bringing spiritual care of patients into mainstream medical practice. Efforts to find ways of easily including assessment of such factors as social support, social network, neuroticism, and spirituality in a brief (10 minute) evaluation for patients in HF programs are being investigated, but no standard quality-of-life evaluation has yet attained widespread acceptance.[119] Martensson et al.[120,121] explored how a total of 24 senior men and women with congestive HF conceived their life situation and found that feelings of being limited and even powerless over their disease created a vicious cycle of anxiety and further limitation. These nurse investigators suggested several interventions as means of providing psychosocial support: having patients verbalize their feelings, set realistic goals/expectations, and increase their knowledge of the disease. Most of the available data suggest that social support and religious involvement (including intrinsic religiousness) act as buffers against anxiety and depression (a notable exception being Jews, who seem to be at increased risk of depression).[122,123]

The spiritual aspect of caring for patients is not so mysterious and foreign as one might think. Most caregivers have had unpleasant times in which medical treatment plans have been thwarted because of a patient's religious beliefs.[113,114] But there will have been the good times of relating closely to a patient and the patient's family and that relationship, often with communication by spiritual inquiry, led to understanding of the patient's values and beliefs. The caring relationship was reflected in the caregiver's service and commitment to the patient, as nurses considered the patient's spiritual practices in scheduling, as social workers who had assessed spiritual needs coordinated resources for the patient, and as chaplains accommodated diverse cultural and religious needs.[124] Spiritual support has to do with relationships, with compassion, with building trust, and with helping patients tap into their inner resources of strength and hope. The focus of spirituality in medicine is on the science of what works best for the patient, as well as on the art of medicine, which involves an understanding of how healing is in post acknowledging the patient's search for answers to difficult existential and spiritual issues in the clinical environment.

Spiritual support takes place in many environments other than the hospital, such as the physician's office, extended-care facilities, community clinics, and HF centers. The latter provide opportunity for ready collaboration of skilled professionals. There is increasingly more information on the importance of spirituality in these settings. Patients with chronic illness, such as HF, face deep suffering. Patients look to caregivers for compassion and for support as they search for meaning, hope, and peace.[125–127]

As patients with life-threatening disease try to make sense of life, one way to bring peace to the spirit is to let go of guilt and grudges. Forgiveness is a way to find that peace. Research efforts have discovered strategies that help persons take the steps in forgiveness of self, others, and sometimes even God.[128,129]

Compassion means suffering with, or being fully present with, our patients as they suffer; it is partnering or being a spiritual companion with them in the midst of their pain.[65] We are not advocating that the caregiver be intrusive and discuss spiritual matters with a patient who does not wish to do so. Some studies indicate that 16–17% of patients do not wish for their physicians to make such a spiritual inquiry.[14,17] It is not the intent that the health-care professional, who is usually not adequately trained to coordinate quality spiritual care, should step over the boundary into the professional area of the chaplain.[47,130]

For those caregivers who wish to provide spiritual care in clinical practice, there are educational opportunities at seminaries, including parish nursing tracks. At least one accredited program of pastoral care training for physicians has been developed.[131,132] There are also continuing medical education courses at some annual medical conferences, training programs at organizations such as Omega, and an online graduate certificate program in spirituality and health that one of us (CMP) developed at the George Washington University.[133]

The caregiver must also give attention to his/her own spiritual needs.[65] Caregivers not only need to 'get literate' in spiritual matters but there is equal need to be 'mindful', in the sense of one's own critical reflection.[134] The intensity and demands of compassionate caregiving require giving attention to one's own physical, emotional, and spiritual health.[135]

Final thoughts

Caregivers have known all along that the journey from heart disease to better health is much more than the repair of a leaking heart valve or giving of the proper medications. Besides the vital scientific understanding and skills required for the modern practice of medicine, there is an art to the practice of medicine that is perhaps learned but that also has something to do with the beliefs and attitudes of mind and heart of the practitioner, and that art has healing power. The doctor's bedside manner, the nurse's caring presence, the social worker's comprehension of the needs, listening to the patient's story, empathizing, giving realistic hope, being there in the hour of need; these are some of the qualities of that healing, compassionate care of the sick.[136]

The experienced, caring physician knows instinctively that there is a time to grasp the patient's hand and that informed clinician knows when he/she has permission to do so. During serious illness, patients are reassured and sometimes pain lessened, or extrasystoles on the monitor diminished, just when a caring nurse touched the patient or while that trusted clinician was present with the patient. It isn't as though the relief of anxiety and stress were imaginary. For example, modern imaging techniques have shown dopamine release with placebo dosing in patients with Parkinson's disease.[137] The 'powerful placebo' response may simply capture the effects of the interaction between caregivers and patients, as spiritual support occurs. Whatever the explanation, caregivers can make a difference in the life experience of an ill patient. Let us acknowledge that the first act of compassion for all caregivers is competence. This is closely followed by service, whether that is in expertly replacing a leaking mitral valve or simply in responding to the patient's urgent call for a bedpan. The goal of competent service-grounded care is that we not only practice modern medicine well, but that we also connect heart to heart with our patients and their families, so that healing may take place.

References

1. Puchalski CM (2001). The critical need for spirituality in our healthcare system. *New Theology Rev* 9–21.
2. Goldman L (1998). Evidence-based medicine. *Primary Cardiology*, p. 2. Philadelphia: W.B. Saunders Company.
3. http://www.acc.org/clinical/guidelines/failure//index.pdf (accessed 8/11/2006).
4. Kohn D (2006). Depression; research shows head, heart linked. *Baltimore Sun*, 30 June 2006.
5. Ferketich AK, Binkley PF (2005). Psychological distress and cardiovascular disease: results from the 2002 National Health Interview Survey. *Eur Heart J* **26**: 1923–9.
6. MacMahon KMA, Lip GYH (2002). Psychological factors in heart failure, a review of the literature. *Arch Intern Med* **162**: 509–16.
7. Lane DA, Chong AY, Lip GYH (2005). Psychological interventions for depression in heart failure. *Cochrane Database of Systematic Reviews*, 2005, Issue 1. Art. No. CD003329. DOI: 10.1002/-14651858.CD003329.pub2.
8. Rustøen T, Howie J, Eidsmo I *et al.* (2005). Hope in patients hospitalized with heart failure. *Am J Crit Care* **14**: 417–25.
9. Ai AL, Peterson C, Tice TN *et al.* (2004). Faith-based and secular pathways to hope and optimism subconstructs in middle-aged and older cardiac patients. *J Health Psychol* **9**: 435–50.
10. Koenig HG, McCullough ME, Larson DB (2001). *Handbook of Religion and Health*, pp. 123, 527–30. New York: Oxford University Press.
11. Kaplan M (1996). Ambushed by spirituality. *Time* 24 June, p. 62.
12. McNichol T (1996). The new faith in medicine. *USA Today*, April 5–7, pp. 4–5.
13. Plotnikoff GA (2000). Should medicine reach out to the spirit? *Postgrad Med* **108**: 19–22, 25.
14. McCord G, Gilchrist VJ, Grossman SD *et al.* (2004). Discussing spirituality with patients: a rational and ethical approach. *Ann Fam Med* **2**: 356–61.
15. Koenig HG (2002). An 83-year-old woman with chronic illness and strong religious beliefs. *J Am Med Assoc* **288**: 478–93.
16. Anandarajah G, Hight E (2001). Spirituality and medical practice: using HOPE questions as a practical tool for spiritual assessment. *Am Fam Physician* **63**: 81–9.
17. Ehman JW, Ott BB, Short TH *et al.* (1999). Do patients want physicians to inquire about their spiritual or religious beliefs if they become gravely ill? *Arch Intern Med* **159**: 1803–6.
18. King DE, Wells BJ (2003). End-of-life issues and spiritual histories. *South Med J* **96**: 391–3.
19. Sloan RP, Bagiella E, Powell T (1999). Religion, spirituality, and medicine. *Lancet* **353**: 664–7.
20. Relman AS, Angell M (2002). Resolved: psychosocial interventions can improve clinical outcomes in organic disease (con). *Psychosom Med* **64**: 558–63.
21. Curlin FA, Chin MH, Sellergren SA *et al.* (2006). The association of physicians' religious characteristics with their attitudes and self-reported behaviors regarding religion and spirituality in the clinical encounter. *Med Care* **44**: 446–53.
22. Monroe MH, Bynum D, Susi B *et al.* (2003). Primary care physician preferences regarding spiritual behavior in medical practice. *Arch Intern Med* **163**: 2751–6.
23. Ellis MR, Vinson DR, Ewigman B (1999). Addressing spiritual concerns of patients: family physicians' attitudes and practices. *J Fam Pract* **48**: 105–9.
24. McCauley J, Jenckes MW, Tarpley MJ *et al.* (2005). Spiritual beliefs and barriers among managed care practitioners. *J Religion Health* **44**: 136–46.
25. The Graduate Center, The City University of New York. *American Religious Identification Survey*. Available at: http://www.gc.cuny.edu/faculty/research_briefs/Aris/key_findings.htm (accessed 30 January 2007).

26. Puchalski C, Romer AL (2000). Taking a spiritual history allows clinicians to understand patients more fully. *J Palliat Med* **3**: 129–37.

27. Koenig HG (2005). Religion, spirituality and medicine: the beginning of a new era. *South Med J* **98**: 1235–6.

28. The Joint Commission (2004). *Setting the Standard of Quality in Health Care, Spiritual Assessment*, 1 January.

29. Hodge DR (2006). A template for spiritual assessment: a review of the JCAHO requirements and guideline for implementation. *Social Work* **51**: 317–26.

30. Keen S (2003). Healing in a time of crises. Presented at the 53rd Institute for Spirituality and Medicine, Johns Hopkins University School of Medicine, Baltimore, Maryland, 13 May 2003.

31. Weaver AJ, Koenig HG (2006). Religion, spirituality, and their relevance to medicine: an update. *Am Fam Physician* **73**: 1336–7.

32. Fonarow GC, Adams KF, Abraham WT *et al.* (2005). Risk stratification for in-hospital mortality in acutely decompensated heart failure. *J Am Med Assoc* **293**: 572–80.

33. Sullivan M, Simon G, Spertus J *et al.* (2002). Depression-related costs in heart failure care. *Arch Intern Med* **162**: 1860–6.

34. Owan TE, Hodge DO, Herges RM *et al.* (2006). Trends in prevalence and outcome of heart failure with preserved ejection fraction. *New Engl J Med* **355**: 251–9.

35. American Heart Association (2006). Heart failure. *Heart Disease and Stroke Statistics, 2006 Update*. Dallas, TX: American Heart Association.

36. King DE, Bushwick B (1994). Beliefs and attitudes of hospital inpatients about faith healing and prayer. *J Fam Pract* **39**: 349–52.

37. Koenig HG (2002). Religion, congestive heart failure, and chronic pulmonary disease. *J Religion Health* **41**: 263–78.

38. Flannelly KJ, Galek K, Handzo GF (2005). To what extent are the spiritual needs of hospital patients being met? *Int J Psychiat Med* **35**: 319–23.

39. Braunwald E *et al.* (ed.) (2001). *Harrison's Principles of Internal Medicine*, 15th edn. New York: McGraw-Hill.

40. Fuster V *et al.* (ed.) (2001). *Hurst's The Heart*, 10th edn, p. 655. New York: McGraw-Hill.

41. Puchalski CM, Kilpatrick SD, McCullough ME *et al.* (2003) A systematic review of spiritual and religious variables in *Palliative Medicine, American Journal of Hospice and Palliative Care, Hospice Journal, Journal of Palliative Care*, and *Journal of Pain and Symptom Management*. *Palliat Support Care* **1**: 7–13.

42. Kilpatrick SD, Weaver A, McCullough M *et al.* (2005). A review of spiritual and religious measures in nursing research journals. *J Religion Health* **44**: 55–66.

43. Weaver AJ, Flannelly KJ, Case DB *et al.* (2004). Religion and spirituality in three major general medical journals from 1998 to 2000. *South Med J* **97**: 1245–9.

44. Bruce E, Shaman MD (2002). *A Plastic Surgeon's Remarkable Journey into the World of Shapeshifting*. Rochester, VT: Destiny Books.

45. Evans AR (1999). *The Healing Church; Practical Programs for Health Ministries*, p. 9. Cleveland, OH: United Church Press.

46. Modjarrad K (2004). Medicine and spirituality. *Student J Am Med Assoc* **291**: 2880.

47. Post SG, Puchalski CM, Larson DB (2000). Physicians and patient spirituality: professional boundaries, competency, and ethics. *Ann Intern Med* **132**: 578–83.

48. Astrow AB, Puchalski CM, Sulmasy DP (2001). Religion, spirituality, and health care: social, ethical, and practical considerations. *Am J Med* **110**: 283–7.

49. Flannelly KJ, Ellison CG, Strock AL (2004). Methodologic issues in research on religion and health. *South Med J* **97**: 1231–41.

50. Berlinger N (2004). Spirituality and medicine: idiot-proofing the discourse. *J Med Phil* **29**: 681–95.
51. Fortin AH, Barnett KG (2004). Medical school curricula in spirituality and medicine. *Student J Am Med Assoc* **291**: 2883.
52. Puchalski CM (Chair) *et al.* (1999). *Contemporary Issues in Medicine: Communication in Medicine*, Medical School Objectives Project. Washington, DC: Association of American Medical Colleges (available at: http://www.aamc.org/meded/msop/msop3.pdf).
53. Garrison FH (1960). *History of Medicine*, p.101. Philadelphia: W. B. Saunders.
54. Cousins N (1981). *Anatomy of an Illness*, p. 139. New York: Bantam Books.
55. Kottke TE, Battista RN, DeFriese GH *et al.* (1988). Attributes of successful smoking cessation interventions in medical practice. *J Am Med Assoc* **259**: 2883–9.
56. Koenig HG, George LK, Cohen HJ *et al.* (1998). The relationship between religious activities and cigarette smoking in older adults. *J Gerontol A: Biol Sci Med Sci* **53**: M426–M434.
57. (1976). *Alcoholics Anonymous*, p.569. New York: Alcoholics Anonymous World Services, Inc.
58. Westlake C, Dracup K (2001). Role of spirituality in adjustment of patients with advanced heart failure. *Prog Cardiovasc Nurs* **16**: 119–25.
59. Galek K, Flannelly KJ, Vane A *et al.* (2005). Assessing a patient's spiritual needs: a comprehensive instrument. *Holistic Nurs Prac* 19: 62–9.
60. Frankl VE (1984). *Man's Search For Meaning; An Introduction to Logotherapy*, p. 116. New York: Simon & Schuster.
61. Daaleman TP, VandeCreed L (2000). Placing religion and spirituality in end-of-life care. *J Am Med Assoc* **284** 2514–17.
62. Callahan H (2003). Families dealing with advanced heart failure: a challenge and an opportunity. *Crit Care Nurs Q* **26**: 230–43.
63. Stillwater M, Malkin G (2000). *Graceful Passages*. Novato, CA: Companion Arts.
64. Gillilan R (2006). Medical science and healing of spirit. *Heart to Heart*, Winter 2006. Baltimore, MD: St Agnes Hospital Heart Services.
65. Puchalski C (2004). Spirituality in health: the role of spirituality in critical care. *Crit Care Clin* **20**: 487–504.
66. Nouwen HJM (1979). *The Wounded Healer*, p. 88. New York: Doubleday Dell Publishing Group.
67. Cassidy S (1999). *Sharing the Darkness; the Spirituality of Caring*, p.6. Maryknoll, NY: Orbis Books.
68. Rozanski A, Blumenthal JA, Kaplan J (1999). Impact of psychological factors on the pathogenesis of cardiovascular disease and implications for therapy. *Circulation* **99**: 2192–217.
69. Benson H (1975). *The Relaxation Response*. New York: Avon Books.
70. Komaroff AL (ed.) (2005). Meditation in psychotherapy. *Harvard Ment Health Lett* **21**: 1–4.
71. Bremner JD, Vythilingam M, Ng CK *et al.* (2003). Regional brain metabolic correlates of α-methyl-paratyrosine-induced depressive symptoms. *J Am Med Assoc* **289**: 3125–34.
72. Canter PH (2003). The therapeutic effects of meditation. *Br Med J* **326**: 1049–50.
73. Krisanaprakornkit T, Krisanaprakornkit W, Piyavhatkul N, Laopaiboon M (2006). Meditation therapy for anxiety disorders. *Cochrane Database of Systematic Reviews* 2006, Issue 1. DOI: 10.1002/-14651858.CD004998.pub2.
74. Eppley KR, Abrams AE, Shear J (1989). Differential effects of relaxation techniques on trait anxiety: a meta-analysis. *J Clin Psychol* **45**: 957–74.
75. Wallis C, McDowell J (1996). Faith and healing. *Time* **147**: 58.
76. Mueller PS, Plevak DJ, Rummans TA (2001). Religious involvement, spirituality, and medicine: implications for clinical practice. *Mayo Clin Proc* **76**: 1225–35.
77. Koenig HG, Idler E, Kasl S *et al.* (1999). Religion, spirituality, and medicine: a rebuttal to skeptics. *Int J Psychiat Med* **29**: 123–31.

78. Koenig HG (2001). Religion, spirituality, and medicine: how are they related and what does it mean? *Mayo Clin Proc* **76**: 1189–91.

79. McCullough ME, Hoyt WT, Larson DB *et al.* (2000). Religious involvement and mortality: a meta-analytic review. *Health Psychol* **19**: 211–22.

80. Bagiella E, Hong V, Sloan RP (2005). Religious attendance as a predictor of survival in the EPESE cohorts. *Int J Epidemiol* **34**: 443–51.

81. Koenig HG, McCullough ME, Larson DB (2001). *Handbook of Religion and Health*, pp. 519–23. New York: Oxford University Press.

82. Oxman TE, Freeman DH, Jr, Manheimer ED (1995). Lack of social participation or religious strength and comfort as risk factors for death after cardiac surgery in the elderly. *Psychosom Med* **57**: 5–15.

83. Beery TA, Baas LS, Fowler C *et al.* (2002). Spirituality in persons with heart failure. *J Holistic Nurs* **20**: 5–25.

84. Murray SA Kendall M, Worth A *et al.* (2004). Exploring the spiritual needs of people dying of lung cancer or heart failure: a prospective qualitative interview study of patients and their carers. *Palliat Med* **18**: 39–45.

85. King M, Speck P, Thomas A (1999). The effect of spiritual beliefs on outcome from illness. *Soc Sci Med* **48**: 1291–9.

86. Koenig HG, McCullough ME, Larson DB (2001). *Handbook of Religion and Health*, pp. 337–8. New York: Oxford University Press,

87. Pargament KI, Koenig HG, Tarakeshwar N, Hahn J (2001). Religious struggle as a predictor of mortality among medically ill elderly patients. *Arch Intern Med* **161**: 1881–5.

88. Fitchett G, Murphy PE, Kim JL *et al.* (2004). Religious struggle: prevalence, correlates and mental health risks in diabetic, congestive heart failure, and oncology patients. *Int J Psychiat Med* **34**: 179–96.

89. Asser SM, Swan R (1998). Child fatalities from religion-motivated medical neglect. *Pediatrics* **101**: 625–9.

90. Rhee SM, Garg VK, Hershey CO (2004). Use of complementary and alternative medicines by ambulatory patients. *Arch Intern Med* **164**: 1004–9.

91. Schuster MA, Stein BD, Jaycox LH *et al.* (2001). A national survey of stress reactions after the September 11, 2001, terrorist attacks. *New Engl J Med* **345**: 1507–12.

92. MacLean CD, Susi B, Phifer N *et al.* (2003). Patient preferences for physician discussion and practice of spirituality. *J Gen Intern Med* **18**: 38–43.

93. Olive KE (1995). Physician religious beliefs and the physician-patient relationship: a study of devout physicians. *South Med J* **88**: 1249–55.

94. Dossey L (1994). *Healing Words*, p. 170. New York: HarperCollins Publishers.

95. Brooke A (1996). *Healing in the Landscape of Prayer*, p. 43. Boston, MA: Crowley Publications

96. Puchalski CM (2001). Spirituality and health: the art of compassionate medicine. *Hosp Physician* **37**: 30–6.

97. Byrd RC (1988). Positive therapeutic effects of intercessory prayer in a coronary care unit population. *South Med J* **81**: 826–9.

98. Harris W, Gowda M, Kolb JW *et al.* (1999). A randomized, controlled trial of the effects of remote, intercessory prayer on outcomes in patients admitted to the coronary care unit. *Arch Intern Med* **159**: 2273–8.

99. Austin JA, Harkness E, Ernst E (2000). The efficacy of "distant healing": a systematic review of randomized trials. *Ann Intern Med* **132**: 903–10.

100. Matthews DA, Marlowe SM, McNutt FS (2000). Effects of intercessory prayer on patients with rheumatoid arthritis. *South Med J* **93**: 1177–86.

101. Krucoff MW, Crater SW, Gallup D *et al.* (2005). Music, imagery, touch, and prayer as adjuncts to interventional cardiac care: the Monitoring and Actualisation of Noetic Trainings (MANTRA) II randomized study. *Lancet* **366**: 211–17.

102. Aviles JM, Whelan SE, Hernke DA *et al.* (2001). Intercessory prayer and cardiovascular disease progression in a coronary care unit population: a randomized controlled trial. *Mayo Clin Proc* **76**: 1192–8.

103. Benson H, Dusek JA, Sherwood JB *et al.* (2006). Study of the therapeutic effects of intercessory prayer in cardiac bypass patients: a multicenter randomized trial of uncertainty and certainty of receiving intercessory prayer. *Am Heart J* **151**: 934–42.

104. Krucoff MW, Crater SW, Green CL *et al.* (2001). Integrative noetic therapies as adjuncts to percutaneous intervention during unstable coronary syndromes: Monitoring and Actualization of Noetic Training (MANTRA) feasibility pilot. *Am Heart J* **142**: 760–7.

105. Krucoff MW, Crater SW, Lee KL (2006). From efficacy to safety concerns: A STEP forward or a step back for clinical research and intercessory prayer?: the Study of Therapeutic Effects of Intercessory Prayer (STEP). *Am Heart J* **151**: 762–4.

106. Roberts L, Ahmed I, Hall S (2007). *Cochrane Database of Systematic Reviews* 2007, Issue 1. Art. No.: CD000368. DOI: 10.1002/14651858.CD000368.pub2.

107. Chibnall JT, Jeral JM, Cerullo MA (2001). Experiments on distant intercessory prayer. *Arch Intern Med* **161**: 2529–35.

108. MacNutt F (2006). Does science now prove that intercessory prayer doesn't work? *The Healing Line*, May/June, pp. 1–6. Jacksonville, FL: Christian Healing Ministries.

109. Myers DG *et al.* (2000). Theme: What happens when we pray? *Reformed Review*, **53**: 93–126.

110. Barr DA (2004). A time to listen. *Ann Intern Med* **140**: 144.

111. Tumulty PA (1973). *The Effective Clinician*, p.14. Philadelphia: W. B. Saunders Company.

112. Crawley LM, Marshall PA, Lo B *et al.* (2002). Strategies for culturally effective end-of-life care. *Ann Intern Med* **136**: 673–9.

113. Brett AS, Jersild P (2003). 'Inappropriate' treatment near the end of life. *Arch Intern Med* **163**: 1649–1649.

114. Alibhai SMH, Gordon M (2004). Muslim and Jewish perspectives on inappropriate treatment at the end of life. *Arch Intern Med* **164**: 916–17.

115. Curlin FA, Lantos JD, Roach CJ *et al.* (2005). Religious characteristics of U.S. physicians: a national survey. *J Gen Intern Med* **20**: 629–34.

116. Lo B, Ruston D, Kates LW *et al.* (2002). Discussing religious and spiritual issues at the end of life: a practical guide for physicians. *J Am Med Assoc* **287**: 749–54.

117. Steinhauser KE, Voils CI, Clipp EC *et al.* (2006). Are You at Peace? *Arch Intern Med* **166**: 101–5.

118. Koenig H, Parkerson GR, Jr, Meador KG (1997). Religion index for psychiatric research. *Am J Psychiat* **153**: 885–6.

119. Westlake C, Dracup K, Creaser J *et al.* (2002). Correlates of health-related quality of life in patients with heart failure. *Heart Lung* **31**: 85–93.

120. Martensson J, Karlsson JE, Fridlund B (1997). Male patients with congestive heart failure and their conception of the life situation. *J Adv Nurs* **25**: 579–86.

121. Martensson J, Karlsson JE, Fridlund B (1998). Female patients with congestive heart failure: how they conceive their life situation. *J Adv Nurs* **28**: 1216–24.

122. Koenig HG, McCullough ME, Larson DB (2001). *Handbook of Religion and Health*, pp. 119, 123, 153. New York: Oxford University Press.

123. Hughes JW, Sketeh MH, Watkins LL (2004). Social support and religiosity as coping strategies for anxiety in hospitalized cardiac patients. *Ann Behav Med* **28**: 179–85.

124. Ai AL, Peterson C, Bolling SF, Koenig H (2002). Private prayer and optimism in middle-aged and older patients awaiting cardiac surgery. *Gerontologist* **42**: 70–81.

125. Kub JE, Nolan MT, Hughes MT *et al.* (2003). Religious importance and practices of patients with a life-threatening illness: implications for screening protocols. *Appl Nurs Res* **16**: 196–200.

126. Davidson PM, Paull G, Introna K *et al.* (2004). Integrated, collaborative palliative care in heart failure: the St. George Heart Failure Service experience 1999–2002. *J Cardiovasc Nurs* **19**: 68–75.

127. Overvold JA (2005). A study of religion, ministry, and meaning in caregiving among health professionals in an institutional setting in New York. *J Pastoral Care Counsel* **59**: 225–35.

128. Worthington E (2001). *Five Steps to Forgiveness.* New York: Crown Publishers.

129. Luskin F (2002). *Forgive for Good.* New York: Harper Collins.

130. Connelly R, Light K (2003). Exploring the "new" frontier of spirituality in health care: identifying the dangers. *J Religion Health* **42**: 35–46.

131. Todres DI, Catlin EA, Thiel MM (2005). The intensivist in a spiritual care training program adapted for clinicians. *Crit Care Med* **33**: 2733–6.

132. http://www.stmarys.edu/ecumenical

133. The George Washington Institute for Spirituality and Health. http://www.gwish.org.

134. Epstein RM (1999). Mindful Practice. *J Am Med Assoc* **282**: 833–9.

135. Nelson RM (2005). The compassionate clinician: Attending to the spiritual needs of self and others. *Crit Care Med* **33**: 2841–2.

136. O'Mathuna DP (2003). The placebo effect and alternative therapies. *Altern Med Alert* **6**(6): 61–9.

137. de la Fuente-Fernandez R, Ruth TJ, Sossi V *et al.* (2001). Expectation and dopamine release: mechanism of the placebo effect in Parkinson's disease. *Science* **293**: 1164–6.

Chapter 17

The elderly patient with heart failure

Christopher Ward and Neil Gillespie

Introduction

Defining older patients

Patients older than 65–70 years were excluded from the original heart failure (HF) treatment trials.[1] This age span also corresponds with the retirement age in many countries and it therefore identifies, at least in the eyes of clinical trialists and the general public, the transition from 'middle aged' to 'elderly'. But this perception is changing: life expectancy and retirement age are increasing and we now recognize that in terms of survival, biological age is more important than chronological age.[2]

In the light of these uncertainties and the lack of an agreed definition of 'elderly' we will use it to mean patients aged about 70 years and above.

The aspirations of patients with HF

The natural history of HF is characterized by a downhill course punctuated by episodes of acute deterioration (and sudden death in approximately 40%), symptoms that are increasingly resistant to conventional treatment, and a progressive reduction in the quality of life. This pattern is independent of age. Conventional treatment can halt this progression and improve prognosis, symptoms, and quality of life for several years but eventually the underlying natural history returns.

The needs and wishes of most elderly patients faced with this scenario are the same as those of younger patients: symptom relief, an improved prognosis, and a better quality of life. The means of achieving these objectives are also the same: guideline-based medication, surgery, interventional treatments when appropriate, and palliative care support. They should therefore be offered optimal conventional treatment while recognizing that their priorities may be different from those of younger patients: When patients are frail and elderly, they may consider a treatment which offers an improvement in quality of life to be more important than any mortality benefit, and in such circumstances 'adding life to years' may be as important as 'adding years to life'. Consequently they may prefer more conservative care, whereas a biologically young elderly patient may wish, and is entitled, to be considered for surgical or interventional treatment (see below)

HF: specific age-related problems

The problems of treating and managing HF in the elderly are different and more complex than in younger patients. They are related to:

♦ demographics and epidemiology

♦ prognosis

♦ diagnostic difficulties

♦ the lack of evidence-based treatment

♦ the implications of age-related physiological changes and co-morbidities for prescribing practice

♦ the burden of hospitalization

♦ quality of life.

Demographics and epidemiology

HF is effectively a disease of middle and old age. The prevalence increases with age, by 27% each decade in men and by 61% in women.[3] The average age at the time of diagnosis is over 75 years.[3–5] In Scotland, the overall prevalence is 10–15/1000 but in those aged over 85 it is 90/1000: 87% of patients are aged over 65 years, of whom 60% are older than 75 years.[5]

The mortality also increases with age: the annual mortality in patients younger than 65 years is 24.2% but is 58.1% in those aged over 84 years.[4]

HF in the elderly is therefore a major health-care problem. It is also an increasingly common problem: The prevalence is increasing, largely because of improved survival following myocardial infarction and more effective treatment for hypertension and because it is predicted that the population of over 85s will double in the next 30 years.[6]

The aetiology of HF in the elderly and the significance of the normal aging process

HF in younger patients usually results from left-ventricular systolic dysfunction (LVSD), which was a pre-requisite for a patient's inclusion in the landmark trials of drug treatment for HF (see Chapters 2 and 4). But with increasing age more patients have preserved or near normal systolic function ['diastolic heart failure', 'heart failure with preserved systolic function' (HF-PSF)]. The reported prevalence of the two patterns varies widely, mainly because of different ages and diagnostic criteria in the populations studied:[7]

♦ The majority of younger HF patients have LVSD, usually caused primarily by coronary artery disease or a dilated cardiomyopathy.

♦ The prevalence of HF-PSF increases with age and is more common in women than in men.[8]

◆ Hypertension, diabetes, obesity, and aortic stenosis are more common in patients with HF-PSF, many of whom also have coronary artery disease, and are regarded as risk factors.

◆ The prognosis of HF-PSF is somewhat better than that of LVSD (See also discussion in Chapter 2).[9]

◆ Patients with HF-PSF are more likely to have atrial fibrillation but are otherwise less symptomatic.[9]

The elderly may be more prone to HF-PSF because the pathological changes associated with it are similar to those of normal cardiovascular aging.[9,10] Other, physiological, changes affect the ability of elderly patients to respond to the onset of HF:

◆ The basic level of fitness (VO_2 max) declines by 50% between the ages of 20 and 80 years.

◆ Age-related decline in activity of the autonomic nervous system is responsible for a reduction in maximum achievable heart rate by a third between the ages of 20 and 85 years.

◆ The maximal achievable cardiac output declines with age.

◆ There is decreased arterial compliance.[11]

Diagnostic difficulties in the elderly

Guidelines for the diagnosis of HF are summarized in Table 17.1.[12] The diagnosis is relatively simple when symptoms are severe, signs are obvious, and there is echocardiographic evidence of LVSD. But it is more difficult in the elderly because symptoms are often mild or difficult to interpret and echocardiography is frequently less informative because of the high prevalence of HF-PSF.

Table 17.2 lists typical and atypical symptoms in the elderly patient with suspected HF and common differential diagnoses.

History

History-taking may be time-consuming and of uncertain value because of cognitive impairment or confusion, although even in younger patients with suspected HF the diagnosis may be difficult with up to 50% of cases being diagnosed incorrectly in a primary-care setting.[13]

Table 17.1 European Society of Cardiology guidelines for the diagnosis of HF

Essential features:	Symptoms of HF at rest or during exercise (for example, breathlessness, fatigue, ankle swelling)
	Objective evidence of cardiac dysfunction at rest (usually by echocardiography)
Non-essential features:	In cases where the diagnosis is in doubt, there is a response to treatment directed towards HF

Table 17.2 Symptoms of HF in the older patient and differential diagnoses

Classical symptoms	Dyspnoea
	Peripheral oedema
	Fatigue
Atypical features	Falls
	Dizziness
	Lethargy
	Syncope
	Immobility
Differential diagnosis	COPD
	Renal disease
	Hypoalbuminaemia
	Depression
	Malignancy

Symptoms and signs

Exertional breathlessness in the elderly is often caused by non-cardiac pathologies, notably chronic obstructive pulmonary disease (COPD), anaemia, or obesity. In others, musculoskeletal and cerebrovascular disease may limit patients' ability to exercise to the point of exertional dyspnoea.[14]

Fatigue and lethargy occur frequently but are subjective and difficult to assess: both may also be caused by depression or anaemia, each of which is common (see Co-morbidities). Symptoms are often erroneously attributed by patients and medical staff to 'getting old'.

A high index of suspicion is therefore required when initially assessing the elderly patient with suspected HF but orthopnoea or paroxysmal nocturnal dyspnoea make the diagnosis likely.[15]

Ankle oedema has many non-cardiac aetiologies: commonly, in elderly women, no cause is found. Many patients are obese[13] but other possible causes are venous insufficiency and/or pelvic obstruction, cor pulmonale, recurrent pulmonary emboli, dependent oedema, and hypoalbuminaemia.

Physical signs can also be unhelpful when assessing a patient with mild HF but are more helpful when it is advanced. Although crepitations are non-specific, and may be present in many chest conditions but absent in chronic HF, a gallop rhythm, a displaced apex beat, and raised jugular venous pressure are highly suggestive.[15]

Simple preliminary investigations such as an ECG or blood sample for B-type natriuretic peptide (BNP) may give early support to the diagnosis of HF, as in younger patients. Likewise, echocardiography is the diagnostic investigation of choice and should be arranged whenever possible to evaluate cardiac structure and function.

Echocardiographic confirmation of HF-LVSD (ejection fraction equal to or less than 45%), is relatively simple but the confirmation of 'diastolic dysfunction' is more difficult as the echocardiographic criteria are still debated.

The diagnosis of HF-PSF is therefore often based on the presence of typical symptoms and signs, as in LVSD, and a normal or near normal ejection fraction on echocardiography.[17] Most patients with HF-PSF have a history of hypertension, diabetes, or aortic stenosis and/or a history of coronary disease. Although echocardiography shows a normal or near normal ejection fraction it, or the ECG, often shows evidence of left-ventricular hypertrophy.

Treatment of HF in the elderly

The recommended treatment for HF in the elderly is, as in younger patients, based on national and international guidelines for medication regimes, non-pharmacological advice, interventional and surgical procedures.

Non-pharmacological advice

The distance walked in 6 min is an objective measure of cardiac performance in HF, often utilized in older patients, and provides a benchmark of an individual patient's functional status and improvement.[17]

Exercise to maintain activities of daily living should be advised, although this may not be possible when co-morbidities such as degenerative arthritis or stroke disease are present. However, in principle, moderate exercise should be encouraged to improve fitness levels: It is less clear whether more vigorous exercise should be encouraged. Other advice, with respect to diet, smoking, and alcohol intake should be given.

Pharmacological treatment

Although effectively excluded from the landmark trials on which treatment guidelines are based[1] data taken from these trials[18] and subsequent studies confined to older patients[19,20] show that most of the originally reported benefits apply equally to the elderly and that side-effects are broadly similar (see Chapter 4 for details).

Despite this evidence, only a third of the over 75s are prescribed an angiotensin-converting enzyme (ACE) inhibitor, a quarter receive a β-blocker, and one in seven spironolactone: many receive lower than the recommended doses, usually for subjective reasons.[5,21,22]

There are several explanations for these disparities:

- the high prevalence of renal failure in the elderly is a relative contraindication to ACE inhibitors, angiotensin receptor blockers and spironolactone;
- a lack of supporting trial data;
- concerns about increased adverse drug reactions in older patients;
- concerns about prescribing for patients with co-morbidities

These concerns are often ill-founded (see Chapter 4).[23,24]

Prescribing for the elderly

Adverse drug reactions are common, resulting from age-related physiological changes in pharmacokinetics, renal function, and the autonomic nervous system[27] and because of polypharmacy and co-morbidities.

- The glomerular filtration rate (GFR) falls by 25% between the ages of 40 and 65 and continues to do so thereafter: this is not signalled by a rise in serum creatinine because of the age-related decline in lean body mass.[25,26]

- The responsiveness of the sympathetic nervous system is reduced, resulting in the well-known age-related reduction in exercise heart rate. There is also a decreased response to β-blockers and to β-agonists.[25]

Co-morbidities, notably renal failure and cognitive impairment (see below), polypharmacy, and non-compliance, are responsible for most adverse reactions. The majority are avoidable with simple measures: stopping unnecessary medicines, educating patients and carers about their treatment, its benefits, and side-effects, and regular medical checks to identify non-compliance and to pre-empt problems.

Adverse drug reactions cause a wide range of non-specific symptoms including confusion, cognitive impairment, ataxia, nausea, constipation, and urinary incontinence. A 'start low–go slow' approach is often adopted, and this facilitates early detection of potential adverse effects.

Inevitably, initiation of treatment may be easier in the hospital setting as there is usually close supervision and blood pressure monitoring. While there are concerns about renal impairment and cognitive function, medication-induced postural hypotension is often a greater problem with the older patient. Although postural hypotension is usually symptomatic, this is not always the case. It is therefore important to have confirmation of structural heart disease in the elderly before commencing patients on potentially potent (and harmful) vasodilator therapy. There is evidence to suggest that if older patients with HF are assessed echocardiographically, they are more likely to receive optimum treatment.[27]

HF management in the elderly should be the same as in younger patients but with safeguards to reflect the age-related changes in pharmacokinetics and the impact of co-morbidities. In many geriatric medicine services, nurse practitioners and clinical pharmacists facilitate optimum dosing and titration of therapies. Where therapy is instigated in hospital practice, multidisciplinary team involvement may improve adherence with therapy. However, in the community setting, such expertise may not be available, with a reluctance to prescribe treatments where back-up services are less well developed. This can be addressed by the more widespread use of geriatric medicine day hospitals for the assessment and management of these patients (see below and Chapter 7).

The rationale for guideline-based medications in elderly patients

ACE inhibitors and angiotensin receptor blockers

ACE inhibitors reduce mortality, symptoms, and hospitalization independent of age.[18,28] They are generally well tolerated but there is an increased risk of hypotension and of causing or worsening renal dysfunction (see above).[29] The benefits and side-effects of the angiotensin receptor blocker candesartan are independent of age.[30]

β-Blockers

The elderly derive the same benefits from β-blockers as younger patients except perhaps for the very oldest.[19] Patients with HF-PSF benefit to the same extent as those with LVSD, a finding not demonstrated in the landmark trials. Older patients are however more at risk of β-blocker-induced hypotension and bradycardia. Despite this, the maximum recommended doses can be achieved in 70% of patients. Fewer than 6% of patients are totally intolerant.[19,20]

Spironolactone

Fifty per cent of the elderly may be precluded from treatment with spironolactone because of the high prevalence of renal dysfunction (see Co-morbidities below). However, the overall incidence of side-effects is independent of age, although they are more serious in the elderly and result in drug discontinuation in 25%.[32,33] Nevertheless, because of the benefits, spironolactone should be prescribed for all eligible patients but with more frequent biochemical monitoring.

Loop diuretics

The regimen for taking loop diuretics should take into account the high prevalence of incontinence in the elderly. Minimizing the dose of loop diuretic will be beneficial for those with incontinence, and also in terms of minimizing postural hypotension.

Digoxin

Digoxin is used to control the heart rate in atrial fibrillation. It also reduces hospitalization irrespective of cardiac rhythm in patients taking the standard medications.[34] But side-effects are common, mainly because of the age-related decline in GFR, especially in those who are not followed up closely. Nausea is common in patients taking multiple medications: digoxin toxicity should always be considered when this occurs. Initial and maintenance doses should be lower than in standard regimens.[12]

Statins

In the elderly, statins prescribed for primary and secondary prevention reduce mortality, including sudden death, non-fatal myocardial infarction, and stroke.[35,36] They should be prescribed on the same basis as in younger patients. Because they reduce the incidence of sudden death, a case can be made their use in all patients not fitted with an implantable cardioverter defibrillator (see Chapter 5).

Warfarin

Achieving a balance between providing protection from an embolic stroke and avoiding a major episode of bleeding is difficult. Warfarin is not usually prescribed for those who remain in sinus rhythm except for those at particular risk of pulmonary thromboembolic disease, but it should always be considered for those in atrial fibrillation.

It is contraindicated in patients with dementia unless close supervision is assured. But the situation is less clear cut in those who have sustained a fall, and especially those prone to falling repeatedly. The dangers of anticoagulation in this situation have to be judged against the devastating impact of a non-fatal stroke, with requirements for percutaneous endoscopic gastrostomy feeding (PEG), on the already poor quality of life of individual patients and their carers. These decisions cannot be made without detailed discussion with the patient and/or their carers.

Non-steroidal anti-inflammatory drugs (NSAIDs)

Of non-cardiac drugs, the NSAIDs are most likely to cause adverse effects. They are often prescribed for the elderly, and many others obtain them without prescription, to treat arthritides, musculoskeletal pains, influenza-like symptoms, and headache.

The cardiovascular system is adversely affected by NSAIDs in three main ways: (1) reduced effectiveness of loop diuretics, (2) inhibition of the action of ACE inhibitors and β-blockers and (3) a reduction of GFR. This may cause worsening HF, impaired control of blood pressure, and may precipitate hospitalization.

In principle NSAIDs should not be prescribed for HF patients. If this is unrealistic, a short-acting NSAID can be prescribed (e.g. ibuprofen or diclofenac) in the lowest effective dose, in combination with paracetemol.[37,38]

Medication for patients with HF with preserved left ventricular systolic function

Patients with HF-PSF are often not prescribed the standard treatment because of diagnostic uncertainties, lack of supportive trial data (see above) and, at least in the UK, non-accreditation of HF nurses to prescribe for patients with HF-PSF. But in practice, doctors are increasingly treating HF-PSF patients as they do those with LVSD. There is certainly evidence of benefit from the angiotensin receptor blocker candesartan[30] and from the β-blocker nebivolol.[19] There is also a general acceptance that the standard drugs recommended for patients with LVSD 'might be effective to minimise symptoms' [in those with HF-PSF].[16]

Interventional treatments

Cardiac resynchronization therapy (CRT), in which there is simultaneous pacing of the right and left ventricles, improves functional capacity and quality of life and reduces the incidence of sudden death.[39] Implantable cardioverter defibrillators (ICDs) reduce sudden death.[40,41] Trials of both have largely excluded the elderly[40,42] and realistically, in some countries, they will be provided for only a minority of the eligible elderly for the foreseeable future (see Chapter 5).

Between 40% and 50% of HF patients die suddenly. This is an added reason for treating the elderly with medications which have been shown to directly or indirectly to reduce sudden death, namely ACE inhibitors, β-blockers, aldosterone receptor blockers, and statins.[43]

Surgery

In all age groups, the operative and post-operative mortality and morbidity for cardiac surgery is higher in patients with HF.[44]

HF caused by valve disease or coronary artery disease is potentially curable, although coronary artery surgery is offered to only a small minority of patients, irrespective of age.

Aortic valve replacement for aortic stenosis in particular improves life expectancy and quality of life in all age groups. Aortic stenosis affects between 2% and 9% of the over 65s.[45] They should be evaluated in precisely the same way as younger patients: by assessing operative risk against improved life expectancy (see Chapter 6).[46,48]

Co-morbidities

The elderly often have several chronic diseases, and for those with HF it is the norm: 75% have three or more significant co-morbidities, the number increasing with age. As a result, morbidity and mortality are higher and recurrent hospitalization more likely.[48] Co-morbidities may dominate the clinical picture and impact in interrelated ways on the patient's health and management. Most are either aetiologically related to HF or to its progression. The commonest are hypertension, atrial fibrillation, diabetes, COPD, renal failure, anaemia, depression, and cognitive impairment. But malignant disease, obesity, arthritis, and cerebrovascular disease are also common. Consequently, in some situations, treatment directed towards improvements in quality of life may be just as important as mortality benefits, especially in patients with severe symptoms.

Co-morbidities cause many problems:

- Symptoms similar to those of HF, for example in COPD, cause confusion and delayed diagnosis of one or other condition.
- They may reduce the quality of life, accelerate the progression of HF, or independently limit prognosis.
- They may limit treatment options.
- Their treatment often results in polypharmacy, increasing the likelihood of non-compliance and of adverse drug reactions.
- Co-morbidities account for as many as 50% of episodes of hospitalization in HF patients.[14]
- A third of patients struggle, or fail to lead an independent existence, frequently because of co-morbidities.[14]

Commonly, in patients with several chronic diseases, the treatment of one is optimized at the expense others being ignored.[49] Because the optimum control of HF and of several co-morbidities are interdependent it is important that they are given equal attention.

Specific co-morbidities

Hypertension

Hypertension is the commonest aetiology of HF-PSF[12] but is often classified as a co-morbidity. Careful control of blood pressure is essential for the optimum management of HF, vascular disease, and diabetes. However, optimum control of blood pressure may be associated with postural hypotension. As a result, guidelines are not always appropriate, and achieving target blood pressure levels may not be possible.

Atrial fibrillation

The prevalence of atrial fibrillation increases with age from 0.2% in the under 35s to 6–10% in the over 80s: in severe HF it is 40–50%[52] and is associated with a worse prognosis and increased morbidity.

Patients often present at the onset of atrial fibrillation and it is also a common cause of hospitalization in established cases.

Cardioversion rarely restores sinus rhythm, and although ablation therapy re-establishes sinus rhythm in selected cases, it is available for only a minority. Rate control using a β-blocker with or without digoxin is therefore appropriate, and is effective in most patients.[12]

Diabetes

The prevalence of diabetes will double in the next 20 years[51] and, like HF, it affects predominantly the elderly.

Their relationship is, however, more than the chance association of two common separate disorders. Diabetes is an independent risk factor for HF: the risk of diabetics developing HF is higher in those with poorly controlled HbA1c[52] and patients with HF are prone to develop insulin resistance.[53] Ten to thirty per cent of HF patients have Type 2 diabetes and the prevalence increases with worsening HF.[53,54] The link between the two is multifactorial: diabetic cardiomyopathy, coronary artery disease, and the metabolic syndrome.[55]

Optimum control of diabetes and its complications improves outcomes in HF: HF patients with poor glycaemic control are more likely to be hospitalized,[56] have more severe HF symptoms, and a worse prognosis.[51,56–58]

The 30–50% of diabetics who develop nephropathy or microalbuminuria[59] have an even higher incidence of cardiovascular events, worsening symptoms of HF, and increased hospitalization. These outcomes are improved by optimum glycaemic control combined with an ACE inhibitor and treatment of the metabolic syndrome.[60]

It is also important to pre-empt the development of overt diabetes by checking for subclinical hyperglycaemia when patients are reviewed.

COPD

Twenty per cent of patients with HF have COPD[61] mainly because smoking is a shared risk factor and because the prevalence of each increases with age.

It may be difficult to differentiate between HF and COPD clinically for several reasons: breathlessness is common to both, routine echocardiography may be unhelpful in the presence of emphysema, and because of the high prevalence of HF-PSF in the elderly. Also, patients with HF may have a variety of abnormalities of pulmonary function, most commonly a restrictive defect, even in the absence of chronic lung disease.[62]

Cough is another shared symptom: it can result from chronic pulmonary congestion and occurs in 10% of patients taking an ACE inhibitor.

Traditionally, β-blockers have been contraindicated in patients with COPD but this is no longer the case: bisoprolol, metoprolol, and carvedilol can be prescribed long term to most patients with fixed COPD (i.e. with less than 15% reversibility) without any reduction in FEV1. But they are contraindicated in patients with reversible airways disease[63] and in those with Type II respiratory failure.

Cognitive impairment

Dementia affects 8% of the over 65s, and cognitive impairment, a defect in the mental activities associated with thinking, learning, and memory, affects 17%.[64] But in patients with HF the prevalence of dementia (a score of less than 24 on the Mini-Mental State Examination) is more than 50%.[65] It is associated with a five-fold increase in mortality, increased hospitalization, and an increased need for social support.[64] Cerebral perfusion and silent cerebral infarction are likely explanations.[64,65]

Progression from mild cognitive impairment to Alzheimer's disease occurs in 10–15% of HF patients annually, compared with 1–2% in the otherwise healthy elderly. Although cognitive impairment is associated with hypotension, anaemia, and hyperglycaemia[67] there is, as yet, no evidence that it can be prevented or modified by addressing these or other factors.[64]

The practical importance of identifying cognitive impairment lies in its impact on the ability to self-medicate, the provision of informed consent and advanced directives, and its effects on carers and the need for additional service provision and for supervision of treatment. (See also Chapter 14.)

Depression

Between 15% and 35% of patients with HF have moderate or severe depression and 20–30% have mild depression: the prevalence increases with the severity of HF symptoms, a perceived lack of personal control, poor social support, co-morbidities, and age.[66]

Symptoms are similar to those of HF and most cases go unrecognized or untreated.[66,67] The severely depressed are repeatedly hospitalized and have a worse quality of life and a poorer prognosis than the non-depressed.[68,69] The diagnosis should therefore be actively sought using the Hospital Anxiety and Depression (HAD) Scale, a simple to use self-administered questionnaire[70] and treated. Treatment should be initiated using a selective serotonin receptor inhibitor (SSRI) commencing with a low dose. Patients and carers should be advised that a response to treatment may take several weeks.

Anaemia

Anaemia occurs in 20–30% of HF patients and the prevalence increases with age,[71,72] the severity of HF, renal dysfunction, and diabetes. The latter two are thought to be aetiological factors.[71] It is associated with a poor prognosis, worsening symptoms, and increased hospitalization.[73] In approximately 50% of cases, many of whom have renal dysfunction, it is normochromic. Other causes are haemodilution, reduced renal perfusion caused by diuretics, increased circulating levels of cytokines, iron deficiency, and hypothyroidism.[74] Between 40% and 50% of elderly patients have a reversible cause, usually iron deficiency.

Some studies report an improvement in symptoms and quality of life of patients treated with a combination of intravenous iron and erythropoietin.[75,76] These findings have not been confirmed by randomized controlled trials. However, those who also have renal failure should be treated with erythropoietin.[75,77]

Renal failure

Chronic renal disease is a marker of cardiovascular risk[78] and the maintenance of normal cardiac and renal function are interdependent, but the onset of HF initiates neuroendocrine responses (notably the renin–angiotensin–aldosterone system and cardiac naturetic peptides) which are not compatible with the maintenance of normal functioning of either.[79]

The prevalence of moderate-severe renal dysfunction (GFR less than 60–75 ml min^{-1}) increases with age and with the severity of HF. It occurs in 25–50% of patients with HF[80,81] and independently predicts mortality. The aetiology is usually hypertension, renal vascular disease, or diabetes. In addition, as part of the normal aging process, renal function decreases by 1% per year after the age of 40.[27]

The optimum treatment of renal disease, irrespective of aetiology, reduces cardiovascular risk,[78] although an improvement in HF has not been the primary outcome in clinical trials.

The monitoring of renal function is integral to the treatment of HF and in routine clinical practice, serum creatinine is accepted as a surrogate for GFR provided cardiac function is reasonably stable. The major trials of drugs for HF[28,30,33] excluded patients with a serum creatinine greater than 177–265 mmol L^{-1}, but in practice patients with higher levels are safely treated—although because of the physiological and pharmacokinetic changes of aging, particular caution is need in the elderly.

Quality of life

Quality of life (QOL) 'the difference between the patient's perceived expectations and achievement',[82] is not exclusively dependent on symptom relief and is worse in HF than in other chronic conditions.[83] Many factors which reduce QOL are common to all age groups. But, for several reasons, it is particularly poor in the elderly, notably those who are female: these reasons include the burden of multiple co-morbidities,[84] a lack of a partner to give support, and family or social isolation. The services provided by disease management programmes (DMPs) improve QOL and have a major role in addressing many patients' supportive needs (see section on 'Models of care') until the advanced stages of the disease (see section on 'End-stage HF'). (See also Chapter 8.)

Hospitalization

Elderly patients with HF are frequently hospitalized,[85–87] and almost 50% are readmitted within 3 months. It is the commonest reason for hospitalization in the elderly[88] and is a major drain on health service resources.[89] It adversely affects patients' quality of life and is associated with a poor prognosis: the in-hospital mortality is 5–15%[91] and 30%, more in the very old, die within 2 months of discharge.[92] Hospitalization therefore has major implications for staff, service providers, patients, and carers: for all concerned, reducing hospitalisation is a priority.

Approximately 50% of cases are admitted because of worsening HF[93] usually precipitated by atrial fibrillation or myocardial ischaemia. But many, perhaps the majority, of admissions are for other, often multiple reasons: co-morbidities, sub-optimal medication, non-compliance with drug regimes or lifestyle advice, drug interactions, inadequate follow-up or discharge arrangements, difficulties with self-care, depression, poor social support, a lack of patient education, incontinence, and a range of musculoskeletal problems.[14,50]

A package of measures provided by DMPs can reduce hospitalization by 50%, as well as readmissions and mortality (see below). These measures include:

- early post-discharge review at a HF clinic or by HF nurses;[94,95]
- continuing medical education for primary and secondary care staff based on working to agreed management protocols;
- hospital clinics, ideally with open access, to deal with problems as they arise;[95]
- day care facilities and day hospitals (see below);
- individually tailored drug regimens;
- training of patients in self-care;
- the identification of non-compliance;
- comprehensive discharge planning
- education and social support for patients and carers.[97]

The most effective interventions are the control of fluid balance, by the adjustment of diuretic dosage, weight monitoring and biochemical checks of renal function, and continuous patient and staff education.[92,96]

Models of care: disease management programmes

The delivery of care is more complex and labour intensive in elderly patients: physical and mental frailty, multiple co-morbidities, and social isolation are commonplace and elderly patients are often less able or willing to travel to obtain treatment.

Strategies for the care of patients with HF should equitably address these and other problems, most of which affect particularly the elderly:

- under diagnosis and suboptimal treatment;[5]
- hospitalization and readmission;

◆ communication with patients about issues important to them, which is currently poor;[98]

◆ poor physical, social, and psychological support for the terminally ill.

There is no 'best way' to address these diverse needs in what are sometimes widely dispersed populations.

Most models of care incorporate two principles:

1. A multidisciplinary team—this being the only way to provide the necessary combination of skills and expertise.[99]

2. The integration of hospital and primary care (community) services.[99,100]

A hospital HF clinic will usually provide:

◆ initial patient assessment

◆ diagnostic facilities

◆ cardiological expertise

◆ management of complications.

The role of the primary care (community) service is to:

◆ optimize treatment

◆ maintain patients' independence

◆ as far as possible, avoid hospitalization.

The primary care team will ideally include primary care physicians (GPs), practice and HF nurses, a community pharmacist, and the community palliative care team. Physiotherapists and occupational therapists, dieticians, and social workers should also be involved in both primary and secondary care.

DMPs based on these principles reduce hospital admissions and mortality.[101] The details of the structure of the service does not significantly affect outcomes: the content of the programme is more important.[100]

The balance, in terms of staffing and financing, between primary and secondary care based services will depend on national or local health service structures, particularly on whether or not there is a well-developed general practice/primary-care service. The frail and elderly are especially dependent on the latter (see Chapter 7).

Geriatric day hospitals

Geriatric day hospitals provide a link between hospital and community services. They can supplement a HF strategy by providing facilities, mainly for primary care, not available in busy hospital wards or outpatient clinics. A forum for the multidisciplinary assessment of patients with multiple problems is a key function, ideal for the optimum management of HF patients. And there is the opportunity to develop the individualized management plans which are needed for patients with competing treatment priorities.

Patients usually attend for 6–20 weeks depending on the nature and complexity of their problems.[102] Table 17.3 highlights some of the conditions evaluated and treated in a day hospital.

Table 17.3 Conditions evaluated and managed in a geriatric day hospital that may co-exist or be associated with HF

Falls secondary to many causes including:	Postural hypotension
	Diabetes/hypoglycaemia
	Poor eyesight
	Parkinson's disease
	Osteoarthritis
Anaemia secondary to:	Gastrointestinal blood loss
	Chronic disease
	B_{12}/folate deficiency
Mood disorders	
Breathlessness/fatigue secondary to:	COPD
	Anxiety
	Pulmonary thromboembolic disease

While the majority of patients attending a day hospital benefit from multidisciplinary assessment and management, there are few randomized controlled trial data evaluating service efficacy. However, of the reported studies, improvements in quality of life and in adherence to treatment regimes are reported.[103] In recent years, attention has been directed to utilizing day hospital facilities to prevent unnecessary admissions to acute care facilities.

Day care centres

There is some overlap between the functions of day hospitals and day care centres. The latter offer a wide range of physical, psychological, and social support. Depending on facilities and staffing, patients usually attend once or twice weekly. They and their carers have the opportunity to agree a care plan with the centre's health-care team who also provide comprehensive palliative care support which is often not otherwise available. Such centres provide an important social 'highlight' for the socially isolated.

Nursing homes and care homes (long-term care facilities)

Patients, usually the elderly, are admitted to long-term care facilities when home care becomes impractical. Nursing home residents in the USA are less frail than those in the UK, despite which those with HF have a high mortality. Compared with the HF population as a whole, residents are older, have more co-morbidities, less often receive standard medication, and are more frequently hospitalized.[104–106] A specific objective of a DMP should be to target residents for improved treatment according to standard criteria. Recent data suggest that geriatricians attending nursing homes on a regular basis improve the management of the older patient with HF.[107]

The role and problems of caregivers in the context of the models of care

Carer education and involvement in patient management is essential for an effective care strategy: most HF patients rely at some stage on their family, friends, or relatives for help with normal daily activities.

The physical, emotional and social support provided by informal caregivers improves the patient's prognosis and quality of life and helps to reduces hospital readmissions.[108] But this increases the carers' own physical and psychological morbidity, which may then result in patients' hospitalization: ensuring the health of caregivers should therefore be seen as part of the patients' disease management programme.[109]

It is relatively easy to provide DMPs described here for urban communities. It is more difficult in rural and remote areas whose populations are increasingly elderly. But this does not preclude comparable levels of health or satisfaction with service provision.[110] Alternative innovative strategies are needed, tailored to changing rural demographics and to locally available or acquired expertise, facilities, communications, transport. and geography.[111-113] The core requirements of a successful rural service are as for urban services: to improve the identification of undiagnosed cases, maximize medications and other treatments, develop palliative care support, and provide continuing education for all involved health-care workers, patients, and carers. Telephone help lines and telemedicine are being increasingly used for this.

End-stage HF and end-of-life care

The term 'end-stage HF' describes patients with marked LVSD and severe symptoms (New York Heart Association Class III/IV) despite receiving 3 months' optimum conventional treatment.[114] The annual mortality in this patient group is at least 50%.

Patients of all ages become increasingly dependent on others for day to day support. This applies particularly to the elderly because of co-morbidities and their social circumstances.

Supportive care should be increasingly implemented during this stage: to ensure that patients and carers fully understand their situation, to agree management plans with them, and to ensure 24-hour availability of medical care, including palliative care if needed.[115] But because of the cumulative effect of co-morbidities, the problems of the elderly are multiple and more complex. Also, as they become increasingly bed bound, they often develop infections and pressure sores.[117] Added to this is the high prevalence of confusion, dementia, social hardship, and social isolation.[118]

The elderly are, in general, more accepting of dying than younger patients, place a higher priority on quality of life than on longevity, and appear to be less interested in euthanasia or assisted suicide.[116] The option to choose where to die is important to patients. Most wish to die at home but usually die elsewhere, especially if elderly and female, often because of a lack of community support services.[119] Specifically with respect to HF, plans to remain at home may be thwarted by an acute, often terminal, event such as a myocardial infarction or arrhythmia which precipitates hospitalization, unless it is anticipated by having in place a home management strategy.[119] Many of the barriers to achieving this aim have been identified.[119] The role of carers, and support for them, is essential if the terminally ill are to die at home:[120] this is more difficult to provide for the elderly for the reasons given above.

References

1. Konstam MA (2000). Progress in heart failure management? Lessons from the real world. *Circulation* **102**: 1076–8.

2. Batchelor WB, Jollis JG, Friesinger GC (1999). The challenge of health care delivery to elderly patients with cardiovascular disease. *Cardiol Clin* **17**: 1–15.

3. Ho KKL, Anderson DM, Kannel WB *et al.* (1993). Survival after the onset of congestive heart failure in Framingham heart study subjects. *Circulation* **88**: 107–15.

4. MacIntyre K, Capewell S, Stewart S *et al.* (2000). Evidence of improving prognosis in heart failure: trends in case fatality in 66,547 patients hospitalised between 1986 and 1995. *Circulation* **102**: 1126–31.

5. Murphy NF, Simpson CR, McAlister FA *et al.* (2004). National survey of the prevalence, incidence, primary care burden and treatment of heart failure in Scotland. *Heart* **90**: 1129–36.

6. Rich MW (1999). Heart failure. *Cardiol Clin* **17**: 123–35.

7. Owan TE, Redfield MM (2005). Epidemiology of diastolic heart failure. *Prog Cardiovasc Dis* **47**: 320–32.

8. Lenzen MJ, Scholte op Reimer WJM, Boersma E *et al.* (2004). Differences between patients with a preserved and depressed left ventricular function: a report from the EuroHeart Survey. *Eur J Heart Fail* **25**: 1214–20.

9. Hogg K, Swedberg K, McMurray J (2004). Heart failure with preserved left ventricular function. *J Am Coll Cardiol* **43**: 317–27.

10. Schulman SP (1999). Cardiovascular consequences of aging. *Cardiovasc Clin* **17**: 35–49.

11. Lakatta EG (2001). Cardiovascular aging without a clinical diagnosis. *Dialogues Cardiovasc Med* **6**: 67–91.

12. The Task Force for the Diagnosis and Treatment of Chronic Heart Failure of the European Society of Cardiology (2005). Guidelines for the diagnosis and treatment of chronic hear failure: full text update (2005). *Eur J Heart Fail* **26**: 1115–40.

13. Remes J, Miettinen H, Rennanen *et al.* (1991). Validity of clinical diagnosis of heart failure in primary health care. *Eur Heart J* **12**: 315–21.

14. Lien CTC, Gillespie ND, Struthers AD *et al.* (2002). Heart failure in frail elderly patients: diagnostic difficulties, co-morbidities, polypharmacy and treatment dilemmas. *Eur J Heart Fail* **4**: 91–8.

15. Stevenson LW (2005). Design of therapy for advanced heart failure. *Eur J Heart Fail* **7**: 323–31.

16. Hunt AS, Abraham WT, Chin MH *et al.* (2005). ACC/AHA 2005 Guideline update for the diagnosis and management of chronic heart failure in the adult. *Circulation* **112**: 154–235.

17. Opasich C, Pinna GD, Mazza A *et al.* (1998). Reproducibility of the six-minute walk test in chronic congestive heart failure patients: practical implications. *Am J Cardiol* **81**: 1497–500.

18. Garg R, Yusuf S (1995). Overview of randomised trials of angiotensin-converting enzyme inhibitors on mortality and morbidity in patients with heart failure. *J Am Med Assoc* **273**: 1450–6.

19. Flather MD, Shibata MC, Coats AJS *et al.* (2005). Randomised trial to determine the effect of nebivolol on mortality and cardiovascular hospital admission in elderly patients with heart failure (SENIORS). *Eur Heart J* **26**: 215–25.

20. Dulin BR Haas SJ, Abraham WT *et al.* (2005). Do elderly systolic heart failure patients benefit from beta blockers to the same extent as the non elderly? Meta-analysis of >12,000 patients in large-scale clinical trials. *Am J Cardiol* **95**: 896–8.

21. Rangaswamy C, Finn JI, Koelliong TM (2005). Angiotensin converting enzyme inhibitor use in elderly patients hospitalised with heart failure and left ventricular systolic dysfunction. *Cardiology* **103**: 17–23.

22. Shibata MC, Soneff CM, Tsuyuki RT (2005). Utilisation of evidence-based therapies for heart failure in the institutionalised elderly. *Eur J Heart Fail* **7**: 1122–5.

23. Hulsman L, Berger R, Mortl D *et al.* (2005). Influence of age and in-patient care on prescription rate and long-term outcome in chronic heart failure: a data-based substudy of the EuroHeart Failure Study. *Eur J Heart Fail* **7**: 657–61.

24. Masoudi AF, Rathore SS, Wang Y *et al.* (2004). National patterns of use and effectiveness of angiotensin-converting enzyme inhibitors in older patients with heart failure and left ventricular systolic dysfunction. *Circulation* **110**: 724–31.

25. Podrazik PM, Schwartz JB (1999). Cardiovascular pharmacology of the aging. *Cardiovasc Clin* **17**: 17–34.

26. Laurence DR, Bennett PN, Brown MJ (1997). General pharmacology. In: *Clinical Pharmacology*, pp. 77–120. New York: Churchill Livingstone.

27. Aronow WS (1994). Echocardiography should be performed in all elderly patients with congestive heart failure. *J Am Geriatr Soc* **42**: 1300–2.

28. The CONSENSUS Study Group (1987). Effects of enalapril on mortality in severe congestive heart failure. *New Engl J Med* **316**: 1429–35.

29. ACE Inhibitor Myocardial Infarction Collaborative Group (1998). Indications for ACE inhibitors in the early treatment of acute myocardial infarction. *Circulation* **97**: 2202–12.

30. Pfeffer MA, Swedberg K, Granger CB *et al.* (2003). Effects of candesartan on mortality and morbidity in patients with chronic heart failure: the CHARM-Overall programme. *Lancet* **362**: 759–66.

31. Krum H (2004). Tolerability of beta-blockers in elderly patients with heart failure: clinical trial experience. *Am J Cardiol* **93**: 58B–63B.

32. Sligl W, McAlister FA, Ezekowitz J *et al.* (2004). Usefulness of spironolactone in a specialised heart failure clinic. *Am J Cardiol* **94**: 443–7.

33. Pitt B, Reeme W, Zannad F *et al.* (1999). The effect of spironolactone; on morbidity and mortality in patients with severe heart failure. *New Engl J Med* **341**: 709–17.

34. The Digitalis Investigation Group (1997). The effects of digoxin on mortality and morbidity in patients with heart failure. *New Engl J Med* **336**: 525–3.

35. The Long Term Intervention with Pravestatin in Ischaemic Disease (LIPID) Study Group (1998). Prevention of cardiovascular events and death with Pravastatin in patients with coronary heart disease and a broad range of initial cholesterol levels. *New Engl J Med* **339**: 1349–57.

36. Packard CJ, Ford I, Robertson M *et al.* (2005). Plasma lipoproteins and apolipoproteins as predictors of cardiovascular risk and treatment benefit in the Prospective Study of Pravastatin in the Elderly at Risk (PROSPER). *Circulation* **112**: 3058–65.

37. Hillis WS (2002). Areas of emerging interest in analgesia: cardiovascular complications. *Am J Ther* **9**: 259–69.

38. Nurmohamed MT, van Halm VP, Dijkmans BAC (2002). Cardiovascular risk profile of antirheumatic agents in patients with osteoarthritis and rheumatoid arthritis. *Drugs* **62**: 1599–609.

39. Cleland JGF, Daubert J-C, Erdman E *et al.* (2005). The effect of cardiac resynchronisation on morbidity and mortality in heart failure (CARE-HF). *New Engl J Med* **352**: 1539–49.

40. Moss AJ, Hall WJ, Cannom DS *et al.* (1996). Improved survival with an implanted defibrillator in patients with coronary disease at high risk for ventricular arrhythmia. *New Engl J Med* **335**: 1933–40.

41. Goldberger Z, Lambert R (2006). Implantable cardioverter-defibrillators. Expanding indications and technologies. *J Am Med Assoc* **295**: 809–18.
42. Abraham WT, Fisher WG, Smith AL *et al.* (2002). Cardiac resynchronisation in chronic heart failure. *New Engl J Med* **346**: 1845–53.
43. Richter S, Duray G, Gronefeld G *et al.* (2005). Prevention of sudden cardiac death: lessons from recent controlled trials. *Circ J* **69**: 625–9.
44. Otto CM (1999). Aortic stenosis. In: *Valvular Heart Disease* (ed. CM Otto), pp. 179–217. Philadelphia: W. B. Saunders Company.
45. Hinchman DA, Otto CM (1999). Valvular disease in the elderly. *Cardiol Clin* **17**: 137–58.
46. Thibault GE (1993). Too old for what? *New Engl J Med* **328**: 946–50.
47. Wong JB, Salem DN, Pauker SG (1993). You're never too old. *New Engl J Med* **328**: 971–75.
48. Braunstein JB, Anderson G, Gestrenblith W *et al.* (2003). Non-cardiac comorbidity increases preventable hospitalisations and mortality among Medicare beneficiaries with chronic heart failure. *J Am Coll Cardiol* **42**: 1226–33.
49. Redeilmeier DA, Tan SH, Booth GL (1998). The treatment of unrelated disorders in patients with chronic medical diseases. *New Engl J Med* **338**: 1516–20.
50. Podrid PJ (1997). Atrial fibrillation in the elderly. *Cardiol Clin* **17**: 173–88.
51. King H, Aubert RE, Herman WH (1998). Global burden of diabetes, 1995–2025. *Diabetes Care* **21**: 1414–31.
52. Nichols GA, Gullion CM, Koro CE *et al.* (2004). The incidence of congestive heart failure in type 2 diabetes: an update. *Diabetes Care* **27**: 1879–84.
53. Kistrop C, Galatius S, Gustaffson F *et al.* (2005). Prevalence and characteristics of diabetic patients in a chronic heart failure population. *Int J Cardiol* **100**: 281–7.
54. Solang L, Malmberg K, Ryden L (1999). Diabetes mellitus and congestive heart failure: further knowledge needed. *Eur Heart J* **20**: 789–95.
55. Expert Panel on Detection, Evaluation, and Treatment of High Blood Cholesterol in Adults (2001). Executive Summary of the Third Report of the National Cholesterol Education Program (NCEP) Expert Panel on Detection, Evaluation, and Treatment of High Blood Cholesterol in Adults (Adult Treatment Panel III). *J Am Med Assoc* **285**: 2486–97.
56. Irebarran C, Karter AJ, Go AS *et al.* (2001). Glycaemic control and heart failure among adult patients with diabetes. *Circulation* **103**: 668–73.
57. Witteles RM, Wilson WH, Jamali AH *et al.* (2004). Insulin resistance in idiopathic dilated cardiomyopathy. *J Am Coll Cardiol* **44**: 78–81.
58. Tenenbaum A, Motro M, Fisman EZ *et al.* (2003). Functional class in patients with heart failure is associated with the development of diabetes. *Am J Med* **114**: 271–5.
59. Gross JL, de Azevedo MJ, Sileiero SP (2005). Diabetic nephropathy: diagnosis, prevention and treatment. *Diabetes Care* **28**: 176–88.
60. Baumelou A, Brukert E, Bagnis C *et al.* (2005). Renal disease in cardiovascular disorders: an under-recognised problem. *Am J Nephrol* **25**: 95–105.
61. Dahlstrom U (2005). Frequency of non-cardiac comorbidities in patients with chronic heart failure. *Eur J Heart Fail* **7**: 309–16.
62. Wagner PD (1997). Involvement of the lungs. In: *Heart Failure* (ed. PA Poole-Wilson, WS Colucci, BM Massie, K Chatterjee, AJS Coats), pp. 247–60. New York: Churchill Livingstone.
63. Kotlyar E, MacDonald PS, McCaffry DJ *et al.* (2002). Tolerability of carvedilol in patients with heart failure and concomitant chronic obstructive pulmonary disease or asthma. *J Heart Lung Transplant* **21**: 1290–5.
64. Taylor J Stott DJ (2002). Chronic heart failure and cognitive impairment: co-existence of conditions or true association? *Eur Heart J* **4**: 7–9.

65. Zuccala G, Cattel C, Manes-Gravina E *et al.* (1997). Left ventricular dysfunction: a clue to cognitive impairment in older patients with heart failure. *J Neurol Neurosurg Psychiat* **63**: 509–12.

66. Havrenek EP, Spertus JA, Masoudi FA *et al.* (2004). Predictors of the onset of depressive symptoms in patients with heart failure. *J Am Coll Cardiol* **44**: 2333–8.

67. Koenig HG (1998). Depression in hospitalised older patients with congestive heart failure. *Gen Hosp Psychiat* **20**: 29–43.

68. Jiang W, Alexander J, Christopher E *et al.* (2001). Relationship of depression to increased risk of mortality and rehospitalisation in patients with congestive heart failure. *Arch Intern Med* **161**: 1849–56.

69. Junger J, Schellberg D, Muller-Tasch T *et al.* (2005). Mortality increasingly predicts the course in congestive heart failure. *Eur J Heart Fail* **7**: 261–7.

70. Bjelland I, Dahl AAS, Haug TT *et al.* (2002). The validity of the Hospital Anxiety and Depression Scale: an updated literature review. *J Psychosom Res* **52**: 69–77.

71. Lindenfeld JA (2005). Prevalence of anaemia and effects on mortality in patients with heart failure. *Am Heart J* **149**: 391–401.

72. Coats AJ (2005). Erythropoietin therapy to treat anaemia in chronic heart failure. ESC *E-J Cardiol Prac* **3**: 36.

73. Rogers WJ, Johnstone DE, Yusuf S *et al.* (1994). Quality of life among 5025 patients with left ventricular dysfunction randomised between placebo and enalapril: the studies of left ventricular dysfunction. *J Am Coll Cardiol* **23**: 393–400.

74. Cromie N, Lee C, Struthers AD (2002). Anaemia in chronic heart failure: what is the frequency in the UK and its underlying cause? *Heart* **87**: 377–8.

75. Silverberg DS, Wexler D, Iaina A (2002). The importance of anaemia and its correction in the management of severe congestive heart failure. *Eur J Heart Fail* **4**: 681–6.

76. Mancini DM, Katz SD, Lang CC *et al.* (2003). Effect of erythropoietin on exercise capacity in patients with moderate to severe chronic heart failure. *Circulation* **107**: 294–9.

77. Ryan E, Devlin M, Prendiville T *et al.* (2004). The prevalence and natural history of anaemia in an optimally treated heart failure population. *Br J Cardiol* **11**: 369–75.

78. Curtis BM, Levin A, Parfrey PS (2005). Multiple risk factor intervention in chronic renal disease: management of cardiac disease in chronic kidney disease patients. *Med Clin North Am* **89**: 511–23.

79. Brandt RR, Burnet JC (1997). Hormonal control of the kidney during congestive cardiac failure. In: *Heart Failure* (ed. PA Poole-Wilson, WS Colucci, BM Massie, K Chatterjee, AJS Coats), pp. 143–72. New York: Churchill Livingstone.

80. Dries DL, Exner DV, Domanski MJ *et al.* (2000). The prognostic implications of renal insufficiency in asymptomatic and symptomatic patients with left ventricular systolic dysfunction. *J Am Coll Cardiol* **35**: 681–9.

81. Hillege HL, Girbes ARJ, de Kam PJ *et al.* (2000). Renal function, neurohormonal activation, and survival in patients with chronic heart failure. *Circulation* **102**: 203–10.

82. Calman KC (1984). Quality of life in cancer patients: an hypothesis. *J Med Ethics* **10**: 124–7.

83. Stewart AL, Hays RD, Ware JE (1988). The MOS short-form general health survey: reliability and validity in a patient population. *Med Care* **26**: 724–35.

84. Gott M, Parke S, Payne C *et al.* (2005). Predictors of the quality of life of older patients with heart failure recruited from primary care. *Age Aging* **35**: 172–7.

85. Grigioni F, Carinci V, Favero L *et al.* (2002). Hospitalisation for congestive heart failure: is it still a cardiology business? *Eur J Heart Fail* **4**: 99–104.

86. Rich MW, Vinson JM, Sperry JC *et al.* (1993). Prevention of readmission in elderly patients with congestive heart failure. *J Gen Intern Med* **8**: 585–90.

87. Schwarz KA, Ellman CS (2003). Identification of factors predictive of hospital readmissions for patients with heart failure. *Heart Lung* **32**: 88–99.

88. Kannel WB (2005). Incidence and epidemiology of heart failure. *Heart Fail Rev* **5**:167–73.

89. McMurray J, Stewart S (2000). Epidemiology, aetiology, and prognosis of heart failure. *Heart* **83**: 596–602.

90. Zumer-Meulenbelt A, Joubert A, Lefort JF *et al.* (2002). Retrospective study of hospitalisations for heart failure in elderly patients in a cardiology service of a general hospital centre. *Arch Mal Coeur Vaiss* **95**: 769–74.

91. Reis SE, Holubkov R, Edmundoeicz D *et al.* (1997). Treatment of patients admitted to hospital with congestive heart failure: speciality-related disparities in practice patterns and outcomes. *J Am Coll Cardiol* **30**: 733–8.

92. Klein L, O'Connor CM, Leimberger D *et al.* (2005). Low serum sodium is associated with increased short term mortality in hospitalised patients with worsening heart failure. *Circulation* **111**: 2454–60.

93. Cowie MR, Fox KF, Wood DA (2002). Hospitalisation of patients with heart failure: A population-based study. *Eur Heart J* **23**: 877–85.

94. Kornowski R, Zeeli D, Averbuch M *et al.* (1995). Intensive home-care surveillance prevents hospitalisation and improves morbidity rates among elderly patients with severe congestive heart failure. *Am Heart J* **29**: 762–6.

95. Stromberg A (2005). Heart failure management programmes: the time for action has arrived. *Eur J Heart Fail* **7**: 1077–8.

96. Shah MR, Flavell CM, Weintraub JR *et al.* (2005). Intensity and focus of heart failure disease management after hospital discharge *Am Heart J* **149**: 715–21.

97. Blue L, Lang E, McMurray JJ *et al.* (2006). Randomised controlled trial of specialist nurse intervention in heart failure. *Br Med J* **323**: 715–18.

98. Murray SA, Kendall M, Boyd K *et al.* (2004). Exploring the spiritual needs of people dying of lung cancer or heart failure: a prospective qualitative interview study of patients and their cares. *Palliat Med* **18**: 39–45.

99. Jaarsma T (2005). Inter-professional team approach to patients with heart failure. *Heart* **91**: 832–8.

100. Roccaforte R, Demers C, Baldassarre F *et al.* (2005). Effectiveness of comprehensive disease management programmes in improving clinical outcomes in heart failure patients. A meta-analysis. *Eur J Heart Fail* **7**: 1133–44.

101. Holland R, Battersby J, Harvey I *et al.* (2005). Systematic review of multidisciplinary interventions in heart failure. *Heart* **91**: 899–906.

102. Gillespie ND, Turpie ID (2006). Geriatric day hospitals. In: *Principles and Practice of Geriatric Medicine*, Vol. 2 (ed. JMS Pathy, AJ Sinclair, JE Morely), pp. 1907–14. New York: John Wiley.

103. Eagle DJ, Guyatt GH, Patterson C *et al.* (1991). Effectiveness of a geriatric day hospital. *Can Med Assoc J* **318**: 699–704.

104. Wang R, Mysore M, Denman S (1998). Mortality of the institutionalised old-old hospitalized with congestive heart failure. *Arch Int Med* **158**: 2464–8.

105. Gambassi G, Forman DE, Lapane KL *et al.* (2000). Management of heart failure among very old persons in long term care: has the voice of trials spread? *Am Heart J* **139**: 85–93.

106. Valle R, Aspromonte N, Barro S *et al.* (2005). The NT-pro BNP assay identifies very elderly nursing home residents suffering from pre-clinical heart failure. *Eur J Heart Fail* **7**: 542–51.

107. Misiaszek B, Heckman Ga, Mirali F *et al.* (2005). Digoxin prescribing for heart failure in elderly residents in long term care facilities. *Can J Cardiol* **21**: 281–6.

108. Luttik ML, Jaarsma T, Moser D *et al.* (2005). The importance and impact of social support on outcomes in patients with heart failure: an overview of the literature. *J Cardiovasc Nurs* **20**: 162–9.

109. Molloy GJ, Johnston DW, Witham MD (2005). Family caregiving and congestive heart failure. Review and analysis. *Eur J Heart Fail* **7**: 592–603.
110. Farmer J, Hinds K, Richards H *et al.* (2004). *Access, satisfaction and expectations: a comparison of attitudes to health care in rural and urban Scotland.* Report to the Scottish Executive Remote and Rural Areas Resource Initiative. University of Aberdeen.
111. Godden D (2005). Providing health services to rural and remote communities. *J R Coll Physicians Edinburgh* **35**: 294–5.
112. Remote and Rural Medicine. http://www.rcpe.ac.uk/publications/remoteandruralmedicine.php
113. Scottish Executive (2005). *Building a Service Fit for the Future* [the Kerr Report]. http://www.scotland.gov.uk/Resource/Doc/924/0012113.pdf
114. Adams KF, Zannad F (1998). Clinical definition and epidemiology of advanced heart failure. *Am Heart J* **135**: S204–S215.
115. http://www.goldstandardframework.nhs.uk/
116. Catt S, Blanchard M, Addington-Hall J *et al.* (2005). Older adults' attitudes to palliative treatment and hospice care. *Palliat Med* **19**: 402–10.
117. Manckoundia P, Mischis-Troussard C, Ramanantsoa M *et al.* (2005). Palliative care in geriatrics: a retrospective study of 40 cases. *Rev Med Int* **26**: 851–7.
118. The National Council for Palliative Care (2005). *The Palliative Care Needs of Older People.* Briefing Bulletin 14 (http://www.ncpc.org.uk/).
119. Thomas K (2003). Evidence-based care. In: *Caring for the Dying at Home: Companions on the Journey* (ed. K Thomas), pp. 63–78. Oxford: Radcliffe Publishing.
120. King N, Bell D, Thomas K (2003). An out-of-hours protocol for community palliative care: practitioners' perspectives. *Int J Palliat Nurs* **9**: 1–6.

Chapter 18

The course to death in heart failure

Jeffrey Teuteberg and Winifred G. Teuteberg

Introduction

The growing epidemic of congestive heart failure (HF) carries substantial social and economic burdens to society. In the United States alone, there are over 5 million patients who have been diagnosed with HF with an additional 550 000 new cases being diagnosed each year, resulting in a total expenditure of almost US$30 billion.[1] The most symptomatic patients are estimated to account for over 60% of this cost and comprise the majority of the 57 000 deaths per year from HF.[1,2] In the past, the most costly aspect of HF care was attributable to hospitalizations; however, with broadening indications and availability of expensive therapies such as biventricular pacing there is increasing interest in understanding the process of the end-stages of HF to better guide the application of these therapies.[3] Furthermore insight into the disease process of HF, especially in its advanced stages, is crucial to properly address the physical and emotional toll of chronic HF on patients and their caregivers. However, even at its end-stage, HF remains a disease of exacerbations and remissions.[4] The persistent clinical challenge whether a patient will have sustained improvement or is on a path of inexorable decline. While specific prognostic models for HF are fully explored elsewhere in this text (see Chapter 21), recognizing the disease course for those with advanced HF provides a context for understanding the timing and rationale of palliative care for these patients.

Unfortunately the course of advanced HF remains somewhat mercurial due to the continued advancements in HF management on those with the most advanced stages of HF. Even for very symptomatic, functionally limited patients, aggressive medical and device-based therapy for HF can have dramatic benefits. The widespread use of such therapies, in turn, has had an impact on the natural history of the disease. For those who nevertheless reach the end-stages of the disease, interventions such as cardiac transplantation and left ventricular assist devices (VAD) still may be appropriate and result in substantial improvements. Aside from the impact of these therapies on the disease course, there is a lack of good data on patients in the terminal phase of HF. Most existing information is inferential and comes from the large randomized trials of medical and device therapies. Unfortunately these trials consist almost exclusively of those with systolic HF and overwhelmingly consist of middle-aged white men. This contrasts with large registries of patients with HF that demonstrate of those who are hospitalized, nearly half will have a normal ejection fraction.[5] Furthermore, as the population ages the vast majority of patients will not only have diastolic HF, but will also predominantly be women.[5,6] There is also little specific data on how the patient experiences the disease state in the medical trials of systolic HF. Despite these limitations, these trials can be quite revealing in that they often have large numbers of NYHA class III and IV patients who are followed closely for many years.

Mode of death in patients with HF

Since the introduction of angiotensin converting enzyme inhibitors (ACE-I), there has been a gradual shift in the mode and timing of death, that paralleled the development of the modern HF regimen. The current standard medical therapy for HF includes beta-blockade,[7–10] aldosterone inhibitors,[11,12] and even angiotensin receptor blockade[13,14] on a background of an ACE-I, diuretics and digoxin. Device-based therapy has also become a cornerstone of HF therapy with implantable cardiac defibrillators (ICD)[15–17] and for class NYHA class III patients, biventricular pacing, also known as chronic resynchronization therapy (CRT).[18–20] Not only has the mode of death shifted over time, but patients are surviving longer with chronic HF. Prior to the current era of HF management, patients were more likely to die suddenly and do so earlier in their disease process when their HF symptoms were only mild to moderate.[21] In contrast, patients are now much more likely to die of progressive pump failure, later in their disease course when their HF symptoms are much more severe and long-standing. This shift is primarily a result of the success of the current HF regimen which has substantially reduced mortality and therefore increased the length of time a patient survives with HF. The shift in the mode of death to progressive HF is in large part due to the ICD's role in primary and secondary prevention of sudden death from ventricular tachyarrhythmias.[15–17,22–25] In addition, medical therapy has also impacted this shift in the cause of death with ACE-I,[18,26] beta-blockers,[7,8] and aldosterone receptor blockers[11] decreasing the rate of sudden death as well as delaying disease progression. The cause of death from several medical and device-based HF trials of patients with systolic HF and NYHA class III and IV symptoms are listed in Table 18.1. All of the patients listed in the table are from the treatment arms of the trials and hence are being treated with a modern HF regimen. Even over the course of 5 years there is a trend toward more deaths from progressive HF and a decrease in the incidence of sudden death. Of note is the relatively higher rate of sudden death in the MERIT-HF trial which may be a consequence of a higher proportion of less sick patients, who are less likely to have progression of HF during follow-up. Another notable feature is that the incidence of sudden death in the defibrillator trials (COMPANION and CARE-HF) can still be substantial. While some of these sudden deaths may still be from refractory ventricular tachyarrhythmias despite having a functioning ICD, many are not, and hence serve as a reminder of the difficulty in accurately attributing an etiology to a mode of death.

Determining the true mode of death in HF can be complicated as the definition of sudden death or death from progressive HF has not been consistent among HF trials.[27] The variability in definitions across studies is mostly attributable to the difficulty in determining the true etiology of death even when witnessed.[28] Sudden death in particular

Table 18. 1 Comparison of the percentage of deaths attributed to sudden death in trials of advanced HF. Adapted from Carson P *et al.* (2005). Mode of death in advanced heart failure: the Comparison of Medical, Pacing, and Defibrillation Therapies in Heart Failure (COMPANION) trial. *J Am Coll Cardiol* **46**: 2329–34, Copyright 2005, with permission from Elsevier.

	MERIT-HF[a]	RALES[a]	BEST	COMPANION[a]	CARE-HF
Deaths					
Sudden (%)	54	29	45	16	33
CHF (%)	21	45	31	50	44
Year	1999	1999	2001	2004	2005
Characteristics					
Age (years)	64	65	60	66	67
EF (%)	28	26	23	22	25
Ischemic (%)	65	55	59	55	40
Male (%)	77	73	77	67	74
NYHA Class(%)					
II	41	0.5	0	0	0
III	56	72	92	86	94
IV	3	27	8	14	6
Medications (%)					
Diuretics	91	100	94	97	-
ACE-I	89	95	91	69	95
β-blockers	100	11	100	68	70
Digoxin	63	75	93	-	40

[a]The treatment group of the study is listed.

Abbreviations: ACE-I, angiotensin-converting enzyme inhibitor; CARE-HF, Cardiac Resynchronization Heart Failure Trial; CHF, congestive heart failure; COMPANION, Comparison of Medical, Pacing, and Defibrillation Therapies in Heart Failure; EF, ejection fraction; MERIT-HF, Metoprolol CR/XL Randomized Intervention Trial in Congestive Heart Failure; NYHA, New York Heart Association; RALES, Randomized Aldactone Evaluation Study.

is problematic as many assume a ventricular tachyarrhythmia, but sudden death may be from a tachycardic, bradycardic, ischemic, or even embolic event.[21,29,30] Furthermore, the context of a death that is labeled sudden differs from trial to trial. In some studies a death may be called sudden only in the absence of worsening HF,[31] whereas some trials allow deaths to be categorized as sudden even on the background of a recent worsening of HF symptoms.[32] In some respects the difficulty in adjudicating these end-points has been assisted with the broad application of ICDs and their ability to store information on terminal dysrhythmias, but even so such information is not always routinely obtained.

Nevertheless, with the current therapies for HF delaying or even preventing sudden death in combination with the growing epidemic of HF there will be a steadily growing population of patients who will die of progressive HF. Current estimates are that anywhere from 5 to 10% of those with HF have end-stage disease.[2] While these patients would benefit the most from palliative interventions, there is a dearth of information about those who have reached this stage of their illness. Beyond mere prognostication lies a complex and debilitating disease course that those with end-stage HF and their care givers experience. Overall quality of life is poor,[33] patients must also cope with multiple co-morbidities,[34] especially in the elderly,[35] which leads to a degree of suffering which exceeds that of patients with cancer.[36]

Death from progressive systolic HF

The final common end point of HF, whether systolic or diastolic is now termed Stage D HF. This stage is defined by the American Heart Association/American College of Cardiology (AHA/ACC) HF guidelines as 'patients who have marked symptoms at rest despite maximal medical therapy'.[37] For this group of patients there are also AHA/ACC guidelines for end-of-life care (see Table 18.2). Practically, however, there can be considerable variability between practitioners as to who meets this definition of end-stage HF. Even at these end-stages some aggressive interventions such as transplantation or VAD may still be appropriate in select populations. Other interventions such as intravenous diuretics and continuous inotropes, though not life-prolonging, may still offer symptomatic relief.[38] This determination is further complicated by the waxing and waning nature of symptoms even at the terminal stages of HF.[4]

Ideally one would be able to foresee who is on a course of irrevocable decline well before their terminal decompensation. However prognostication is complicated

Table 18.2 The 2005 ACC/AHA chronic HF guidelines—end-of-life recommendations

Class I	(1) Ongoing patient and family education regarding prognosis for functional capacity and survival is recommended for patients with HF at the end of life
	(2) Patient and family education about options for formulating and implementing advance directives and the role of palliative and hospice care services with re-evaluation for changing clinical status is recommended for patients with HF at the end of life
	(3) Discussion is recommended regarding the option of inactivating ICDs for patients with HF at the end of life
	(4) It is important to ensure continuity of medical care between inpatient and outpatient settings for patients with HF at the end of life
	(5) Components of hospice care that are appropriate to the relief of suffering, including opiates, are recommended and do not preclude the options for use of inotropes and intravenous diuretics for symptom palliation for patients with HF at the end of life
	(6) All professionals working with HF patients should examine current end-of-life processes and work toward improvement in approaches to palliation and end-of-life care
Class III	(1) Aggressive procedures performed within the final days of life (including intubation and implantation of a cardioverter-defibrillator in patients with NYHA functional Class IV symptoms who are not anticipated to experience clinical improvement form available treatments) are not appropriate

by the lack of robust data to determine who is entering the final stages of their disease course.[35,39] Despite the inability to accurately predict who may be entering the end-stages of HF, many recommendations about care at the end-of-life rest on such a determination. The AHA/ACC guidelines for ICDs proscribe their placement if life expectancy is less than 6 months.[40] In addition the Medicare hospice benefit requires a prognosis of less than 6 months.[35]

There are many large randomized trials of HF patients with systolic dysfunction and advanced symptoms; however most still do not fully clarify this issue. In a trial such as COMPANION, which randomized 1520 patients, 86% of whom were NYHA Class III, to optimal medical therapy, CRT or CRT with an ICD in addition to a modern HF regimen, approximately 75% of patients survived after 2 years.[19]. Even in other trials with a preponderance of NYHA Class III patients, the annual mortality is only about 15–20%.[41] The very sickest patients are usually not entered into these large trials and the few that are generally do not represent the overall population of patients who have end-stage disease. Even the National Hospice Organization's own guidelines for determining prognosis are poor predictors of 6-month survival.[39].

Prediction models

Prediction models have been developed to assist in risk stratifying patients with HF. The outpatient models have been found to have good predictive capacity, however they often include variables which are not always routinely available[41,42] or are based on a less symptomatic population of patients prior to the current era of HF therapy.[43] Two large community-based, in-hospital mortality predictors have also been developed that include patients with both systolic and diastolic failure.[44,45] Both use widely available clinical and laboratory data and can identify a very high risk group with a 1-year mortalities of about 75%,[45] but again are limited in their derivation from a hospitalized cohort. Lastly, the most recent and most versatile survival predictor for systolic HF is the Seattle Heart Failure Model.[46] It was validated from past clinical trials of 1125 HF patients and tested on cohorts from five other trials totaling nearly ten thousand patients who were mostly NYHA Class II and III. There were a small group of very sick patients and the highest scores by this model correspond to a 2-year survival of only 10.8%. The web-based calculator relies on fairly common clinical and laboratory data, plots a survival curve and calculates a mean life expectancy over the next 5 years rather than giving a single survival percentage. This model also will plot a second survival curve that allows the patient and physician to see the survival advantage, or lack thereof, for medical and device-based interventions. Such information will hopefully facilitate communication about end-of-life issues and help to avoid unnecessary interventions. However, these models still fall somewhat short in fully describing the course and characteristics of those with refractory HF (see Chapter 21).

Inotrope dependent and transplant eligible patients

While many of the most symptomatic patients have been excluded from most large clinical trials, there have been a few involving exclusively Stage D patients. Many of these trials involved patients who were inotrope dependent or eligible for cardiac transplantation. In examining groups of such severely ill patients a number of similar characteristics emerge. One of the most recent studies of patients on inotropes was the Care Processes and Clinical Outcomes of Continuous Outpatient Support with Inotropes (COSI) trial by Herschberger *et al.* who followed 36 inotropic dependent patients. In this series, progressive HF accounted for 80% of patient deaths as would be expected for such a group of patients. Their HF was long-standing and recurrent with a mean duration of symptoms of 5.4 years and a mean of almost two hospitalizations within the 6 months preceding initiation of inotropes. Prior to initiation of inotropes patients were hospitalized for a mean of 21 days. Eventually over half of the patients died at home and nearly 70% had documented wishes not to be resuscitated. Their continued deterioration can be inferred by their last recorded creatinine having increased to a mean of 2.5 mg dl^{-1} from 1.5 mg dl^{-1} upon study entry. Overall median survival was only 3.4 months and 12-month survival was 6% (see Figure 18.1). This poor survival for patients on inotropes mirrors other published series[38,47–57] with over 60% mortality at 6 months and near universal mortality at 1 year[58] as noted in Figure 18.2.

Another recent study was the Randomized Evaluation of Mechanical Assistance for the Treatment of Congestive Heart Failure (REMATCH) which followed a group of patients who were sick enough to merit transplantation, but had a contraindication to transplantation.[57] This group of 129 patients was randomized to a VAD or optimal medical management (OMM). The OMM group had 61 patients and provides valuable insights

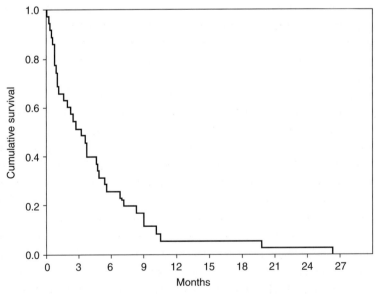

Fig. 18.1 Survival in months for those patients determined to be inotrope dependent in COSI. Reprinted from: Hershberger RE *et al.* (2003). Care processes and clinical outcomes of continuous outpatient support with inotropes (COSI) in patients with refractory end-stage heart failure. *J Card Fail* **9**: 184, Copyright 2003, with permission from Elsevier.

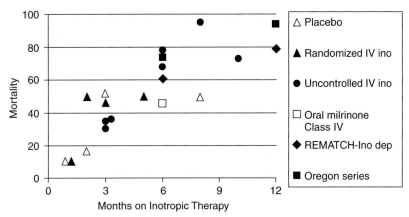

Fig. 18.2 Mortality over time based on published studies of patients on inotropic (ion) therapy. Reproduced from Stevenson LW (2003). Clinical use of inotropic therapy for heart failure: looking backward or forward? Part II: chronic inotropic therapy. *Circulation* **108**: 492–7, with permission from Lippincott, Williams and Wilkins.

into this extremely sick group of patients rigorously followed in a trial setting. About half of the patients were still able to tolerate ACE-I and only 20% were still on beta-blockers. Of note these patients also had documented baseline quality-of-life assessments (Minnesota Living with Heart Failure), SF-36, and Beck's Depression Inventory, which showed significant impairment that worsened by 1 year. After 1 year the survivors in the OMM group remained limited with activities such as walking up one flight of stairs or even bathing or dressing. Overall survival in the OMM group was dismal with a 6-month, 12-month, and 1-year mortality of approximately 50%, 75%, and 100%, respectively. Median survival was 150 days, of which the median number of days spent hospitalized was 24.

The characteristics of patients in COSI, the OMM group of REMATCH and the inotropic dependent patients in REMATCH are compared in Table 18.3. Similar to many trials of advanced HF the patients were older, male, and had systolic HF about half of which had an ischemic etiology. As would be expected patients were relatively hypotensive and had elevated left-sided filling pressures with a marginal cardiac index. Renal dysfunction and perturbations of sodium homeostasis are also common in this group of patients. Studies have shown that both inotrope dependence and renal insufficiency are independent markers of patients at risk for death from progressive HF in advanced HF.[59] This is especially evident in REMATCH where 50 of the 54 deaths in the OMM group were from progressive HF, none of the remaining were categorized as arrhythmic deaths.

While patients who are inotrope dependent may represent a definable group of patients who have a particular poor prognosis, there is not a universally accepted definition of inotrope dependency, but rather generally accepted guidelines for such therapy. Like the patients in COSI such patients have often been monitored and had their therapies adjusted as part of a long hospitalization, often with concomitant right heart

Table 18. 3 Characteristics of patients with advanced HF

	COSI (*n* = 36)	REMATCH OMM (*n* = 61)	REMATCH inotrope dependent[a] (*n* = 64)
Clinical characteristics			
Age (years)	55	68	67
Male (%)	66	82	–
Ischemic (%)	47	69	–
EF (%)	20	17	18
Hemodynamics			
SBP (mmHg)	97	103	98
Wedge (mmHg)	28	24	26
Cardiac index (L min $^{-1}$ m^{-2})	1.9	2.0	2.0
Laboratory data			
Sodium (mmol L^{-1})	132	135	133
Creatinine (mg dl^{-1})	1.5	1.8	1.8

[a] At baseline for all patients whether eventually randomized to medical management or ventricular assist device.

Abbreviations: COSI. Continuous Outpatient Support with Inotropes; REMATCH, Randomized Evaluation of Mechanical Assistance for the Treatment of Congestive Heart failure; OMM, optimal medical management; EF, ejection fraction; SBP, systolic blood pressure.

catheterization.[60] They have also likely failed several prior attempts to wean from inotropy due to hemodynamic instability, refractory volume overload, or worsening renal insufficiency. Such failures to wean can occur within hours or over the course of days to weeks, which can be manifested in frequent subsequent hospitalizations. These patients are either on no beta-blockade or a small dose which is stopped around the time that inotropic therapy is instituted. Furthermore, hypotension, renal insufficiency, or hyperkalemia often necessitate discontinuing aldosterone inhibitors, lowering the doses of ACE-I or stopping them altogether, or substituting a combination of nitrates and hydralazine.[60] However, inotropy per se, is not the *sine quo non* of end-stage HF. When the inotrope and non-inotrope dependent patients in the OMM group of REMATCH were compared, their survival was not statistically significantly different (see Figure 18.3).[61]

Studies of patients at the end-of-life

In a study of the 160 HF deaths at a tertiary referral institution since the year 2000, Teuteberg *et al.*[62] examined the baseline clinical characteristics of the decedants and the evolution of their laboratories over the last 6 months of their lives. The patients had a long-standing disease course with an overall duration of HF of about 5 years, over 2 years of which included follow-up in a specialized HF clinic. During the last 6 months of life, fully 79% were NYHA Class IV at some time, but no patient had NYHA Class I symptoms at any time. Sixty percent of the patients had moderate or severe mitral regurgitation while

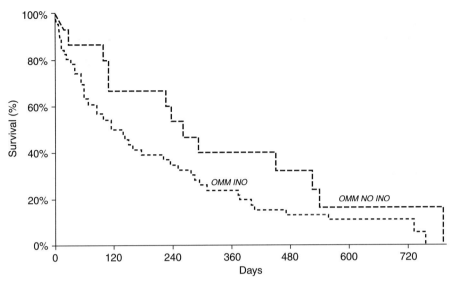

Fig. 18.3 Survival for patients randomized to optimal medical therapy (OMM) in the REMATCH. Ino = on inotropes at the time of randomization. No ino = not on inotropes at the time of randomization. From Stevenson LW *et al.* (2004). Left ventricular assist device as destination for patients undergoing intravenous inotropic therapy: a subset analysis from REMATCH (Randomized Evaluation of Mechanical Assistance in Treatment of Chronic Heart Failure). *Circulation* **110**: 975–81 with permission from Lippincott, Williams and Wilkins.

53% had moderate to severe right ventricular dysfunction in addition to a mean left ventricular ejection fraction of 20%. Only 55% were on ACE-I prior to death, 35% were deemed ACE-I intolerant, and only 38% were able to tolerate beta-blockers. In the 6 months prior to death, 74% of the patients had been hospitalized at least once and over 40% were hospitalized two or more times. Half of the patients studied died while ambulatory and the other half died either while hospitalized or enrolled in hospice, however there were few differences in the baseline characteristics between these two groups.

In order to assess the disease course, laboratory data were examined over the last 6 months of life. The last known laboratory values were compared to the worst laboratory values in the past 6 months. For serum sodium, blood urea nitrogen, and creatinine the worst values in the last 6 months were 128 mmol l^{-1}, 87 mg dl^{-1}, and 3.1 mg dl^{-1}, respectively, all of which were statistically significantly worse than the last known values of 135 mmol l^{-1}, 62 mg dl^{-1}, and 2.2 mg dl^{-1}. Hence the renal function and hyponatremia at death usually reflected an improvement from a prior exacerbation, rather than progressive dysfunction. These exacerbations were a median of 19 days before death in the hospitalized patients and a median of 71 days prior to death in the outpatients. Consistent with the findings in COSI and REMATCH, perturbations of renal function and sodium homeostasis are common in this group of patients with 55% of patients having a serum sodium of less than 130 mmol l^{-1} and 75% having a creatinine of over 2.0 mg dL^{-1} sometime in the last 6 months of life. The improvement in these preterminal exacerbations of sodium homeostasis and renal function likely also reflects the ongoing interventions for HF such as changes in diuretic regimes and the use, dosage, or number of inotropic agents.

Overall the large studies of patients with advanced systolic HF have shown that patients who are inotrope dependent or eligible for cardiac transplant have high 6-month mortality. The HF is long-standing and accompanied by advanced ventricular and valvular dysfunction. The loss of homeostatic mechanisms is evident by the presence of hyponatremia and renal dysfunction. This syndrome of worsening renal function that accompanies worsening HF, or the cardiorenal syndrome, is consistent with multiple prior studies that have shown renal insufficiency as a strong predictor of poor outcomes in HF.[63,64] As the disease course advances patients are less able to tolerate the dosages or classes that make up the modern HF regimen. This is consistent with prior studies that have shown an increase in mortality for those unable to tolerate ACE-I or ARBs.[65] Patients also consistently demonstrate poor levels of functioning and their general health status continues to decline over time. Lastly, death is almost exclusively a result of progression of HF rather than as a sudden event.

Other studies have attempted to better understand the disease course by retrospective review of HF deaths. In the last 6 months of life breathlessness was the most common of over twenty symptoms. Despite the documentation of these symptoms, care givers rarely provided therapies directed toward their alleviation. A subgroup analysis of the 539 patients in the SUPPORT trial who had an acute exacerbation of HF was performed. The caveat to this study was that the patients were enrolled through January 1994, so the patients may not as accurately reflect the current population with HF. The baseline characteristics are similar to the above studies in that the mean age was close to 70 years, about 65% were men, and over 80% were white. Dyspnea and pain in the last three days of life, as reported by patient's families, was common, but in the group that died during the index hospitalization, the rates of dyspnea and pain were even higher, occurring in 42% and 35% respectively. As the time prior to death decreased, patients had greater dependencies for activities of daily living, worse Duke Activity Status and a poorer perceived quality of life (see Table 18.4). Patients who lived for less than 1 month spent a median of 28% of that time hospitalized. The incidence of pain, confusion, and dyspnea also increased as the time to death decreased (see Figure 18.4). However, there was little change in the perceived quality of life with the nearness to death, approximately a third of those less than a month from death reported a good to excellent quality of life. The impact of advanced HF on families was also profound, the incidence of a family member having to quit work was 13% and about one quarter of the families lost the majority of their savings.

Despite long-standing nature of the disease and the often intractable renal insufficiency seen in this population the overall goal of HF medical management remains the same, relief of congestion. While increases in diuretics may lead to worsening of baseline renal dysfunction, this is often the price to be paid to alleviate symptoms. Worsening renal insufficiency in the face of inadequate diuresis despite increasing doses of diuretics may necessitate the institution of inotropy. Given the incidence of concomitant right HF,

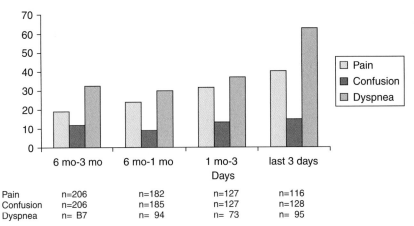

	6 mo-3 mo	6 mo-1 mo	1 mo-3 Days	last 3 days
Pain	n=206	n=182	n=127	n=116
Confusion	n=206	n=185	n=127	n=128
Dyspnea	n= B7	n= 94	n= 73	n= 95

Fig. 18.4 Physical symptoms during the last 6 months of life in patients with congestive HF from the SUPPORT study. *P*-values for trends: pain, *P* < 0.001; confusion, *P* = 0.151; dyspnea, *P* < 0.001. From Levenson JW *et al.* (2000). The last six months of life for patients with congestive heart failure. *J Am Geriatr Soc* **48**: S101–S109 with permission from Blackwell Publishing.

symptoms such as abdominal distension, early satiety, and edema may be as if not more prominent than left-sided symptoms such as dyspnea and orthopnea. Co-existing mitral and tricuspid valve regurgitation may only exacerbate symptoms and further complicate efforts to relieve conjestion. Patient may still be quite symptomatic as a result of advanced HF even without elevated filling pressures. Poor cardiac output can lead to confusion, lethargy, fatigue, and abdominal discomfort in addition to worsening end-organ function.[66] Such patients may enjoy symptomatic relief from the institution of inotropy, but over time as their cardiac function progressively declines they may have more difficulty weaning from such therapies and may eventually become inotrope dependent.

Diastolic HF

Unfortunately most of the clinical information that exists for HF, especially in its advanced stages, has been derived from cohorts of patients with systolic dysfunction. Those with the clinical syndrome of HF, but with a normal ejection fraction have historically been said to have 'diastolic dysfunction'. There is a movement within the HF community to more precisely describe this entity as 'HF with a normal ejection fraction' or 'HF with preserved systolic function'; however, these terms have still not gained widespread acceptance and hence for simplicity this text, for the most part, will refer to it simply as diastolic HF. The prevalence of HF increases as the population ages and diastolic HF represents over 50% of the incident cases of HF and comprise an even larger proportion in older cohorts.[67–69] As compared with the male predominance in systolic HF, in diastolic HF, women predominate.[69] In the older cohort of patients with HF, the mortality rates of those with systolic versus diastolic dysfunction are not significantly different.[70–72] In addition their quality of life and level of functioning are similar to

Table 18. 4 Patients with congestive HF from the SUPPORT study. Adapted from Levenson *et al.*[4] with permission

	Time before death			
	3–6 months	1–3 months	3 days–1 month	P-value for trend
% of days hospitalized	8	13	28	< 0.001
Number of dependences in ADL s				
In hospital	98	111	109	< 0.001
Out of hospital	125	96	52	< 0.001
Duke Activity Status index				
In hospital	17.4	154.	16.4	0.026
Out of hospital	16.0	17.5	15.0	0.416
Perceived QOL (%)				
Poor	25	29	30	n.s.
Fair	42	44	41	n.s.
Good	21	27	22	n.s.
Very good or excellent	12	31	7	n.s.
Anxiety				
In hospital	0.8	0.8	0.8	0.001
Out of hospital	0.8	0.8	1.3	0.333
Depression				
In hospital	0.6	0.7	–	< 0.001
Out of hospital	0.6	0.6	1.2	0.035

All values except for quality of life (QOL) are the median values. Activities of Daily Living (ADL): range 0–7 with higher scores indicating more functional impairment. Duke Activity Status: range 0–35, lower scores indicate greater functional impairment. Anxiety and depression scores: range 0–4, measured with Profile of Mood State, with increasing scores representing increasing severity of symptoms.

patients with systolic dysfunction.[73,74] A large national database of over 100 000 hospitalizations for congestive HF has shed some light onto the prognosis of those with HF and preserved systolic function.[75] Patients admitted with diastolic HF were found to be more likely to have rales and edema and to be hypertensive than those with systolic HF. However the level of dyspnea and renal dysfunction were similar in the two groups. Overall in hospital mortality was low, but was lower, 2.8% in the diastolic group, than the 3.9% mortality in those with systolic dysfunction. For those with diastolic failure the median length of hospitalization was 4.9 days and about 19% were admitted to an ICU during their hospitalization. Similar to the observations in systolic HF, renal insufficiency was a major independent risk factor for poor outcomes. Patients with diastolic HF are likely to have some aspects of their management that is different from those with systolic failure as their disease course progresses, but many of the limitations and symptoms clusters are likely to overlap with those found in systolic HF. Thus caregivers will have to rely somewhat on these commonalities to help guide care for those with diastolic HF until more data is forthcoming.

Barriers to supportive care

The perception that HF is a life-limiting condition still does not have wide acceptance among patients or physicians.[76] Examining the survival curves after a first hospitalization for HF as compared to various forms of cancer demonstrate that HF is almost a universally more lethal condition (see Figure 18.6).[77] Moreover, once the disease state reaches its end-stages, survival is worse than even metastatic lung cancer (see Figure 18.7).[57,58].

However, in contrast to many chronic progressive diseases, patients with highly symptomatic HF can sometimes have dramatic recoveries with aggressive medical care, hence the symptom burden does not necessarily relate to prognosis. Even excluding those with acute inflammatory or ischemic myopathies, patients with chronic disease may enjoy substantial symptomatic benefit from a variety of specific therapies. At its most symptomatic stages introducing or aggressively titrating HF medications can still result in substantial clinical improvement and improved survival.[79] Chronic ischemic or valvular heart disease may have dramatic improvements from percutaneous or surgical intervention. Patients with NYHA Class III symptoms who undergo biventricular pacing not only can have significant improvements in their symptoms, but in their cardiac function as well.[80] Some interventions, such as destination VAD and cardiac transplantation can completely remove an otherwise moribund patient from their prior illness trajectory as

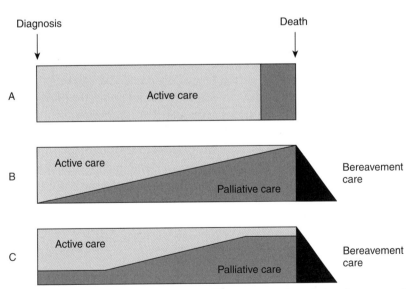

Fig. 18.5 Models for the involvement of palliative care in cancer (A and B) and a proposed model for HF (C). From JS Gibbs *et al.* (2002). Living with and dying from heart failure: the role of palliative care. *Heart* **88**(Suppl. 2): ii36–ii39 with permission from the BMJ Publishing Group.

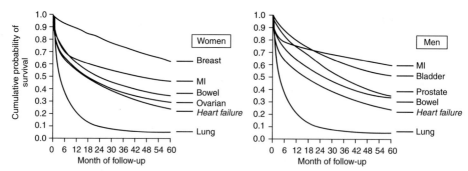

Fig. 18.6 Survival by gender after the first admission for HF, myocardial infarction, and the four most common gender-specific cancers. Reprinted from Stewart S *et al.* (2001). More 'malignant' than cancer? Five-year survival following a first admission for heart failure. *Eur J Heart Fail* **3**: 315–22, Copyright 2001, with permission from Elsevier.

seen in Figure 1.2, Chapter 1. In contrast, patients with advanced cancer might be enrolled in clinical trial or offered second or third round chemotherapy, neither of which has a high likelihood of extending their lives as dramatically as these interventions for HF.

Supportive care and the course of illness in HF

As outlined above, the course to death from HF is variable, can be significantly altered by HF therapies and has a timeline that is extremely difficult to predict. However, patients with HF may benefit significantly from supportive care. Given the ambiguities in disease course, it is important to examine when supportive care might be introduced for patients with HF, what should constitute supportive care in this population, how it might impact disease course and barriers to providing this type of care.

Current models of supportive care are based on experience primarily with cancer patients. In these models, supportive care plays a minor role at the time of diagnosis and increases linearly, completely replacing active care entirely during the final weeks to months of life. As mentioned in the introduction to this text, an alternate model of supportive care has been suggested for HF.[81] This model is outlined in Figure 18.5. Supportive care intervention would consist primarily of improved communication and assistance in decision-making early in the disease course and some active HF therapies would be continued, even for patients whose goal of care is not prolonged survival.[82,83]

Very little data exists on what currently constitutes supportive or hospice care provided to HF patients and the characteristics of the patients who receive it. A recent retrospective chart review looked at all patients referred for HF who died in a metropolitan hospice with both a rural and urban catchment area.[84] Patients were primarily Caucasian and elderly and their average ejection fraction was 25%. On average patients had a poor functional status, 52% were bed bound and on admission, only 25% reported pain. During the last week of life, primary symptoms included shortness of breath, edema,

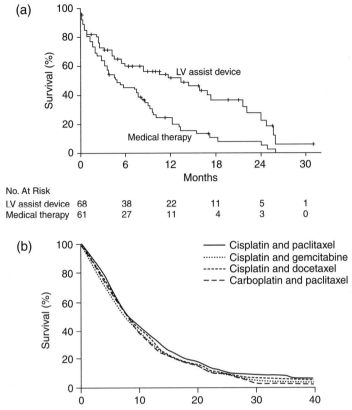

Fig. 18.7 Survival curves for REMATCH (A) and a randomized controlled trial of four different chemotherapeutic agents for advanced lung cancer. Note that 12-month survival between the medically managed end-stage HF patients and those with advanced lung cancer are nearly identical. From Rose EA *et al.* (2001). Long-term mechanical left ventricular assistance for end-stage heart failure. *New Engl J Med* **345**: 1435–53 and Schiller JH *et al.* (2002). Comparison of four chemotherapy regimens for advanced non-small-cell lung cancer. *New Engl J Med* **346**: 92–8. Copyright (c) 2001/2002 Massachusetts Medical Society.

incontinence of bowel or bladder, and confusion. There was no significant improvement in symptoms between hospice admission and the time of death.

The median hospice length of stay for those patients was only 10 days, although 25% were in hospice for longer than 2 months. Nine percent of those referred were actively dying and only survived in hospice for 1–2 days. Fifty seven percent of patients were admitted directly from an acute care hospital and an additional 31% had been hospitalized in past 6 months. Seventeen percent were referred from long-term care facilities. The settings for hospice delivery included home (42%), long-term care facility (31%) and an inpatient hospice unit (21%).

In general, patients made use of the multidisciplinary team, primarily using social workers, chaplains and home health aides. Care also involved patient and family education.

Medications prescribed included anxiolytics (79%), morphine (74%), antidepressants (26%), haloperidol (24%) and scopolamine (21%). The specific HF medications prescribed diuretics (68%), nitrates (49%), digoxin (32%), angiotensin converting enzyme inhibitors (24%) and beta blockers (20%). The types of medications prescribed may reflect the large number of patients referred during the final days of life. This data gives us some idea of the HF hospice population, but was a very elderly population, many of whom were in their final days of life.

Although there is little data on symptoms experienced by HF patients referred for supportive care, we do have some information on symptoms experienced by patients with advanced HF. From the SUPPORT study we know that family members of patients dying from HF reported the presence of significant dyspnea, pain and confusion during the last three days of life.[85] Another study reported that approximately half of patients dying from HF experience pain, dyspnea, low mood and anxiety.[36] In the population described early, hospice intervention did not significantly improve symptoms.[84] We also know that patients dying from HF suffer an earlier functional decline than do patients dying from cancer.[86] Currently there is insufficient data available to determine whether or not supportive care might alter patient symptom burden during their disease course and this area warrants further research.

While there is not yet direct evidence to demonstrate how supportive care for HF affects patient symptoms, there is some evidence to suggest that it might affect disease course with regards to what interventions occur in the months leading up to death and the site of death. In the hospice population discussed above, almost all patients died outside of the hospital. Only 8 of the 90 patients were unaccounted for and may have died in the hospital. All other patients died at home (40%), in an inpatient hospice unit (30%) or at a long-term care facility (26%). This is vastly different from location of death from other studies of HF patients. In a study described earlier of patients dying with advanced HF at a tertiary referral center, 44% died in the hospital.[62] Furthermore, a recent study looking at patients with end-stage HF cared for in a specialized HF program consisting of patient education, day-care and home-care elements and intravenous drug administration demonstrated a significant decrease in number of patient hospital days.[87]

In addition to dying outside of the hospital, we can surmise that the patients in the hospice population mentioned avoided many of the interventions that occur late in disease course in other settings. We know that patients dying from HF undergo invasive and often costly interventions during the final days, weeks and months of life. In the SUPPORT study during last 3 days of life, approximately 15% of HF patients received CPR, mechanical ventilation or tube feedings.[85] Moreover, the study of patients dying from HF at a tertiary referral center reported that the terminal hospitalization was long, with a mean length of stay of 17.1 days. These admissions were marked by many invasive interventions including intubation (60%) and hemodialysis (21%). Forty-five percent of these patients died in the intensive care unit.[88] In a smaller study of patients who died with advanced HF found that 18% of defibrillators were placed during the last

6 months of life, many for primary prevention.[88] A proportion of these patients were likely far enough along in their course of illness to recognize that death might be approaching.

When we put the information about location of death and interventions late in the disease course together with our knowledge that patients with HF often have a strong preference for either quality of life or prolonged survival[89,90] one can infer that earlier supportive care for patients with advanced HF might decrease late hospital admissions and invasive therapies in those patients preferring quality of life. Supportive care could provide assistance in complex decision making surrounding invasive and potentially disease-altering therapies for patients during the middle of their HF course, such as ICD, CRT, VAD, or transplantation. These decisions are even more critical for some patients at the very beginning of their course, as in patients who develop cardiogenic shock as their first presentation of HF. In these cases, complex decisions regarding VAD or transplant fall on the heels of relative health, rather than after a prolonged disease course. In any case, a decision between complex and potentially morbid therapies must be weighed against the continuing burdens and mortality of advanced HF. Ideally, patient and care-giver decisions should be as informed and balanced as possible to avoid unnecessary or potentially unwanted prolongation of life or continuation of suffering.

Although more people die from heart disease than from any other cause and there are many reasons why supportive care might benefit patients with HF, the majority of HF patients do not receive supportive care. There are numerous theories to explain this apparent discrepancy, including attitudes and expectations of patients and clinicians, variable disease course, difficulties in prognosis and poor communication, which are discussed elsewhere in the text. It is likely that HF patients require a very different approach to symptom management than do patients with cancer. This would include more active management of HF therapies, including continuation and titration of HF medications as well as management of volume status. Many active therapies for HF also provide symptom relief and improve quality of life. Some of these, such as intravenous diuretics and inotropes can be quite costly and are often not covered by hospice, leading many patients to defer hospice enrollment in favor of continuing these therapies. Hospital admission for many HF patients can lead to improvement of their symptoms of congestion and dramatic improvement of their quality of life,[91] but in the United States, hospices must pay for inpatient care under a 'general inpatient care' contract when they are admitted. These issues of reimbursement, as well as earlier functional decline in HF, require some re-examination of systems for providing supportive care for HF that are different than for cancer. New systems would provide continued reimbursement for sometimes costly therapies that improve quality of life as well as improved home care or long term care for patients, even when their goals are no longer focused on prolonged survival.

In summary, supportive care may likely benefit patients throughout the course of HF, even as early as the time of diagnosis. Ideally, this would involve an ongoing accessibility to and reimbursement for supportive care resources throughout the course of illness in combination with strong communication between the various clinical disciplines caring for these patients.

References

1. Thom T, Haase N, Rosamond W, et al (2006). Heart disease and stroke statistics—2006 update: a report from the American Heart Association Statistics Committee and Stroke Statistics Subcommittee. *Circulation* **113**, e85-151.
2. Miller LW, Lietz K (2006). Candidate selection for long-term left ventricular assist device therapy for refractory heart failure. *J Heart Lung Transplant* **25**, 756-64.
3. Mackowiak J (1998). Cost of heart failure to the healthcare system. *Am J Manag Care* **4**, S338-42.
4. Levenson JW, McCarthy EP, Lynn J, Davis RB, Phillips RS (2000). The last six months of life for patients with congestive heart failure. *J Am Geriatr Soc* **48**, S101-9.
5. Adams KF, Jr., Fonarow GC, Emerman CL, et al (2005). Characteristics and outcomes of patients hospitalized for heart failure in the United States: rationale, design, and preliminary observations from the first 100,000 cases in the Acute Decompensated Heart Failure National Registry (ADHERE). *Am Heart J* **149**, 209-16.
6. Galvao M (2005). Reshaping our perception of the typical hospitalized heart failure patient: a gender analysis of data from the ADHERE Heart Failure Registry. *J Cardiovasc Nurs* **20**, 442-50.
7. Packer M, Bristow MR, Cohn JN, et al (1996). The effect of carvedilol on morbidity and mortality in patients with chronic heart failure. U.S. Carvedilol Heart Failure Study Group. *N Engl J Med* **334**, 1349-55.
8. The CIBIS II Investigators (1999). The Cardiac Insufficiency Bisoprolol Study II (CIBIS-II): a randomised trial. *Lancet* **353**, 9-13.
9. The MERIT-HF Investigators (1999). Effect of metoprolol CR/XL in chronic heart failure: Metoprolol CR/XL Randomised Intervention Trial in Congestive Heart Failure (MERIT-HF). *Lancet* **353**, 2001-7.
10. Packer M, Coats AJ, Fowler MB, et al (2001). Effect of carvedilol on survival in severe chronic heart failure. *N Engl J Med* **344**, 1651-8.
11. Pitt B, Zannad F, Remme WJ, et al (1999). The effect of spironolactone on morbidity and mortality in patients with severe heart failure. Randomized Aldactone Evaluation Study Investigators. *N Engl J Med* **341**, 709-17.
12. Pitt B, Gheorghiade M, Zannad F, et al (2006). Evaluation of eplerenone in the subgroup of EPHESUS patients with baseline left ventricular ejection fraction ≤ 30%. *Eur J Heart Fail* **8**, 295-301.
13. Pfeffer MA, Swedberg K, Granger CB, et al (2003). Effects of candesartan on mortality and morbidity in patients with chronic heart failure: the CHARM-Overall programme. *Lancet* **362**, 759-66.
14. Krum H, Carson P, Farsang C, et al (2004). Effect of valsartan added to background ACE inhibitor therapy in patients with heart failure: results from Val-HeFT. *Eur J Heart Fail* **6**, 937-45.
15. Moss AJ, Zareba W, Hall WJ, et al (2002). Prophylactic implantation of a defibrillator in patients with myocardial infarction and reduced ejection fraction. *N Engl J Med* **346**, 877-83.
16. Bardy GH, Lee KL, Mark DB, et al (2005). Amiodarone or an implantable cardioverter-defibrillator for congestive heart failure. *N Engl J Med* **352**, 225-37.

17. Kadish A, Dyer A, Daubert JP, et al (2004). Prophylactic defibrillator implantation in patients with nonischemic dilated cardiomyopathy. *N Engl J Med* **350**, 2151-8.

18. Abraham WT, Fisher WG, Smith AL, et al (2002). Cardiac resynchronization in chronic heart failure. *N Engl J Med* **346**, 1845-53.

19. Bristow MR, Saxon LA, Boehmer J, et al (2004). Cardiac-resynchronization therapy with or without an implantable defibrillator in advanced chronic heart failure. *N Engl J Med* **350**, 2140-50.

20. Cleland JG, Daubert JC, Erdmann E, et al (2005). The effect of cardiac resynchronization on morbidity and mortality in heart failure. *N Engl J Med* **352**, 1539-49.

21. Packer M (1992). Lack of relation between ventricular arrhythmias and sudden death in patients with chronic heart failure. *Circulation* **85**, I50-6.

22. Moss AJ, Hall WJ, Cannom DS, et al (1996). Improved survival with an implanted defibrillator in patients with coronary disease at high risk for ventricular arrhythmia. Multicenter Automatic Defibrillator Implantation Trial Investigators. *N Engl J Med* **335**, 1933-40.

23. Buxton AE, Lee KL, Fisher JD, Josephson ME, Prystowsky EN, Hafley G (1999). A randomized study of the prevention of sudden death in patients with coronary artery disease. Multicenter Unsustained Tachycardia Trial Investigators. *N Engl J Med* **341**, 1882-90.

24. Connolly SJ, Gent M, Roberts RS, et al (2000). Canadian implantable defibrillator study (CIDS): a randomized trial of the implantable cardioverter defibrillator against amiodarone. *Circulation* **101**, 1297-302.

25. Kuck KH, Cappato R, Siebels J, Ruppel R (2000). Randomized comparison of antiarrhythmic drug therapy with implantable defibrillators in patients resuscitated from cardiac arrest: the Cardiac Arrest Study Hamburg (CASH). *Circulation* **102**, 748-54.

26. Cleland JG, Puri S (1994). How do ACE inhibitors reduce mortality in patients with left ventricular dysfunction with and without heart failure: remodelling, resetting, or sudden death? *Br Heart J* **72**, S81-6.

27. Narang R, Cleland JG, Erhardt L, et al (1996). Mode of death in chronic heart failure. A request and proposition for more accurate classification. *Eur Heart J* **17**, 1390-403.

28. Ziesche S, Rector TS, Cohn JN (1995). Interobserver discordance in the classification of mechanisms of death in studies of heart failure. *J Card Fail* **1**, 127-32.

29. Luu M, Stevenson WG, Stevenson LW, Baron K, Walden J (1989). Diverse mechanisms of unexpected cardiac arrest in advanced heart failure. *Circulation* **80**, 1675-80.

30. Cleland JG, Massie BM, Packer M (1999). Sudden death in heart failure: vascular or electrical? *Eur J Heart Fail* **1**, 41-5.

31. The SOLVD Investigators (1991). Effect of enalapril on survival in patients with reduced left ventricular ejection fractions and congestive heart failure. The SOLVD Investigators. *N Engl J Med* **325**, 293-302.

32. Cohn JN, Archibald DG, Ziesche S, et al (1986). Effect of vasodilator therapy on mortality in chronic congestive heart failure. Results of a Veterans Administration Cooperative Study. *N Engl J Med* **314**, 1547-52.

33. Gibbs LM, Addington-Hall J, Gibbs JS (1998). Dying from heart failure: lessons from palliative care. Many patients would benefit from palliative care at the end of their lives. *Bmj* **317**, 961-2.

34. Hauptman PJ, Havranek EP (2005). Integrating palliative care into heart failure care. *Arch Intern Med* **165**, 374-8.

35. Goodlin SJ, Hauptman PJ, Arnold R, et al (2004). Consensus statement: Palliative and supportive care in advanced heart failure. *J Card Fail* **10**, 200-9.

36. McCarthy M, Lay M, Addington-Hall J (1996). Dying from heart disease. *J R Coll Physicians Lond* **30**, 325-8.

37. Hunt SA, Abraham WT, Chin MH, et al (2005). ACC/AHA 2005 Guideline Update for the Diagnosis and Management of Chronic Heart Failure in the Adult: a report of the American College of Cardiology/American Heart Association Task Force on Practice Guidelines (Writing Committee to Update the 2001 Guidelines for the Evaluation and Management of Heart Failure): developed in collaboration with the American College of Chest Physicians and the International Society for Heart and Lung Transplantation: endorsed by the Heart Rhythm Society. *Circulation* **112**, e154-235.

38. O'Connor CM, Gattis WA, Uretsky BF, et al (1999). Continuous intravenous dobutamine is associated with an increased risk of death in patients with advanced heart failure: insights from the Flolan International Randomized Survival Trial (FIRST). *Am Heart J* **138**, 78-86.

39. Fox E, Landrum-McNiff K, Zhong Z, Dawson NV, Wu AW, Lynn J (1999). Evaluation of prognostic criteria for determining hospice eligibility in patients with advanced lung, heart, or liver disease. SUPPORT Investigators. Study to Understand Prognoses and Preferences for Outcomes and Risks of Treatments. *Jama* **282**, 1638-45.

40. Gregoratos G, Abrams J, Epstein AE, et al (2002). ACC/AHA/NASPE 2002 guideline update for implantation of cardiac pacemakers and antiarrhythmia devices: summary article: a report of the American College of Cardiology/American Heart Association Task Force on Practice Guidelines (ACC/AHA/NASPE Committee to Update the 1998 Pacemaker Guidelines). *Circulation* **106**, 2145-61.

41. Aaronson KD, Schwartz JS, Chen TM, Wong KL, Goin JE, Mancini DM (1997). Development and prospective validation of a clinical index to predict survival in ambulatory patients referred for cardiac transplant evaluation. *Circulation* **95**, 2660-7.

42. Lund LH, Aaronson KD, Mancini DM (2003). Predicting survival in ambulatory patients with severe heart failure on beta-blocker therapy. *Am J Cardiol* **92**, 1350-4.

43. Brophy JM, Dagenais GR, McSherry F, Williford W, Yusuf S (2004). A multivariate model for predicting mortality in patients with heart failure and systolic dysfunction. *Am J Med* **116**, 300-4.

44. Fonarow GC, Adams KF, Jr., Abraham WT, Yancy CW, Boscardin WJ (2005). Risk stratification for in-hospital mortality in acutely decompensated heart failure: classification and regression tree analysis. *Jama* **293**, 572-80.

45. Lee DS, Austin PC, Rouleau JL, Liu PP, Naimark D, Tu JV (2003). Predicting mortality among patients hospitalized for heart failure: derivation and validation of a clinical model. *Jama* **290**, 2581-7.

46. Levy WC, Mozaffarian D, Linker DT, et al (2006). The Seattle Heart Failure Model: prediction of survival in heart failure. *Circulation* **113**, 1424-33.

47. Hershberger RE, Nauman D, Walker TL, Dutton D, Burgess D (2003). Care processes and clinical outcomes of continuous outpatient support with inotropes (COSI) in patients with refractory endstage heart failure. *J Card Fail* **9**, 180-7.

48. Applefeld MM, Newman KA, Sutton FJ, et al (1987). Outpatient dobutamine and dopamine infusions in the management of chronic heart failure: clinical experience in 21 patients. *Am Heart J* **114**, 589-95.

49. Erlemeier HH, Kupper W, Bleifeld W (1992). Intermittent infusion of dobutamine in the therapy of severe congestive heart failure—long-term effects and lack of tolerance. *Cardiovasc Drugs Ther* **6**, 391-8.

50. Harjai KJ, Mehra MR, Ventura HO, et al (1997). Home inotropic therapy in advanced heart failure: cost analysis and clinical outcomes. *Chest* **112**, 1298-303.

51. Krell MJ, Kline EM, Bates ER, et al (1986). Intermittent, ambulatory dobutamine infusions in patients with severe congestive heart failure. *Am Heart J* **112**, 787-91.

52. Miller LW (1991). Outpatient dobutamine for refractory congestive heart failure: advantages, techniques, and results. *J Heart Lung Transplant* **10**, 482-7.

53. Oliva F, Latini R, Politi A, et al (1999). Intermittent 6-month low-dose dobutamine infusion in severe heart failure: DICE multicenter trial. *Am Heart J* **138**, 247-53.

54. Packer M, Carver JR, Rodeheffer RJ, et al (1991). Effect of oral milrinone on mortality in severe chronic heart failure. The PROMISE Study Research Group. *N Engl J Med* **325**, 1468-75.

55. Roffman DS, Applefeld MM, Grove WR, et al (1985). Intermittent dobutamine hydrochloride infusions in outpatients with chronic congestive heart failure. *Clin Pharm* **4**, 195-9.

56. Sindone AP, Keogh AM, Macdonald PS, McCosker CJ, Kaan AF (1997). Continuous home ambulatory intravenous inotropic drug therapy in severe heart failure: safety and cost efficacy. *Am Heart J* **134**, 889-900.

57. Rose EA, Gelijns AC, Moskowitz AJ, et al (2001). Long-term mechanical left ventricular assistance for end-stage heart failure. *N Engl J Med* **345**, 1435-43.

58. Stevenson LW (2003). Clinical use of inotropic therapy for heart failure: looking backward or forward? Part II: chronic inotropic therapy. *Circulation* **108**, 492-7.

59. Derfler MC, Jacob M, Wolf RE, Bleyer F, Hauptman PJ (2004). Mode of death from congestive heart failure: implications for clinical management. *Am J Geriatr Cardiol* **13**, 299-304; quiz 305-6.

60. Stevenson LW (2003). Clinical use of inotropic therapy for heart failure: looking backward or forward? Part I: inotropic infusions during hospitalization. *Circulation* **108**, 367-72.

61. Stevenson LW, Miller LW, Desvigne-Nickens P, et al (2004). Left ventricular assist device as destination for patients undergoing intravenous inotropic therapy: a subset analysis from REMATCH (Randomized Evaluation of Mechanical Assistance in Treatment of Chronic Heart Failure). *Circulation* **110**, 975-81.

62. Teuteberg JJ, Lewis EF, Nohria A, et al (2006). Characteristics of patients who die with heart failure and a low ejection fraction in the new millennium. *J Card Fail* **12**, 47-53.

63. Schrier RW (2006). Role of diminished renal function in cardiovascular mortality: marker or pathogenetic factor? *J Am Coll Cardiol* **47**, 1-8.

64. Stevenson LW, Nohria A, Mielniczuk L (2005). Torrent or torment from the tubules? Challenge of the cardiorenal connections. *J Am Coll Cardiol* **45**, 2004-7.

65. Kittleson M, Hurwitz S, Shah MR, et al (2003). Development of circulatory-renal limitations to angiotensin-converting enzyme inhibitors identifies patients with severe heart failure and early mortality. *J Am Coll Cardiol* **41**, 2029-35.

66. Nohria A, Lewis E, Stevenson LW (2002). Medical management of advanced heart failure. *Jama* **287**, 628-40.

67. Senni M, Tribouilloy CM, Rodeheffer RJ, et al (1998). Congestive heart failure in the community: a study of all incident cases in Olmsted County, Minnesota, in 1991. *Circulation* **98**, 2282-9.

68. Senni M, Tribouilloy CM, Rodeheffer RJ, et al (1999). Congestive heart failure in the community: trends in incidence and survival in a 10-year period. *Arch Intern Med* **159**, 29-34.

69. Vasan RS, Larson MG, Benjamin EJ, Evans JC, Reiss CK, Levy D (1999). Congestive heart failure in subjects with normal versus reduced left ventricular ejection fraction: prevalence and mortality in a population-based cohort. *J Am Coll Cardiol* **33**, 1948-55.

70. Senni M, Redfield MM (2001). Heart failure with preserved systolic function. A different natural history? *J Am Coll Cardiol* **38**, 1277-82.

71. McAlister FA, Teo KK, Taher M, et al (1999). Insights into the contemporary epidemiology and outpatient management of congestive heart failure. *Am Heart J* **138**, 87-94.

72. Pernenkil R, Vinson JM, Shah AS, Beckham V, Wittenberg C, Rich MW (1997). Course and prognosis in patients or = 70 years of age with congestive heart failure and normal versus abnormal left ventricular ejection fraction. *Am J Cardiol* **79**, 216-9.

73. Jaarsma T, Halfens R, Abu-Saad HH, Dracup K, Stappers J, van Ree J (1999). Quality of life in older patients with systolic and diastolic heart failure. *Eur J Heart Fail* **1**, 151-60.

74. Smith GL, Masoudi FA, Vaccarino V, Radford MJ, Krumholz HM (2003). Outcomes in heart failure patients with preserved ejection fraction: mortality, readmission, and functional decline. *J Am Coll Cardiol* **41**, 1510-8.

75. Yancy CW, Lopatin M, Stevenson LW, De Marco T, Fonarow GC (2006). Clinical presentation, management, and in-hospital outcomes of patients admitted with acute decompensated heart failure with preserved systolic function: a report from the Acute Decompensated Heart Failure National Registry (ADHERE) Database. *J Am Coll Cardiol* **47**, 76-84.

76. Murray SA, Boyd K, Kendall M, Worth A, Benton TF, Clausen H (2002). Dying of lung cancer or cardiac failure: prospective qualitative interview study of patients and their carers in the community. *Bmj* **325**, 929.

77. Stewart S, MacIntyre K, Hole DJ, Capewell S, McMurray JJ (2001). More 'malignant' than cancer? Five-year survival following a first admission for heart failure. *Eur J Heart Fail* **3**, 315-22.

78. Schiller JH, Harrington D, Belani CP, et al (2002). Comparison of four chemotherapy regimens for advanced non-small-cell lung cancer. *N Engl J Med* **346**, 92-8.

79. Krum H, Roecker EB, Mohacsi P, et al (2003). Effects of initiating carvedilol in patients with severe chronic heart failure: results from the COPERNICUS Study. *Jama* **289**, 712-8.

80. Bax JJ, Abraham T, Barold SS, et al (2005). Cardiac resynchronization therapy: Part 1—issues before device implantation. *J Am Coll Cardiol* **46**, 2153-67.

81. Gibbs JS, McCoy AS, Gibbs LM, Rogers AE, Addington-Hall JM (2002). Living with and dying from heart failure: the role of palliative care. *Heart* **88 Suppl 2**, ii36-9.

82. Tanvetyanon T, Leighton JC (2003). Life-sustaining treatments in patients who died of chronic congestive heart failure compared with metastatic cancer. *Crit Care Med* **31**, 60-4.

83. Haydar ZR, Lowe AJ, Kahveci KL, Weatherford W, Finucane T (2004). Differences in end-of-life preferences between congestive heart failure and dementia in a medical house calls program. *J Am Geriatr Soc* **52**, 736-40.

84. Zambroski CH, Moser DK, Roser LP, Heo S, Chung ML (2005). Patients with heart failure who die in hospice. *Am Heart J* **149**, 558-64.

85. Lynn J, Teno JM, Phillips RS, et al (1997). Perceptions by family members of the dying experience of older and seriously ill patients. SUPPORT Investigators. Study to Understand Prognoses and Preferences for Outcomes and Risks of Treatments. *Ann Intern Med* **126**, 97-106.

86. Lunney JR, Lynn J, Foley DJ, Lipson S, Guralnik JM (2003). Patterns of functional decline at the end of life. *Jama* **289**, 2387-92.

87. Roig E, Perez-Villa F, Cuppoletti A, et al (2006). [Specialized care program for end-stage heart failure patients. Initial experience in a heart failure unit]. *Rev Esp Cardiol* **59**, 109-16.

88. Teuteberg JJ, Tedrow U, Lewis EF, et al (2004). Deaths from heart failure in the era of the implantable defribrillator. *J Am Coll Cardiol* **43S**, 178.

89. Lewis EF, Johnson PA, Johnson W, Collins C, Griffin L, Stevenson LW (2001). Preferences for quality of life or survival expressed by patients with heart failure. *J Heart Lung Transplant* **20**, 1016-24.
90. Stanek EJ, Oates MB, McGhan WF, Denofrio D, Loh E (2000). Preferences for treatment outcomes in patients with heart failure: symptoms versus survival. *J Card Fail* **6**, 225-32.
91. Steimle AE, Stevenson LW, Chelimsky-Fallick C, et al (1997). Sustained hemodynamic efficacy of therapy tailored to reduce filling pressures in survivors with advanced heart failure. *Circulation* **96**, 1165-72.

Chapter 19

The last few days of life

John Ellershaw and Miriam Johnson

The last few days of life

The achievement of a dignified and peaceful death for a patient, with their carers well supported in the final days and hours of life, should be a universal goal for all health-care professionals. The modern hospice movement together with specialist palliative care expertise has developed a framework for best care for the dying patient.[1,2] Hospices are regarded as models of excellence in caring well for dying patients by both health-care professionals and by society in general. However, this model of care is not universal throughout our health-care system. In order to address this, the Liverpool Care of the Dying Pathway (LCP) was developed to transfer best practice for the care of dying patients into the hospital setting. It has subsequently been adapted to the community and nursing home setting.[3–5] This chapter will overview the care of the dying within the framework of the LCP and then look specifically at the care of the patient who is dying of heart failure (HF).

There are generally four phases of care identifiable within the dying trajectory:

1. diagnosing dying
2. initial assessment and care
3. ongoing care
4. care after death.

Diagnosing dying

Diagnosing dying is a complex area within palliative care. However, experienced clinicians can recognize specific signs and symptoms that suggest a patient is entering the dying phase. Within the cancer population the following signs are commonly associated with the dying phase:[6]

- the patient becomes bed-bound
- the patient is semi-comatose
- the patient is only able to take sips of fluid
- the patient is no longer able to take oral medication.

Signs and symptoms specific to HF will be dealt with later in the chapter. However, the importance of diagnosing dying is that it allows the clinical team to move away from a cure model to a care model including the physical, psychological, social, and spiritual aspects of care and support for the relatives. Underpinning this is sensitive and timely communication.

Initial assessment and care

Once the patient is diagnosed as dying the needs of the patients and family over the next hours and days can be anticipated. These are represented as goals of care within the LCP (Fig. 19.1). It is traditionally at this moment that the clinical team may withdraw from interacting with the patient and relatives, yet it is at this very moment that the clinical team need to be proactive if the management of the dying phase is to be optimized.

Physical care

As the patient's condition deteriorates and they become weaker it becomes increasingly difficult for them to take their medication. Therefore non-essential medication should be discontinued and essential medication should continue via a parenteral route. This can usually be achieved by a continuous subcutaneous infusion delivered by a syringe driver.[7] Key symptoms and drugs to be considered in the dying phase are shown in Table 19.1.

As well as ensuring continuity of symptom control by prescribing an equivalent subcutaneous dose to the previously prescribed oral dose, patients should also have 'as required medication' written up for the symptoms highlighted in the table. This is to ensure that if the patient develops one of these symptoms in the dying phase that they

Goal 1: Current medication assessed and non essentials discontinued

Goal 2: PRN subcutaneous medication written up for list below as per protocol
- Pain   - Analgesia
- Agitation   - Sedative
- Respiratory tract secretions   - Anticholinergic
- Nausea & vomiting   - Anti-emetic
- Dyspnoea   - Anxiolytic / Muscle relaxant

Goal 3: Discontinue inappropriate interventions

Goal 3a: Decisions to discontinue inappropriate nursing interventions taken

Goal 3b: Syringe driver set up within 4 hours of doctors orders

Goal 4: Ability to communicate in English assessed as adequate

Goal 5: Insight into condition assessed

Goal 6: Religious/spiritual needs assessed

Goal 7: Identify how family/other are to be informed of patient's impending death

Goal 8: Family/other given hospital information via facilities leaflet

Goal 9: G.P Practice is aware of patient's condition

Goal 10: Plan of care explained & discussed with:
- Patient
- Family/Other

Goal 11: Family/other express understanding of planned care

Fig. 19.1 Initial assessment. From the Liverpool Care Pathway for the Dying Patient, Version 11 (http://www.lcp-mariecurie.org.uk).[5]

Table 19.1 Key symptoms and drugs in the dying phase

Symptom	Drug type
Pain	Analgesic
Agitation	Sedative
Respiratory tract secretions	Anticholinergic
Nausea and vomiting	Anti-emetic
Dyspnoea	Anxiolytic/muscle relaxant

will immediately receive the correct medication from the nurse, and there will be no delay in prescribing.

Any inappropriate investigations and treatment should be discontinued. This includes blood tests, routine turning regimes, and monitoring vital signs. In some circumstances it may be less clear, for example, whether antibiotics should be discontinued or continued for a further 24 or 48 hours. If this is the case then the decision should be clearly documented with the clinical rationale.

Evidence is limited, but suggests that the continuation of artificial fluid in the dying phase is of limited benefit and in general artificial hydration can be discontinued. If it is to be continued then the maximum recommended is 1 L of fluid over 24 hours. The symptoms related to hydration, in particular that of dry mouth, are often best relieved by local measures and family members can be encouraged to participate in this type of care.[8]

The issue of cardiopulmonary resuscitation should also be addressed. This must be dealt with in a sensitive manner, but in the same way that burdensome treatments and interventions are withdrawn at this phase of life, cardiopulmonary resuscitation is not appropriate.[9]

Psychological care

The importance of good communication cannot be emphasized highly enough in this emotionally charged and sometimes distressing phase of care.[10] These skills include:

- Being able to break bad news; for example, the family need to be able to understand that the patient is now in the dying phase.
- Dealing with difficult questions; for example, the patient may want to know why no further treatment is being undertaken.
- Addressing existential questions such as 'why me' and 'why now'.
- Giving information in a clear and sensitive manner regarding previous interventions and outcomes of treatment.

It is also important that the needs of the wider family are encompassed, including those of any children who may be involved (see Chapter 22).

Social care

The support for the family at this time is crucial if their experience of the death of their loved one is to be positive. If the patient is being cared for at home there may be a need for increased practical support. This can range from a contact number which enables carers to obtain help and advice on a 24-h basis to 24-h nursing care. The family will also need information on what to do if the patient dies and a health-care professional is not present.

In a hospital setting it is important to ensure that the family are made aware of the facilities available to support them, for example whether they can stay overnight and where they can obtain meals. They may also need to know how they can gain access to the hospital if they are called in the middle of the night. An information sheet to outline these facilities should be provided for relatives.

Spiritual care

Sensitivity to the patient's cultural and religious background is essential. This may require formal religious traditions to be observed in the dying phase and may influence care of the body after death.[11]

In the hospital setting access to information and support for the various religious and spiritual traditions is essential to meet the needs of patients in the dying phase. This information needs to be coordinated and made available at ward level. In the patient's home it is often a local contact who is familiar to the family who will support them at this time (see Chapters 16 and 25).

Ongoing care

The period following the initial assessment and care of the patient in the dying phase is often an active time for the doctors and nurses on the team and includes providing clear information and communication to the patient and family. Ongoing care includes regular review of the physical symptoms including pain, respiratory tract secretions, agitation, nausea and vomiting, dyspnoea, and mouth care. It is also important to relieve urinary retention or urinary incontinence and catheterization may be indicated. Bowel intervention is rarely necessary in the last days and hours of life.

Review of the patient's symptom control and review of the safe administration of the drugs, particularly if there is a subcutaneous syringe driver *in situ*, should be done on a 4-hourly basis.

During this ongoing phase of care, regular communication with the family regarding their insight, adequate support, and any spiritual needs should continue. This is often very welcome to the relatives who can feel isolated and may be spending long periods of time with their loved ones.

Care after death

Following the patient's death relatives should be dealt with in a compassionate manner. They are often at their most vulnerable at this time and need clear concise information regarding the practice and procedures that must be followed. A bereavement leaflet explaining issues related to grief can also be helpful. The specific goals in this section of the pathway support staff in delivering consistent bereavement care.

The Liverpool Care of the Dying Pathway (LCP)

The four phases of care within the dying trajectory are contained within the LCP. This document replaces all other documentation for the multidisciplinary team, and becomes the focus for the patient's management. It has attached symptom control guidelines and associated information leaflets to support health-care professionals and relatives.

The LCP forms part of a continuous quality improvement programme for care of the dying, which can promote care of the dying as a quality indicator within the clinical governance framework of organizations. The LCP framework has been highlighted at a national level in England for widespread dissemination[12,13] and is forming the basis of a National Care of the Dying Audit in hospitals in England. A number of international collaborations in both English-speaking and non-English-speaking countries have been established.

The dying phase—heart failure

The skills required to care for a patient dying from HF are similar to those required to care for a patient dying from cancer. Many centres using the LCP routinely use it unchanged for patients dying with HF. However, there are several specific issues in relation to HF that can make both recognition and management of the dying potentially difficult.

Recognition of the dying phase

The criteria for 'diagnosing' dying (see above) appear to be appropriate for HF patients. A pilot study of the LCP with minor modifications only is currently under way in HF. However, problems arise in several circumstances.

Recognition that this episode is the terminal decompensation

A significant number of HF patients die suddenly without a preceding deterioration in health, particularly those patients with greater functional status (New York Heart Association Class I or II). This discussion refers to those who continue on the expected trajectory of a slowly deteriorating condition interspersed by episodes of decompensation. These may be triggered by intercurrent infection, ischaemic episodes, worsening co-morbidities, suboptimal medication, or inappropriate medication such as non-steroidal anti-inflammatory drugs. Hence patients often respond to treatment and return to somewhere near their previous level of health. At first this may be a relatively simple matter of intravenous diuretics and fluid balance with treatment of any underlying infection, metabolic imbalance, and optimization of medication. As the patient's cardiac function worsens, or in the event of a major insult, more intensive treatment may be needed. Typically, as the patient's condition worsens, there is no obvious precipitant for the decompensation. Even with the 'last' deterioration, the patient may appear to initially respond to treatment encouraging the team to continue a very active approach, only for the patient to worsen and die apparently unexpectedly.

Professional team factors

It can be very hard for the professional team to realize that a patient is nearing the stage where further aggressive treatment is either futile or not in accordance with the patient's wishes, who may well rather trade quality for quantity. The patient may have repeated readmissions to the same hospital but to different receiving teams where lack of continuity leads to lack of recognition and poor communication with the patient. Even if the patient is cared for by the same team there is a risk that the doctors and nurses cannot let themselves see that a patient they have come to care for has reached such a point. This situation can also be hard for a patient who respects, likes, and is very grateful to his or her doctors, but who does not wish for further active treatment. Alternatively, the patient may not realize that their condition is so poor because of their previous experience, and skilled communication is required to discuss the aims of further management. If this is not done then potentially they are denied a chance to plan issues surrounding the end of life.[14]

Hospice and home factors

This situation is one of several reasons why very few patients with HF have the opportunity to die in a hospice. There may be little time between realizing that a patient is not responding to treatment, and death. Unless hospices consider admitting patients who do not wish to have inotropic support or cardiopulmonary resuscitation but still want one more try at correcting fluid balance, the patient is likely to die in the hospital by default. If hospices only admit patients for terminal care when it is clear that they are dying, it may be too late.

For patients wishing to die at home, the situation is equally difficult. If a patient deteriorates out of hours, the call centre, depending on its triage strategy, may routinely send an emergency ambulance. Even if the patient is visited by a doctor it is likely to be one unfamiliar with the patient, and they will be admitted to hospital instead having comfort measures put into place. Considerable planning is required by the patient's own family practitioner and primary-care team as well as good communication between hospital and community teams, such as that seen in the Gold Standards Framework.[15] Even with the best planning and communication, there may be insufficient support for the patient's informal carers and admission becomes inevitable.

Younger patients and those awaiting transplantation

All the issues outlined above seem to be exacerbated in this patient group. It can be emotionally difficult for staff caring for deteriorating younger patients. Seeing the distress of parents who never expected to outlive their children, and the distress of a patient who will leave young children, is costly. These are the patients most likely to be awaiting transplantation, which continues to keep hope alive but which can also lead to a feeling of being 'cheated', or 'if only', if a transplant is not forthcoming in time. It is unsurprising that under these circumstances both patients and staff find it difficult to recognize the dying phase. Such patients may therefore die, possibly a long way from home, family and friends, in a tertiary centre still receiving active treatment.

Recognition of the dying phase then, is difficult unless the team and patient have seen that the illness has become end-stage before the patient is imminently dying.

Although the 'Holy Grail' of clear prognostic factors has yet to be found, patients with worsening symptoms and hospital admissions despite optimal cardiac medication are likely to be reaching the terminal phase. This situation is suggested as a trigger for inclusion on a Gold Standards palliative care register.[16] Honest communication regarding the stage of disease and exploration of the patient's wishes would allow end-of-life planning for more patients than currently have that opportunity, without denying optimal treatment as necessary for their HF.

Signs that the HF patient is now dying include:

◆ previous admissions with worsening HF despite optimum tolerated medication

◆ no identifiable reversible precipitant

◆ deteriorating renal function

◆ failure to respond within 2–3 days with appropriate diuretic or vasodilator management.[17]

Implantable cardioverter defibrillators (ICDs)

Electrical device therapy is discussed in Chapter 5. This discussion relates to the dying phase. Although ICDs reduce the risk of sudden death, there will come a time when the heart is likely not to respond to cardioversion, and thus it becomes a futile intervention. Also, as the patient's HF worsens there is increasing risk that a successful cardioversion would result in serious morbidity due to hypoxic cerebral or renal damage. Potentially clear awareness of shocks in a dying patient would be very distressing to the patient, carer, and professionals.[18] It is important to recognize deterioration so that calm discussion with all concerned about the implications of a 'do not attempt resuscitation'[19–24] decision can be had before a crisis situation. If the patient is still able to travel, then a visit to the tertiary centre which placed the device for reprogramming to pacing mode (withdrawal of cardioverter support) is possible. Some district general pacemaker clinics provide a local service. Some local and tertiary centres (depending upon distance) will supply a technician who will visit a patient in the hospice, their own home, or hospital ward. Some manufacturer's representatives will also provide this service. It is highly recommended that local protocols are agreed. In an emergency situation strong magnets (usually available from pacemaker departments or coronary care units) held directly over the ICD will prevent activation, but will only work whilst in place.

Good communication is vital as patients may hold erroneous beliefs about the ICD's efficacy; possibly believing it will keep them alive indefinitely. Inevitably the discussion involves talking about death and dying and can be difficult. Conversely many are relieved to discuss the situation, realizing that they have deteriorated and concerned that it will activate.

Pacemakers

A patient with a pacemaker, may request that it be 'turned off'. It is thought that that the myocardium becomes less and less responsive to pacing and so pacemaking ultimately becomes ineffective. It is possible to reduce the pacemaker rate to 30 beats per minute. If the patient is pacemaker dependent it is likely then to hasten death, but also carries the risk of exacerbating symptoms. If the patient is not pacemaker dependent, turning down the rate may make little difference. Ethically, reducing pacemaker activity constitutes withdrawal of treatment and thus would be permitted at the request of a competent patient,[21] but it is difficult to be certain that this would be in the best interest of the patient and there is little literature to guide the clinician. The patient's underlying concern may be that the pacemaker would greatly prolong the dying phase, and reassurance that this is unlikely to be the case may be all that is needed.

Use of diuretics, oxygen, and sedation

The general principles of stopping oral medication and providing analgesics, anti-emetics, anti-secretory drugs, and sedatives as appropriate via the subcutaneous route is just as applicable to patients dying with HF as to other patients. In the dying phase where the patient is unlikely to be able to take oral medication, the decision to stop angiotensin-converting enzyme inhibitor therapy, β-blockers, spironolactone, and statin is self evident compared with earlier on in the illness. The patient may need no specific cardiac measures, and peripheral and pulmonary oedema may not be an issue as the patient drinks less and less or nothing at all. However, sometimes this is a problem. Peripheral oedema can be severe, unsightly, and uncomfortable and lead to lymphorrheoa, cellulitis, and pressure sores. Pulmonary oedema can lead to a severely distressing death including the 'textbook' pink frothy respiratory secretions and severe breathlessness. Diuretics and oxygen are therefore sometimes required.

Diuretics

The intravenous route may be undesirable because venous access is difficult or impossible, or because the patient finds the cannula uncomfortable or irritating. Depending on the clinical staff available it also may affect the timeliness of injection if the nurses on duty are not qualified to administer intravenous drugs. Also it is less likely to be possible to use if the patient wishes to die at home. In these circumstances furosemide can be administered by intramuscular injection, but this is often uncomfortable. Therefore there are benefits in administering furosemide subcutaneously, either intermittently or by continuous infusion.[25,26] If peripheral oedema is extensive, care must be taken to site the needle in an area of non-oedematous skin if possible as absorption may be affected.

Oxygen

Patients with HF do not usually desaturate unless there is pulmonary oedema or co-morbid pulmonary pathology. There is little and conflicting evidence that oxygen palliates breathlessness in ambulatory HF patients.[27,28,29] In the dying phase, due to the above reasons, the patient may be hypoxic. However, any potential benefits from oxygen should be weighed up against the visual impact for relatives, discomfort from nasal cannulae/face mask, and the practical problems of obtaining home oxygen. If the patient is conscious and the hypoxia is affecting cognition, then a trial of oxygen may be helpful.

Likewise a trial of oxygen to help breathlessness is sensible, but a clear therapeutic target is important for staff, patient, and relatives so oxygen therapy is not continued merely by default. Once the patient is unconscious, then there is little benefit in its continuation. However, as there is no evidence base to guide the clinician, each patient should be assessed on their own merits.[30]

Sedation

Breathlessness can often be controlled with opioids and diuretics. However, it can be severe and distressing, particularly if there is resistant pulmonary oedema. Anxiety may also be present and a benzodiazepine required. Rarely, sedation sufficient to render the patient asleep may be the only option to make the breathlessness bearable for the patient in the dying phase. In these circumstances it is useful to have discussed this in advance with the patient and relatives.

Cheyne–Stokes respiration

Cheyne–Stokes, or periodic, respiration is often seen in the dying phase from any disease. HF patients may have periodic respiration earlier on in their illness particularly at night-time when it may aggravate daytime somnolence and fatigue. Daytime periodic respiration can occur, and indicates a poor prognosis. Again there is a paucity of literature regarding therapeutic options and none in the dying phase itself. There is one paper describing the effectiveness of dihydrocodeine on periodic respiration in HF patients[31] and another on the use of oxygen.[32] It would therefore be reasonable to use opioids in the dying phase if the amplitude of the periodic respiration is distressing the patient (see Chapter 10).

Palliative care service provision for dying patients with HF

Over the last few years the increasing call for a palliative care approach and access to specialist palliative care (SPC) services,[33] has stimulated pockets of collaborative working between palliative care and cardiology in both the UK and USA. However, the majority of hospice units in the UK have grown up in the independent sector and are often funded through cancer charities. Hence it remains that 95% of hospice patients have cancer, and there are still a few hospice services that do not accept referrals for patients with HF.[34]

The LCP has brought the hospice approach and skills of care of the dying into the acute hospital setting, and this has gone a considerable way, where it is used, to extending good care for HF patients dying in hospitals if the dying phase is recognized. However, dying at home or in the hospice, if that is the patient's expressed preferred place of death, can prove difficult because of the issues discussed above. Even where there are collaborative services, the chance of dying in hospital remains high. Barriers that contribute to difficult access to SPC services are outlined in Table 19.2.

However, where collaborative services have developed, many of these fears have not been realized and each discipline has brought their own skills to complement those of others.[35,36] In doing so, there has also been considerable transfer of skills. Where there are Heart Failure Nurse Specialists (HFNS), these appear to function as key-workers,

Table 19.2 Barriers to accessing specialist palliative care (SPC) services

From cardiology	From SPC
Little or no contact with, or understanding of SPC services	Fear of overwhelming often precariously funded services
Perception that SPC services are for the end of life only ('prognostic paralysis')	Little or no contact with cardiology services
Lack of communication skills required to discuss stage of disease and aim of care, including death and dying	Fear of lack of skills
Lack of acknowledgement that HF is likely to be a terminal illness	Perception that treatment is complex and highly technological
Perception that patients will not wish for SPC involvement	Fear of being involved 'too early' thus blocking places/beds ('prognostic paralysis')
Lack of recognition of dying phase	Lack of recognition of dying phase

liaising between primary, secondary, and SPC as needed, but provision and role is patchy. Likewise, other initiatives such as 'care of long term conditions' or the 'community matrons', which aim to prevent hospital admissions, are variable in skills, resources, and joint working across sectors.

Hence the problem appears to be two-fold; firstly SPC services may not be involved early enough, and secondly, when they are, the dying phase may still not be recognized in time for the patient to have a choice about their place of death.

Conclusion

For patients with HF who do not suffer sudden death, it is possible to have a planned, symptom-controlled death with support for patient, family, and friends. Principles of care for patients dying with malignant disease are transferable and generic skills can be learnt by the ward or community team with support from SPC. Recognition of deteriorating illness is the trigger for communication with the patient and family about the patient's wishes, whilst continuing optimum tolerated therapy. Clear discussion between all services is needed to support the patient with regard to these wishes. Significant challenges remain for the community services to provide home support and liaison with out-of-hours services to prevent unwanted hospital admission. Similarly, a challenge faces hospices regarding their willingness and capability to accept decompensated patients for a trial of intravenous diuretics. Hospital teams face a major challenge of recognizing the stage of illness and developing the communication skills required to discuss preferred place of death, and speedy discharge planning in the event of a deteriorating patient's request to die at home.

If these challenges can be met, then patients with heart failure may have better deaths than those observed by Hinton:[37] 'Discomfort was not necessarily greatest in those dying from cancer; patients dying of heart failure, or renal failure, or both, had most physical distress'.

References

1. Twycross R, Lichter I (1998). The terminal phase. In: *Oxford Book of Palliative Medicine*, 2nd edn (ed. D Doyle, GWC Hanks, N MacDonald). Oxford: Oxford University Press.

2. Higginson IJ, Sen-Gupta G, Dunlop D (1997). *Changing Gear: Guidelines for Managing the Last Days of Life in Adults. The Research Evidence.* London: National Council for Hospice and Specialist Palliative Care Services.

3. Ellershaw JE, Murphy D, Shea T, Foster A, Overill S (1997). Development of a multiprofessional care pathway for the dying patient. *Eur J Palliat Care* **4**: 203–8.

4. Ellershaw JE, Wilkinson S (ed.) (2003). *Care for the Dying: a Pathway to Excellence.* Oxford: Oxford University Press.

5. The Marie Curie Palliative Care Institute Liverpool. http://www.lcp-mariecurie.org.uk

6. Ellershaw JE, Sutcliffe J, Saunders CM (1995). The dying patient and dehydration. *J Pain Symptom Manage* **10**: 192–7.

7. Dickman A, Littlewood C, Varga J (2002). *The Syringe Driver.* Oxford: Oxford University Press.

8. Joint Working Party between the National Council for Hospice and Specialist Palliative Care Services and the Ethics Committee of the Association for Palliative Medicine of Great Britain and Ireland (1997). Ethical decision making in palliative care: artificial hydration for people who are terminally ill. *J Eur Assoc Palliat Care* July/August: 12.

9. Joint Working Party between the National Council for Hospice and Specialist Palliative Care Services and the Ethics Committee of the Association for Palliative Medicine of Great Britain and Ireland (2002). *Ethical Decision Making in Palliative Care: Cardiopulmonary Resuscitation for People Who are Terminally Ill.* London: National Council for Hospice and Specialist Palliative Care Services.

10. Fallowfield LJ, Jenkins VA, Beveridge HA (2002). Truth may hurt but deceit hurts more: communication in palliative care. *Palliat Med* **16**: 297–303.

11. Neuberger J (2004). Caring for Dying People of Different Faiths, 3rd edn. Oxford: Radcliffe Medical Press.

12. National Institute for Clinical Excellence (2004). Key recommendation 14. P11. In: *Guidance on Cancer Services: Improving Supportive and Palliative Care for Adults with Cancer. The Manual.* London: NICE.

13. Department of Health (2006). *Our Health, Our Care, Our Say: a New Direction for Community Services.* London: HMSO.

14. Murray SA, Boyd K, Kendall M *et al.* (2002). Dying of lung cancer or cardiac failure: prospective qualitative interview study of patients and their carers in the community. *Br Med J* **325**: 929–932.

15. Department of Health. The gold standards framework. A programme for community palliative care. http://www.goldstandardsframework.nhs.uk (accessed November 2007).

16. Free A (2005). Using the Gold Standards Framework for non-cancer patients. http://www.goldstandardsframework.nhs.uk/content/spread_and_developments/Extending_the_GSF_to_non_17_10_05.pdf (accessed November 2007).

17. Ellershaw J, Ward C (2003). Care of the dying patient: the last hours or days of life. *Br Med J* **326**: 30–4.

18. Nambisan V, Chao D (2004). Dying and defibrillation: a shocking experience. *Palliat Med* **18**: 482–3.

19. Goldstein NE, Lampert R, Bradley E *et al.* (2004). Management of implantable cardioverter defibrillator in end-of-life care. *Ann Intern Med* **141**: 835–8.

20. Berger JT (2005). The ethics of deactivating implanted cardioverter defibrillators. *Ann Intern Med* **142**: 631–4.

21. Mueller PS, Hook CC, Hayes DL (2003). Ethical analysis of withdrawal of pacemaker or implantable cardioverter–defibrillator support at the end of life. *Mayo Clin Proc* **78**: 959–63.

22. Ross HM (2005). Deactivating implantable cardioverter defibrillators/in response [letter]. *Ann Intern Med* **143**: 690.

23. Berger JT (2005). Deactivating implantable cardioverter defibrillators/in response [letter]. *Ann Intern Med* **143**: 691.

24. Beattie JM, Connolly MJ, Ellershaw JE (2005). Deactivating implantable cardioverter defibrillators/in response [letter]. *Ann Intern Med* **143**: 690.

25. Verma AK, da Silva JH, Kuhl DR (2004). Diuretic effects of subcutaneous furosemide in human volunteers: a randomised pilot study. *Ann Pharmacother* **38**: 544–9.

26. Goenaga MA. Millet M, Sanchez E *et al.* (2004). Subcutaneous furosemide [comment]. *Ann Pharmacother* **38**: 1751.

27. Moore DP, Weston AR, Hughes JM *et al.* (1992). Effects of increased inspired oxygen concentrations on exercise performance in chronic heart failure. *Lancet* **339**: 850–3.

28. Restrick LJ, Davies SW, Noone L *et al.* (1992). Ambulatory oxygen in chronic heart failure. *Lancet* **340**: 1192–3.

29. Russell SD, Koshkarian GM, Medinger AE *et al.* (1999). Lack of effect of increased inspired oxygen concentrations on maximal exercise capacity or ventilation in stable heart failure. *Am J Cardiol* **84**: 1412–16.

30. Booth S, Wade R, Johnson MJ *et al.* (2004). The use of oxygen in the palliation of breathlessness. A report of the expert working group of the scientific committee of the Association for Palliative Medicine. *Resp Med* **98**: 66–77.

31. Ponikowski P, Anker SD, Chua TP *et al.* (1999). Oscillatory breathing patterns during wakefulness in patients with chronic heart failure: clinical implications and role of augmented peripheral chemosensitivity. *Circulation* **100**: 2418–24.

32. Franklin KA, Eriksson P, Sahlin C, Lundgren R (1997). Reversal of central sleep apnoea with oxygen. *Chest* **111**: 163–9.

33. Department of Health. *National Service Framework for Coronary Heart Disease*. Available from http://www.doh.gov.uk/nsf/coronary.htm.

34. Gibbs LME, Khatri AK, Gibbs JSR (2006). Survey of specialist palliative care and heart failure: September 2004. *Palliat Med* **20**: 603–9.

35. Davidson PM, Paull G, Introna K *et al.* (2004). Integrated, collaborative palliative care in heart failure: the St. George Heart Failure Service experience 1999–2002. *J Cardiovasc Nurs* **19**: 68–75.

36. Johnson MJ, Houghton T (2006). Palliative care for patients with heart failure – description of a service. *Palliat Med* **20**: 211–14.

37. Hinton JM (1963). The physical and mental distress of the dying. *Q J Med* **32**: 1–21.

Chapter 20

Bereavement support for patients and families

Diane Snyder Cowan and Karen Hatfield

Introduction

Grief is a normal and necessary process associated with any loss. It is a blend of physical, emotional, behavioral, intellectual, and spiritual responses that is unique to each person. The range of normal reactions is vast, and it can be challenging for grieving persons to understand and cope with what they are experiencing. The goal of bereavement professionals is to assist clients in understanding and moving through their grief reactions.

For patients with heart failure (HF) and their families, grief is an unseen and often unnoticed companion. Although medical advancements have increased the life expectancy associated with HF, the course of the illness is often unpredictable. In the early stages of HF, patients concurrently must cope with physical symptoms, anticipated losses, and other concerns associated with the disease progression. All of these factors contribute to the grief of both patients and families. With the diminution of abilities, and deterioration, remissions, and relapses, the patient and family continue to experience grief, and this grief will increase as the loved one declines.

The words grief and mourning are commonly interchanged. Simply, grief refers to an internal response, while mourning is the outward expression of the loss (Table 20.1). In this chapter we will refer to both. This chapter explores the grief of the patient and family, including the primary caregiver, during the disease as well as that which occurs after the patient's death. It will also offer suggestions on how to support the grieving patient and family.

Table 20.1 Grief: definitions

Grief	A natural, normal and necessary response to a loss
Anticipatory grief	Normal grief that occurs when a patient or family is expecting a death. Anticipatory grief has many of the same symptoms as those experienced after a death has occurred
Complicated grief	Extended duration of grief symptoms resulting in interference in normal functions or characterized by the intensity of the symptoms. Complicated grief may appear as a complete absence of grief and mourning, an ongoing inability to experience normal grief reactions, delayed grief, conflicted grief, or chronic grief

The challenges of living with HF

Illness presents an emotionally challenging time for patients and families, and treating the patient and family as a unit, while also considering the individual needs of each, is helpful. Inherent in any chronic illness are both physical and secondary losses. The losses associated with HF, and a person's response to them, will affect that individual's experience of the disease. In addition, these losses will affect the family during the illness and may have an impact on the family's grief after the death.

Sotile and Miller[1] suggest that the age of the patient and primary caregiver need to be considered. Elderly patients are often coping with the effects of other illnesses in addition to HF. Often, middle-aged patients are taking care of their own elderly parents. The psychosocial aspects of the family members have an impact on both the support system and also the grief that is experienced after the death. When working with patients and caregivers, it is important to seek information about the family unit, dynamics, and relationships, and to be prepared to handle complicated situations. Available support will vary from family to family, and the lack of formal and informal support may give rise to feelings of guilt and anger that can complicate the grief reaction.

A common symptom of HF is fatigue. At its worst, fatigue makes performing everyday tasks such as dressing or putting away groceries difficult. While rest and lower extremity exercises are helpful, weakness and fatigue are identifiable losses that patients and families experience. The patient recognizes that he or she can no longer climb the stairs, take out the garbage, or play with youngsters on the floor. The caregiver may need more and more assistance to meet the loved one's every day needs. (See also Chapter 11) In advanced HF, hospice and palliative care teams become increasingly important. By anticipating the patient's needs, the hospice and palliative care team can increase nursing assistant services, volunteer visits and other supportive services to provide respite for the caregiver (see Table 20.2).

Anxiety, anger, and longing are common factors contributing to the grief of patients with HF. Some people may feel anxious about the future or have regrets about the past. Anxiety can also be related to other life stressors such as financial concerns or estranged relationships.

Table 20.2 Losses, challenges, and coping strategies

Losses and challenges	Loss of independence
	Loss of control
	Lifestyle changes
	Altered relationships
	Occupational/monetary impact
	Loss of future dreams
Coping strategies	Increased use of health-care services
	Increased family caregiving
	Use of medical technology and equipment
	Anticipatory grieving
	Advance care planning/living wills/power of attorney

Physical concerns such as shortness of breath, fear of suffocation, and thoughts of impending death increase anxiety and can intensify the grief reaction. Dyspnea is one of the most anxiety-producing symptoms and is more common in patients with a co-morbid diagnosis of depression.[2] In addition, Gibbs et al.[3] report that the symptom of breathlessness was more difficult to manage than pain, with 63% of patient surrogates reporting that patients were severely short of breath during the 3 days before death. Clearly, stress and anxiety can exacerbate physical and emotional symptoms, leading to a vicious cycle that is difficult to interrupt without adequate support and education (see also Chapter 15).

Providing care for a person with advanced HF can be difficult, stressful, and complicated. Families often grieve the loss of their previous roles and relationships. As symptoms increase and the patient's health declines, the caregiver experiences emotional and physical stress and discomfort.

Offering education and information to the patient and family about the disease process is valuable. Family members should be assessed on their perception of the illness and what will happen as the disease advances. Knowing what may happen as well as techniques to manage symptoms can provide some sense of control at an emotionally difficult time. Family members often express feeling better prepared as they gain knowledge from the hospice team regarding what to expect as a loved one declines.

Anticipatory grief

Anticipatory grief (Table 20.3) refers to grief that occurs when there is an opportunity to anticipate the death of a loved one or of oneself. It includes feelings associated with losses over the course of the disease. For patients, losses may be physical, psychosocial, or symbolic. Physical losses are tangible, such as the removal of a breast for a cancer patient or the diminished exertional capacity for a patient with HF. Psychosocial losses are intangible, and often include the loss of future dreams. For family members there may be secondary losses that develop as a consequence of the disease progression and, later, the death of the patient. These secondary losses can be both physical and psychosocial and will affect the roles of both patients and families, such as chauffeur, cook, lover, parent, partner, and breadwinner. According to Rando,[4] all of the various losses must be acknowledged and grieved.

Anticipatory grief includes past, present, and future losses. The past refers to experiences in the past that one has had or shared, and which can never be regained.

Table 20.3 Characteristics of anticipatory grief

Relates to past, present and future losses

Opportunity to prepare emotionally for the patient's death

Catalyst for life closure activities and resolution of relationships

Can be related to grieving past deaths

Does not take the place of grief after the patient's death

A caregiver may mourn the loss of her vibrant, healthy partner as well as unwanted changes in the relationship resulting from the illness. Patients and caregivers alike may experience grief surrounding the realities of an altered lifestyle. Both might reminisce over activities that were shared when the patient was stronger, and mourn the loss of things that have now been taken away.[4]

Present losses include changes that occur and are experienced as a patient's abilities dwindle and eventually cease. There may be frequent hospitalizations, as well as recoveries and relapses. Experiencing the erosion that accompanies the disease progression is part of the mourning of what is currently being lost. The inability to realize hopes and future goals adds another dimension to the anticipatory grief reaction. If anticipated, death is an impending loss and includes related losses such as loneliness and of future events that will never be shared.

Many factors influence the grief of the patient with HF. Lifestyle changes and diminishing abilities are just two of the losses experienced. In addition to anticipatory grief regarding their own situation, many elderly patients are also still grieving the deaths of others they have loved. Because this segment of the population is less likely to receive grief education or counseling,[1] their grief experiences can often become complicated. The acute pains of grief may continue for 2 years after the death of a loved one and there is an increase in mortality for more than 2 years after widowhood.[5] One can literally die of broken heart syndrome.

For families, the cyclical pattern of crisis and recovery that is characteristic of HF can often make the actual death of the patient seem unexpected. Sudden death takes on new meaning when the crisis pattern of recovery is interrupted and death occurs unexpectedly.[6] When there have been multiple rebounds with HF, death may not seem as imminent as it is with patients with cancer or other life-limiting illnesses. These families have become accustomed to living in crisis and recovery mode. Inability to predict the time of death for patients with HF can lead to hope for these families and make it difficult to accept the transition from gravely ill to terminally ill.[7] Due to the unpredictable trajectory of the illness, families may delay seeking hospice or palliative care where they would have bereavement support. The family may have repeatedly experienced grief during multiple crises, but this may or may not mitigate the grief process when death finally occurs. In fact, complications associated with the unpredictability of the disease process may include the bereaved second-guessing decisions made during times of crisis or feeling guilty if they feel their response to a crisis was too slow. This supports the assertion of Goodlin et al.[8] that families would benefit from information to assist them in responding in the event of an emergency.

Many physicians continue to be reluctant to talk about death, dying, and end-of-life care. However, as approximately half of HF patients die within 5 years of diagnosis, some suddenly, physicians must play a part in assisting patients and families in planning for the future.[9] Goodlin et al.[8] state that most patients and families want an active role in decision-making and are interested in receiving information to assist them with understanding and responding to the disease process, although some may chose not to receive information or participate in decisions (see also Chapter 22).

Gottleib[10] notes that for surviving family members the last weeks and moments of a patient's life may be filled with frustration and anger that can hinder the bereavement process. On the other hand, the final days and weeks may be a source of inspiration and strength. Health-care professionals need to skillfully and unhurriedly communicate with patients and their families about death and dying. Rather than experiencing the advanced disease as a time wrought with aggravation and resentment, coping with anticipatory grief can afford families precious time to do end-of-life work. Relationships can be re-established, celebrated, or reconciled, unspoken words may be expressed, and legacy work can be initiated or completed.

For many individuals the task of providing care evolves into a full-time responsibility. Persons in the role of caregiver frequently experience secondary losses as a result of the advanced HF and impending death. Employment, recreation, and social activities may be suspended due to the perceived and real needs of the patient and caregiver. Twenty-four hours a day, caregivers are meeting the needs of their loved one. With the patient's death, grief changes for the caregiver, and feelings associated with the recent responsibilities of caregiving may complicate the grief response. This will be discussed later in the chapter.

Anticipatory grief, being multidimensional and chronological, provides the family with an opportunity to reflect and work through some of the losses that have occurred in the past as well as losses related to the loved one dying and the element of future loss (Table 20.3). The mourning experienced during this time can assist family members to emotionally prepare for a loved one's death. It is important to remember, however, that while anticipatory grief can include a series of significant grieving episodes, it does not negate the existence of grief after the death.[4]

Reactions of bereaved families

To help corroborate the literature, anecdotal information was ascertained from 15 Hospice of the Western Reserve families who had a loved one with a diagnosis of HF who died in 2005. Bereavement counselors assessed these family members as having an uncomplicated grief reaction. After explaining the purpose of the call, the family member was asked some or all of the following questions:

- How well did you understand your loved one's illness?
- What did the hospice team do to help you cope during your loved one's illness?
- What have you continued to think about since your loved one's death?
- Some people have told us they were not ready for their loved one's death while others have expressed a sense of relief. What are your thoughts on this?
- The literature talks about periods of crisis followed by stretches of relief or feeling better, which can lead families to feel that the death is unexpected. Was this true in any way for you?
- What were some of the hard decisions you had to make during your loved one's illness?
- What things do you think have affected your ability to grieve?
- What advice would you give others in a similar situation?

Based on the answers, the authors allowed the bereaved to share their stories, which is a critical part of the healing process. While each individual's experience was unique in some way, several common themes were shared by most or all of those interviewed. These are found in Table 20.4.

Every family interviewed expressed appreciation for the support from the hospice team. They felt comforted, as the hospice team often seemed to appear 'out of nowhere'. Hospice support described included reassurance to the family members and education regarding care and what to expect. Families appreciated knowing what might happen as well as what was occurring during the dying process. Some families expressed knowing that something 'wasn't right', but were unable to articulate the symptomology. Those familiar with the progression of HF were often surprised to learn that their loved one died from kidney failure or had early signs of dementia. They had expected a heart attack. Most felt they would have benefited from hospice care sooner. More than one family expressed that individuals must advocate for themselves and ask the physician about all options in order to receive adequate information. For many reasons, physicians may not always present all available information to the family. Prior to the involvement of the hospice team, one family had obtained most of their information regarding the disease and treatment options from sources on the Internet. Others had also researched disease process and the medications prescribed to their loved one in this manner. This illustrates the need for frank discussions among physicians, patients, and families.

A common trend among several families was the feeling that the patient's death was unexpected. For some, the patient had lived with HF for years and experienced multiple relapses and periods of recovery. Still, many felt they were not ready for the death. One family described a sense of shock when the physician called the entire family into the hospital. They had expected instructions on how to get a bed and to care for their loved one and instead learned that they would returning home with hospice. In contrast, others expressed a sense of relief at the completion of the journey. Older adults who had been providing care for a number of years felt they were prepared for the death and experienced some relief, which validates the study for caregivers of dementia by Schulz et al.[11] Others had experienced past losses, which they felt gave them the strength to cope with this death.

Table 20.4 Common themes of bereaved families

Need for education regarding the disease process

Need for education regarding the grief reaction

The role of support systems

Adjusting to new roles

Anger

Ambivalence

Guilt

Negligence

Family members often discussed their lingering feelings regarding hard decisions that were made during the patient's life. Often, these decisions were made without the benefit of addressing the topic with the patient directly. The feelings related to these choices can complicate the grief reaction. Nursing facility placement was a common topic for some of our families. They described their own inability to adequately care for their loved ones at home, as well as their feelings of remorse or satisfaction with their respective choices. Not surprisingly, this was often related to the quality of care provided by various facilities as well as families' feelings of whether or not the dignity of their loved ones had been maintained. Teno *et al.*[12] concluded that families of persons who were able to remain in their homes until death were more likely to perceive the dying experience as favorable, and reported higher levels of satisfaction and fewer concerns with the care provided to their loved ones. In other settings, families' concerns involved adequate treatment and respect for the dying person, emotional support for the family, and coordination of services. This supports the findings of our interviews.

The loss of relationship was a common theme shared by all families interviewed. All spoke of the qualities of the relationships as they had evolved over the years and throughout the course of the illness. They all spoke often of missing the person who had died, and most mentioned changes to other relationships as a result of the death of the patient. One bereaved spouse indicated that his relationship with his daughter had been strengthened by their shared grief. Other individuals noted the strain on certain relationships brought about by variations in grieving and coping styles. Some people found support through family, friends, church, and lodges. Many utilized the bereavement counseling offered through the hospice, and received home and telephone visits or attended support groups. Just as grief is unique, individuals used varying coping skills including writing a journal, gardening, pet therapy, prescribed medications, and cognitive psychotherapy, among others.

Some of the adult children interviewed had no other family members. While they had friends and other supports, they repeatedly mentioned how others did not want to hear about their grief. Grief counselors and support groups may provide a setting for this aspect of grief work. Table 20.5 shows the determinants of grief after a death.

Table 20.5 Determinants of grief after death

Educational preparedness
Satisfaction regarding difficult decisions
Sudden death versus anticipated death
Level of patient comfort at the time of death
Adequacy of support systems
Quality of the relationship between the patient and the bereaved
Quality of the caregiving experience

Grief reactions and clinical interventions

There is little literature related specifically to bereavement in families of HF patients; however, the concepts of normal grief and interventions appropriate to those experiencing the death of a loved one after other chronic illnesses apply.

We have said that grief is a normal, necessary, and natural response to a loss. Normal grief reactions cover an enormous continuum and individuals' responses will vary

Table 20.6 Reactions in the normal grief experience

Physical reactions in the normal grief experience	Appetite—loss or increase
	Backaches
	Breathing difficulties
	Hyperventilation
	Shallow or shortness of breath
	Chest tightness
	Cold hands
	Dizziness or fainting spells
	Dry mouth
	Fatigue
	Constipation
	Gas
	Diarrhea
	Nausea
	High blood pressure
	Hives, rashes, itching
	Indigestion
	Insomnia
	Low resistance to infection and minor illness
	Muscle tightness
	Nightmares
	Numbness or tingling
	Pounding or rapid heartbeat
	Shaking or trembling
	Altered sleep patterns
	Sighing
	Slowed speech
	Stuttering
	Sweating
	Tearfulness
	Frequent urination
	Voice—change of pitch
	Weakness
	Weight gain or loss
Behavioral and emotional reactions in the normal grief experience	Absent mindedness
	Accident proneness
	Agitation
	Crying
	Fear
	Fingernail biting
	Hair twisting
	Hyper-mobility

Table 20.6 (continued) Reactions in the normal grief experience

	Nightmares
	Indecisiveness
	Grinding teeth
	Treasuring objects of the deceased
	Visiting places of the deceased
	Lack of coordination
	Searching and calling out
	Withdrawal from feelings
	Restlessness
	Irritability
	Loneliness
	Mood swings
Intellectual/cognitive reactions in the normal grief experience	Difficulty concentrating
	Errors in judging distances
	Mispronunciation of words
	Errors in grammar
	Lack of attention to details
	Over-attention to details
	Perfectionism
	Loss of productivity
	Lack of awareness of external events
	Mental 'blocking'
	Forgetfulness
	Confusion

(see Table 20.6). In addition, there is no timetable for grief or predictable steps to follow. While the experience of grief is difficult, we know that, with support, the feelings associated with normal grief typically soften over time, allowing the individual the ability to move forward successfully with his or her life.

Strategies for clinicians to interact with those who are grieving

Validating an individual's grief often normalizes the response. Educating patients and family members about grief responses lets them know that their feelings are common. Health-care providers are often not only hesitant to use the words *death* and *dying*, they are also cautious with the word *grief*. Using these words as part of conversation normalizes their presence. Talking about the losses associated with HF is a good way to begin and can occur prior to death. These losses are more tangible and familiar; not being able to climb the stairs is a recognizable loss. This discussion will assist in the transition towards more symbolic losses that have been and will be experienced. It will also allow opportunities to speak openly about feelings associated with the progression of the disease and eventual death.

Rando[4] suggests several interventions for the bereaved whose loved one has died after a lengthy illness. These would apply to individuals grieving the death of HF patients as well. Strategies include:

- providing the mourner with psychoeducational material to promote understanding of the loss;

- working through guilt and ambivalence that come from the experiences of an extended illness;
- explaining that it is not uncommon for family members to feel surprised when the end comes;
- working through any lingering anger;
- providing extra support and facilitating assumptions of new roles for the mourner.

Because normal grief reactions encompass such a wide range of feelings, the practice of providing psychoeducational material describing the grief process is key. Awareness of what to expect is as helpful in grief recovery as knowledge of the disease process was during the illness of the patient. Most hospice programs provide bereavement literature to the family soon after a death to assist in validating and normalizing the feelings that occur. Family members commonly express the need for reassurance that they are not 'going crazy'. After accepting the loss, working through the pain of grief can be difficult. Grief hurts. The deep feelings of sadness can collide with feelings of anger, ambivalence, and guilt that may accompany families when a loved one has been living for many years with HF. Bereavement counselors can accompany caregivers as they gain insight into these feelings. Counselors can also help individuals process any feelings of surprise for those who experienced the death as unexpected despite enrollment in the hospice. Most importantly, bereavement specialists are able to assess the grief reaction, identify complications, and determine the need for more aggressive treatment.

Assisting family members in the recognition of and response to secondary losses may enable them to adjust to these changes more successfully. As mentioned previously, caregiving has an effect on the anticipatory grief of the caregiver as well as the grief experienced after the patient's death. For some, the role of caregiver was a cherished honor; an opportunity to serve and demonstrate love for the person dying. For others it was a burden fraught with guilt and anger. The qualities of that experience will have an impact on the grief of the caregiver after the patient's death. Some caregivers may feel that the grief experienced prior to death was adequate for their needs and find that they are able to return to life much as it was prior to the advanced stage of the illness. The ability to come and go freely, or to return to work or socialize may be healing. For others, the loss of the caregiving role itself may be a cause for grieving. In addition to missing the person who died, they may now be unsure of their role or how to spend their days. Part of the grief process will be to identify and adjust to a new role after the patient's death.

Assisting individuals with the identification and utilization of support systems is an important function of the bereavement professional. The theme of loneliness is prevalent with many bereaved caregivers, who frequently find support with family, friends, faith communities, and sometimes pets. However, when the grief presented is complicated, it is best to augment that support with a bereavement specialist or counselor. Grief support groups offer an opportunity for members to share their stories, express their feelings, and develop coping strategies. Grief reactions are normalized and members learn that they are not alone.

Table 20.7 Recommended clinical interventions

Normalize and validate grief reaction(s)

Provide bereavement literature and educate on the grieving process

Facilitate sharing of events surrounding the loss and life stories

Encourage life and relationship review

Facilitate discussion of coping strategies

Facilitate development and acceptance of new role

Refer as appropriate for additional counseling

Helping families plan realistically for the future allows for a sense of control. They can advance problem-solving skills and research available resources. People often discuss the need to learn new skills that were unfamiliar to them during the life of their loved one. Financial management, home repair, and car maintenance are just a few of the practical areas bereaved individuals often feel unprepared to face. Support group members often speak with pride about buying a car, balancing a checkbook, or redecorating their homes for the first time without their partners. In contrast, others may express anger and frustration at having to assume new roles. The hospice team can help support and facilitate the development of new skills and acceptance of new roles.

Table 20. 7 provides a summary of the clinical interventions discussed here.

Complicated grief and depression

While even normal grief can be difficult to define, signs of complicated grief and/or depression can be identified and require increased bereavement support and/or involvement of other mental health professionals. Table 20.8 lists the characteristics of complicated grief. Table 20.9 illustrates a comparison between normal grief and depression.

It is important to note that while depression can include grief, grief can also mimic depression. Recognizing the characteristics of each is critical. Grief encompasses a broad spectrum of behaviors and feelings that are common after a loss, which can make differentiating between normal grief, complicated grief, and depression challenging.

Table 20.8 Complicated grief reactions

Absence of grief reaction

Maladaptive behavior and distortion of normal grief reaction

Prolongation or extensive interruption of healing

Minimal or total lack of emotional expression

Prolonged inability to recognize that loss has happened

Extreme reactions (usually anger or guilt) that persist over time

Marked or gradual change in health status (especially symptoms of the deceased)

Prolonged depression

Table 20. 9 Grief versus depression

Normal grief	Clinical depression
Responds to comfort and support	Unable to accept support
Exhibits feelings of sadness and emptiness	Exhibits a pervasive sense of doom
Relates depressed feelings to the loss	Displays a sense of helplessness and chronic emptiness
May have transient physical complaints	Unable to relate feelings and experiences to a particular life event
May express guilt over a specific aspect of the loss	Has generalized feelings of guilt
Rarely suicidal	May have suicidal plans or attempts

Summary and future concerns

Grief and loss for patients with HF and their families is multidimensional and occurs over the continuum of the disease. Hope is often experienced through the subsiding of symptoms during the course of the illness, and families may often feel that the death is a shock. When hospice and palliative care teams are involved, families are educated about what to expect and consequently may feel more prepared.

Physicians and other health-care professionals who are willing to engage in open dialogue about the progression of HF can pave the way for patients and families. This facilitates anticipatory mourning, which can help the patient and family 'rehearse' their grief. It affords time for the entire family to do important end-of-life work, such as life review, reminiscence, completion of unfinished business, and reconciliation. After the death, bereavement support offers the family an opportunity to work through the pain of grief and sort out feelings of lingering anger, ambivalence, and the rollercoaster of emotions that accompany grief. Bereavement support facilitates the adjustment of caregivers learning new skills and gaining experience in new roles.

Grief will accompany the death of a loved one. While it is primarily seen as an unwanted visitor, it can also be an opportunity for growth. Emotional support from family, friends, and health-care providers through this life-altering journey is paramount to healing.

References

1. Sotile W, Miller H (1998). Helping older patients to cope with cardiac and pulmonary disease. *J Cardiopulmon Rehab* **18**: 124–8.
2. Artiman N (2003). The psychosocial aspects of heart failure. *Am J Nurs* **103**: 32–43.
3. Gibbs J, McCoy A, Gibbs A, Addington-Hall JM (2002). Living with and dying from heart failure: the role of palliative care. *Heart* (Suppl II): **88**: ii 36–9.
4. Rando TA (1993). *Treatment of Complicated Mourning*. Champagne, IL: Research Press.
5. Schaefer C, Quesenberry CP, Jr, Wi S (1995). Mortality following conjugal bereavement and the effects of a shared environment. *Am J Epidemiol* **141**: 1142–52.
6. Doka KJ (ed.) (2002). *Disenfranchised Grief: New Directions, Challenges, and Strategies for Practice.* Champagne, IL: Research Press.

7. Quaglietti S, Lovett S, Hawthorne C, Byler A, Atwood JE (2004). Management of the patient with congestive heart failure in the home care and palliative care setting. *Ann Long-Term Care* **12**: 33–7.

8. Goodlin SJ, Hauptman PJ, Arnold R *et al.* (2004). Consensus statement: Palliative and supportive care in advanced heart failure. *J Card Fail* **10**: 200–9.

9. Pantilat SZ, Steimle AE (2004). Palliative care for patients with heart failure. *J Am Med Assoc* **291**: 2476–82.

10. Gottlieb S (2003). Palliative care in heart failure. *Adv Stud Med* **3**: 456–63.

11. Schulz R, Mendelsohn A, Haley W *et al.* (2003). End-of-life care and the effects of bereavement on family caregivers of persons with dementia. *New Engl J Med* **349**: 1934–42.

12. Teno JM, Clarridge BR, Casey V *et al.* (2004). Family perspectives on end-of-life care at the last place of care. *J Am Med Assoc* **291**: 88–93.

Part 3

Prognostication and communication

Chapter 21

Mortality risk assessment and prognostication

Maral Ouzounian, Jack V. Tu, Peter C. Austin, and Douglas S. Lee

Introduction

Heart failure (HF) is a clinical syndrome associated with decreased quality of life and substantial rates of morbidity and mortality.[1–6] The incidence of HF is increasing: more than 550,000 new cases are diagnosed in the United States each year,[5] accounting for an estimated $29.6 billion in direct and indirect costs in 2006.[1] Over 80% of patients hospitalized with HF are more than 65 years old and HF is the number one discharge diagnosis in this age group.[5] From 1993 to 2003, the number of deaths from HF in the United States increased by 20.5% whereas deaths from coronary heart disease were reduced by 14.7% in the same time period.[1]

Despite important advances in its treatment, most patients with clinically evident HF suffer from inexorable disease progression and eventually die a HF-related death. For patients and health-care providers dealing with this chronic and lethal disease, the benefits of reliable estimates of death are considerable. There are, however, several challenges in estimating the likelihood of survival for an individual patient with HF. First, annual mortality rates for HF vary dramatically with the severity of the disease.[7–10] Second, the ultimate mode of death for a given HF patient remains unpredictable, despite a general increase in pump failure deaths as compared to sudden cardiac deaths when progressing from mild to advanced HF.[11–15] Third, the most commonly used estimate of survival, left-ventricular ejection fraction (LVEF), is unreliable for predicting death when it is greater than 45%.[16,17] Finally, the intuitive judgment of physicians in predicting mortality for their HF patients is an inadequate metric for accurate prognostication.[18–20]

Accurate prognostication is a crucial aspect of disease management in HF. As the demand for improved supportive care at the end of life grows, there is a need for physicians to identify the 'terminally ill' and to communicate openly with patients and their families.[21] This may help patients complete advance directives, attend to financial and legal matters, avoid futile interventions, and make better-informed decisions regarding all aspects of their care (see also Chapter 22).[22] A small proportion of patients with advanced HF will benefit from more aggressive intervention with the goal of prolonging life, including mechanical support and cardiac transplantation. For the many patients with HF, however, the emphasis will become symptom control and quality of life.

A clinical prediction rule (CPR) is a risk assessment tool that uses elements of the history, physical examination, or diagnostic tests to aid a clinician in making a diagnosis, predicting an outcome, or taking a therapeutic course of action.[23–27] CPRs may help overcome the limitations of physician intuition by providing a more rational means by which to solve a complex clinical problem.

Risk assessment and prognostication using clinical prediction methods

Methodological standards for developing and evaluating CPRs have been devised by Wasson *et al.*[25] and further modified by Laupacis *et al.*[26] and Reilly and Evans.[27] In brief, the evidentiary standards for a CPR can be categorized from level 1 to level 5, with an increase in level of evidence by the demonstration of wider applicability and clinical impact. The derivation of a CPR (level 1) should include clearly described outcomes, predictive variables, patient characteristics, study sites, statistical techniques, and results. The rule should be reproducible and clinically sensible. Prospective validation in a narrow (level 2) and broad (level 3) setting supports the soundness of the rule in diverse populations. Finally, narrow (level 4) and broad (level 5) impact analyses demonstrate the effect of these clinical tools on patient care.

Ultimately, a CPR may have the potential to 'inform clinical judgment' and to 'change clinical behavior'.[23] Reilly and colleagues evaluated the use of a CPR in helping to triage patients seen in the emergency department with suspected acute cardiac ischemia.[24] They found that the use of a previously developed[28] and validated CPR[29,30] reduced unnecessary admissions to inpatient, monitored beds without compromising patient safety. This type of rigorous impact analysis of a CPR is uncommon and does not exist currently in the HF literature.

Clinicians and researchers need simple and rational ways to assess their patients' prognosis, and, in particular, the risk of death. In this chapter, we review the available clinical methods for mortality risk assessment and prognostication in HF.

Classical predictors of HF mortality

Numerous studies have attempted to determine which factors predict mortality in HF.[31–68] These studies differ in important attributes, which may account for the diversity of the findings. The patients studied vary from those enrolled in highly selective clinical trials to unselected consecutive HF patients in the community, and this wide variance has contributed greater insights into the determinants of prognosis. The potential variables analyzed range from demographic traits available through administrative databases to specialized echocardiographic measurements and neurohormonal levels. Broad knowledge of potential predictors provides the mechanistic insights that underlie the biological rationale for mortality risk prediction tools. Such knowledge may be important for the interpretation of epidemiological observations that are generated by various statistical methods, which delineate associations rather than demonstrate causation.

Nevertheless, despite the heterogeneity of the research available, useful information may be gleaned from a closer examination of these studies. Many potential predictors of HF mortality have been identified (see Table 21.1) and certain variables have been found to be consistently predictive, such as age and renal dysfunction. Several factors reflect the severity of the disease, such as functional class, low ejection fraction, and peak oxygen consumption, whereas others indicate poor peripheral vascular or pathogenic cardiorenal interactions. Despite the high lethality of HF, other coexisting co-morbid conditions and the attendant occurrence of end-organ damage are frequently implicated in mortality prediction models.

Large randomized trials of pharmacological therapy in HF have confirmed the association of poor functional class, most commonly described by New York Heart Association (NYHA) criteria, with decreased survival. Symptoms range from NYHA Class I, with no limitation during ordinary activity, to NYHA Class IV, an inability to carry out any activity without symptoms, or symptoms at rest. Annual mortality rates have been found to range from 5% for NYHA Class I patients,[8] to 75% with advanced (NYHA Class III–IV) symptoms;[9,10] however, there may be large variations in mortality within each group. Although NYHA class seems practical as a tool for risk assessment, more

Table 21.1 The spectrum of potential predictors of HF mortality

Clinical data (history and physical examination)	Demographic factors: age, sex Clinical characteristics: functional class, prior decompensation, duration of HF, ischemic etiology Co-morbidity: diabetes, hypertension, peripheral vascular disease, depression, cerebrovascular disease, chronic obstructive pulmonary disease, cirrhosis, dementia, cancer Physical examination: tachycardia, tachypnea, low blood pressure (systolic or diastolic), low body mass index, cachexia, S3, pulmonary rales, peripheral edema
Basic assessment	Routine laboratory values: urea nitrogen, creatinine, hyponatremia, anemia, per cent lymphocytes, uric acid, cholesterol Electrocardiogram: long QRS duration, left-ventricular hypertrophy Chest X-ray: cardiothoracic ratio, pulmonary edema, pleural effusion Global function: health status questionnaire, 6-min walk
Specialized assessment	LV function: radionuclide angiography, echocardiogram, ventriculography Echocardiogram: chamber dimensions, diastolic function, mitral regurgitation, right-ventricular function Assessment of VO₂max Coronary angiogram: presence and extent of coronary disease Invasive hemodynamics: cardiac index, pulmonary artery pressure, pulmonary capillary wedge pressure, right-atrial pressure, systemic vascular resistance Electrophysiology testing: non-sustained ventricular tachycardia, other ventricular arrhythmias, T wave alternans, low heart rate variability, QTc dispersion, atrial fibrillation/flutter Biomarkers: BNP, norepinephrine, troponin, inflammatory markers

objective measures of functional capacity, such as oxygen consumption at peak exercise (VO_2 max), may be more reliable. HF patients with a VO_2 max of less than 10–12 ml kg^{-1} min^{-1} have consistently been shown to have a poor prognosis.[35,69] Thus, this measure is used routinely as a selection criterion for cardiac transplantation.

Reduced LVEF, as measured by echocardiography, radionuclide angiography, or ventriculography, has long been recognized as a predictor of mortality. Although LVEF is a powerful prognostic tool, a multivariate approach is more likely to yield predictive instruments with greater discriminative ability for a given individual. There is also no predictable correlation between symptoms or exercise tolerance and LVEF, and its relationship to mortality is not linear when LVEF exceeds 45%.[16,17] Additionally, like most variables, LVEF can lose discriminatory power when a very narrow range of values is studied, for example in patients with severe systolic dysfunction. Other factors, such as concomitant diastolic dysfunction, particularly a restrictive pattern by mitral inflow, can add to the prediction of mortality in patients with HF and reduced LVEF.[70,71] Other echocardiographic findings, including left-ventricular dilatation, left-ventricular mass, the severity of mitral regurgitation, and right-ventricular dysfunction have also been associated with reduced survival in HF.[72–74]

Neurohormonal activation, principally through the closely linked sympathetic and renin–angiotensin systems, has been proposed as a key mechanism underlying the progression of HF. Patients with HF have increased sympathetic tone resulting in increased plasma norepinephrine levels, which is thought to contribute directly to the pathogenesis of HF.[35,75,76] Sympathetic stimulation also reduces vagal activity, contributing to the prognostically important manifestations of autonomic dysfunction seen in HF. Resting tachycardia, reduced heart rate variability, and a blunted heart rate response to exercise each predict increased mortality in these patients.[34,58–62] Hyponatremia and increased levels of plasma renin, angiotensin II, aldosterone, atrial natriuretic factor, and endothelin-1 are other indicators of neurohormonal activation that reflect worsened HF prognosis (see also Chapter 3).[68,77,78]

The predictive value of B-type natriuretic peptide (BNP) in HF has been systematically reviewed by Doust and colleagues[63] who found it to be a consistently strong predictor of mortality and adverse cardiac events. They estimated an overall increase in risk of death by 35% per 100 pg ml^{-1} increment in serum levels of BNP. Interestingly, BNP was also found to predict mortality in several studies of asymptomatic patients. BNP is released from the ventricles in response to volume expansion or pressure overload and may be an indicator of an adaptive response to the pathophysiological sequelae of HF.[64] The functional properties of BNP may affect both pump failure and arrhythmogenesis as mechanisms of death in HF.[63–66]

Several studies have highlighted the contribution of ischemic etiology to HF mortality. A significant proportion of sudden deaths may be the arrhythmic consequence of an ischemic event, and progressive pump failure over time may reflect recurrent ischemic insults. The extent of coronary disease contributes more prognostic information than its presence.[37] Hypertension and diabetes may importantly predict prognosis via their association with ischemic heart disease as well as their direct myocardial effects.[37]

Impaired renal function is one of the strongest predictors of mortality in HF.[44–47,79] Renal function has been quantified by serum creatinine concentration, blood urea nitrogen concentration, creatinine clearance, or estimated glomerular filtration rate. Among the potential contributory factors, impaired renal function may reflect the compromised hemodynamics of severe cardiac failure or it may be a marker of coexistent disease, such as hypertension, diffuse vascular disease or potentially drug-related toxic effects. Renal dysfunction may limit the use of therapies such as angiotensin-converting enzyme (ACE) inhibitors and prevent symptom relief from diuresis. Many of the neurohormones discussed earlier, including endothelin-1 and the natriuretic peptides, modulate renal perfusion independent of central hemodynamics.[80,81] Finally, data supporting the cardiorenal interaction suggest that renal insufficiency may play a causative role in progressive ventricular dysfunction, possibly through impaired clearance of sodium and fluid, leading to elevated cardiac filling pressures and ventricular dilation.[45]

Anemia is common in HF patients and is associated with increased mortality.[48–51,82,83] Reduced hemoglobin may be partly caused by hemodilution secondary to volume overload, malnutrition from cardiac cachexia, renal insufficiency, or it may be a direct effect of drugs such as ACE inhibitors.[51] Increased levels of cytokines that are components of the HF milieu may also interfere with erythropoiesis.[83] The Randomized etanercept North American Strategy to Study Antagonism of Cytokines (RENAISSANCE) trial randomized patients with moderate to severe HF to receive either placebo or the tumour necrosis factor-alpha antagonist etanercept. Patients with lower levels of hemoglobin enrolled in RENAISSANCE had an increased left-ventricular mass index, one of the earliest indications of a potential causal relationship of anemia to HF progression through adverse left-ventricular remodeling.[82]

Additionally, global measures reflecting quality of life have gained attention as potential indicators of prognosis in HF,[54–57] providing additional information to standard biological measures. How a patient perceives the impact of the disease, for example on daily activity level or satisfaction with social life, may influence mortality.[56] The association of major depression with mortality in HF may be mediated by poor social contact, a lack of support networks, non-compliance with medications, and the poor functional status of these patients.[38–41] A small study of outpatients with systolic dysfunction found that social support, exemplified by the quality of a patient's marital life, may have a significant impact on survival.[36] Further probing into the impact of health status and social constructs may broaden our classic treatment strategies, focusing more on patient-centered care and outcome measures.

HF mortality scores

Risk stratification of patients based on a single clinical or laboratory parameter is likely to have limited accuracy and reproducibility. It is impractical to rank the predictive variables discussed in the previous section by relative importance unless all such predictors can be assessed simultaneously in one overarching statistical model. Potentially more accurate prognostication for HF patients may result from multivariable

CPRs, and many have been developed and published.[84–93] There are several considerations when choosing a CPR for potential clinical use. An ideal CPR would: (1) incorporate several easily obtainable, independent, non-invasive variables; (2) have maximum discriminatory power; and (3) have been reliably derived and validated in representative target populations. A temporally adaptable CPR could potentially permit the incorporation of newly discovered prognostic variables, treatments, and changes in clinical status to the model.[94] An ideal CPR should be user-friendly and may identify a clinically useful threshold such as the need for transplantation, hospital admission, or an alternative approach to management.

General comments on mortality prediction in HF

In this section we review 10 published HF mortality scores (see Tables 21.2 and 21.3), and in this overview we have attempted to capture diverse populations and methodologies in order to portray the breadth of available prognostic models. The user of these CPRs should bear in mind that each of these predictive instruments has been developed for use in distinct clinical circumstances and patient populations, since none of these have as yet demonstrated the wide spectrum transportability required to be a universal measure of HF risk. Of equal importance is the need for the user to heed the particular outcome and the time horizon of predicted risk when evaluating a score for potential clinical use. Finally, it is anticipated that any CPR will be more effectively utilized when the applications are tempered by good clinical judgment.

Among the published HF mortality prediction methodologies, notable differences exist in study settings and patient selection methods. Hospitalized HF patients represent, by definition, a more acute, decompensated state of HF than ambulatory patients, who have more stable, chronic HF. Hospitalized patients with acute decompensated HF are potentially more symptomatic, having warranted more careful observation or aggressive treatment than could be provided as an outpatient. There are also likely to be marked dissimilarities between patients enrolled in randomized controlled trials (RCTs) and the patient samples available in community-based studies. Patients in RCTs are often younger and have less co-morbidity. Thus far, RCTs have typically focused on patients with systolic HF and depressed LVEF, and thus there is a growing emphasis on experimental trial designs incorporating a distinct set of enrollees with diastolic HF.[95] RCTs have also generally tended to exclude patients with less common secondary causes of HF, such as infiltrative disease, valvular dysfunction, and viral or toxin-induced cardiomyopathy. The end result of these restrictions is to create a relatively homogeneous group of HF patients, which is desirable when determining the effect of specific treatment interventions but which may limit the wide applicability of a CPR derived from such a randomized trial population.

The outcome of interest should be considered carefully when assessing a CPR for use. Short-term (in-hospital or 30-day) mortality estimates may be useful for physicians involved in triaging HF patients to an inpatient bed of varying monitoring intensity or a researcher designing a trial interested in short-term outcomes. In one study, 'serious medical complications that occurred during the index hospitalization' were added as

Table 21.2 Broadly validated HF mortality clinical prediction rules

Study	Population studied[a]	Outcome	Predictive variables	Methodology, performance measured in external validation[b]
Heart Failure Survival Score, 1997[84]	Outpatient Community-based SHF	Death or urgent transplantation	Ischemic cardiomyopathy, ↑resting heart rate LVEF, QRS duration ≥ 0.12 s, ↓ mean resting BP, VO₂max, hyponatremia	Logistic regression. AUC (1-year): 0.76 ± 0.04
EFFECT-HF model, 2003[85]	Inpatient Community-based SHF and DHF	30-day and 1-year mortality	↑Age, ↓systolic BP, ↑RR, hyponatremia, ↑BUN, cerebrovascular disease, COPD, cirrhosis, dementia, and cancer. Anaemia only for 1-year model	Logistic regression. AUC: 0.79 (30day), 0.76 (1-year)
ADHERE Registry, 2005[86]	Inpatient Community-based SHF and DHF	In-hospital mortality	By CART: ↑BUN, ↓systolic BP, and ↑creatinine. By multivariate logistic regression: ↑BUN, ↓systolic BP, ↑heart rate, ↑and age	Logistic regression and CART. AUC CART: 0.67, Logistic regression: 0.76
Seattle Heart Failure Model, 2006[87]	Outpatient Mostly RCTs Mostly SHF	1-, 2-, and 3-year survival free of death, LVAD, or transplantation	↑NYHA class, ischemic etiology, ↑diuretic dose, ↓LVEF, ↓systolic BP, hyponatrema, anamia, per cent lymphocytes, ↑uric acid, ↓cholesterol, ↓statin use, ↑allopurinol use	Logistic regression. Overall: AUC 0.729 (95% CI 0.714 to 0.744)
Digitalis Group Study, 2004[91]	Outpatient RCT SHF	1-year mortality	↓LVEF, ↑creatinine, cardiothoracic ratio >50%, ↑NYHA class, signs or symptoms of HF, ↓BP, ↓BMI, diabetes–ischemic etiology interaction	Bayesian approach. Goodness of fit test for predicted vs. observed mortality at 1 year: P = 0.14

[a] Ambulatory vs. outpatient; randomized controlled trial (RCT) vs. community-based; systolic HF (SHF) vs. systolic and diastolic HF (DHF).

[b] Externally validated cohort.

Abbreviations: BBB, bundle branch block; BMI, body mass index; BP, blood pressure; BUN, blood urea nitrogen; CAD, coronary artery disease; CI, confidence interval; COPD, chronic obstructive pulmonary disease; CVA, cerebrovascular accident; CXR, chest X-ray; EKG, electrocardiogram; Hb, hemoglobin; LVAD, left-ventricular assist device; LVEF, left-ventricular ejection fraction; LVH, left-ventricular hypertrophy; MI, myocardial infarction; MR, mitral regurgitation; NSVT, non-sustained ventricular tachycardia; NYHA, New York heart Association; PTCA, percutaneous transluminal coronary angioplasty; RR, respiratory rate; SDNN, standard deviation of all normal-to-normal RR intervals; WBC, white blood cell.

Table 21.3 Internally validated HF mortality clinical prediction rules

Study	Population studied[a]	Outcome	Predictive variables[b]	Methodology, performance measures†
BNP Score, 2005[88]	Outpatient Community-based SHF and DHF	Death from any cause	↑ BNP, age, CVA, male, diabetes, abnormal EKG	Logistic regression Corrected by bootstrap: 0.748
CHARM Score, 2006[89]	Outpatient RCT SHF and DHF	Death from any cause (primary outcome was CV death or hospitalization)	↑Age, diabetes, ↓ LVEF, ↓BMI, male, NYHA class III or IV, current smoker, BBB, ↑ cardiothoracic ratio, prior HF hospitalizations, ↓diastolic BP, HF diagnosis > 2 yrs, prior MI, edema, tachycardia, pulmonary rales, pulmonary edema on CXR, MR, atrial fibrillation, shortness of breath at rest	Logistic regression. Corrected by bootstrap: 0.74
OPTIME-CHF 2004[90]	Inpatient RCT SHF	60-day mortality	↑ Age,↓ systolic BP, NYHA class IV, ↑BUN, hyponatremia	Logistic regression Corrected by bootstrap: 0.76
UK-HEART, 2003[92]	Outpatient Community-based Mostly SHF	Death from any cause	Hyponatremia ↑ creatinine, cardiothoracic ratio ≥ 0.52 ↓SDNN, ↓ QTc, ↑ QRS dispersion, NSVT, LVH voltage criteria on EKG	Logistic regression Dichotomous model: C-statistic 0.74 C-Parameter estimates: statistic 0.78
ER Study, 2005[93]	Inpatient Community-based SHF and DHF	In-hospital mortality or serious complication	Male, history of CAD, angina, PTCA, diabetes, lung disease, ↓ systolic BP, ↑ heart rate, ↑ RR, ↑ temperature, ↑ BUN, ↓ sodium, ↑ potassium, ↑ creatinine, ↑ glusoce, ↑ WBC, ↓ pH, MI or ischemia on EKG, pleural effusion or pulmonary edema	CART Not described

a Ambulatory vs. outpatient; RCT vs. community-based; systolic vs. systolic and diastolic HF.

b Internally validated cohort.

† Abbreviations: BBB, bundle branch block; BMI, body mass index; BP, blood pressure; BUN, blood urea nitrogen; CAD, coronary artery disease; COPD, chronic obstructive pulmonary disease; CV, cardiovascular; CVA, cerebrovascular accident; CXR, chest X-ray; EKG, electrocardiogram; Hb, hemoglobin; LVH, left ventricular hypertrophy; MI, myocardial infarction; MR, mitral regurgitation; NSVT, non-sustained ventricular tachycardia; NYHA, New York Heart Association; PTCA, percutaneous transluminal coronary angioplasty; RR, respiratory rate; SDNN, standard deviation of all normal-to-normal RR intervals; WBC, white blood cell.

composite outcomes to in-hospital mortality, in order to better aid emergency department physicians when deciding upon admission or discharge for a patient with HF.[93] Longer-term (1-, 2-, and 3-year) mortality outcomes may be more relevant for physicians who are assessing outpatients in HF clinics or in general practice. Other groups have included treatments into a risk score, which could potentially result in confounding when the biases related to treatment are not fully considered. The inclusion of other potentially important endpoints such as left-ventricular assist device placement or cardiac transplantation may also be of potential clinical interest.[84,87]

HF mortality prediction methodologies

The variables included in a CPR can vary widely in their practicality. Specifically, invasive diagnostic tests, such as electrophysiological assessment and right-heart catheterization, carry a small but significant degree of risk inherent in the procedure. Aaronson et al.[84] compared two models that incorporated either non-invasive or invasive variables which were each derived from among a total of 80 clinical variables, and found that discrimination of the models was similar. A limitation of models that require invasive variables is that some facilities may not offer certain biochemical assays or diagnostic tests, therefore limiting general use. For example, despite the utility of maximal VO_2 information, patients may not be able to perform such testing.

The Heart Failure Survival Score (HFSS) was the first report that studied patients with advanced HF, in which a CPR for survival was derived and then prospectively validated in a separate group of patients.[84] The study sample included ambulatory patients who were young [mean age, 50 ± 11 (standard deviation, SD) years], mostly male (80%), with systolic HF (mean LVEF, 20 ± 8%), and were being considered for cardiac transplantation. The model was developed prior to the wider adoption of current therapies with mortality implications, such as β-adrenoreceptor antagonists (10% of study patients were on such therapy) and cardiac resynchronization therapy. These factors could have a direct impact on predictors (e.g. heart rate and intraventricular conduction delay) that were included in the final HFSS model. Notably, the HFSS is one of the few CPRs that imply a clinical decision. The authors suggest that 'transplantation (could) be safely deferred in patients in the low-risk group', in whom the 1-year event-free survival rates in the validation sample were 88 ± 4%—a survival rate that could be considered to be better than that expected with heart transplantation.

The investigators of the Enhanced Feedback For Effective Cardiac Treatment (EFFECT) study examined a broad sample of patients who were hospitalized with a primary diagnosis of HF.[85] The authors chose candidate variables routinely available at the time of hospital presentation, and the final model predictors included age, vital signs, standard laboratory values, and co-morbid conditions. The population used to derive and validate the model reflected a broad, community-based HF study, with elderly patients (mean age, 76.3 ± 11.2 years), women (50.5%), and a substantial inclusion of patients with diastolic HF (47.2%). The mortality prediction model stratified patients into quintiles of risk for both 30-day and 1-year mortality, with potential utility for acute-care decisions and longer-term planning based on expected mortality up to 1 year of follow-up (http://www.ccort.ca/CHFriskmodel.aspx).

The Seattle Heart Failure Model was derived using patients from the Prospective Randomized Amlodipine Survival Evaluation (PRAISE-1) trial and was validated across five additional cohorts from 46 countries.[87] This model evaluated ambulatory patients, mostly from RCTs, although validation was performed in one cohort of HF clinic patients (University of Washington) and another of general cardiology clinic patients (Italian Heart Failure Registry). The Seattle model is potentially most relevant for outpatients with systolic HF. Only about 2% of the patients studied had diastolic HF (approximately 300 of 11,067 patients evaluated). Although age and renal function were univariate predictors of mortality, they were not independent predictors in the final multivariable model. Co-morbid conditions were not available and may potentially add prognostic value to this score. The Seattle model incorporates a wide range of clinical variables and, unlike most scores, incorporates medications and device therapies. In addition to risk stratification, this CPR allows health-care providers to calculate the predicted benefit of a therapy if added (http://depts.washington.edu/shfm/).

Despite the strong evidence supporting the prognostic value of BNP, it has been incorporated into HF CPRs to only a limited degree. The population studied by Adlam et al.[88] was 75 ± 10 years of age, 41% male, with an LVEF ranging from less than 25% to greater than 55%. As a continuous variable, BNP was found to be an independent predictor of mortality, although the cause of death was non-cardiac (e.g. lung disease, cancer) in 43% of cases. As acknowledged by the study authors, interpretation of the BNP scoring system is potentially limited by the selection methods used in designing the model. The investigators included all patients prescribed loop diuretics in general practice, and therefore may have enrolled patients treated with diuretics for indications other than HF.

The model created by the UK-HEART investigators attempted to integrate the autonomic, electrical, mechanical, and neurohormonal factors known to affect HF prognosis.[92] In this study, the mean age of the patients was 62.7 ± 9.7 years, 76% were male, and the mean LVEF was $42 \pm 17\%$. All patients underwent 24-h electrocardiographic monitoring as well as echocardiography. NYHA Class IV HF patients were excluded from the study, and 79% of patients had an ischemic HF etiology. In the UK-HEART model, six of the nine final variables were electrical, including low standard deviation of all normal-to-normal RR intervals (an estimate of heart rate variability), increased QTc interval duration, increased QRS dispersion, the presence of non-sustained ventricular tachycardia, and left-ventricular hypertrophy. Interestingly, age and LVEF were not independently predictive of mortality.

Considerations in the development of HF risk prediction models

As progressive developments in HF care occur and as new needs for prediction are identified, refinement or development of novel risk prediction models may be needed. In such cases, there are several methodological considerations involved in creating a new

CPR. The first point of consideration in the development of a CPR is the clinical context and the patient population to which the rule would apply. Identification of an appropriate source of data for patients who are at a well-defined inception point in their disease is of importance for future clinical applications and subsequent model validation. The selection of candidate predictor variables for risk assessment models should be based on a review of the literature and should be clinically and biologically plausible markers of prognosis. Careful consideration should also be given to covariates that may be indicators of treatment. For example, use of a pharmacological agent may be an important indicator of future prognosis, but is, as expected, often confounded as a prognostic factor since more severely ill patients may not be able to tolerate treatment. Risk assessment methods that include treatments as a predictor cannot be used to determine the relationship between risk and treatment rates.[96]

The majority of the 10 CPRs in Tables 21.2 and 21.3 used multivariable regression analysis to create their prognostic indices. This technique quantifies the relationship between multiple covariates (i.e. predictors) and the outcome of interest (i.e. mortality).[97–99] The selection of a limited number of predictors for inclusion in the model should be based on both statistical and clinical significance. The limitations of multivariable models which select covariates based on stepwise selection methods have been well described and are beyond the scope of this chapter.[100] The selection of potential covariates that are biologically plausible in the model design stage may improve its performance and face validity. Model performance can be improved by determining the shape and strength of associations of continuous variables with outcomes of interest by examining polynomial splines.[101] Ultimately, parsimonious models with high predictive accuracy are more likely to be used in clinical practice. An excessive number of model covariates may result in overfitting of multiple regression models, resulting in decreased likelihood of withstanding external validation.[101,102]

Although multiple regression analysis is commonly used for predictive modeling, other methods have also been applied to create prognostic indices. The Acute Decompensated Heart Failure Registry (ADHERE) study investigators derived their model through both classification and regression tree (CART) analysis and multiple logistic regression, providing readers with a choice of two different models.[86] The authors proposed that the CART method is well suited to generating CPRs because it can handle numerical data that are highly skewed or multimodal and categorical predictors with either an ordinal or non-ordinal structure.[86] CART is based on recursive partitioning analysis and produces decision trees composed of progressive binary splits.[86] However, recent research has shown that, in the context of predicting mortality from acute myocardial infarction, CART did not perform as well as conventional logistic regression.[103] The Digitalis Investigators' Group (DIG) used Bayesian model averaging, suggesting that 'stepwise approaches often have difficulty distinguishing between competing models, ignore the uncertainty involved in multivariate model selection, and may overfit models'.[91]

Model performance is evaluated through measures of discrimination and calibration. Discrimination refers to the ability to distinguish between patients who do or do not develop an event and is commonly quantified by a concordance statistic (c, c-statistic or c-index). In logistic regression, c is equivalent to the area under the receiver operating characteristic curve (AUC).[104] The c-index ranges from 0.5 to 1.0, the former meaning no discriminative ability and the latter representing perfect ability to distinguish between patients with and without an event. Calibration refers to whether the predicted probabilities agree with the observed probabilities and may be quantified by goodness-of-fit statistics. Performance measures were described for all of the HF CPRs with the exception of the ER study.[93]

Predictive models should be assessed for their internal and external validity.[105] Internal validity is assessed using the same sample from which the model was derived, whereas external validity examines the model in external population samples. The established methodological standards for CPRs underscore the importance of validation. Five of the ten models reviewed in this chapter achieved level 3 evidence as detailed by Reilly and Evans, meaning that they have been broadly validated (see Table 21.2).[27] The CPRs of the HFSS, EFFECT, ADHERE, Seattle, and DIG studies[84–87,91] have been validated internally and externally.[23] Other studies (e.g. BNP, CHARM, OPTIME-CHF, UK-HEART, ER Study[88–90,92,93]) have yet to be validated and therefore achieve only the level 1 evidentiary standard (see Table 21.3). Reproducibility or internal validation of a predictive model requires the system to 'replicate its accuracy in patients who were not included in development of the system but who are from the same underlying population'.[106] This reflects the potential for models to be overfitted to random noise, rather than true associations. The methods of internal validation for clinical risk prediction include split-sample, cross-validation, jackknife, and bootstrapping techniques, all of which estimate how model performance is affected when applied to a resampling of *similar* patients as the derivation sample. Among these, bootstrap resampling may be preferable because of the low bias compared with other internal validation methods.[107] In general, CPRs that are only internally validated should be applied, preferably prospectively, to a different population before being widely used.

External validity pertains to generalizability or transportability of the model.[106] Transportability requires that the model be able to produce accurate predictions in a sample drawn from a different but plausibly related population, using slightly different methods from those used in the derivation sample. Reduced transportability can result from omission of important outcome predictors from the model, or historical or geographical differences between the derivation sample and the newly tested sampled. Follow-up transportability implies that the model retains its predictive accuracy when applied to different durations of observation for outcome events. Spectrum transportability implies that the model predicts outcome in a broad range of disease severities. Among the HF mortality prediction models, the AUCs generally deteriorated with external validation and ranged from a low of 0.73 (95% CI 0.71, 0.74) in the Seattle HF model to a high of 0.79 (30-day EFFECT-HF model). For the externally validated cohorts in ADHERE, the accuracy of the CART model (AUC 0.67) was less than that of the more complicated logistic regression model (AUC 0.76).

Summary of HF mortality prediction

In summary, before implementing a CPR, a physician or researcher should consider a number of factors: the characteristics of the population, the feasibility of obtaining the specified variables, and the relevance of the primary outcome. The level of evidence (as per the methodological standards described above) and the performance statistics of the model are also important attributes. Some older CPRs do not incorporate what is now considered standard HF therapy and may already be outdated. A balance of parsimony and accuracy must exist for a model to be useful from the clinical and research standpoint. Some HF CPRs offer normograms for risk estimation whereas others require a computer-based calculation and provide online links with a web-based interface. Finally, it should be noted that none of the published HF CPRs have undergone any form of impact analysis. Therefore, it is unclear whether implementing these CPRs would have a measurable effect on patient care.

Special populations

Unlike the more uniform risk factors and mechanisms underlying ischemic heart disease, HF is a clinical syndrome that represents an eventual maladaptive response to a diverse array of etiologies and hemodynamic stresses. As such, mortality risk assessment and prognostication must consider the heterogeneity of the disease. HF with preserved LVEF, also referred to as diastolic HF (DHF), is increasingly recognized as an important clinical entity, representing up to half of all HF patients.[108–111] Recent publications have countered the commonly held belief that patients with DHF have better outcomes than patients with systolic HF.[112,113] The morbidity and mortality associated with DHF are substantial, and better tools for prognostication are important in this subgroup.

The majority of the scores developed from RCTs focus predominantly on systolic HF (Seattle, OPTIME-CHF, the Digitalis Study[87,90,91]), whereas most of the community based CPRs include a significant proportion of patients (up to half) with DHF (EFFECT, ADHERE, BNP[85,86,88]). As the molecular mechanisms contributing to DHF become better understood, there is some evidence supporting DHF as a separate pathophysiological entity.[114,115] Mortality CPRs limited to patients with DHF could identify unique risk factors and potentially modifiable therapeutic targets for the development of new treatment strategies. CPRs with well-defined or substantial proportions of patients with known secondary causes of HF, such as valvular disease, are currently unavailable.

There are data to suggest that despite recognized concerns regarding the need to diversify, clinical trials continue to poorly represent women, the elderly, and non-white ethnic populations.[116–119] A review of RCTs of interventions for chronic HF published in Medline between 1985 and 1999 found that many government-funded trials underrepresented the populations that carry the burden of the disease.[116] Only two trials (3%) during the study period achieved a mean age and gender distribution (75 years and at least 50% respectively) approximating that of the general HF population; only four trials (7%) included at least 25% non-white participants. The pathophysiology of HF as well as its outcomes vary as a function of age, sex, and race, and CPRs based on RCTs that under-represent these subgroups may not be generalizable.

HF is a disease of the elderly and it is anticipated that the occurrence of this condition in the aging population will become more prevalent in the next decade.[120] More than 80% of HF deaths and prevalent cases are among people over 65 years of age, and HF is the most common reason for hospitalization in elderly patients.[121] The prevalence of HF rises from 2–3% at age 65 to more than 15% in persons older than 80 years of age.[122–125] Age also remains one of the strongest independent predictors of mortality. Changes in left-ventricular relaxation and filling also occur with age, and therefore HF with preserved systolic function is common in the elderly. The cumulative effects of age-related co-morbid conditions further complicate HF care in the elderly, with an increasing prevalence of coexistent hypertension, coronary artery disease, dyslipidemia, atrial fibrillation, and diabetes mellitus in elderly patients. The clinical presentation of HF in the elderly may also present a diagnostic challenge, with greater likelihood of presenting with non-specific symptoms such as fatigue and decreased exercise tolerance (see also Chapter 17).[126,127] Additionally, cognitive impairment, frailty, and depression are more prevalent in the elderly and are independently associated with increased mortality (see also Chapters 14 and 15).[128–130] Given the above, predictive models for elderly patients in intensive care units have incorporated measures of nutritional, cognitive, and functional status.[131] In sum, HF in the elderly is underdiagnosed, undertreated, and poorly studied.[120,132] Models for HF mortality in the elderly are lacking and could guide clinicians, patients, and their families in determining appropriate approaches to care.

Although the overall prevalence of HF is similar among men and women, male patients significantly outnumber female patients younger than 75 years of age, but opposite trends are observed in HF patients older than 75 years.[133] Women account for a greater proportion of those with diastolic HF, which may partly account for their under-representation in large HF trials of systolic dysfunction. Hypertension, diabetes mellitus, and smoking may be more potent risk factors for the development of HF in women than in men.[134] The effect of gender on survival in HF is a topic of some debate.[135–138] Some large epidemiological studies, including the Framingham Heart Study[7] and the National Health and Nutrition Examination Survey Epidemiological Follow-Up Study (NHANES1),[139] have found a protective effect of female gender on survival in HF; however, counter observations have been reported.[8] Mechanistically, there is biological rationale for an improved prognosis in women because they have a more favorable response to pressure overload, reduced myocyte necrosis and apoptosis, and less maladaptive activation of the sympathetic and renin–angiotensin systems.[135] Further work will clearly be required to elucidate the mechanisms behind possible gender-determined differences in HF survival. As with DHF and elderly populations, representation of women in CPRs derived from community-based studies is greater than those based on RCTs.

Population differences in health-care outcomes exist across ethnic groups.[140] Ethnic minorities have poorer overall health status than non-minorities and differences in the quality of health care as well as access to health care also exist. Outcomes in HF have been noted to differ between ethnic groups, with variations in mortality, treatment-seeking behavior, and hospitalizations (See Chapter 25).[141–146] Further research is needed in order to dissect the contributing causes of these disparities including interactions between social, genetic, environmental, and lifestyle factors. Only by studying these differences can we identify measures which can reduce the disparities to improve health in all populations. Currently, CPRs do not distinguish between ethnicities, and predictive tools derived from RCTs have traditionally underrepresented minority populations.

In order to broaden the representation of women and ethnic minority groups, mandates were issued by the National Institutes of Health in 1994 to increase these participant groups in clinical trials, and by the Food and Drug Administration to include geriatric and pediatric subjects.[147–149] These factors relating to generalizability of CPRs may need to be considered when such tools are developed and applied in practice.

Impact of HF prognostication on supportive care

There is a clear need for knowledge that allows one to determine whether a patient with HF is entering a pre-terminal phase of illness.[21,22,150–152] Once a terminal condition is identified, reducing the burden of illness for patients and their families may take precedence over the sometimes competing goal of prolonging life. Symptom relief and quality of life have been identified as a vital aspect of care by patients and their families (see Chapter 19).[153,154] From the Study to Understand Prognoses and Preferences for Outcomes and Risks of Treatment (SUPPORT), we learned that during exacerbations of HF, a patient's functional status declines dramatically, but often improves through the ensuing months.[155] In SUPPORT, 36% of seriously ill hospitalized patients felt the care they received was inconsistent with their preferences.[156] Open discussions with patients regarding care preferences must be had when considering treatment strategies. Given the possibility of sudden death and the imperfect nature of current tools for prognostication, communication regarding end-of-life planning should start soon after a diagnosis of HF.

Identifying patients near death is a necessary step in the referral of HF patients to hospice care. Only about 10% of patients enrolled in hospice have a diagnosis of HF.[22] To be eligible, patients must have a physician who will direct their care and must be expected to survive for 6 months or less. Goodlin and colleagues[157] have identified barriers to hospice care for HF patients, including a lack of staff knowledge and expertise in HF as well as inadequate identification of palliative treatments. Hospice care is an underused service that may provide important support for patients and respite for caregivers. Tools for mortality risk assessment may improve physicians' confidence in their prognostic ability and readiness to refer patients to a hospice.

Patients and caregivers must understand the life-limiting nature of HF. Physicians may be reluctant to discuss prognosis, potentially because they may be errant in their predictions [19,158] Most patients, however, welcome the opportunity to discuss end-of-life issues,[159] and armed with more information, they may be able to plan appropriately for their future (see Chapter 19). Recent HF guidelines have stressed the importance of integrating optimal medical management with palliative care, including frank discussion regarding prognosis, cardiopulmonary resuscitation, advance directives, symptom management, and hospice care.[4,6]

Conclusion

HF mortality risk assessment and prognostication is an area of rapid evolution. Common predictors of mortality include demographic factors and characteristics that reflect the severity of HF, neurohormonal activation, co-morbid conditions, and measures of quality of life. Univariate predictors have limited accuracy and reproducibility when used alone. Multivariable clinical prediction rules for HF mortality have been developed that attempt to mathematically combine several parameters to aid physicians and researchers in prognostication. In assessing these CPRs, one must consider the setting of the study as well as the selection of patients, variables, and the outcome of interest. The techniques used to create the model, performance statistics, and internal and external validity must be evaluated. Established methodological standards for evaluating CPRs have been developed and may guide this assessment. Finally, the need for CPRs relevant to those with diastolic HF, women, elderly, and non-white populations should be acknowledged.

HF is a chronic disease that has a high rate of progression to death, and as such demands supportive care. Accurate prognostication and mortality risk assessment is a challenging yet crucial component of providing compassionate and comprehensive care to the growing numbers of patients with HF.

References

1. Thom T, Haase N, Rosamond W et al. (2006). Heart disease and stroke statistics–2006 update: a report from the American Heart Association Statistics Committee and Stroke Statistics Subcommittee. *Circulation* **113**: e85–e151.
2. McAlister FA, Teo KK, Taher M et al. (1999). Insights into the contemporary epidemiology and outpatient management of congestive heart failure. *Am Heart J* **138**: 87–94.
3. O'Connell JB, Bristow MR (1994). Economic impact of heart failure in the United States: time for a different approach. *J Heart Lung Transplant* **13**: S107–S112.
4. Hunt SA, Baker DW, Chin MH et al. (2002). ACC/AHA guidelines for the evaluation and management of chronic heart failure in the adult: executive summary. *J Heart Lung Transplant* **21**: 189–203.
5. DeFrances CJ, Podgornik MN (2006). 2004 National Hospital Discharge Survey. *Adv Data* May 4(371): 1–19.
6. Arnold JM, Liu P, Demers C et al. (2006). Canadian Cardiovascular Society consensus conference recommendations on heart failure 2006: diagnosis and management. *Can J Cardiol* **22**: 23–45.
7. Ho KK, Anderson KM, Kannel WB, Grossman W, Levy D (1993). Survival after the onset of congestive heart failure in Framingham Heart Study subjects. *Circulation* **88**: 107–15.
8. Effect of enalapril on mortality and the development of heart failure in asymptomatic patients with reduced left ventricular ejection fractions. The SOLVD Investigators (1992). *N Engl J Med* **327**: 685–91.
9. Califf RM, Adams KF, McKenna WJ et al. (1997). A randomized controlled trial of epoprostenol therapy for severe congestive heart failure: the Flolan International Randomized Survival Trial (FIRST). *Am Heart J* **134**: 44–54.

10. Rose EA, Gelijns AC, Moskowitz AJ *et al.* (2001). Long-term mechanical left ventricular assistance for end-stage heart failure. *N Engl J Med* **345**: 1435–43.

11. Carson P, Anand I, O'Connor C *et al.* (2005). Mode of death in advanced heart failure: the Comparison of Medical, Pacing, and Defibrillation Therapies in Heart Failure (COMPANION) trial. *J Am Coll Cardiol* **46**: 2329–34.

12. Derfler MC, Jacob M, Wolf RE, Bleyer F, Hauptman PJ (2004). Mode of death from congestive heart failure: implications for clinical management. *Am J Geriatr Cardiol* **13**: 299–304.

13. Poole-Wilson PA, Uretsky BF, Thygesen K, Cleland JG, Massie BM, Ryden L (2003). Mode of death in heart failure: findings from the ATLAS trial. *Heart* **89**: 42–8.

14. Hofmann T, Meinertz T, Kasper W *et al.* (1988). Mode of death in idiopathic dilated cardiomyopathy: a multivariate analysis of prognostic determinants. *Am Heart J* **116**: 1455–63.

15. Uretsky BF, Sheahan RG (1997). Primary prevention of sudden cardiac death in heart failure: will the solution be shocking? *J Am Coll Cardiol* **30**: 1589–97.

16. Solomon SD, Anavekar N, Skali H *et al.* (2005). Influence of ejection fraction on cardiovascular outcomes in a broad spectrum of heart failure patients. *Circulation* **112**: 3738–44.

17. Curtis JP, Sokol SI, Wang Y *et al.* (2003). The association of left ventricular ejection fraction, mortality, and cause of death in stable outpatients with heart failure. *J Am Coll Cardiol* **42**: 736–42.

18. Poses RM, Smith WR, McClish DK *et al.* (1997). Physicians' survival predictions for patients with acute congestive heart failure. *Arch Intern Med* **157**: 1001–7.

19. Christakis NA, Iwashyna TJ (1998). Attitude and self-reported practice regarding prognostication in a national sample of internists. *Arch Intern Med* **158**: 2389–95.

20. Smith WR, Poses RM, McClish DK *et al.* (2002). Prognostic judgments and triage decisions for patients with acute congestive heart failure. *Chest* **121**: 1610–17.

21. Goodlin SJ, Hauptman PJ, Arnold R *et al.* (2004). Consensus statement: Palliative and supportive care in advanced heart failure. *J Card Fail* **10**: 200–9.

22. Pantilat SZ, Steimle AE (2004). Palliative care for patients with heart failure. *J Am Med Assoc* **291**: 2476–82.

23. McGinn TG, Guyatt GH, Wyer PC, Naylor CD, Stiell IG, Richardson WS (2000). Users' guides to the medical literature: XXII: how to use articles about clinical decision rules. Evidence-Based Medicine Working Group. *J Am Med Assoc* **284**: 79–84.

24. Reilly BM, Evans AT, Schaider JJ *et al.* (2002). Impact of a clinical decision rule on hospital triage of patients with suspected acute cardiac ischemia in the emergency department. *J Am Med Assoc* **288**: 342–50.

25. Wasson JH, Sox HC, Neff RK, Goldman L (1985). Clinical prediction rules. Applications and methodological standards. *New Engl J Med* **313**: 793–9.

26. Laupacis A, Sekar N, Stiell IG (1997). Clinical prediction rules. A review and suggested modifications of methodological standards. *J Am Med Assoc* **277**: 488–94.

27. Reilly BM, Evans AT (2006). Translating clinical research into clinical practice: impact of using prediction rules to make decisions. *Ann Intern Med* **144**: 201–9.

28. Goldman L, Cook EF, Johnson PA, Brand DA, Rouan GW, Lee TH (1996). Prediction of the need for intensive care in patients who come to the emergency departments with acute chest pain. *New Engl J Med* **334**: 1498–504.

29. Reilly B, Durairaj L, Husain S *et al.* (1999). Performance and potential impact of a chest pain prediction rule in a large public hospital. *Am J Med* **106**: 285–91.

30. Durairaj L, Reilly B, Das K *et al.* (2001). Emergency department admissions to inpatient cardiac telemetry beds: a prospective cohort study of risk stratification and outcomes. *Am J Med* **110**: 7–11.

31. Campana C, Gavazzi A, Berzuini C *et al.* (1993). Predictors of prognosis in patients awaiting heart transplantation. *J Heart Lung Transplant* **12**: 756–65.

32. Cohn JN, Rector TS (1988). Prognosis of congestive heart failure and predictors of mortality. *Am J Cardiol* **62**: 25A–30A.

33. Parameshwar J, Keegan J, Sparrow J, Sutton GC, Poole-Wilson PA (1992). Predictors of prognosis in severe chronic heart failure. *Am Heart J* **123**: 421–6.

34. Kearney MT, Fox KA, Lee AJ *et al.* (2002). Predicting death due to progressive heart failure in patients with mild-to-moderate chronic heart failure. *J Am Coll Cardiol* **40**: 1801–8.

35. Cohn JN, Johnson GR, Shabetai R *et al.* (1993). Ejection fraction, peak exercise oxygen consumption, cardiothoracic ratio, ventricular arrhythmias, and plasma norepinephrine as determinants of prognosis in heart failure. The V-HeFT VA Cooperative Studies Group. *Circulation* **87**(Suppl.): VI5–V16.

36. Coyne JC, Rohrbaugh MJ, Shoham V, Sonnega JS, Nicklas JM, Cranford JA (2001). Prognostic importance of marital quality for survival of congestive heart failure. *Am J Cardiol* **88**: 526–9.

37. Bart BA, Shaw LK, McCants CB, Jr *et al.* (1997). Clinical determinants of mortality in patients with angiographically diagnosed ischemic or nonischemic cardiomyopathy. *J Am Coll Cardiol* **30**: 1002–8.

38. Sullivan MD, Levy WC, Crane BA, Russo JE, Spertus JA (2004). Usefulness of depression to predict time to combined end point of transplant or death for outpatients with advanced heart failure. *Am J Cardiol* **94**: 1577–80.

39. Jiang W, Alexander J, Christopher E *et al.* (2001). Relationship of depression to increased risk of mortality and rehospitalization in patients with congestive heart failure. *Arch Intern Med* **161**: 1849–56.

40. Murberg TA, Bru E, Svebak S, Tveteras R, Aarsland T (1999). Depressed mood and subjective health symptoms as predictors of mortality in patients with congestive heart failure: a two-years follow-up study. *Int J Psychiat Med* **29**: 311–26.

41. Faris R, Purcell H, Henein MY, Coats AJ (2002). Clinical depression is common and significantly associated with reduced survival in patients with non-ischaemic heart failure. *Eur J Heart Fail* **4**: 541–51.

42. Anker SD, Ponikowski P, Varney S *et al.* (1997). Wasting as independent risk factor for mortality in chronic heart failure. *Lancet* **349**: 1050–3.

43. Kalantar-Zadeh K, Block G, Horwich T, Fonarow GC (2004). Reverse epidemiology of conventional cardiovascular risk factors in patients with chronic heart failure. *J Am Coll Cardiol* **43**: 1439–44.

44. Gottlieb SS, Abraham W, Butler J *et al.* (2002). The prognostic importance of different definitions of worsening renal function in congestive heart failure. *J Card Fail* **8**: 136–41.

45. Dries DL, Exner DV, Domanski MJ, Greenberg B, Stevenson LW (2000). The prognostic implications of renal insufficiency in asymptomatic and symptomatic patients with left ventricular systolic dysfunction. *J Am Coll Cardiol* **35**: 681–9.

46. Smith GL, Vaccarino V, Kosiborod M *et al.* (2003). Worsening renal function: what is a clinically meaningful change in creatinine during hospitalization with heart failure? *J Card Fail* **9**: 13–25.

47. Forman DE, Butler J, Wang Y *et al.* (2004). Incidence, predictors at admission, and impact of worsening renal function among patients hospitalized with heart failure. *J Am Coll Cardiol* **43**: 61–7.

48. Felker GM, Gattis WA, Leimberger JD *et al.* (2003). Usefulness of anemia as a predictor of death and rehospitalization in patients with decompensated heart failure. *Am J Cardiol* **92**: 625–8.

49. Mitka M (2003). Researchers probe anemia–heart failure link. *J Am Med Assoc* **290**: 1835–8.

50. Szachniewicz J, Petruk-Kowalczyk J, Majda J *et al.* (2003). Anaemia is an independent predictor of poor outcome in patients with chronic heart failure. *Int J Cardiol* **90**: 303–8.

51. Ezekowitz JA, McAlister FA, Armstrong PW (2003). Anemia is common in heart failure and is associated with poor outcomes: insights from a cohort of 12 065 patients with new-onset heart failure. *Circulation* **107**: 223–5.

52. Bode-Schnurbus L, Bocker D, Block M *et al.* (2003). QRS duration: a simple marker for predicting cardiac mortality in ICD patients with heart failure. *Heart* **89**: 1157–62.

53. Iuliano S, Fisher SG, Karasik PE, Fletcher RD, Singh SN (2002). QRS duration and mortality in patients with congestive heart failure. *Am Heart J* **143**: 1085–91.

54. Heidenreich PA, Spertus JA, Jones PG *et al.* (2006). Health status identifies heart failure outpatients at risk for hospitalization or death. *J Am Coll Cardiol* **47**: 752–6.

55. Rodriguez-Artalejo F, Guallar-Castillon P, Pascual CR *et al.* (2005). Health-related quality of life as a predictor of hospital readmission and death among patients with heart failure. *Arch Intern Med* **165**: 1274–9.

56. Konstam V, Salem D, Pouleur H *et al.* (1996). Baseline quality of life as a predictor of mortality and hospitalization in 5,025 patients with congestive heart failure. SOLVD Investigations. Studies of Left Ventricular Dysfunction Investigators. *Am J Cardiol* **78**: 890–5.

57. Roul G, Germain P, Bareiss P (1998). Does the 6-minute walk test predict the prognosis in patients with NYHA class II or III chronic heart failure? *Am Heart J* **136**: 449–57.

58. Jiang W, Hathaway WR, McNulty S *et al.* (1997). Ability of heart rate variability to predict prognosis in patients with advanced congestive heart failure. *Am J Cardiol* **80**: 808–11.

59. La Rovere MT, Pinna GD, Maestri R *et al.* (2003). Short-term heart rate variability strongly predicts sudden cardiac death in chronic heart failure patients. *Circulation* **107**: 565–70.

60. Olshausen KV, Stienen U, Schwarz F, Kubler W, Meyer J (1988). Long-term prognostic significance of ventricular arrhythmias in idiopathic dilated cardiomyopathy. *Am J Cardiol* **61**: 146–51.

61. Schoeller R, Andresen D, Buttner P, Oezcelik K, Vey G, Schroder R (1993). First- or second-degree atrioventricular block as a risk factor in idiopathic dilated cardiomyopathy. *Am J Cardiol* **71**: 720–6.

62. O'Neill JO, Young JB, Pothier CE, Lauer MS (2004). Severe frequent ventricular ectopy after exercise as a predictor of death in patients with heart failure. *J Am Coll Cardiol* **44**: 820–6.

63. Doust JA, Pietrzak E, Dobson A, Glasziou P (2005). How well does B-type natriuretic peptide predict death and cardiac events in patients with heart failure: systematic review. *Br Med J* **330**: 625.

64. Koglin J, Pehlivanli S, Schwaiblmair M, Vogeser M, Cremer P, von Scheidt W (2001). Role of brain natriuretic peptide in risk stratification of patients with congestive heart failure. *J Am Coll Cardiol* **38**: 1934–41.

65. Berger R, Huelsman M, Strecker K *et al.* (2002). B-type natriuretic peptide predicts sudden death in patients with chronic heart failure. *Circulation* **105**: 2392–7.

66. Cheng V, Kazanagra R, Garcia A *et al.* (2001). A rapid bedside test for B-type peptide predicts treatment outcomes in patients admitted for decompensated heart failure: a pilot study. *J Am Coll Cardiol* **37**: 386–91.

67. Horwich TB, Patel J, MacLellan WR, Fonarow GC (2003). Cardiac troponin I is associated with impaired hemodynamics, progressive left ventricular dysfunction, and increased mortality rates in advanced heart failure. *Circulation* **108**: 833–8.

68. Marcucci R, Gori AM, Giannotti F *et al.* (2006). Markers of hypercoagulability and inflammation predict mortality in patients with heart failure. *J Thromb Haemost* **4**: 1017–22.

69. Ross H, Hendry P, Dipchand A *et al.* (2003). 2001 Canadian Cardiovascular Society Consensus Conference on cardiac transplantation. *Can J Cardiol* **19**: 620–54.

70. Pinamonti B, Di LA, Sinagra G, Camerini F (1993). Restrictive left ventricular filling pattern in dilated cardiomyopathy assessed by Doppler echocardiography: clinical, echocardiographic and hemodynamic correlations and prognostic implications. Heart Muscle Disease Study Group. *J Am Coll Cardiol* **22**: 808–15.

71. Xie GY, Berk MR, Smith MD, Gurley JC, DeMaria AN (1994). Prognostic value of Doppler transmitral flow patterns in patients with congestive heart failure. *J Am Coll Cardiol* **24**: 132–9.

72. Grayburn PA, Appleton CP, DeMaria AN *et al.* (2005). Echocardiographic predictors of morbidity and mortality in patients with advanced heart failure: the Beta-blocker Evaluation of Survival Trial (BEST). *J Am Coll Cardiol* **45**: 1064–71.

73. Wong M, Staszewsky L, Latini R *et al.* (2004). Severity of left ventricular remodeling defines outcomes and response to therapy in heart failure: Valsartan heart failure trial (Val-HeFT) echocardiographic data. *J Am Coll Cardiol* **43**: 2022–7.

74. de Groote P, Millaire A, Foucher-Hossein C *et al.* (1998). Right ventricular ejection fraction is an independent predictor of survival in patients with moderate heart failure. *J Am Coll Cardiol* **32**: 948–54.

75. Sigurdsson A, Amtorp O, Gundersen T, Nilsson B, Remes J, Swedberg K (1994). Neurohormonal activation in patients with mild or moderately severe congestive heart failure and effects of ramipril. The Ramipril Trial Study Group. *Br Heart J* **72**: 422–7.

76. Simpson P (1983). Norepinephrine-stimulated hypertrophy of cultured rat myocardial cells is an alpha 1 adrenergic response. *J Clin Invest* **72**: 732–8.

77. Aronson D, Burger AJ (2003). Neurohormonal prediction of mortality following admission for decompensated heart failure. *Am J Cardiol* **91**: 245–8.

78. Swedberg K, Eneroth P, Kjekshus J, Wilhelmsen L (1990). Hormones regulating cardiovascular function in patients with severe congestive heart failure and their relation to mortality. CONSENSUS Trial Study Group. *Circulation* **82**: 1730–6.

79. Hillege HL, Nitsch D, Pfeffer MA *et al.* (2006). Renal function as a predictor of outcome in a broad spectrum of patients with heart failure. *Circulation* **113**: 671–8.

80. Friedrich EB, Muders F, Luchner A, Dietl O, Riegger GA, Elsner D (1999). Contribution of the endothelin system to the renal hypoperfusion associated with experimental congestive heart failure. *J Cardiovasc Pharmacol* **34**: 612–17.

81. Abassi Z, Gurbanov K, Rubinstein I, Better OS, Hoffman A, Winaver J (1998). Regulation of intrarenal blood flow in experimental heart failure: role of endothelin and nitric oxide. *Am J Physiol* **274**: F766–F774.

82. Anand I, McMurray JJ, Whitmore J *et al.* (2004). Anemia and its relationship to clinical outcome in heart failure. *Circulation* **110**: 149–54.

83. Iversen PO, Woldbaek PR, Tonnessen T, Christensen G (2002). Decreased hematopoiesis in bone marrow of mice with congestive heart failure. *Am J Physiol Regul Integr Comp Physiol* **282**: R166–R172.

84. Aaronson KD, Schwartz JS, Chen TM, Wong KL, Goin JE, Mancini DM (1997). Development and prospective validation of a clinical index to predict survival in ambulatory patients referred for cardiac transplant evaluation. *Circulation* **95**: 2660–7.

85. Lee DS, Austin PC, Rouleau JL, Liu PP, Naimark D, Tu JV (2003). Predicting mortality among patients hospitalized for heart failure: derivation and validation of a clinical model. *J Am Med Assoc* **290**: 2581–7.

86. Fonarow GC, Adams KF, Jr, Abraham WT, Yancy CW, Boscardin WJ (2005). Risk stratification for in-hospital mortality in acutely decompensated heart failure: classification and regression tree analysis. *J Am Med Assoc* **293**: 572–80.

87. Levy WC, Mozaffarian D, Linker DT *et al.* (2006). The Seattle Heart Failure Model: prediction of survival in heart failure. *Circulation* **113**: 1424–33.

88. Adlam D, Silcocks P, Sparrow N (2005). Using BNP to develop a risk score for heart failure in primary care. *Eur Heart J* **26**: 1086–93.

89. Pocock SJ, Wang D, Pfeffer MA *et al.* (2006). Predictors of mortality and morbidity in patients with chronic heart failure. *Eur Heart J* **27**: 65–75.

90. Felker GM, Leimberger JD, Califf RM *et al.* (2004). Risk stratification after hospitalization for decompensated heart failure. *J Card Fail* **10**: 460–6.

91. Brophy JM, Dagenais GR, McSherry F, Williford W, Yusuf S (2004). A multivariate model for predicting mortality in patients with heart failure and systolic dysfunction. *Am J Med* **116**: 300–4.
92. Kearney MT, Nolan J, Lee AJ *et al.* (2003). A prognostic index to predict long-term mortality in patients with mild to moderate chronic heart failure stabilised on angiotensin converting enzyme inhibitors. *Eur J Heart Fail* **5**: 489–97.
93. Auble TE, Hsieh M, Gardner W *et al.* (2005). A prediction rule to identify low-risk patients with heart failure. *Acad Emerg Med* **12**: 514–21.
94. De Marco T, Goldman L (1997). Predicting outcomes in severe heart failure. *Circulation* **95**: 2597–9.
95. Yusuf S, Pfeffer MA, Swedberg K *et al.* (2003). Effects of candesartan in patients with chronic heart failure and preserved left-ventricular ejection fraction: the CHARM-Preserved Trial. *Lancet* **362**: 777–81.
96. Lee DS, Tu JV, Juurlink DN *et al.* (2005). Risk-treatment mismatch in the pharmacotherapy of heart failure. *J Am Med Assoc* **294**: 1240–7.
97. Feinstein AR (1996). *Multivariable Analysis*. New Haven: Yale University Press.
98. Kleinbaum DG, Morgenstern H (1982). *Epidemiologic Research: Principles and Quantitative Methods*. Belmont: Lifetime Learning Publications.
99. Rothman KJ, Greenland S (1998). *Modern Epidemiology*, 2nd edn. Philadelphia: Lippincott-Raven.
100. Steyerberg EW, Eijkemans MJ, Harrell FE, Jr, Habbema JD. Prognostic modelling with logistic regression analysis: a comparison of selection and estimation methods in small data sets. *Stat Med* 2000 April 30;19(8):1059–79.
101. Harrell FE, Jr, Lee KL, Mark DB (1996). Multivariable prognostic models: issues in developing models, evaluating assumptions and adequacy, and measuring and reducing errors. *Stat Med* **15**: 361–87.
102. Van Houwelingen JC, Le Cessie S (1990). Predictive value of statistical models. *Stat Med* **9**: 1303–25.
103. Austin PC (2007). A comparison of regression trees, logistic regression, generalized additive models, and multivariate adaptive regression splines for predicting AMI mortality. *Stat Med* **26**: 2937–57.
104. Hanley JA, McNeil BJ (1982). The meaning and use of the area under a receiver operating characteristic (ROC) curve. *Radiology* **143**: 29–36.
105. Terrin N, Schmid CH, Griffith JL, D'Agostino RB, Selker HP (2003). External validity of predictive models: a comparison of logistic regression, classification trees, and neural networks. *J Clin Epidemiol* **56**: 721–9.
106. Justice AC, Covinsky KE, Berlin JA (1999). Assessing the generalizability of prognostic information. *Ann Intern Med* **130**: 515–24.
107. Steyerberg EW, Harrell FE, Jr, Borsboom GJ, Eijkemans MJ, Vergouwe Y, Habbema JD (2001). Internal validation of predictive models: efficiency of some procedures for logistic regression analysis. *J Clin Epidemiol* **54**: 774–81.
108. Owan TE, Redfield MM (2005). Epidemiology of diastolic heart failure. *Prog Cardiovasc Dis* **47**: 320–32.
109. Vasan RS, Benjamin EJ, Levy D (1995). Prevalence, clinical features and prognosis of diastolic heart failure: an epidemiologic perspective. *J Am Coll Cardiol* **26**: 1565–74.
110. Zile MR, Brutsaert DL (2002). New concepts in diastolic dysfunction and diastolic heart failure: Part I: diagnosis, prognosis, and measurements of diastolic function. *Circulation* **105**: 1387–93.
111. Hogg K, Swedberg K, McMurray J (2004). Heart failure with preserved left ventricular systolic function; epidemiology, clinical characteristics, and prognosis. *J Am Coll Cardiol* **43**: 317–27.
112. Bhatia RS, Tu JV, Lee DS *et al.* (2006). Outcome of heart failure with preserved ejection fraction in a population-based study. *New Engl J Med* **355**: 260–9.
113. Owan TE, Hodge DO, Herges RM, Jacobsen SJ, Roger VL, Redfield MM (2006). Trends in prevalence and outcome of heart failure with preserved ejection fraction. *New Engl J Med* **355**: 251–9.

114. Katz AM, Zile MR (2006). New molecular mechanism in diastolic heart failure. *Circulation* **113**: 1922–5.

115. van Heerebeek L, Borbely A, Niessen HW *et al.* (2006). Myocardial structure and function differ in systolic and diastolic heart failure. *Circulation* **113**: 1966–73.

116. Heiat A, Gross CP, Krumholz HM (2002). Representation of the elderly, women, and minorities in heart failure clinical trials. *Arch Intern Med* **162**: 1682–8.

117. Hall WD (1999). Representation of blacks, women, and the very elderly (aged > or = 80) in 28 major randomized clinical trials. *Ethn Dis* **9**: 333–40.

118. Gurwitz JH, Col NF, Avorn J (1992). The exclusion of the elderly and women from clinical trials in acute myocardial infarction. *J Am Med Assoc* **268**: 1417–22.

119. Harris DJ, Douglas PS (2000). Enrollment of women in cardiovascular clinical trials funded by the National Heart, Lung, and Blood Institute. *New Engl J Med* **343**: 475–80.

120. Goodlin SJ (2005). Heart failure in the elderly. *Expert Rev Cardiovasc Ther* **3**: 99–106.

121. Rich MW (2001). Heart failure in the 21st century: a cardiogeriatric syndrome. *J Gerontol A Biol Sci Med Sci* **56**: M88–M96.

122. Wolinsky FD, Overhage JM, Stump TE, Lubitz RM, Smith DM (1997). The risk of hospitalization for congestive heart failure among older adults. *Med Care* **35**: 1031–43.

123. Philbin EF, Rocco TA, Jr, Lynch LJ, Rogers VA, Jenkins P (1997). Predictors and determinants of hospital length of stay in congestive heart failure in ten community hospitals. *J Heart Lung Transplant* **16**: 548–55.

124. Candlish P, Watts P, Redman S, Whyte P, Lowe J (1998). Elderly patients with heart failure: a study of satisfaction with care and quality of life. *Int J Qual Health Care* **10**: 141–6.

125. Krumholz HM, Parent EM, Tu N *et al.* (1997). Readmission after hospitalization for congestive heart failure among Medicare beneficiaries. *Arch Intern Med* **157**: 99–104.

126. Jarrett PG, Rockwood K, Carver D, Stolee P, Cosway S (1995). Illness presentation in elderly patients. *Arch Intern Med* **155**: 1060–4.

127. Tresch DD (1997). The clinical diagnosis of heart failure in older patients. *J Am Geriatr Soc* **45**: 1128–33.

128. Kerzner R, Gage BF, Freedland KE, Rich MW (2003). Predictors of mortality in younger and older patients with heart failure and preserved or reduced left ventricular ejection fraction. *Am Heart J* **146**: 286–90.

129. Rockwood K, Fox RA, Stolee P, Robertson D, Beattie BL (1994). Frailty in elderly people: an evolving concept. *Can Med Assoc J* **150**: 489–95.

130. Almeida OP, Flicker L (2001). The mind of a failing heart: a systematic review of the association between congestive heart failure and cognitive functioning. *Intern Med J* **31**: 290–5.

131. Bo M, Raspo S, Massaia M *et al.* (2003). A predictive model of in-hospital mortality in elderly patients admitted to medical intensive care units. *J Am Geriatr Soc* **51**: 1507–8.

132. Ko DT, Tu JV, Masoudi FA *et al.* (2005). Quality of care and outcomes of older patients with heart failure hospitalized in the United States and Canada. *Arch Intern Med* **165**: 2486–92.

133. Jessup M, Pina IL (2004). Is it important to examine gender differences in the epidemiology and outcome of severe heart failure? *J Thorac Cardiovasc Surg* **127**: 1247–52.

134. Pina IL, Buchter C (2003). Heart failure in women. *Cardiol Rev* **11**: 337–44.

135. Grigioni F, Barbieri A, Russo A *et al.* (2006). Prognostic stratification of women with chronic heart failure referred for heart transplantation: relevance of gender as compared with gender-related characteristics. *J Heart Lung Transplant* **25**: 648–52.

136. De Feo S, Opasich C (2003). Comparison of the outcome in men and women with chronic heart failure. *Ital Heart J* **4**: 511–13.

137. Tandon S, Hankins SR, Le Jemtel TH (2002). Clinical profile of chronic heart failure in elderly women. *Am J Geriatr Cardiol* **11**: 318–23.

138. Richardson LG, Rocks M (2001). Women and heart failure. *Heart Lung* **30**: 87–97.

139. Schocken DD, Arrieta MI, Leaverton PE, Ross EA (1992). Prevalence and mortality rate of congestive heart failure in the United States. *J Am Coll Cardiol* **20**: 301–6.

140. Groman R, Ginsburg J (2004). Racial and ethnic disparities in health care: a position paper of the American College of Physicians. *Ann Intern Med* **141**: 226–32.

141. Philbin EF, DiSalvo TG (1998). Influence of race and gender on care process, resource use, and hospital-based outcomes in congestive heart failure. *Am J Cardiol* **82**: 76–81.

142. Dries DL, Exner DV, Gersh BJ, Cooper HA, Carson PE, Domanski MJ (1999). Racial differences in the outcome of left ventricular dysfunction. *New Engl J Med* **340**: 609–16.

143. Ghali JK (2002). Race, ethnicity, and heart failure. *J Card Fail* **8**: 387–9.

144. Philbin EF, DiSalvo TG (1998). Influence of race and gender on care process, resource use, and hospital-based outcomes in congestive heart failure. *Am J Cardiol* **82**: 76–81.

145. Alexander M, Grumbach K, Remy L, Rowell R, Massie BM (1999). Congestive heart failure hospitalizations and survival in California: patterns according to race/ethnicity. *Am Heart J* **137**: 919–27.

146. Lafata JE, Pladevall M, Divine G, Ayoub M, Philbin EF (2004). Are there race/ethnicity differences in outpatient congestive heart failure management, hospital use, and mortality among an insured population? *Med Care* **42**: 680–9.

147. King TE, Jr (2002). Racial disparities in clinical trials. *New Engl J Med* **346**: 1400–2.

148. NIH guidelines on the inclusion of women and minorities as subjects in clinical research (1994). *Federal Register* **59**: 14508–13.

149. (2003). *Public Law No. 108–155. Pediatric Research Equity Act of 2003.*

150. Fried TR, Bradley EH, Towle VR, Allore H (2002). Understanding the treatment preferences of seriously ill patients. *New Engl J Med* **346**: 1061–6.

151. Mast KR, Salama M, Silverman GK, Arnold RM (2004). End-of-life content in treatment guidelines for life-limiting diseases. *J Palliat Med* **7**: 754–73.

152. Workman S (2003). End-of-life care and congestive heart failure. *Arch Intern Med* **163**: 737.

153. Walden JA, Dracup K, Westlake C, Erickson V, Hamilton MA, Fonarow GC (2001). Educational needs of patients with advanced heart failure and their caregivers. *J Heart Lung Transplant* **20**: 766–9.

154. Lewis EF, Johnson PA, Johnson W, Collins C, Griffin L, Stevenson LW (2001). Preferences for quality of life or survival expressed by patients with heart failure. *J Heart Lung Transplant* **20**: 1016–24.

155. A controlled trial to improve care for seriously ill hospitalized patients. The study to understand prognoses and preferences for outcomes and risks of treatments (SUPPORT). The SUPPORT Principal Investigators (1995). *J Am Med Assoc* **274**: 1591–8.

156. Teno JM, Fisher ES, Hamel MB, Coppola K, Dawson NV (2002). Medical care inconsistent with patients' treatment goals: association with 1-year Medicare resource use and survival. *J Am Geriatr Soc* **50**: 496–500.

157. Goodlin SJ, Kutner JS, Connor SR, Ryndes T, Houser J, Hauptman PJ (2005). Hospice care for heart failure patients. *J Pain Symptom Manage* **29**: 525–8.

158. Lamont EB, Christakis NA (2003). Complexities in prognostication in advanced cancer: 'to help them live their lives the way they want to'. *J Am Med Assoc* **290**: 98–104.

159. McCormick TR, Conley BJ (1995). Patients' perspectives on dying and on the care of dying patients. *West J Med* **163**: 236–43.

Chapter 22

Communication between clinicians and their heart failure patients and families

Sarah J. Goodlin and Timothy E. Quill

Introduction

Heart failure (HF) is a chronic illness that has a broad impact on the patient and family, and in which monitoring of the patient's clinical status, diet, and fluids plays a critical role. For many patients, HF is also life-limiting. 'Patient-centered care', identified by the Institute of Medicine and others,[1] emphasizes the active participation of the patient and patient's family in health care, particularly for chronic illness. Patient-centered care integrates patient preferences into plans for care, manages symptoms to the level of comfort desired by the patient, and attempts to reduce the burden of illness on the patient and their family. Communication between clinicians and HF patients and their families is integral to patient-centered care.

Comprehensive HF care provides concurrent HF care and supportive care (see Fig. 1.2 in Chapter 1). 'HF care' is evidence-based or guideline-directed pharmacological, interventional, and surgical treatment related to cardiovascular pathophysiology. This care has been best defined in early and mid-phases of the disease course, and is least clear for advanced HF and at the end of life. 'Supportive care' (also called 'palliative care' with which it is synonymous[2]) includes a broad range of multidisciplinary interventions directed at improving the patient's quality of life, including education for the patient and family about the illness and its prognosis, symptom management, assistance with difficult medical decision-making, and holistic care that integrates psychosocial and spiritual support as needed by patients and their families throughout the illness from diagnosis to death. Communication to define the goals of care for an individual patient in the light of full knowledge of their clinical condition, and then to identify options and make decisions about interventions, lies at the interface of supportive care and HF care. The patient's preferences and values must be integrated with an understanding of HF care options and their likely benefits and burdens to the patient given the patient's overall health status. HF treatments that are optimal may differ from the patient's preferences at each phase of HF depending on the patient's burden of illness, prognosis, and personal experience with and without added treatment. Similarly, the information needs of patients and their families will change over the course of the illness or with the patient's perceived health status and preferences.

Communication between physicians and patients has not been well studied in HF care. We lack data specific to HF about barriers to effective communication for both patient and clinician and about the information needed by patients and families to facilitate self-care and decision-making. This chapter will review what is known about communication between clinicians and HF patients (and families), and will propose approaches to important aspects of communication, based on literature developed largely in oncology and general medical care.

Using the 'model of comprehensive HF care' pictured in Fig. 1.2, we have attempted to identify issues that will be confronted in communication with HF patients at five phases of the illness, from the initial diagnosis to the end of life. Although these phases are not always distinct and many of the decision-making issues identified may be postponed or considered earlier depending on individual preferences and circumstances, the series of tables will identify guidelines for conversation and potential decision-making. Based on knowledge from the communication literature from other medical fields, we recommend approaches to these issues and language that might be used in each phase.

General principles of physician communication with patients

Several decades of research have identified issues in and approaches to the improvement of physician–patient communication in cancer care, general medical care, and, recently, human immunodeficiency virus (HIV) disease care. The discussion below attempts to apply knowledge gained from these disciplines to patient–physician communication in HF. Multidisciplinary teams are increasingly used in HF care, and while it has not been studied, it is probably appropriate to apply knowledge about physicain–patient communication to communication between other clinicians and patients.

In general, patients understand and speak a different language regarding health care than their physicians. Clear communication from clinicians that uses 'plain language' rather than medical terminology is most effective. Medical terms or labels should be defined in lay language as they are employed. Issues of 'health literacy' or patient beliefs may further modify a patient's understanding of what they are told. A fundamental model for communication is 'ask–tell–ask'. The physician asks the patient what they would like to know and how they want to receive information, then gives the information in small digestible amounts in accordance with their preferences. Once delivered, the physician can check the patient's comprehension by asking them to explain what they understood. Finally, the physician should ask 'What are your questions?'. Asking 'what are' rather than 'do you have' gives encouragement to ask questions. Often patients and their families require time to process new information. Providing written summaries of key points and directing patients to written, internet, or other resources may help them assimilate information given to them. A major challenge is to keep the information straightforward enough to be understood by patients for whom this is an emotionally loaded, intellectually challenging new domain of learning.

Phase 1: Communication issues at initial diagnosis of 'HF'

Ethical principles and patient-centered care require honest communication with patients about their diagnosis, about what they can expect during the course of their illness, and about prognosis. At the time of initial diagnosis there is often a temptation to overload the patient with information that he or she will not be able to remember. Patients who receive a new, serious diagnosis may be so emotionally overwhelmed that they do not remember much of the details of the conversation. Some patients will not understand what HF is or its potentially life-limiting nature,[3] whereas others will experience it as a death sentence from the outset. For many, the term 'HF' will require some explanation. Some have proposed that 'failure' is too frightening or blameworthy a term, and have suggested a change in language to 'impairment' or 'insufficiency'.[4,5] Regardless of the appeal of less direct language, usually the HF label should be used when giving the diagnosis. Calling the illness 'Heart Failure' and providing information will permit the patient and family to access resources with additional information.

Use of euphemisms to describe HF may leave the patient with misperceptions about the seriousness and longevity of the illness; in the long run it may provoke more anxiety and depression than a more straightforward expression of the condition does.[6] A physician's avoidance of clear honest language may have the adverse effect of reducing the trust of the patient and family in the physician. In fact, many British patients with chronic symptomatic HF felt physicians were not honest or avoided discussing death. In this same study, patients requested information about prognosis from the research assistant. Half of patients saw death as inevitable while others were unaware of their prognosis or did not want to acknowledge it.[7] In another study, patients with advanced HF felt poorly informed about the course of their illness and prognosis, and felt uninvolved in decision-making.[8] Patient preferences for information and for involvement in treatment or decision-making vary greatly.[9]

Delivering bad news

The delivery of a diagnosis of HF probably represents 'bad news' for patients. Not labeling the illness HF or not telling the patient that life expectancy with HF is limited may not be ethical, unless the patient has said they do not want to know their diagnosis. Because understanding the diagnosis is critical to subsequent management of the illness, patients who do not wish to have information should be asked to designate someone who can communicate on their behalf. The delivery of bad news generally follows predictable steps:[10]

1. Sit down to meet with patient and key family members.

2. Find out, and build your conversation on, what the patient already knows.

3. Ask the patient if he or she is ready to discuss your findings. If they are, first give a warning 'I am afraid I have some bad news for you. . . .'.

4. Tell the diagnosis clearly, using language that is unlikely to be misunderstood 'You have heart failure'.

Table 22.1 Comprehensive HF care

	Phase 1	Phase 2	Phase 3	Phase 4	Phase 5
	Initial symptoms of HF develop and HF treatment is initiated	Plateaus of variable length may be reached with initial medical management, or following mechanical support or heart transplant	Functional status declines with variable slope, with intermittent exacerbations of HF that respond to rescue efforts	Stage D HF, with refractory symptoms and limited function	End of life
NYHA classification	II–III	II–IV	IIIB	IV	IV
Communication	Understand patient concerns and fears Identify life-limiting nature of HF Elicit preferences for care in emergencies or sudden death Elicit symptoms and assess quality of life (QOL) Elicit preferences for knowledge and role in decision-making	Elicit symptoms and assess QOL Re-evaluate resuscitation preferences for care in emergencies Advise durable power of attorney for health care	Elicit symptoms and QOL Elicit values and re-evaluate preferences Identify present status and likely course(s) Re-evaluate goals of care	Elicit symptoms Acknowledge present status Elicit preferences and reset goals of care Identify worries Review appropriate care options and likely course with each Explore suitability and preferences about invasive options	Elicit desired symptom relief and identify appropriate medications Assistance with delivery of care Preferences for end-of-life care, site of care, family needs, and capabilities

©Sarah Goodlin, modified with permission

Language to use				
'Tell me what you understand about your heart disease' 'I'm afraid I have bad news…You have heart failure' 'I talk to all patients when I first meet them (or there is a change in their status) about what treatment they want when their heart or breathing stop' 'While I hope you have years to live, we need to plan how to respond should you have a sudden abnormal heart rhythm or suddenly die. We can allow you to die naturally or try to revive you'	'How are things going for you? How do you feel?' 'What are your biggest concerns or worries?….' 'We talked earlier about your preferences for what to do when your heart or breathing stop— I'd like to make certain I understand what you'd like to happen' 'All adults should have someone who has the legal authority to make health-care decisions for them if ever they cannot speak for themselves'	'How do you feel you are doing?' 'I'm afraid I have bad news ' 'That must feel frightening' or 'I can see you are worried' 'When there is a change, I review the approach to care as well as what to do when your heart and breathing stop' 'Looking back, what has been most important to you?' 'We are going to do everything we can to stabilize your HF with medications and diet, but it is possible that we will not be successful. What do you need to take care of in case things don't go as we hope?'	'How do you feel you are doing?' 'As you think about the next period of time, what is most important to you? What are your biggest worries?' 'What do you hope for at this time? How can we prepare should things not go as you hope?' 'We have some new invasive treatments for HF that have serious risks, but also potential benefits. We want to talk to you in depth so you fully understand all aspects of this decision' 'We need to finally understand what path is best for you'	'What are your biggest concerns or worries?' 'Tell me what is most distressing for you' 'What is important to you at this point?' 'We can offer you some treatment for advanced HF which won't prolong your life, but may help you feel better. It would require continuous intravenous treatment at home. Is that something you would like to try?' 'I wish there were more effective treatments' 'We should be able to relieve serious shortness of breath if it occurs toward the end without putting you on machines by using morphine or related medications'

QOL, quality of life.

5. Give additional information that is key for immediate management and that is as asked for by the patient, in small amounts; ask–tell–ask.

6. Respond and generally normalize the associated emotions 'Anyone hearing this news would feel frightened and upset. . . '.

7. Make a clear plan for follow-up and next steps.

8. Reinforce your commitment to ongoing treatment and care.

Framing the conversation as a dichotomy ('HF is a chronic illness for which there is no cure, and careful management with medications and diet often permits patients to live years with good quality of life') allows patients to hope for positive outcomes while acknowledging that HF is likely to be life-limiting. Occasional HF patients recover normal or near normal function with appropriate medical management, so hope is not unreasonable, yet the conversation can be structured to ensure that patients understand the seriousness of the condition, and the importance of learning about new medications, diet, and lifestyle. This approach also sets up a partnership between the physician and the patient and family. Providing a diagnosis of HF and simultaneously setting goals for care with the patient based on what they value may reduce anxiety or discouragement associated with the diagnosis. Many times these complex tasks may need to be accomplished over several visits, or if operating in a multidisciplinary team, elements can be delegated to a nurse practitioner, physician assistant, or nutritionist.

Phases 1–2: Communication issues during the early phases

Discussing resuscitation preferences

Because sudden death is a potential outcome after diagnosis or during initiation of medications, it is important to talk with patients and their families around the time of the initial HF diagnosis about resuscitation preferences. Discussing preferences for resuscitation and other interventions with all patients early in care or routinely around the time of initial diagnosis normalizes the topic and permits the clinician to honestly state that this is a conversation they have with all HF patients. Initial discussions can be introduced by talking about 'what to do in an emergency', specifically addressing whether a sudden death event or cardiac arrest should be attended to with an attempt at resuscitation or by allowing natural death. Discussing resuscitation preferences requires the physician to acknowledge that HF patients die. Again, such a conversation can be made more palatable by assuring patients that you will 'Hope for the best' (work with them to take full advantage of all effective treatments of which there are many), and, at the same time, 'Plan for the worst'[11] (so you know their views and wishes in case they die or worsen suddenly despite your best efforts). Thus, you can encourage the patient that with appropriate medications the risk of sudden death is lessened, while simultaneously identifying whether they would want an attempt at cardiopulmonary resuscitation (CPR) should they have a sudden death event, as well as whether they are candidates for an implantable defibrillator. Families of patients desiring CPR attempts should receive basic life support training.

Advance care planning

Part of the 'planning for the worst' conversation should include plans for an alternate decision-maker to speak for him- or herself should the patient lose capacity in the future. The topic of advance care planning might be addressed at the time of HF diagnosis for some patients, particularly when patients have considered the subject previously. For other patients, advance care planning is new or has been avoided. The topic can be introduced and the patient and family can be provided written material,[12] and a promise that the subject will be revisited at a later date. If not clarified during initial HF care, once their status has stabilized and the patient has reached a plateau of improved function it is appropriate to review their preferences, make advance care plans and set goals of care.

Many patients will want all potentially effective therapeutic measures as long as they have a chance to return to a condition where they are mentally intact and able to make decisions for themselves. However, many patients also draw a line at conditions where they would not be cognitively intact, for example having had significant brain injury after CPR. For such patients, completing an advance directive early on in their treatment can be reassuring rather than frightening. Advance directives are of two types:

1. Health-care proxy—a person designated by the patient to make decisions on the patient's behalf (using what is known of the patient's views and values, or 'substituted judgment') should they lose capacity in the future.

2. Living will—the patient sets out his or her philosophy for medical treatment if they lose capacity in the future and are not likely to regain it (e.g. 'If I am unable to make decisions for myself, I would want all life-sustaining therapy to be discontinued and to receive only comfort oriented measures').

Only about 20% of patients nationally have completed advance directives, but such documents are especially critical for HF patients who are at higher than normal risk for arrhythmias from which they might recover but be left with significant cognitive impairment.

Phases 1–5: Communication issues that cut across all phases of HF

Discussing HF medical management

HF is complex, and is best managed in all phases by meticulous monitoring of weight, adherence to a low-sodium diet, complying with multiple medications and an exercise regimen. Despite having received HF education, patients frequently have a poor understanding of the illness, their medications, and diet.[13] Education about HF management requires ongoing coaching and re-education over time. Specific detailed instructions about diet or exercise are much more effective than general directions, and allow patients to invest in self-management of their HF.[14] Coaching about HF care may be achieved through group classes,[15] telephone review and management of medications, outpatient multidisciplinary care, or home care. A review of interventions for HF care found that telephone contact with advice to see their physician for deterioration did not reduce

HF hospitalization. In contrast, multidisciplinary team follow-up with regular visits for monitoring in the clinic or at home, and programs that enhance patients' self-care activity significantly reduce hospitalization for HF decompensation (see also Chapter 7).[16]

Eliciting the patient's symptoms and addressing issues that affect their quality of life are important throughout HF care. Some symptoms and issues should be screened for, such as depression, present in 30% or more of persons with HF, and cognitive impairment, also present in 30% or more of HF patients (see Chapters 14 and 15). Depression and cognitive impairment may both affect the patient's ability to manage their HF. Recognizing cognitive problems, especially with executive function (the ability to apply and process information) may require the clinician to set up systems to help patients identify changes in status and titrate medications. Pain is common in persons with HF and it is important to identify this, given many patients' reluctance to report pain and the importance of avoiding self-medication with non-steroidal anti-inflammatory drugs (see Chapter 12).

Helping patients and families correlate their HF-specific symptoms, such as dyspnea and fatigue, with their volume status is likely to improve their self-care skills and foster the partnership between them and their clinicians.[17] Eliciting symptoms also opens an opportunity to provide empathetic support to patients. Phrases such as 'That must be difficult' or 'I can see that upsets you' are simple empathetic responses that make patients feel heard.[18] The relationship that develops over time with patients and their families also facilitates conversations and decision-making when HF worsens.

Phase 3: Exacerbations and remissions; gradual functional decline

Many of the communication challenges of earlier care need to be revisited when the patient declines clinically. For example, each exacerbation will be experienced as 'bad news', potentially signifying deterioration in the patient's condition and reawakening concerns about mortality. With a decline in status or a hospitalization, the patient and family will probably meet new providers who must revisit the patient's and their family's understanding and preferences, using the ask–tell–ask strategy. As functional status and quality of life potentially decline, the patient's preferences about CPR may change, as may the probabilities of it being successful. If advance care planning has been avoided earlier in care, then it certainly should be reopened at the time of any deterioration. With each exacerbation, careful exploration of compliance with diet and medicinal therapies should be reviewed with the patient and family, given the prevalence of non-compliance as a root cause.[19]

Begin an exploration of advanced therapies

If the patient begins to have more frequent exacerbations, and it is confirmed with a reasonable degree of certainty that the issue is disease progression and not non-compliance, the clinician must begin to explore the patient's views and values with regard to the advanced therapies that are possible later. This exploration often begins with another 'bad news' discussion, as the patient and family are once again being informed that the patient's clinical condition is worsening, as is the prognosis. These discussions often begin with an exploration of the patient's view of his or her quality of life between exacerbations, and their views about potentially utilizing invasive medical technologies to improve quality of life or potentially extend life in the future. The range of potential options is rapidly expanding, such that in addition to cardiac transplantation it now includes the possibility of ventricular assist devices as destination therapies for those who may not be candidates for transplantation (See Chapter 6).[20] The task here has several facets: 1) to inform patients about the kinds of medical options that may be down the road for them, 2) to learn about their views of using invasive medical technology to potentially prolong life, 3) to integrate the patient's views about risk taking.

When the patient declines in functional status or HF clinically worsens, a discussion about the worsened status should accompany a review of the patient's values and preferences for treatment. Goals for the general direction of care should be identified anew and options for technological or other HF interventions identified. Decision-making about interventions when HF status worsens should be guided by the identification of goals. These conversations must be guided by the physician, with knowledge of what options for care are available and what their likely course would be for that individual patient. Guidance and recommendations from physicians should integrate the patient's values and preferences as much as possible.[21]

Communicating about prognosis

Communication with HF patients about their prognosis differ depending on the phase of their illness, so it is often an ongoing discussion that must be revised and updated with each phase of illness. At the time of diagnosis, much of the communication will be about the underlying cause, medications for HF, and how to manage the illness, but even then the physician should acknowledge that HF is a life-limiting illness. Limited data suggest that these conversations rarely occur, even with hospitalized HF patients.[22]

A sample of community-dwelling patients with life-limiting HF, chronic obstructive lung disease, or cancer frequently reported not being told they could die from their illness and not having discussed prognosis with their clinician, despite the clinician having reported doing so.[23] Forty per cent of those who reported not discussing life expectancy did not want such a discussion; however, more than four out of five patients who believed they had a year or less to live did wish to discuss prognosis. An 'ask–tell–ask' approach might yield better concordance between clinician and patient understanding when discussions about prognosis and dying from HF are initiated ('Would it be useful to you for us to discuss your prognosis?').

When HF status worsens, because of the inevitable uncertainty about prognosis in any individual HF patient, a return to the 'hope for the best, and prepare for the worst' conversation is appropriate. On the 'hope' side, there is a return to optimization of the medical and dietary regimen, a discussion about devices or other interventions if appropriate, and information that some patients with even advanced disease can live for several years. On the 'preparation for the worst' side, the clinician must provide information that unfortunately death could come rather suddenly at any time, so if there are unfinished issues (such as a will, unresolved financial issues, or family matters that need attention) they should be attended to quickly. Patients living with this uncertainty should be encouraged to attend to the most important matters in their lives now, and if they can return to them later, all the better.

Exploring tradeoffs in treatment

Most chronically ill persons with HF would choose aggressive inpatient care or treatments that might require prolonged hospitalization rather than die, unless the interventions are very likely to leave them with significant functional or cognitive deficits.[24] Understanding conditions in which prolonging life would be unacceptable ('unacceptable health states') as well as general preferences for treatment are important aspects of advance care planning. As illness progresses or function declines, ill persons often reset their acceptance of more functional limitation when defining quality of life, so physicians should expect that patients' preferences might change over time. Most people would prefer a long life with good quality of life. As illness progresses, patients may decide a given focus is most important to them. Among advanced HF patients, there is significant variability in patients' willingness to trade quality of life for longevity. Patients with more symptom distress may be most willing to trade quantity for quality of life, yet clinical status does not correlate well with preferences,[25] so clinicians must ask about the patient's preferences and values, and revisit them frequently as the patient's condition deteriorates.

Phases 4 and 5: Exploring invasive measures, maximizing quality of life, and preparing for the likelihood of death

When HF status has worsened despite appropriate medical or other therapy, the clinician should again have a conversation that might begin, 'Unfortunately we are at that point [we previously discussed] and we need to consider what path to take in therapy'. The likely course with a given intervention for a given patient with advanced HF is not optimally defined unless the patient meets the limited description of persons enrolled in HF clinical trials.[26] Moreover, even with advanced HF, the prognosis for a given patient is uncertain. Three-quarters of persons with New York Heart Association (NYHA) Class III or IV HF eventually die from progressive HF or sudden cardiac death (see also Chapter 18).[27] While NYHA classification is associated with risk of dying, some patients with NYHA Class IV symptoms live for 2 or more years, particularly when their fluid status can be optimized and euvolemia maintained.[28] Dependence on intravenous inotropes suggests a prognosis of 3 to 6 months.[29,30] Predictive models or 'risk scores' identify profiles that make death likely in 30 days, 60 days, or 1 year,[31,32] but no data have been published about the prospective application of these models to clinical practice. In REMATCH, 20% of medically treated patients hospitalized with advanced HF died within a month of enrollment, and about half of patients lived 6 months or less, but several patients lived 24 months or more (prognostication is reviewed in detail in Chapter 21).[20]

The physician is thus left with uncertainty as to what the likely course of the advanced HF patient will be with or without many interventions, with acute hospital care or with hospice care.[33] While uncertainty is difficult for many patients and families to understand, most eventually accept it and often desire their physician's assessment or recommendation in decision-making about their care.[34,35] Counseling a patient with advanced HF thus requires acknowledgement of uncertainty as well as the physician's best estimate of the patient's course. The physician's role in such conversations is to share their expertise, while learning the patient's concerns and perspective. General goals for the direction of care should be set, and then interventions discussed in the context of these goals. Discordance between the patient's understanding and what is reasonable to expect from the physician's perspective can be identified and discussed.[36] Both the potential benefits and burdens of advanced interventions should be explored with the patient, along with the clinician's recommendations about whether such interventions are indicated given what is known about the patient's views and values, as well as the particulars of their medical condition.

Despite uncertainty, the prognosis for HF is poor and most patients with Stage D HF die in 1 to 2 years even with aggressive medical and device therapy,[37] so general statements about HF prognosis are warranted. Although the topic seems difficult to initiate, avoiding a conversation about dying may cause unease or anxiety for both the patient and the physician.[38] Sudden death is proportionally less likely to be the cause of death for advanced HF patients than it is for those with NYHA Class II symptoms; however, revisiting the conversation about allowing natural death versus attempting resuscitation is warranted as HF worsens.

Discussing end-of-life issues

When patients are very ill, asking them about their concerns or biggest fears often helps to initiate the conversation. Usually patients or their families recognize they are not doing well. Sometimes patients will directly ask if they are dying, and the physician can acknowledge that there is unfortunately a good chance that is happening, though it is impossible to pinpoint exactly when. This acknowledgement opens the door to ask how they feel about dying, and what fears and concerns they have about the process. Sometimes the biggest fear will be how to handle the sensation of shortness of breath if one is not to go on a ventilator, and the physician can discuss the potential efficacy of opioids in easing the sensation of dyspnea, and state that the clinician will use all that would be needed to relieve that suffering. Sometimes the fears are more complex, including fear of death, what to expect after death, or concerns about family members who are left behind. Physicians or nurses may not always be the best members of the team to address such concerns, and involving clergy, psychiatry, or social work colleagues may be important at these times. With advanced HF, considerable uncertainty about the exact timing of death inevitably remains. Here the physician can acknowledge the uncertain course, but the likelihood that death will occur in a given time period ('days to weeks',

'weeks to months', or 'months to a year or more' depending on the patient's condition). If the patient wants a purely palliative approach at this phase, a referral to hospice may be appropriate. If the patient wants to continue to 'hope for the best' by continuing some or all advanced medical interventions, then they can still do some of the preparatory work for the possibility (and even likelihood) of dying at the same time as they are holding on to hope to beat the probabilities and get more time than expected. These patients are best managed by experienced HF clinicians with the goals of achieving a reasonable quality of life for several years, while simultaneously planning for both sudden death and for worsened function with a metabolic death. The patient's health status, co-morbidities, and preferences can direct the physician's recommendations about the course of care.

Conclusion

Although few data exist to inform communication between physicians, or other healthcare providers, and their HF patients, approaches to physician–patient communication from research in other conditions can be applied to HF care. HF is not immediately recognized by most as a life-limiting illness, so the inherent risk of sudden death and potential for chronic progressive disease until death must be acknowledged in early phases of illness by physicians when they communicate with patients. The uncertainty about the course and prognosis for individual HF patients presents significant challenges to clinicians. Throughout the course of HF, an 'ask–tell–ask' approach should direct communication. Emotional responses to new information about a patient's condition and prognosis should be solicited, and responded to honestly and empathetically.

Communicating with patients about their prognosis or changes in their clinical status should follow the basic steps of a 'bad news' conversation. The physician should provide recommendations based on their expertise about the patient's clinical condition and what they know about the patient's personal values, while simultaneously soliciting the patient's perspective about each potential decision. Clinicians and their HF patients face a series of communication challenges at each phase of illness, from diagnosis to death. Working through these challenges in partnership with patients and their families is at the heart of the management of advanced HF.

References

1. Corrigan JM, Donaldson MS, Kohn LT *et al.* (2001). *Crossing the Quality Chasm: a New Health System for the 21st Century*. Washington, DC: Institute of Medicine, National Academy of Sciences, National Academies Press.
2. World Health Organization. *WHO Definition of Palliative Care* (http://www.who.int/cancer/palliative/definition/en/).
3. Remme WJ, McMurray JJ, Rauch B *et al.* (2005). Public awareness of heart failure in Europe: first results from SHAPE. *Eur Heart J* **22**: 2413–21.
4. Lehman R, Doust J, Glasziou P (2005). Cardiac impairment or heart failure? *Br Med J* **331**: 415–16.
5. Mitchell JD (2005). Cardiac impairment or heart failure?: what about 'cardiovascular insufficiency syndrome'? *Br Med J* **331**: 577.
6. Tayler M, Ogden J (2005). Doctors' use of euphemisms and their impact on patients' beliefs about health: an experimental study of heart failure. *Patient Educ Counsel* **57**: 321–6.

7. Rogers AE, Addington-Hall JM, Abery AJ *et al.* (2000). Knowledge and communication difficulties for patients with chronic HF: qualitative study. *Br Med J* **321**: 605–7.

8. Murray SA, Boyd K, Kendall M, Worth A, Benton F, Clausen H (2002). Dying of lung cancer or cardiac failure: prospective qualitative interview study of patients in the community. *Br Med J* **325**: 929–34.

9. Levinson W, Kao A, Kuby A, Thisted RA (2005). Not all patients want to participate in decision making. A national study of public preferences. *J Gen Intern Med* **20**: 531–5.

10. Quill TE, Townsend P (1990). Bad news: delivery, dialogue and dilemmas. *Arch Intern Med* **151**: 463–8.

11. Back AL, Arnold M, Quill TE (2003). Hope for the best, and prepare for the worst. *Ann Intern Med* **128**: 439–43.

12. Heart Failure Society of America. *Advance Care Planning* (http://www.hfsa.org/pdf/module9.pdf).

13. Ni H, Nauman D, Burgess D *et al.* (1999). Factors influencing knowledge of and adherence to self-care among patients with heart failure. *Arch Intern Med* **159**: 1613–19.

14. Costlow J. Personal communication (see http://www.chfpatients.com/).

15. Flynn KJ, Powell LH, Mendes de Leon CF (2005). Increasing self-management skills in heart failure patients: a pilot study. *Congest Heart Fail* **11**: 297–302.

16. McAlister FA, Stewart S, Ferrua S, McMurray JJ (2004). Multidisciplinary strategies for the management of heart failure patients at high risk for admission. A systematic review of randomized trials. *J Am Coll Cardiol* **44**: 810–19.

17. Reigel B, Carlson B (2002). Facilitators and barriers to heart failure self-care. *Patient Educ Counsel* **46**: 287–95.

18. Coulehan JL, Platt FW, Egener B *et al.* (2001). 'Let me see if I have this right . . . ': words that help build empathy. *Ann Intern Med* **135**: 221–7.

19. Michalsen A, König G, Thimme W (1998). Preventable causative factors leading to hospital admission with decompensated heart failure. *Heart* **80**: 437–41

20. Rose EA, Gellins AC, Moskowitz AJ *et al.* for the Randomized Evaluation of Mechanical Assistance for the Treatment of Congestive Heart Failure (REMATCH) Study Group (2001). Long-term use of a left ventricular assist device for end-stage heart failure. *New Engl J Med* **345**: 1435–43.

21. Quill TE, Brody H (1996). Physician recommendations and patient autonomy: Finding a balance between physician power and patient choice. *Ann Intern Med* **125**: 763–9.

22. Krumholz HM, Phillips RS, Hamel MB *et al.* (1998). Resuscitation preferences among patients with severe congestive heart failure: results from the SUPPORT project. *Circulation* **98**: 648–55.

23. Fried TR, Bradley EH, O'Leary J (2003). Prognosis communication in serious illness: perceptions of older patients, caregivers and clinicians. *J Am Geriatr Soc* **51**: 1398–403.

24. Fried TR, Bradley EH, Towle VR, Allore H (2002). Understanding the treatment preferences of seriously ill patients. *New Engl J Med* **346**: 1061–6.

25. Lewis EF, Johnson PA, Johnson W *et al.* (2001). Preferences for quality of life or survival expressed by patients with heart failure. *J Heart Lung Transplant* **20**: 1016–24.

26. Heiat A, Gross CP, Krumholz HM (2002). Representation of the elderly, women, and minorities in heart failure clinical trials. *Arch Intern Med* **162**: 1682–8.

27. Carson P, Anand I, O'Connor C (2005). Mode of death in advanced heart failure: the Comparison of Medical, Pacing, and Defibrillation Therapies in Heart Failure (COMPANION) trial. *J Am Coll Cardiol* **46**: 2329–34.

28. Lucas C, Johnson W, Hamilton MA *et al.* (2000). Freedom from congestion predicts good survival despite previous Class IV symptoms of heart failure. *Am Heart J* **140**: 840–7.

29. Hershberger RE, Nauman D, Walker TL *et al.* (2003). Care processes and clinical outcomes of continuous outpatient support with inotropes (COSI) in patients with refractory end-stage heart failure. *J Card Fail* **9**: 180–7.

30. Stevenson LW, Miller LW, Desvigne-Nickens P *et al.* (2004). Left ventricular assist device as destination for patients undergoing intravenous inotropic therapy: a subset analysis from REMATCH (Randomized Evaluation of Mechanical Assistance in Treatment of Chronic Heart Failure). *Circulation* **110**: 975–81.

31. Lee DS, Austin PC, Rouleau JL *et al.* (2003). Predicting mortality among patients hospitalized with heart failure, derivation and validation of a clinical model. *J Am Med Assoc* **290**: 2581–7.

32. Felker GM, Leimberger JD, Califf RM *et al.* (2004). Risk stratification after hospitalization for decompensated heart failure. *J Card Fail* **10**: 460–6.

33. Fox E, Landrum-McNiff K, Zhong Z *et al.* (1999). for the SUPPORT investigators. Evaluation of prognostic criteria for determining hospice eligibility in patients with advanced lung, heart, or liver disease. *J Am Med Assoc* **282**: 1638–45.

34. Daley HM, Armstrong BK, Butow PN (2005). An exploratory study of cancer patients' views on doctor-provided and independent written prognostic information. *Patient Educ Counsel* **56**: 349–55.

35. Fried TR, Bradley EH, O' Leary J (2006). Changes in prognostic awareness among seriously ill older persons and their caregivers. *J Palliat Med.* **9**: 61–9.

36. Quill TE, Brody H (1996). Physician recommendations and patient autonomy: finding a balance between physician power and patient choice. *Ann Intern Med* **125**: 763–9.

37. Frankel DS, Piette JD, Jessup M, *et al.* (2006). Validation of prognostic models among patients with advanced heart failure. *J Card Fail* **12**: 430–8.

38. Quill TE (2000). Initiating end-of-life discussions with seriously ill patients: addressing the 'elephant in the room'. *J Am Med Assoc* **284**: 2502–7.

Chapter 23

Decision-making in advanced heart failure

Clyde W. Yancy

Introduction

The burden of heart failure (HF) is steadily increasing and the characteristic of the patient population has shifted to an older cohort affected by more co-morbidity and more advanced symptoms. Despite the significant advances made with evidence-based medical and device therapies and the subsequent improvement in relevant outcomes such as survival, hospitalizations, and quality of life, an increasing number of patients are now chronically ill and constitute a patient population best characterized as having 'advanced HF'. This emerging group of patients typically has New York Heart Association (NYHA) Class III, 'IIIB' or IV disease severity, i.e. symptoms at rest or symptoms with truly minimal activity. Unfortunately, a NYHA Class IIIB or IV designation is quite plastic and any given patient can vacillate between NYHA Class II, III, or IV HF depending on the state of clinical compensation/decompensation. This definition has now been enhanced by the relatively recent introduction of the new American College of Cardiology/American Heart Association (ACC/AHA) staging classification.[1] ACC/AHA Stage D HF now refers to patients, *already on appropriate medical therapy or otherwise intolerant of evidence-based therapy* with persistent symptoms of HF and at high risk for rehospitalization and/or death.[1] As this is a stage that describes the chronic condition, it is this group that most closely comprises the patient population with 'advanced HF'. Thus, patients with ACC/AHA Stage D HF will be the focus of this chapter.

Natural history of advanced HF

The annual risk of death for ambulatory HF patients on appropriate medical therapy is now about 10% per year or less.[2,3] Though much improved, this is still a considerable disease burden that is even more compelling for patients with advanced HF. It is suspected that the annual rate of death for patients with advanced HF varies from at least 50% to greater than 75%. As there are very few trials in this patient population and virtually no registry data, only inferences can be made regarding the risk of death in this cohort. The clinical trial data that are available, especially CONSENSUS (the Cooperative North Scandinavian Enalapril Survival Study)[4] and REMATCH (the Randomized Evaluation of Mechanical Assistance for the Treatment of Congestive Heart Failure),[5] are alarming.

These trials would place the annual risk of death for patients with NYHA Class IV HF (CONSENSUS) or advanced HF sufficient to warrant consideration of heart transplantation (REMATCH) at about 50% *or greater*. Surgical databases would also suggest that for patients with significant left-ventricular (LV) dysfunction and coronary artery disease, outcomes on conventional medical therapy are poor with 1-year mortality risks of about 30–40%.[6] The more recent β-blocker trials would perhaps lower that risk to around 20%[7] but over a brief 1–3-year time period, the risk of death for these patients is almost a certainty and easily rivals the risk of death associated with some of the more common malignancies.

An even greater burden resides in the risk for rehospitalization, as it is this group in whom the greatest experience with repeat hospitalization is realized. Unfortunately, the euphemism, 'frequent flyer', is not misapplied to many of these patients. It is not uncharacteristic for these patients to experience more than three hospitalizations in a 12-month period, and many of those hospitalizations represent prolonged experiences. The ADHERE (Acute Decompensated Heart Failure Registry) database identified that nearly 40% of hospitalizations for decompensated HF represent repeat events.[8] Moreover, outcomes after hospitalization for HF are associated with a worrisome increase in the risk of death, approximately 33%, at 1-year post index HF hospitalization.[9]

In one small pilot study of patients with chronic decompensated HF (two or more recent hospitalizations), the risk of death or rehospitalization in a group of patients with LV systolic dysfunction and Class IV HF or Class III HF and concomitant renal insufficiency [estimated glomerular filtration rate (GFR) < 60 ml min^{-1}] was 50% at 6 months.[10,11] The REMATCH data regarding patients with HF sufficiently severe to warrant consideration for transplantation clearly set the bar as the risk of death at 1 year in the 'optimal' medically treated group was 75% and at 24 months virtually all of the medically treated patients had succumbed.[5]

What is the evidence that guides management of ACC/AHA Stage D HF?

The 2005 ACC/AHA 'Guidelines for the Care of Chronic Heart Failure' recommend management for this patient population to include all of the evidence-based strategies for ACC/AHA Stages A–C HF. This is an important statement, as even the ACC/AHA staging scheme is subject to interpretation and without insisting on optimal exposure to proven treatment strategies, patients may be classified as being more ill than the actual condition would justify. It is imperative that patients with advanced HF be exposed to best efforts to achieve optimal medical therapy. This may require the expertise of sophisticated disease management programs and referral to such is appropriate before declaring that someone has advanced or end-stage disease. At minimum, truly effective HF clinics are able to reduce morbidity and it is likely that HF-related risks of death are similarly reduced.[1,12]

It has been previously noted that even among patients referred for consideration of heart transplantation more than 50% of these referrals do not in fact have advanced HF but rather are decompensated and are thus likely to respond to medically appropriate interventions. Thus, appropriate use of blockers of the renin–angiotensin–aldosterone system and the sympathetic nervous system are imperative treatment options (see also Chapter 4). Failure to be treated with an angiotensin-converting enzyme (ACE) inhibitor identifies patients with a worse prognosis,[13] and in this group of patients with advanced disease the use of an ACE inhibitor should be given the highest imperative.

ACE inhibitors

There are few definitive trials of medical therapy that have been completed in an ambulatory patient population with advanced HF, and virtually none recently. The CONSENSUS trial was the first randomized controlled trial to clearly demonstrate a significant survival advantage of medical therapy in advanced HF. This trial of an ACE inhibitor compared with placebo with background therapy consisting of digoxin and diuretics conducted in a small number of patients with NYHA Class IV HF was dramatically positive. However, even in those patients treated with enalapril, the residual annual mortality rate was nearly 50%.[4]

β-Blockers

The Carvedilol Prospective Randomized Cumulative Survival (COPERNICUS) trial established a clear mortality benefit of a β-blocker added to background therapy consisting of diuretics and an ACE inhibitor in patients with at least NYHA Class III HF symptoms. An important subgroup of patients in this trial either had recent symptoms, prior exposure to inotropes, Class IV HF, and/or a LV ejection fraction (LVEF) < 0.15. In this clearly higher-risk group, the use of carvedilol was associated with a similar relative risk reduction in mortality as that seen in the overall trial.[7] Even though the primary results of COPERNICUS may be debated as being applicable to a Class IV patient population, this subgroup truly represented a patient population with worse HF and established a precedent for the use of β-blocker therapy even for patients with more advanced HF.

Digoxin

The Digitalis Investigation Group (DIG) trial randomized 6800 patients with symptomatic HF to digoxin or placebo. Although the primary results were neutral, the subgroup with advanced disease realized a significant 27% lower rate of HF-related hospitalizations on digoxin but an increased rate of hospitalization for arrhythmias and digoxin-related toxicity. The real reduction in hospitalizations was a net effect of 6%. The decision to prescribe digoxin must be based on a risk–benefit assessment and, if administered, the target serum level should be kept at < 1.0 ng dl^{-1}.[14]

Aldosterone blockade

The Randomized Aldactone Evaluation Study (RALES) is an important trial in the context of treatment of advanced HF. Patients with advanced HF, either NYHA Class III or IV, defined by evidence of recent hospitalization (within 12 months) were randomized to the aldosterone antagonist spironolactone or placebo with background therapy consisting primarily of digoxin, diuretics, and ACE inhibitors. Fewer than 10% of the patients were treated with β-blockers or had device therapy. A striking mortality benefit was noted which was primarily driven by a reduction of sudden cardiac events.[15] Significant concerns have since emerged that care must be exercised in the use of these agents as drug-associated hyperkalemia may occur. If pre-existing renal insufficiency or a high normal serum potassium level is present, therapy with an aldosterone antagonist should not be considered.[1,12]

LV assist device (LVAD) therapy

Perhaps the most compelling data regarding therapy of advanced HF have come from the REMATCH study.[5] Patients in this study had chronic end-stage HF and were sufficiently ill to be considered for heart transplant candidacy but had overt contraindications to transplantation. Patients were randomized to chronic therapy with a LVAD, i.e. destination therapy, or maximal medical therapy as determined by the investigator. A number of the patients randomized to maximal medical therapy received chronic inotropic support. At 1 year, the mortality rate in the medically treated group was 75%, and by 2 years it was nearly absolute. This very high mortality rate was probably influenced by the concomitant use of continuous inotropic support.[5]

Taken together, all of the foregoing comments indicate that a clear mandate for evidence-based therapy does exist for patients with advanced HF. This therapy should encompass the optimal use of ACE inhibitors, β-blockers, aldosterone antagonists, and perhaps digoxin.

Inotropic support

Several therapies for advanced HF may actually increase the risk of events and the use of these therapies should be applied judiciously and with the awareness that the primary benefit of such is to relieve symptoms. Intravenous inotropes, whether administered in the hospital setting or chronically in an out-of-hospital environment, are associated with an exaggerated risk of death.[16,17] This is both because of the provocation of serious heart rhythm disturbances and exacerbation of the neurohormonal activation cascade with further deleterious effects on the left ventricle.

Diuretic therapy

Additional concerns have also been raised regarding the potential risks associated with high-dose diuretic therapy.[18,19] Despite being the mainstay of therapy for persistently symptomatic patients with advanced HF, the consequences of chronic exposure to high doses of loop diuretics have become a concern. Analyses from several studies raise the provocative possibility that higher doses of loop diuretics are associated with a higher risk of death.[20] These observational data cannot discern whether the need for higher diuretic doses is simply an indicator of greater illness severity, or if the diuretics per se have a direct adverse effect. Animal data are consistent with the development of renal tubular hypertrophy[21] (i.e. 'renal tubular remodeling') after chronic exposure to loop diuretics. The cardiorenal syndrome remains an ill-defined but worrisome observation in the care of patients with advanced HF. The constellation of worsening renal function, progressive requirements for loop diuretics, and lesser efficacy of diuresis constitutes the phenotype described as the cardiorenal syndrome. The exact etiology and/or precipitating factors are yet to be identified and it is difficult to diagnose prospectively. However, the cardiorenal syndrome clearly identifies a higher-risk patient population. This dreadful combination of advanced HF and concomitant renal insufficiency is a harbinger of poor outcomes.[22] In addition to diuretic resistance, several other factors including concomitant anemia, a reduction in estimated GFR, or an elevation in markers of renal function (e.g. serum creatinine and cystatin C levels) appear to characterize this syndrome. Much more research is required, but the appearance of the cardiorenal syndrome in the setting of advanced HF may ultimately represent the best marker of a poor prognosis. Given that the cardiorenal syndrome is associated with the need for higher-dose diuretics, it is possible that the need for higher diuretic doses may identify a high-risk population.

Finally, the ACC/AHA chronic HF guidelines support the use of palliative measures as needed for Stage D HF to provide comfort, and those guidelines de-emphasize the need to prolong survival when symptoms persist and quality of life deteriorates despite the best applied medical and device therapies.[1] Provocative analyses have now emerged suggesting that patients with advanced HF may willingly trade time for quality[23] and thus the value of prolonged survival in patients with advanced HF may not supersede the desire for a better quality of life. This, however, is a very individualized consideration and broad generalizations should not be applied to all patients with advanced HF (see Chapter 22). Figure 23.1 summarizes the treatment options for ACC/AHA Stage C/D HF.

Despite this portfolio of therapies for HF many patients with advanced HF remain severely and persistently ill. It is clear that an unmet clinical need exists for patients with advanced HF. The aggregate burden of morbidity and mortality is excessive and it is unfortunately only modestly impacted by standard evidence-based strategies. Therefore, certain decisions must be made in the setting of advanced HF.

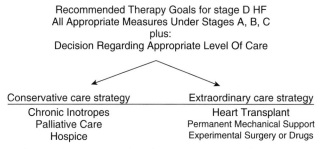

Fig. 23.1 How can chronic decompensated HF (ACC/AHA Stage C/D) be treated?

When to use inotropes?

Inotropes have represented a treatment option for HF for more than 20 years. Chronic continuous inotrope administration with or without concomitant hospice care is considered a reasonable comfort measure to implement in patients with advanced HF, persistent symptoms, and a short-term certainty of death.

Since symptomatic HF is largely driven by hemodynamic perturbations, the correction of abnormal hemodynamics typically results in an improvement of symptoms. Not unexpectedly, patients feel better. However, the benefit of feeling better must be juxtaposed with the inherent risks now shown to be associated with inotrope use whether it be short-term, intermittent, or chronic administration.[16,17]

It should be stated clearly that inotropes remain strongly indicated for cardiogenic shock or impending shock. In clinical states of low perfusion where vasodilator therapy is ineffective in improving a patient's status, inotropes should also be considered.[1,12] If, however, a patient has a complaint of dyspnea only but with good blood pressure, has known adequate cardiac output and has already exhibited adverse sensitivity to inotropic therapy, the use of inotropes should be rigorously avoided.

Despite an apparent sense of convenience and anecdotal evidence of responsiveness, intermittent outpatient exposure to inotropes does not result in an improvement in clinical status and any improvement in symptoms is short-lived. As such, the ACC/AHA chronic HF guidelines have given the use of intermittent exposure to inotropes a Class III recommendation, i.e. *this should not be done.*[1] Ultimately, the decision to be made regarding inotropic support for advanced HF is a judgment call that is at best a palliative care approach. The only acceptable route of administration is via continuous administration of inotropes. This should only be done to relieve chronic Class IV symptoms associated with a low-output state that is not ameliorated with conventional medical therapy. A careful discussion needs to be held with the patient and relevant family members and/or significant others to understand that initiation of inotropic support is associated with a brief respite from symptoms, a more encumbered lifestyle due to chronic parenteral access and the requirement for a continuous infusion pump, and, most importantly, a life expectancy measured in months. Additionally, it should be clear that certain logistics must be addressed, specifically home care, management of the infusion site, insurance support for therapy, and a declaration of resuscitation wishes. Whether or not this therapy may occur under the auspices of hospice varies by agency. Some agencies view continuous administration of inotropes as life-sustaining only and inconsistent with the principles of hospice care while others consider the use of continuous inotropes to be palliative. The best expected outcomes after initiation of continuous inotropes are some measure of improvement in quality of life, likely relief from dyspnea at rest, but compromised survival as previously noted. Death may occur sooner if there is not rigorous control of electrolytes and/or the concomitant presence of an implantable defibrillator.

Is device therapy with a defibrillator and/or cardiac resynchronization pacemaker appropriate?

Cardiac resynchronization therapy (CRT) is indicated in 'ambulatory Class IV' HF and may result in significant functional improvements, an increase in LVEF, and a survival advantage as well, but the routine use of implantable cardiac defibrillators in patients with advanced disease and limited life expectancy is problematic and involves ethical issues of cost–benefit ratios and end-of-life decision-making (see also Chapters 5 and 24).[1,12,24–28]

How is the decision to proceed with CRT made? In real-life practice, the risk profile of the patient population is likely different from the cohort studied in clinical trials; specifically age, co-morbidities, and concomitant therapy for HF are likely to differ. Given that approximately 25–40% of patients who undergo CRT fail to respond, a very thoughtful decision-making process should precede the decision to apply such a device in a patient with advanced HF. If true dyssynchrony of ventricular contraction is demonstrable by echocardiography, especially if significant mitral insufficiency is present, the decision should likely be made in favor of CRT placement, and occasionally quite remarkable improvements in clinical status may follow. If dyssynchrony is not demonstrable, the expected benefit from CRT may be low and this intervention should be considered very carefully. Use of CRT is not appropriate as a 'bailout' strategy, and when used it must be applied in the context of optimal and stable medical therapy. For the patient with advanced HF and an indication for CRT, a device without defibrillation capabilities (see below) may be a reasonable approach.

The issues regarding placement of an implantable defibrillator (ICD) are even more troublesome. For survivors of cardiac arrest or those with syncope and ventricular tachycardia, a device is indicated. However, patients with Class IV HF have not been studied to any significant extent in published primary prevention ICD trials.[26] The benefit of ICD placement takes several years to be realized. Also, if an appropriate shock is delivered, the relative risk of death or hospitalization in the next 2 years is 1.97 *as determined from patients with a baseline NYHA classification of I–III.*[29] This risk is unknown, but might be even higher in patients with baseline NYHA Class IV HF. Note also that as HF disease severity progresses, the mode of death changes so that death due to pump failure is the predominant cause of death in advanced HF. Finally, repetitive ICD discharges are troublesome. Both the natural history of the disease and the patient's quality of life are adversely affected by repetitive shocks. Thus, use of an ICD in advanced HF represents a difficult and uncertain area of clinical practice and the decision should be very much patient specific. Use of the ICD should prompt a discussion that elicits the patient's wishes should the ICD shocks become intolerable. A decision referable to when to turn off or deactivate an ICD is a difficult but necessary process to endure. It is best to have the discussion regarding ICD deactivation at the time of implant so as to avoid the extra stress associated with end-of-life decision-making.

Are we ready for LVADs?

Ventricular replacement therapy, through heart transplantation or LVAD placement as destination therapy, remains the only truly effective therapy for advanced HF.[1,12] However, these therapies are only applicable to a small select patient population due to resource limitations and very restrictive indications for LVAD support. Yet appropriate application of ventricular replacement therapies results in dramatic improvements in longevity and functional status. Virtually every patient with advanced HF should have some thought given to a ventricular replacement regimen, i.e. heart transplantation or placement of a LVAD—and, in the future, cell regeneration or replacement strategies should they ever become clinically appropriate. Most will not qualify, but the number of patients who might benefit from a ventricular replacement regimen is almost assuredly greater than the 2000 annual heart transplant recipients and the several hundred (or fewer) applications of LVAD systems. The issues related to candidacy for ventricular replacement therapy begin with the presence of NYHA Class IV disease but are more challenging with regard to: advanced age, co-morbidities, psychosocial status, and socioeconomics.

In some regards, the selection of candidates for permanent LVAD support is more restrictive than determining candidacy for heart transplantation. Family support is critical. Significant perioperative problems do occur, including risk of stroke, bleeding, and infection; and recovery and rehabilitation may be daunting. Expectations need to be managed accordingly. In the REMATCH trial, the 1-year survival on LVAD support was 52% and at 2 years, 25%, i.e. the risk of death was 48% at 1 year and 75% at 2 years. Newer devices that are smaller and perhaps more durable may expand this technology to more patients but the machine–person interface, living life tethered to a mechanical device, will remain and many patients struggle psychologically with the permanent application of mechanical support.

Transplantation still works for some

Ventricular replacement therapy challenges the patient's psyche, the family dynamic, and financial and personal resources. Transplantation is especially challenging due to the necessary transplant-related longitudinal medical therapies. The inability to tolerate long-term immunosuppression, afford complex medical follow-up, and/or resume a meaningful quality of life represents the usual reasons why transplant candidacy is denied. However, for the patient with repetitive hospitalizations and a high short-term risk of death, transplantation is currently the best and preferred option. After successful heart transplantation, the 1- and 5-year survival rates are approximately 90% and 70%, respectively, and are vastly superior to persistent medical therapy for advanced HF.[30] No patient younger than 70 years of age should be declared 'end-stage' without consideration of heart transplant candidacy.

Available data demonstrate that transplantation of older patients (older than 65–70) is associated with less good outcomes.[30] If advanced age or the confluence of co-morbidities is compelling, transplantation is not an option. Available financial resources may not support transplantation and, importantly, established patient preferences or lifestyle choices may make transplantation considerably less attractive. Thus, the realistic application of heart transplantation for advanced HF is quite modest and transplantation fails to represent a viable treatment option for the majority of patients with advanced HF.

Handling difficult treatment discussions

Patients and significant others

Patients with advanced HF face a sobering moment in their clinical course. The point at which the realization of a poor prognosis occurs is a moment of pause, concern, despair, grief, and eventually resolution. It is both terrifying and relieving as most patients experience angst over 'not knowing' and are relieved when they know the prognosis. Often this is a moment to engage the entire family and it is also a moment where undisclosed family tensions may emerge. Many families will bond and resolve outstanding issues at this time, with the singular focus being on the support of the ill member. For others, this may be an especially troublesome time for patients and an awkward moment for family members. The physician's guidance at this time is critical.

Concomitant with the revelation of the patient's prognosis is a need to address both secular and spiritual concerns. There is no handbook to follow regarding the secular to-do list but consideration should be given to creating or reviewing a last will and testament, declaring beneficiaries of insurance products, trusts, and other inheritable assets, and resolving any outstanding financial issues. Some patients may want to actively participate in funeral planning, but this is a highly individualized experience. All patients should express their desires regarding resuscitation efforts and proceed to enact living wills and advance directives so that their desires may be followed exactly as hoped. Certainly, family attorneys, financial planners, and insurance agents should be apprised of the circumstances and engaged to create any relevant documents. Though a macabre area, all of these issues become so much more troublesome if addressed after the death and it actually becomes a highly valued exercise by all to do this pre-emptively and not at a time of true crisis (see also Chapter 22).

How one handles the spiritual aspect of finally knowing and accepting a poor prognosis addresses the core of human belief. Great reverence and respect should be held for the patient's wishes and expressed preferences. The support of clergy is helpful but should not be foisted on those for whom such an interface would be uncomfortable or unwelcome. For those who express a strong spiritual connection, the embrace of clergy and religious support personnel can become uplifting and gratifying. This is one area where a simple 'What are your wishes?' represents the correct place to start (see also Chapter 16).

Once the correct network is engaged with the awareness of disease severity and prognosis and after the security blanket created by secular and spiritual preparedness is in place, true decision-making can begin. It is at this point where patients will identify themselves as risk tolerant or risk averse. Some will express their tolerance of risk overtly while others will demonstrate their preference through the decision-making process.

As there are very few strong treatment recommendations for this patient population and the few truly effective strategies represent dramatic interventions (transplantation and LVAD support), there should be very little coaxing of decision-making. The patient's expressed choices and decisions, hopefully made in the context of adequate explanations of risks and benefits, should stand unchallenged.

Many patients may be reluctant to address resources out of fear or embarrassment. A discussion should be prompted by health-care providers that proactively offers social work involvement, financial counseling, and as needed interaction with insurance managers. Although different from establishing optimal medical therapy, addressing the information needs, secular and spiritual concerns, defining boundaries of therapies, and discussing these sensitive topics is as important in optimizing care as medical therapy and should not be overlooked.

Providers

Health-care providers are especially challenged by advanced disease states and advanced HF may be one of the more challenging conditions. Given that patients are typically lucid and conversant throughout the entire experience, the health-care provider remains actively engaged even when the treatment options are few, minimally effective, or untoward. Accepting defeat is an odd dynamic for some physicians and perhaps especially so for specialists. The specialist as well as other health-care providers needs to keep the inevitability of death in context and not view far advanced disease as a defeat or failure but as the final phase of a treatment cycle. The physician's care in this final phase is as important as the initial diagnosis and early treatment decisions. Having the skill to shepherd a patient with advanced disease through the terminal period of life is a unique skill set and really defines the highest calling of a physician or other health-care provider.

Sharing bad news is a challenge and disrupts the sense of order and equanimity that is usually characteristic in ordinary practice. Striking a balance between expressing empathy while not being overcome with sympathetic feelings is a challenge. Expressing concern is healthy while showering a struggling family with pity is not beneficial. It is important to maintain objectivity, as certain decisions will be deferred to the health-care provider, and in the midst of a crisis that professional will be expected to behave calmly, rationally, and compassionately.

Clearly, the professional who deals with death and dying must have a personal support network, secular or spiritual support resources, healthy diversions, or other constructive 'check-off' valves. Loss and bereavement takes a toll on all, including the health-care provider. Do not be afraid to seek counsel and/or care. For especially daunting situations, have a rapport with ethics boards or ethic specialists as needed (see also Chapter 27).

It is expected that once a poor prognosis is confirmed, practitioners will shy away and 'disengage'. It is at this time that the practitioner should make 'staying engaged' a priority. Simpler issues like pain, dyspnea and depression control, addressing dietary preferences, and providing other conveniences as requested by the patient and/or patient's family may mark the difference between despair and dignity. Every practitioner has experienced the death of a patient. Unless there is a compelling reason to avoid contact, appropriate professional availability at the time of impending death and afterwards is likely to be welcomed by family members. Avoid the expression of pity and/or guilt as neither is healthy, but do offer to answer questions, express your own sense of loss, triage care as needed for family members, and again, 'stay engaged'.

Medicine is an art and the best practitioners are humble students of science, clinical practice, and life experiences. The real test of a physician is not how tall one stands at the time of triumph but how gracious one bows at the time of death.

References

1. Hunt SA, Abraham WT, Chin MH *et al.* (2005). ACC/AHA 2005 Guideline Update for the Diagnosis and Management of Chronic Heart Failure in the Adult: a report of the American College of Cardiology/American Heart Association Task Force on Practice Guidelines (Writing Committee to Update the 2001 Guidelines for the Evaluation and Management of Heart Failure): developed in collaboration with the American College of Chest Physicians and the International Society for Heart and Lung Transplantation: endorsed by the Heart Rhythm Society. *Circulation* **112**: e154–e235.

2. Cohn J (2002). Lessons learned from the valsartan heart failure trial (VAL-HeFT): angiotensin receptor blockers in heart failure. *Am J Cardiol* **90**: 992–3.

3. Cohn JN, Tognoni G for the Valsartan Heart Failure Trial Investigators (2001). A randomized trial of the angiotensin-receptor blocker valsartan in chronic heart failure. *New Engl J Med* **345**: 1667–75.

4. The CONSENSUS Trial Study Group (1987). Effects of enalapril on mortality in severe congestive heart failure. Results of the Cooperative North Scandinavian Enalapril Survival Study (CONSENSUS). *New Engl J Med* **316**: 1429–35.

5. Rose EA, Gelijns, AC, Moskowitz AJ *et al.* (2001). Randomized evaluation of mechanical assistance for the treatment of congestive heart failure. *New Engl J Med* **345**: 1435–43.

6. Ferguson TB, Hammill BG, Petersen ED, Delong ER, Grover SL (2002). A decade of change – risk profiles and outcomes for isolated coronary artery bypass grafting procedures, 1990–1999: a report from the STS National Database Committee and the Duke Clinical Research Institute. Society of Thoracic Surgeons. *Ann Thorac Surg* **73**: 480–9.

7. Packer M, Coats AJ, Fowler MB *et al.* (2001). Effect of carvedilol on survival in severe chronic heart failure. *New Engl J Med* **344**: 1651–8.

8. Fonarow GC, ADHERE Scientific Advisory Committee (2003). The Acute Decompensated Heart Failure National Registry (ADHERE): opportunities to improve care of patients hospitalized with acute decompensated heart failure. *Rev Cardiovasc Med* **4**: S21–S30.

9. Shahar E, Lee S, Kim J *et al.* (2004). Hospitalized heart failure: rates and long-term mortality. *J Card Fail* **10**: 374–9.

10. Yancy CW, Saltzberg MT, Berkowitz RL *et al.* (2004). Safety and feasibility of using serial infusions of nesiritide for heart failure in an outpatient setting (from the FUSION I trial). *Am J Cardiol* **94**: 595–601.

11. Yancy CW, Singh A (2006). Potential applications of outpatient nesiritide infusions in patients with advanced heart failure and concomitant renal insufficiency (from the Follow-Up Serial Infusions of Nesiritide [FUSION I] trial). *Am J Cardiol* **98**: 226–9.

12. Adams KF, Lindenfeld J, Arnold J *et al.* (2006). Executive summary: HFSA 2006 Comprehensive Heart Failure Practice Guideline. *J Card Fail* **12**: 10–38.

13. Kittleson M, Hurwitz S, Shah MR *et al.* (2003). Development of circulatory-renal limitations to angiotensin-converting enzyme inhibitors identifies patients with severe heart failure and early mortality. *J Am Coll Cardiol* **41**: 2029–35.

14. The Digitalis Investigation Group (1997). The effect of digoxin on mortality and morbidity in patients with heart failure. *New Engl J Med* **336**: 525–33.

15. Pitt B, Zannad F, Remme WJ *et al.* (1999). The effect of spironolactone on morbidity and mortality in patients with severe heart failure. Randomized Aldactone Evaluation Study Investigators. *New Engl J Med* **341**: 709–17.

16. O'Connor CM, Gattis WA, Uretsky BF *et al.* (1999). Continuous intravenous dobutamine is associated with an increased risk of death in patients with advanced heart failure: insights from the Flolan International Randomized Survival Trial (FIRST). *Am Heart J* **138**: 78–86.

17. Krell MJ, Kline EM, Bates ER *et al.* (1986). Intermittent, ambulatory dobutamine infusions in patients with severe congestive heart failure. *Am Heart J* **112**: 787–91.

18. Cotter G, Weissgarten J, Metzkor E *et al.* (1997). Increased toxicity of high-dose furosemide versus low-dose dopamine in the treatment of refractory congestive heart failure. *Clin Pharmacol Ther* **62**: 187–93.

19. Ikram H, Chan W, Espiner EA *et al.* (1980). Haemodynamic and hormone responses to acute and chronic furosemide therapy in congestive heart failure. *Clin Sci* **59**: 443–9.

20. Domanski M, Norman J, Pitt B *et al.* (2003). Diuretic use, progressive heart failure, and death in patients in the studies of left ventricular dysfunction (SOLVD). *J Am Coll Cardiol* **42**: 705–8.

21. Ellison DH (1994). Diuretic drugs and the treatment of edema from clinic to bench and back again. *Am J Kidney Dis* **23**: 623–43.

22. McCullough PA (2002). Cardiorenal risk: an important clinical intersection. *Rev Cardiovasc Med* **3**: 71–6.

23. Lewis EF, Johnson PA, Johnson W *et al.* (2001). Preferences for quality of life or survival expressed by patients with heart failure. *J Heart Lung Transplant* **20**: 1016–24.

24. Mark DB, Nelson CL, Anstrom KJ *et al.* (2006). Cost-effectiveness of defibrillator therapy or amiodarone in chronic stable heart failure: results from the Sudden Cardiac Death in Heart Failure Trial (SCD-HeFT). *Circulation* **114**: 135–42.

25. Stevenson LW (2006). Implantable cardioverter-defibrillators for primary prevention of sudden death in heart failure: are there enough bangs for the bucks? *Circulation* **114**: 101–3.

26. Bardy GH (2005). Amiodarone or implantable cardioverter defibrillator for congestive heart failure. *New Engl J Med* **352**: 225–37.

27. Bristow MR, Saxon LA, Boehmer J *et al.* (2004). Comparison of medical therapy, pacing and defibrillation in heart failure [COMPANION] Investigators. Cardiac-resynchronization therapy with or without an implantable defibrillator in advanced chronic heart failure. *New Engl J Med* **350**: 2140–50.

28. Cleland JG, Daubert JC, Erdmann E, *et al.* Tavazzi L, Cardiac Resynchronization-Heart Failure [CARE HF] Study Investigators (2005). The effect of cardiac resynchronization on morbidity and mortality in heart failure. *New Engl J Med* **352**: 1539–49.

29. McAlister FA, Ezekowitz J, Hooton N *et al.* (2007). Cardiac resynchronization therapy for patients with left ventricular systolic dysfunction: a systematic review. *J Am Med Assoc* **297**: 2502–14.

30. Taylor DO, Edwards LB, Boucek MM *et al.* (2006). Registry of the International Society of Heart and Lung Transplantation: twenty-third official adult heart transplantation report – 2006. *J Heart Lung Transplant* **25**: 869–79.

Chapter 24

Ethical dilemmas in therapy withdrawal

Katrina A. Bramstedt

Introduction

The care and treatment of heart failure (HF) exists amid a broad spectrum of technologies, some of which are simple (diuretics) and others of which are highly complex (ventricular assist devices). In the setting of clinical decompensation and poor prognosis, discussions about withholding and withdrawal of interventions often ensue and such can be ethically troubling for all parties involved. This chapter explores the concept of therapy withdrawal and offers guidance for the resolution of ethical dilemmas that can occur in such situations.

Burdens, benefits, and futility

The utility of any intervention must be based on reflection of its burdens and anticipated benefits for each unique patient. While the intent of a medical or surgical intervention is clinical benefit, this is not always realized, and such intervention is not always without concurrent burdens to the patient. For example, ventricular assist devices are a proven technology for bridging patients to transplant, as well as destination therapy (permanent use without a transplant); however, the use of these devices entails a significant risk of infection[1] and cerebrovascular events.[2] These devices can also be noisy, with bulky external power supplies. Patients and families need to be informed about and comprehend the burdens and benefits of proposed therapies so that they can make informed choices about whether or not to consent to them.

Clinical benefit can consist of many forms including life extension, relief of suffering, halting of disease progression, reversal of disease progression, improvement of functional status, and improvement of quality of life. This said, expectations of clinical benefit must reflect on each patient's co-morbidities. There are situations in which a proposed technology is likely to offer benefit to one patient but not another. In these latter situations, the proposed technology could be deemed futile.[3] Not only do futile interventions not benefit patients, they subject them to harm and potentially worsen their quality of life. Additionally, futile interventions are wasteful of medical resources. If a technology is judged to be futile for a specific patient, there is no ethical obligation to offer it. Further, it is ethically appropriate to discontinue interventions that become futile after they have been initiated (e.g. dialysis, ventricular assist support). Even if patients or families demand futile therapies there is no ethical obligation to provide them.[4,5]

There may be situations in which the patient, the family, and the medical team are in disagreement about whether or not a therapy is futile. In such situations patients should be offered a second opinion regarding the utility of the therapy. If the second opinion concludes that the therapy is futile yet the patient or family still demands it, considera- tion should be given to transferring the patient to a facility that will agree to provide such treatment. If the patient is not stable for transfer or no transfer facility exists, no ethical obligation is created for the current facility to provide the demanded treatment.[5] In these situations, consultation with a hospital ethicist or ethics committee is advised. Additionally, documentation of family discussions should be placed in the patient's medical record.

Patient's treatment preferences

When making clinical decisions, it is optimal to have a treatment partnership (alliance) in which the medical team has an understanding of the patient's values about life and health care. These values are often influenced by a patient's personal life experiences (e.g. prior medical events), role as spouse/parent, educational level, and religious and cultural beliefs. For patients who have the functional capacity for medical decision-making, enquiries should be made by the medical team about their values and health-care preferences.

Some people explicitly desire to forgo 'aggressive' interventions such as dialysis, artificial feeding, and cardiopulmonary resuscitation if they become terminally ill or in a permanent vegetative state. Exclusive of a preference for futile therapy, these values should be respected by the medical team, even when the values might seem odd or irrational. As an example, some patients with decision-making capacity reject therapy that other patients (or their physicians) would accept. These informed refusals must be respected.[6]

Surrogate decision-making

At the end of life, some patients lose the functional capacity for medical decision- making. This loss of capacity can be temporary or permanent. In these situations, it is important for the medical team to ascertain if the patient had declared his/her values about medical treatment and end-of-life care prior to losing decision-making capacity. Some patients record their values in a document called an advance directive or living will.[7] Others use a values history form.[8] Regardless of what documentation is used (formal or informal), this paperwork speaks the values of the patient when the patient cannot speak for him/herself. As such, the words of these patients, recorded at a time when they evidenced decision-making capacity, are just as valid as if the patients were verbally speaking to the medical team. Usually, the patient's spouse, adult child, or family physician will have a copy of these documents. Sometimes, they are already on file at the hospital as a routine part of the patient's medical chart or they have been inserted into the medical record during a prior hospital admission.

When patients lack decision-making capacity, surrogates may intervene and make medical decisions for the patient using one of two methods: (1) expressed preferences or (2) best interests. Surrogates are usually spouses, adult children, or siblings; however, others such as friends or clergy can also function in this role. Lacking these, a member of the health-care team such as a physician, social worker, or ethicist can perform as a surrogate. Decision-making based on 'expressed preferences' involves honoring the values and preferences that the patient specified in written documents such as an advance directive, or the verbally expressed wishes that the surrogate was privy to. Decision-making based on 'best interests' involves making decisions for the patient that would likely contribute most to the patient's welfare (in the absence of knowing the patient's values).

Surrogate decision-making can be difficult for many reasons.[9] Some surrogates are anxious about making 'life-and-death' medical decisions when they do not explicitly know the values of the patient. Some surrogates are emotionally stressed due to the patient's clinical status and the time pressure of critical situations. Additionally, some surrogates feel overwhelmed by the technology and medical terminology related to the situation. Amid all these stressors, surrogates need to understand their role in the decision-making process. Specifically, surrogates are to honor the values and preferences of the patient when they know these values and preferences. This can be difficult when the values and preferences of the patient conflict with those of the surrogate. In cases of divergence, the medical team must be wary of surrogates who attempt to make medical decisions that reflect their own views (projection), and not that of the patient—especially when these decisions involve with withholding or withdrawal of life-saving therapy.[9]

It some cases the solution to this dilemma is educating surrogates as to their duty. In fact, this can provide emotional relief to surrogates as they come to understand their role is to reinforce the values of the patient. This, in essence, removes themselves from personal responsibility for the clinical outcome of the decisions made. If the surrogate is unable or unwilling to perform their medical decision-making duties, the medical team should take steps to switch to an alternate surrogate who will function in accordance with the patient's health-care values and goals. Surrogates who themselves lack decision-making capacity or evidence significant conflict of interest should not be allowed to make medical decisions for the patient. Use of a ethicist or ethics committee can be helpful in resolving such dilemmas.[9]

Terminating implantable interventions

As discussed, clinical situations sometimes require the termination of life support, such as when the burdens outweigh the benefits, the intervention is futile, or the patient with decision-making capacity requests such withdrawal. In cardiovascular medicine, several interventions are implantable and this can increase the complexity of decision-making. Overall, cardiac interventions should be viewed as ethically no different from pulmonary or other interventions. The fact that an intervention is implanted is ethically irrelevant. Further, no device should be seen as facilitating immortality. Patient values and his/her capacity to benefit from the intervention should be foundational to decisions about withdrawal of therapy (see Chapter 5).

As discussed earlier, when patients cannot speak for themselves, medical teams should refer to the patients' prior expressed values (written and verbal). To this end, at the time of device implantation, physicians should discuss the concept of end-of-life care and device inactivation with patients and families. A summary of this discussion should be documented in the medical chart and patients should be asked to complete an advance directive. The physician's summary note is important because patients cannot be forced to complete an advance directive. When decisions are made to withdraw therapy, the patient should never be abandoned, but rather the care plan should shift to patient comfort, including control of physical symptoms and emotional stress. Consultation with a palliative care specialist is suggested.[10]

In all cases of cardiac device inactivation, the cause of death is not the act of stopping the functioning of the device, but rather the patient's underlying cardiac disease taking its natural course to death. This philosophy is no different from that elemental to the discontinuation of dialysis or artificial ventilation. In the case of dialysis, ceasing to perform mechanical blood filtration does not cause the death of the patient, but rather death is caused by the accumulation of toxins due to impaired kidney function. In the case of artificial ventilation, ceasing to perform mechanical inflation and deflation of the lungs does not cause the patient's death, but rather lack of effective gas exchange due to impaired lung function.

Pacemakers

The termination of pacemaker support has proved to be an ethically troubling concept to many physicians, occasionally triggering the assistance of ethicists and ethics committees to resolve specific case dilemmas.[11,12] The root of this ethical discomfort often relates to the manner in which these devices work. If the patient is pacemaker dependent the device can be considered a form of life support and death would quickly follow its deactivation. For a pacemaker that is not working by way of continual pacing but rather providing intermittent electrical activity, device inactivation could result in prolonged, uncomfortable symptoms associated with congestive HF, followed by death. This latter example could be viewed (inappropriately) by some as euthanasia if they envision device inactivation, rather than the underlying disease (which elicited device implantation), as the cause of death. Regardless of device design and programming, pacemaker termination is ethically permissible and is not a form of euthanasia, as the patient's death is related to his/her underlying cardiac disease. Termination of support is accomplished by way of external application of a magnet or device reprogramming, depending on device design.

Defibrillators

As with pacemakers, it is clinically and ethically appropriate to terminate the function of defibrillators in certain situations. Some patients request deactivation of their device due to episodes of painful shocks or anticipatory anxiety about being shocked.[13] Some patients have do not resuscitate (DNR) orders, and the action of implantable defibrillators is contrary to their desire to forgo resuscitation.[14] Even in the absence of a DNR order, a patient should not be subjected to the shock of a defibrillator if the harm outweighs the benefit or such is determined to be futile. For patients who are terminal, defibrillator shocks in the last months, weeks, or days of life prolong inevitable death and can be stressful for patients and their families, worsening the death experience.[15] In fact, some hospice programs require DNR orders and deactivation of implanted defibrillators as a condition of admission. This is because at the end of life the actions of defibrillators are inconsistent with the philosophy of palliative care and the promotion of a 'good death'. Similar to pacemakers, deactivation of implanted defibrillators is by way of application of an external magnet or device reprogramming, depending on device design.

Ventricular assist devices, total artificial heart

The most invasive and complex cardiac technologies are implantable heart pumps. These therapies occur as ventricular assist devices (single or bi-ventricular pumps) and total artificial heart replacement devices. Use of any of these devices makes the patient 'pump dependent'. This means that the pump will function until it malfunctions or is turned off. Also, these pumps function without regard to the patient's co-morbidities and quality of life (see Chapter 6).

The use of ventricular assist devices, as well as total artificial heart replacement devices, often give rise to clinical complications that can impair a patient's quality of life. Examples are chronic infection[1] and cerebrovascular events.[2] Patients developing multi-organ failure or devastating neurological damage evidence little benefit and significant burden from these device technologies. Also, a cardiac pump that is 'working perfectly' can be working in a clinical situation that is futile. Using the same arguments described earlier in this chapter, it is ethically permissible to discontinue ventricular assist devices and total artificial heart replacement devices at the request of patients who have decision-making capacity, when device burdens outweigh the benefits, or in futile situations.[3,16] Further, it is ethically inappropriate to force patients to linger, pump-dependent, when their health-care values and goals indicate a desire for withdrawal of life support. No patient should be at the mercy of their implant, and no medical team should be forced to provide futile therapy.

Ventricular assist devices function by implantation into the ventricle. In this way, the assist device and the native heart are present together, both functioning at the same time, yet in different ways. This partnership of device and organ can create ethical complexity when considering termination of device support. This is because some devices, when turned off, still remain implanted in the heart apex, potentially disrupting the heart's native contractility. Also, because the device is still in place yet not pumping, there is the potential for blood backflow and pooling (leading to thrombosis), as well as inefficient regurgitant blood flow.[16] Notwithstanding all of these scenarios, termination of device support can still be viewed as ethically permissible, as the root of the clinical picture (stimulating the initial need for device support) is incurable cardiac disease.

Similar to pacemakers and implantable defibrillators, consent discussions prior to implantation of a cardiac pump should include a detailed conversation about the concept of pump dependence, as well as the patient's values about health care at the end of life. A summary note should be placed in the patient's chart and he/she should be advised to complete an advance directive that reflects treatment wishes in light of having a cardiac implant that is a form of life support.

Conclusion

All therapies, whether implantable or not, should be regularly evaluated to ascertain their burdens and the patient's capacity to benefit from them. Patients with decision-making capacity should be routinely invited to comment on their quality of life, as well as their health-care goals. When advance directive documentation exists, it should be reviewed by the health-care team and decision-making surrogates. All treatment decisions should reflect the burdens, benefits, and values of the patient or the patient's best interests when discrete values are unknown.

References

1. Gordon RJ, Quagliarello B, Lowy FD (2006). Ventricular assist device-related infections. *Lancet Infect Dis* 6: 426–37.
2. Lazar RM, Shapiro PA, Jaski BE *et al.* (2004). Neurological events during long-term mechanical circulatory support for heart failure: the Randomized Evaluation of Mechanical Assistance for the Treatment of Congestive Heart Failure (REMATCH) experience. *Circulation* 109: 2423–7.
3. Bramstedt KA (2003). Contemplating total artificial heart inactivation in cases of futility. *Death Stud* 27: 295–304.
4. American Medical Association (1994). *Ethical Opinion E-2.035 Futile Care.* Chicago, IL: American Medical Association.
5. American Medical Association (1996). *Ethical Opinion E-2.037 Medical Futility in End-of-Life Care.* Chicago, IL: American Medical Association.
6. Bramstedt KA, Nash PJ (2005). When death is the outcome of informed refusal: dilemma of rejecting ventricular assist device therapy. *J Heart Lung Transplant* 24: 229–30.
7. Hickman SE, Hammes BJ, Moss AH, Tolle SW (2005). Hope for the future: achieving the original intent of advance directives. *Hastings Cent Rep* Nov-Dec: S26–S30.
8. Rudd M (2004). *Life Planning in New Mexico.* Albuquerque, NM: Abogada Press.
9. Bramstedt KA (2003). Questioning the decision-making capacity of surrogates. *Intern Med J* 33: 257–9.
10. Hauptman PJ, Havraneh EP (2005). Integrating palliative care into heart failure care. *Arch Intern Med* 165: 374–8.
11. Mueller PS, Hook CC, Hayes DL (2003). Ethical analysis of withdrawal of pacemaker or implantable cardioverter-defibrillator support at the end of life. *Mayo Clin Proc* 78: 959–63.
12. Mueller PS, Hayes DL, Bramstedt KA, Barnes SA, Harris AM (2006). *Ethical Aspects of Deactivating Pacemakers and ICDs in Terminally Ill Patients.* Oral presentation, Heart Rhythm Society 27th Annual Scientific Sessions (Boston, MA), 18 May 2006. Available on-line at http://www.heartrhythm2006.org/. Accessed 27 June 2006.
13. Fricchione GL, Olson LC, Vlay SC (1989). Psychiatric syndromes in patients with the automatic internal cardioverter defibrillator: anxiety, psychological dependence, abuse, and withdrawal. *Am Heart J* 117: 1411–14.

14. Bramstedt KA (2001). The use of advance directives and do not resuscitate orders when considering the inactivation of implantable cardioverter defibrillators in terminal patients. *Cardiovasc Rev Rep* 22: 175–6.

15. Sears SF, Sowell LV, Kuhl EA *et al.* (2006). Quality of death: implantable cardioverter defibrillators and proactive care. *Pacing Clin Electrophysiol* 29: 637–42.

16. Bramstedt KA, Wenger NS (2001). When withdrawal of life-sustaining care does more than allow death to take its course: the dilemma of left ventricular assist devices. *J Heart Lung Transplant* 20: 544–8.

Chapter 25

Challenges of cultural diversity

Cynthia R. Goh

Introduction

Much of human activity is influenced by the culture in which it occurs. The practice of medicine is necessarily affected by the culture of both the patient and family and that of the health-care provision team. With globalization and increasing migration of individuals and populations, health professionals are less and less likely to find themselves working in monocultural situations.[1] Many feel uneasy about dealing with patients and families of a different ethnicity or religion from their own, especially if they belong to the dominant cultural group within their communities. Yet there are those who function in multicultural environments who seem to sail through the quagmires of cultural diversity with apparent ease.

Culture may be defined as a 'set of distinctive spiritual, material, intellectual and emotional features of society or a social group, and that it encompasses, in addition to art and literature, lifestyles, ways of living together, value systems, traditions and beliefs'.[2] While historians, anthropologists, and sociologists may define culture differently, for the purpose of patient care health professionals need to have some understanding of the worldview, values, beliefs, norms, and customs of their patients, especially if these differ significantly from their own.[3]

Ethnicity and religion may be perceived to provide the greatest diversity in culture between groups. Yet even within the same ethnic and religious group, there may be many cultural differences arising from social class, education, and generational views.[4-7] A family also has its own culture. For example, some families are very open in expressing emotion, with tears, hugs, and kisses. Other families avoid the expression of emotion, suppressing it from their conversations and interactions, and even their thoughts. Certain topics may be taboo. Families have their own way of expressing approval or otherwise, which may be unspoken. Health-care providers have to respect these variations, but first they must be aware of them.

Value systems

Values comprise ideas about the things that are important in life and they guide the rest of the manifestations of culture. Values include basic concepts, such as the sanctity of life, and the relative importance of self versus the family or social group.

Most of the great religions of the world uphold the concept of the sanctity of life, with Christianity and Islam holding that life is in the hands of God, and Buddhism prohibiting the taking of all life, including one's own.[8–11] Suicide is prohibited and euthanasia is equivalent to murder.[12]

Yet within the same society, there may be other views and other traditions. For example, in Chinese culture, several strands of philosophy interact, chief among which are Confucianism and Taoism.[13] These exert their influence to different extents on individuals, and even on the same individual under different life circumstances. For example, one of the greatest Chinese poets, Li Bai, who lived in the Tang dynasty, initially followed Confucianism when he studied to become a court official, but when his ambitions were thwarted he embraced Taoism and started leading the carefree life of a bohemian, often getting drunk while writing some of his best poetry.[14] Confucianism stresses filial piety and duty to emperor, family, and friends.[15] Taoism encourages 'non action', letting go of all that would prevent the self from merging with the universe or Supreme Being.[16] A third major school of Chinese philosophy, also dating back to the time of Confucius and Lao Tzu, is Mohism, which teaches universal love and encourages utilitarianism motivated by altruism.[17] This continues to exert its influence in Chinese society. For example, many elderly, and some younger persons, do not wish to be a burden, and some would prefer to die rather than to drain family and societal resources in keeping them alive or searching for a cure.[12] Suicide and euthanasia may be viewed positively in this light. Without strong religious prohibition, the risk of suicide or a request for euthanasia has to be considered seriously among people holding such views.

Cultural considerations in illness disclosure

There have been many studies in different cultural groups about disclosure of diagnosis and prognosis.[18–20] Much of this is related to the importance placed on the individual's right to know and right to make treatment decisions. In Anglo-Saxon, North European, and North American cultures, individual autonomy is highly valued, and the healthcare team's efforts are directed largely to protecting this. In contrast, disclosure and decision-making by the family is preferred in many cultures other than these, for example in southern and eastern Europe, Latin America, and many parts of Asia and Africa.[18,21–24]

Truth disclosure has been a source of tension in the practice of palliative care in non-Western cultures. Because traditionally Western palliative care practice has always stressed the patient's right to know the diagnosis and prognosis in order to make treatment decisions and to prepare for the end of life, practitioners in non-Western cultures are caught between opposition from the family to tell the patient the diagnosis, and guilt from within the palliative care team whose members may feel they have let the patient down by non-disclosure. Only in recent years has it been more generally recognized that cultural differences in diagnosis disclosure are acceptable, and that there is no absolute right or wrong. Truth should be disclosed judiciously, in a timely manner, and with sensitivity to the wishes of the patient, as well as their family.[5,6,18]

Perhaps one difference in truth-telling between East and West lies in how literal or graphic one's description of a situation has to be. In Western scientific thought, accuracy of description of facts and figures is the preferred norm. But with older and possibly more traditional-thinking folk, graphic description of a situation may be repugnant, and gentler language that puts across the essential ideas, without going into details, may be more acceptable.[7,21] One may reflect that if a patient realizes that he is going to die soon, how necessary is it for him to know the exact name of the condition or the manner in which it will kill him?

The above situation is perhaps much more of a dilemma in cancer palliative care, where the 'cancer' word may mean a death sentence to many patients. In cardiac palliative care, the difficulty lies not in telling the patient that he/she has heart disease, but in putting across the seriousness of the situation. Because heart conditions are commonplace, it is often difficult to explain and to put in perspective the high risk of death without seeming overdramatic and totally pessimistic. Discussions of a pacemaker, or even cardiac transplantation, may still for some patients not signify serious disease. There is great individual variation in conceptualizing risk.

Individual versus family decision-making also has to be respected. Many older patients may delegate decision-making to their children. When this is clearly expressed, there is usually no problem. But tacit understanding may be preferred in some Eastern cultures, where the need to spell out everything clearly, such as on a contractual basis, is not desired.[7,25,26]

Interface between different systems and concepts of disease

In both East and West, there are alternative concepts of physiology and disease to the Western scientific tradition. In the West, homoeopathy is well established, with its principle of 'like should be cured with like'.[27] The traditional Chinese view of health and disease is based on harmony and balance between the negative and the positive, the Yin and Yang. Disease is seen as a disruption of this balance, which affects the flow of life energy or qi, and treatment consists of its restoration.[28]

Many common foods are designated to be 'heaty', adding to the Yang, or 'cooling' adding to the Yin. Depending on the symptom, these foods are taken to restore the balance. Heaty foods include fried foods, spicy or chilli-hot foods, strong-tasting meats such as mutton, and certain fruits, such as the durian. Symptoms of 'heatiness' include constipation as well as dryness of the mouth and sore throat. To counteract these symptoms, 'cooling' drinks and foods are taken. Examples include infusions of cooling herbs, tea, green bean soup, most fruits like apples, pears, oranges, and especially mangosteen.

Many Western drugs are also considered 'heaty' or, less commonly, 'cooling'. Common cardiac drugs such as calcium channel blockers, which predispose to constipation, are considered 'heaty', as are the B vitamins, and morphine. A similar complicated system of food balances is found in India, according to the Ayurvedic system of medicine.[29]

Understanding of symptoms

The Western medical view of the significance of symptoms or the manifestation of disease may be very different from a common layperson's view. While it is common for the layperson with disseminated cancer to attribute any new symptom to progression of disease, there are local idiosyncrasies. Believers in the traditional Chinese view of health and disease would attribute symptoms like constipation, sore throat, and skin rashes to excessive 'heatiness', and symptoms like cough, sputum, rhinorrhoea, diarrhoea, and asthmatic attacks to excessive 'coolness' in the system.[30] Other symptoms like swollen feet, a common manifestation of heart failure (HF) or hypoalbuminaemia, may be viewed with alarm by elderly Chinese men in Singapore because it is considered a harbinger of death. Interestingly, this local myth is not applicable to women.

Fear of morphine

Fear of morphine seems to be universal in most cultures, and not only among patients but among health professionals as well.[31] In Western cultures, morphine may conjure up images of maladapted drug addicts. In East Asia, the 19th-century enslavement of populations to drugs to sustain the tea trade to Europe, culminating in the Opium Wars of 1842 and 1860, is a constant reminder of the ills of narcotic drugs. Ongoing public education campaigns on the dangers of drug addiction add to the negative impact of opioids. Yet morphine is an essential drug, both for pain and for dyspnoea. Before starting morphine, not only is there a need for education about the side-effects and their control, but reassurance about safety and lack of addictive qualities of morphine when used for the relief of symptoms have to be emphasized.

Gender issues

There is much cultural diversity with regard to how gender differences are viewed. In both Eastern and Western cultures, women tend to take the major role in caregiving. But there are differences in who can do what. In many Eastern cultures, it would be unthinkable to have male nurses look after female patients. In some conservative Muslim cultures, this segregation may extend to doctors as well. Not only is there gender segregation in wards, but whole wings of hospitals may be segregated by gender.

It is noticeable that the status of nurses in non-Western societies is often lower than in developed Western societies. Partly, one can speculate that the influence of Florence Nightingale, who came from the highest stratum of British society, was stronger in the West. There is also a greater gap in hierarchy between doctors, who have tended to be male, and nurses, who are mostly female, which has to be overcome when functioning within a team.

Societal norms of behaviour expected of men and women are also influential. In many societies it is not becoming for women to be assertive, at least not outside the home or in mixed company. That does not necessarily mean that women are not influential within both society and the family, just that they are not seen to be so. Many languages have different forms when spoken by men and by women, denoting respect and place in society.

Religious rituals

Many religious and customary rituals are associated with the end of life.[32,33] It is useful for health professionals to be familiar with the different cultural practices found locally. It is important to note that many religious rituals are also affected by local customs.

Christian practices may be familiar to many Western-trained doctors and nurses, yet even among Christians there are differences. Some Roman Catholics may place great importance on the Sacrament of the Sick, sometimes called the Last Rites, or Anointing of the Sick. Other Roman Catholic practices include wearing a crucifix or mementoes of various saints, holding of the rosary beads, and sprinkling, or even drinking, of holy water which has been blessed or brought from a shrine. Yet certain Protestant Christians may find some of this offensive, for example seeing a crucifix with a dying Christ as opposed to an empty cross which symbolizes Christ's victory over death. Charismatic Christians may practise the laying on of hands for the healing of the sick. Christian practices are also influenced by the ethnic origin of the patient and family, be it African, African-American, Indian, or Chinese. A Chinese Christian family may observe local Chinese practices, such as holding a wake for an odd number of days. They may adapt practices like paying respects to the dead by bowing three times while standing upright, instead of kowtowing and burning incense and paper offerings, which Christians would consider idol worship.

For Muslims, death marks the transition from life on earth, which is considered a time of testing, to eternal life where one reaps the rewards of this life. Death is to be accepted as part of the divine plan.[34] For a dying patient, being able to continue daily prayers is very important, which includes being able to perform ablutions before praying. Having a colostomy may sometimes interfere with a patient's view of ritual cleanliness. There is need for patients and family members to ask each other for forgiveness, so there is much visiting when a person is ill or close to death. Reading of the Koran and saying of prayers should ideally continue up to the moment of death. For this reason, Muslims usually prefer to be at home during a terminal illness or immediately before death, unless they can be constantly attended by family members or fellow Muslims in hospital. After death, ritual washing of the body is performed by family members of the same sex, usually at home, and burial takes place before sundown on the same day if possible.[35–37]

Hindus believe in a single life-force, or Supreme Being, called Brahman, which connects all existence and pervades everything, animate or inanimate. Humans are caught in the endless cycle of birth and reincarnation with its inherent suffering, which is affected by karma, which is one's actions in the past and the present reincarnations. The goal is to seek enlightenment, in order to free the soul to be at unity with the Universe.[38]

Hinduism is more a way of life than an organized religion. There is little in the way of pastoral care, and the priests or 'pandits' are mostly involved in rituals at the temple, including marriages and funerals. Hindus believe that a dying individual's thoughts and words should be focused on God, and this determines the destination of the departing soul. Family members recite prayers or hymns and place holy water or a holy leaf on the person's tongue. After death, the body is disposed of within 24 h by burning, on a pyre by the river in India, or at a crematorium, and the ashes dispersed.[39] The family is in deep mourning for 10 to 16 days, receiving condolences from friends, listening to readings of scripture or singing hymns. The most important rituals and prayers are performed on the 10th to 12th day.[32,35]

Buddhism was founded in the 6th century BC by Siddhartha Gautama, an Indian prince who renounced his royal status to seek enlightenment after seeing the suffering in the world. Buddhists are taught the impermanence of all created things. Suffering is an inescapable part of life and the cause of suffering is desire or attachment. The way to end suffering is to cease to desire, by right action according to the Eightfold Path. The goal is to escape from the cycle of birth, death, and reincarnation and reach Nirvana.[32,40]

There are many different Buddhist practices surrounding death, depending on the type or sect of Buddhism, and these are again influenced by local custom in different parts of the world.[11] Followers of the Theravada tradition of Buddhism, such as is found in Cambodia, Laos, Thailand, and Sri Lanka, practise meditation and take up righteous living according to Buddhist precepts. A very different tradition, found in a large subset of Mahayana Buddhism in China, Korea, Japan, and Vietnam and called Pure Land Buddhism, teaches that for those not very practised in the faith, or whose occupation in this life would not allow them to progress towards Nirvana, such as fishermen, hunters, and prostitutes, by concentrating on the Amitabha Buddha and repeating his name, the soul would be taken to the Pure Land where there is no suffering, and where conditions are more conducive to their reaching Nirvana.[40,41] Families may chant or place a tape recording of the name of Amitabha Buddha at the ear of the imminently dying patient in order to facilitate this.

Many Buddhists wish to be very clear-headed at the point of death. Sedatives are not desired and titration of analgesics or morphine for dyspnoea has to be carefully done to avoid sedation. The belief is that the very last thought, described by one patient as 'like the last frame of a television image' has to be a good one, in order to achieve the best possible outcome in reincarnation. Crying around the bedside is discouraged because this would make the soul cling to present relationships and desires and be unable to let go, which may also affect the next reincarnation.

Some Buddhists also believe that the soul or consciousness may not have completely left the body when a patient is pronounced dead.[35] Interference with the body immediately after death may have an effect on the exit of the consciousness from this body and its reincarnation into the next body. Families may request no disturbance of the body for up to 8 hours after death, which may cause practical difficulties in hospital, hence the desire of families with this belief to take the patient home for the death to occur at home.

Tibetan Buddhism, which is the Vajrayana branch of Mahayana Buddhism, focuses on training of the mind and stresses the right preparation for death, because Nirvana can be achieved through this.[42] *The Tibetan Book of the Dead*[43,44] describes each step of the dying process in detail. Tibetan Buddhists believe that the consciousness can remain in the body for up to 3 days after death, and should not be disturbed.

Chinese traditional beliefs often consist of a mixture of Buddhist, Taoist, and Chinese folk religion or so-called animalistic beliefs.[13,30,45] They include belief in reincarnation, together with a diverse mixture of other beliefs which may vary between communities, dialect groups, or even families. Commonly there is the belief that meritorious deeds would accrue to a better reincarnation, while evil deeds do the opposite. However, merit can be accumulated and also transferred from others,[40] so family members can make prayers and donations to temples or charity on behalf of the patient or the deceased. There is belief in hell, where different kinds of torture are meted out for different transgressions. These are often graphically illustrated in comic books, around temples, or even at one time as a theme park in Singapore called Haw Par Villa. Fear of death is often associated with fear of hell and retribution. Dead spirits are believed to require everyday things such as money, clothes, food, houses, servants, cars—even credit cards, computers, and cell phones nowadays. Paper effigies of these items are offered as burnt offerings to the dead, as part of funeral rites and at regular intervals afterwards, such as the first day of each lunar month, on birthday and death day anniversaries, and at the main Chinese festivals. This is part of so-called ancestor worship, which may be considered the continuing care of dead relatives or ancestors by burning paper money and other paper artefacts for their use in other world. The ancestors in turn would bring blessings on the descendants.

Included among these beliefs is the wandering of the human soul around the time of death. Related to the Buddhist beliefs of the consciousness still hovering around the body after death, traditional Chinese beliefs include the soul having to return to visit the corpse. Overseas Chinese in Singapore and Malaysia usually hold wakes before the funeral, which may last an odd number of days, three, five or seven, very occasionally nine, depending on wealth and the practicalities of waiting for family members to gather. The wake is often held at the home of the patient or an offspring, or at a funeral parlour. Some families believe that if the patient dies anywhere other than at home, the soul has to make its way to the location of the corpse. This gives rise to worries that the soul may get lost and become a wandering spirit, or so-called 'hungry ghost', which has no one to feed or provide burnt offerings for it. The risk of the soul getting lost is highest during the lunar seventh month, which is called the 'Hungry Ghosts Month'. It is believed that the gates of Hell are opened on the first night of the month to allow all the hungry ghosts to wander upon the face of the earth for a month until the gates of Hell close again at the end of the seventh month.[40,45] This is the month when believers will shun hospital, even if they are very sick, in case they die there, and many elective operations are postponed.

These beliefs are also held by many Vietnamese, whose culture was strongly influenced by some 900 years of Chinese rule. Yet interestingly, these practices are far less observed in modern China. Pragmatism rules in Hong Kong where few people opt to die at home because the homes are often very cramped. Wakes are rarely held at home for practical reasons, and bodies may have to be held in mortuaries run by funeral parlours for up to several weeks while awaiting a time-slot for cremation.

The time to burial and mode of disposal of the body is often governed by religion. Buddhists and Hindus are usually cremated, the latter preferably by evening of the day of death. Parsees are traditionally exposed. Muslims and Jews are buried. But traditional practices may be impractical in immigrant populations or in large cities. While Chinese traditional beliefs favour burial, preferably on the spur of a hill facing the sea, which has the best feng shui, people in large cities like Singapore and Hong Kong have been forced to opt for cremation because of the scarcity of burial plots, which have to be vacated after a certain number of years, and exhumation has to be done with subsequent disposal of the remains. Lack of space for burial is an ongoing problem in modern China.

The provision of palliative care in these communities has to take these beliefs into account. For patients whose religions require expeditious cremation for the Hindus or burial for Muslims, issuing of the death certificate has to be prompt. Time has to be allowed for religious rites to be performed at home or at the mortuary before the funeral. If the rituals include a wake, and burial or cremation is delayed, then embalming has to be considered in a warm climate. The funeral wake may present opportunities for the palliative care team to pay their respects to the dead and to minister to the family.

Interactions between religions

In the current day of physically and socially mobile populations, generational differences in education and religion occur. In many developing nations, the younger generation may have had a Western education, sometimes at missionary schools. So a family may have members with different religions. With the advent of a life-threatening illness, spiritual issues surface. Sometimes this produces tensions within a family when certain members may be anxious to 'save the souls' of their loved ones by converting them to another faith. This may give rise to confusion and conflict within the person concerned and within the family. Well-meaning Christian children may wish their elderly Taoist parent to be baptized. The patient may bargain with several religions, vowing to believe in whichever deity that would cure them. In Singapore, it is not uncommon to come across a patient who has prayed at a famous Buddhist/Taoist Goddess of Mercy shrine, who then goes next door to the Hindu temple to worship, and on another day attend a Roman Catholic healing service. Providing care for such patients will include journeying with them, wherever they are at. It is best to avoid complicating the situation further by stressing one religion rather than another, or by introducing a different faith. Some of the most challenging family situations may arise from such cases (see Chapter 16).

Interaction of cultures

Providing care for a patient and family who are of a different faith or ethnic group from that of the health professional may be a challenge. Knowledge and understanding of the different cultures cannot be more useful. Some Western practices promote the expression of emotion, especially grief, believing that pent-up emotions may lead to complicated bereavement and grieving. Yet such ideas may clash with certain beliefs. One example is that of a Christian, Western-trained nurse trying to encourage the spouse of a dying patient to talk about her grief. She expressed surprised to find another family member trying to distract the wife by bouncing a baby on her lap while she was trying to have a serious conversation with the nurse. It was later realized that the family member was a staunch Buddhist who was working on getting the patient to let go, believing that grieving would tie the patient to this life and affect reincarnation.

Practical considerations

Working with patients and families from different cultures can be both fascinating and challenging. It is important for all health-care staff to have some knowledge and understanding of the cultural norms of the communities they have to serve. Practical points like understanding dietary practices in the various religions is essential—no beef for Hindus, no pork for Muslims and Jews, halal or kosher food for the more strict Muslims and Jews, respectively, vegetarian for certain groups of Indians according to caste or religious vows or days of observance, vegetarian for certain groups of Mahayana Buddhists, either on New Moon, Full Moon, and festivals only, or long-term. Certain types of foods may also have different significance with certain patients, according to their system of beliefs in how the body works.[28,29] There may also be many local myths about foods, for example avoidance of prawns, crabs, and even chicken after an operation for the Chinese.

A palliative care team in a multicultural society has its strength in being multicultural itself. It is useful to have on the team people of different religions, ethnicity, and language skills. Team members can learn from one another as well as from the patients they meet. Such a team may be able to match a team member to a patient who speaks the same language or dialect, or of the same religion. But being able to match language or religion is a bonus, and not always possible.

When a palliative care team is wholly unable to communicate with a patient or family member verbally, the use of interpreters is essential. Interpreters may come from the family of the patient, or there may be professional or volunteer interpreters within a health service. But the quality of translation may be very variable. Not only is there a need for factual accuracy in the translation, but it is also important to put across the correct emotional context. Some interpreters are able to do this, but others may just translate literally. Worse, some interpreters may put an expression into their own cultural context. For example, an interpreter may feel that an English expression, say, concerning death, may be too blunt, and change it to something more socially acceptable, which may have a different nuance. Without being able to double-check, one can be misled. Having some degree of bilingual skill, even if not fluent in the language in question, is often very helpful. Non-verbal cues from the patient may also help in gauging the accuracy of what is being translated.

Finally, self-awareness and self-knowledge is essential in the practice of palliative care.[46] In working across cultures one must be aware of one's knowledge gaps, presuppositions, and cultural baggage. Being able to understand the effect of one's own culture on one's judgment of situations is crucial. Various guidelines and strategies have been recommended on how to work with patients in a multicultural setting.[5,6,47–49] The essentials consist of respect for diversity, willingness to listen and to learn about the other, and a non-judgmental approach. Whatever the colour or creed, the patient and family are in essence human beings, with qualities of being human which are universal. The effects of culture form merely a veneer over the manifestation of emotions, needs, and aspirations that are common to all.

References

1. Barker J (1992). Cultural Diversity – changing the context of medical practice. [Cross-cultural medicine a decade later (Special Issue)] *West J Med* **157**: 248–54.
2. UNESCO Universal Declaration on Cultural Diversity, 2002
3. Brislin R (1993). *Understanding Culture's Influence on Behavior*. New York: Harcourt Brace.
4. Braun KL, Piersch JH, Blanchette PL (2000). An introduction to culture and its influence on end-of-life decision making. In: *Cultural Issues in End-of-life Decision Making* (ed. KL Braun, JH Pietsch, PL Blanchette), pp. 1–9. Thousand Oaks, CA: Sage Publications.
5. Hern EH, Jr, Koenig BA, Moore LJ *et al.* (1998). The difference that culture can make in end-of-life decision making. *Camb Q Healthcare Ethics* **7**: 27–40.
6. Koenig BA, Gates-Williams J (1995). Understanding cultural difference in caring for dying patients. [Caring for patients at the end-of-life (Special Issue)] *West J Med* **163**: 244–9.
7. Kagawa-Singer M, Blackhall LJ (2001). Negotiating cross-cultural issues at the end-of-life. *J Am Med Assoc* **286**: 2993–3001.
8. Rowell M (2000). Christian perspectives on end-of-life decision making: faith in a community. In: *Cultural Issues in End-of-life Decision Making* (ed. KL Braun, JH Pietsch, PL Blanchette), pp. 147–63. Thousand Oaks, CA: Sage Publications.
9. Alexander MR (2000). Catholic perspectives on euthanasia and assisted suicide: the human person and the quest for meaning. In: *Cultural Issues in End-of-life Decision Making* (ed. KL Braun, JH Pietsch, PL Blanchette), pp. 165–79. Thousand Oaks, CA: Sage Publications.
10. Hai H, Husain A (2000). Muslim perspectives regarding death, dying and end-of-life decision making. In: *Cultural Issues in End-of-life Decision Making* (ed. KL Braun, JH Pietsch, PL Blanchette), pp. 199–211. Thousand Oaks, CA: Sage Publications.
11. Keown D (2005). End-of-life: the Buddhist view. *Lancet* **366**: 952–5.
12. Klessig J (1992). The effect of values and culture on life-support decisions. [Cross-cultural medicine a decade later (Special Issue)] *West J Med* **157**: 316–22.
13. Kemp C, Chang BJ (2002). Culture and the end-of-life: Chinese. *J Hosp Palliat Nurs* **4**: 173–8.
14. Wikipedia. *Li-Bai* http://en.wikipedia.org/wiki/Li_Bai (accessed 18 January 2007).
15. Wikipedia. *Confucianism* http://en.wikipedia.org/wiki/Confucianism (accessed 24 January 2007).
16. Wikipedia. *Taoism* http://en.wikipedia.org/wiki/Daoism (accessed 18 January 2007).
17. Wikipedia. *Mohism* http://en.wikipedia.org/wiki/Mohism (accessed 16 January 2007).
18. Blackhall LJ, Murphy ST, Frank G *et al.* (1995). Ethnicity and attitudes toward patient autonomy. *J Am Med Assoc* **274**: 820–5.
19. Centeno-Cortes C, Nunez-Olarte JM (1994). Questioning diagnosis disclosure in terminal cancer patients: a prospective study evaluating patients' responses. *Palliat Med* **8**: 39–44.
20. Mitchell JC (1998). Cross cultural issues in disclosure of cancer. *Cancer Pract* **6**: 153–60.
21. Olarte JMN, Guillén DG (2001). Cultural issues and ethical dilemmas in palliative and end-of-life care in Spain. *Cancer Control* **8**: 46–54.
22. Lin CC, Wang P, Lai YL *et al.* (2000). Identifying attitudinal barriers to family management of cancer pain in palliative care in Taiwan. *Palliat Med* **14**: 463–70.
23. Lapine A, Wang-Cheng R, Goldstein M *et al.* (2001). When cultures clash: physician, patient, and family wishes in truth disclosure for dying patients. *J Palliat Med* **4**: 475–80.
24. Muller JH, Desmond B (1992). Ethical dilemmas in a cross-cultural context: a Chinese example. [Cross-cultural medicine a decade later (Special Issue)] *West J Med* **157**: 323–7.

25. Kimura R (1998). Death, dying, and advance directives in Japan: socio-cultural and legal point of view. In: *Advance Directive and Surrogate Decision Making in Transcultural Perspective* (ed. HM Sass, RM Veatch, R Kimura) Baltimore, MD: Johns Hopkins University Press.

26. Tong KL, Spicer BJ (1994). The Chinese palliative patient and family in North America: a cultural perspective. *J Palliat Care* **10**: 26–28.

27. Vickers A, Zollman C (1999). Homoeopathy. *Br Med J* **319**: 1115–18.

28. TMN Philosophy of Chinese Medicine (2001). The causes of disease in Chinese medicine. http://www.traditionalmedicine.net.au/chinsynd.htm (accessed 16 January 2007).

29. Dharmananda S (1997). *Basics of Ayurvedic Physiology.* http://www.itmonline.org/arts/ayurbasics.htm (accessed 16 January 2007).

30. Ong KJ, Back MF, Lu JJ *et al.* (2002). Cultural attitudes to cancer management in traditional South-East Asian patients. *Aust Radiol* **46**: 370–4.

31. Lin CC (2000). Barriers to the analgesic management of cancer pain: a comparison of attitudes of Taiwanese patients and their family caregivers. *Pain* **88**: 7–14.

32. Kemp C, Bhungalia S (2002). Culture and the end-of-life: a review of major world religions. *J Hosp Palliat Nurs* **4**: 235–42.

33. Clarifeld AM, Gordon M, Markwell H *et al.* (2003). Ethical issues in end-of-life geriatric care: the approach of three monotheistic religions – Judaism, Catholicism, and Islam. *J Am Geriatr Soc* **51**: 1149–54.

34. Sheikh A (1998). Death and dying – a Muslim perspective. *J R Soc Med* **91**: 138–40.

35. Firth S (2000). Cross-cultural perspectives on bereavement. In: *Death, Dying and Bereavement* (ed. D Dickenson, M Johnson, J Samson Katz), 2nd edn, pp. 339–46. Thousand Oaks, CA: Sage Publications.

36. Lawrence P, Rozmus C (2001). Culturally sensitive care of the Muslim patient. *J Transcult Nurs* **12**: 228–33.

37. Rassool GH (2000). The crescent and Islam: healing, nursing and the spiritual dimension. Some considerations towards an understanding of the Islamic perspectives on caring. *J Adv Nurs* **32**: 1476–84.

38. Deshpande O, Reid MC, Rao AS (2005). Attitudes of Asian-Indian Hindus toward end-of-life care. *J Am Geriatr Soc* **53**: 131–5.

39. Hindu Way of Life. http://mailerindia.com/hindu/veda/index.php?death (accessed 18 January 2007).

40. Nakasone RY (2000). Buddhist issues in end-of-life decision making. In: *Cultural Issues in End-of-life Decision Making* (ed. KL Braun, JH Pietsch, PL Blanchette), pp. 213–28. Thousand Oaks, CA: Sage Publications.

41. Wikipedia. *Pure Land Buddhism* http://en.wikipedia.org/wiki/Pure_Land (accessed 18 January 2007).

42. Smith-Stoner M (2005). End-of-life needs of patients who practice Tibetan Buddhism. *J Hosp Palliat Nurs* **7**: 228–33.

43. Freemantle F, Trungpa C (1992). *The Tibetan Book of the Dead.* Boston: Shambhala.

44. Sogyal R (2001). *The Tibetan Book of Living and Dying.* New York: Harper Collins.

45. Tong D (2003). *A Biblical Approach to Chinese Traditions and Beliefs.* Singapore: Armour Publishing Pte Ltd.

46. Lock M (1993). Education and self reflection: teaching about culture, health and illness. In: *Health and Cultures: Exploring the Relationships* (ed. R Masi *et al.*), p. 139. Oakville, Ontario: Mosaic Press.

47. Berlin EA, Fowkes WC (1983). A teaching framework for cross-cultural health care. *West J Med* **139**: 934–8.

48. Crawley LM, Marshall PA, Lo B *et al.* (2002). Strategies for culturally effective end-of-life care. *Ann Intern Med* **136**: 673–9.

49. Freedman B (1993). Offering truth. *Arch Intern Med* **153**: 572–6.

Chapter 26

Palliative care research in the face of uncertainty

Angie E. Rogers and Julia M. Addington-Hall

Introduction

There is growing recognition that supportive and specialist and generalist palliative care should be provided on the basis of need rather than diagnosis.[1–4] Recognition of the high symptom burden for people with chronic heart failure (HF) in the last months, weeks, and days of life, and the lack of appropriate care for this group has been central in arguments for the extension of palliative and supportive care beyond cancer,[5–8] and is perhaps one of the key conditions outside HIV/AIDS and motor neuron disease that (specialist) palliative care itself has embraced.[9–12]

The research literature has shown that people with chronic HF have a similar symptom burden to many cancer patients and that for many patients their symptoms are longer-lasting and have a greater impact on their quality of life.[13–15] Depression is an important problem for many and there is evidence that it is under-treated.[16,17] Communication with patients about their illness and its consequences is often limited, despite evidence that at least some would like to be able to talk about their prognosis and eventual death.[7,18] The prognosis in HF has been shown to be worse than that for people with lung or bowel cancer.[19] However, prognostication in HF is difficult; this is in part due to the risk of sudden death among patients with less severe HF and relatively stable symptoms.[20,21] Difficulties in prognostication present one of the key challenges to undertaking research in end-of-life care for people in general but are especially pronounced in researching the needs of those with HF.

Despite the growing literature on the palliative or supportive care needs of people with advanced HF[5–9] as in many other areas of palliative care there is a lack of evidence on effective interventions, best practice, and/or service delivery.[22] The role of the specialist HF nurse is possibly an exception to this, with robust evaluations being undertaken of their impact on patient care, but these have not focused specifically on palliative or supportive care needs.[23] More recently a study has begun to test the effectiveness and appropriateness of the Liverpool Care Pathway[24] in HF that will inevitably focus on care in the last days of life.[25]

We will address some of these issues in this chapter. Firstly we will discuss the ethics of researching in this area. Secondly we will outline some of the more common research methods and approaches used in end-of-life care research with reference, where possible, to work undertaken in HF. Finally, we address some of the more specific challenges of working with people with this condition.

Ethical issues

There is a belief, although no evidence, to suggest that it is unethical to undertake research with people who are likely to die in the near future due to an incurable medical condition. There appear to be three key areas of concern regarding the potential unethical nature of undertaking research with people who are close to death or are indeed dying. Firstly, Janssens and Gordijn[26] have suggested that it is unethical to invite people who are nearing the end of their lives to take part in research as they are unlikely to benefit directly from any resultant changes in treatments or interventions. Secondly there is a less well documented but more common belief that it is unacceptable and unethical to ask dying people to take part in research as it uses up their time that could be more usefully spent on other activities.[27] Thirdly some may object to research at this time as such patients are a 'captive audience' who are often reliant on care staff for all their personal and medical needs and may well be concerned that a refusal to participate may impact on their care.[28] However, none of these arguments is unique to undertaking research with patients towards the end of their lives. Many patients taking part in research are unlikely to benefit directly from improved care; they are also likely to face a number of demands on their time and by definition may be reliant on care staff for their personal and medical needs. However, there seems to be less concern about the ethics of undertaking research with other patient groups who may, albeit for different reasons, be just as vulnerable as those nearing the end of their lives. Recent work from Edinburgh indicates that research workers find working with other groups just as problematic and challenging as working with people towards the end of life or those who are living with an incurable disease. In this way the ethical and methodological issues raised in end-of-life research may in fact be very similar to those raised in other so-called 'sensitive' research areas such as domestic violence. The paper from Kendall et al.[29] also indicates that at least some patients with cancer and their carers would like to contribute to research in this area.

It might be argued that the comparatively low response rates for many research studies undertaken with patients known to be suffering from a life-limiting illness or bereaved relatives reflects peoples' unwillingness to take part in research concerned with end-of-life care. While it is true that response rates for end-of-life research are often low this may be a reflection of two key factors. Firstly research in this area by its very nature requires us to work with people who may feel too ill to participate in research. Secondly when asked to take part in these studies, patients and/or those caring for them have felt able to refuse to do so, which in itself is an important indication that the consent process is valid and implies that the research workers involved have correctly stressed the voluntary nature of participation.

It has been suggested that many people take part in health-related research because they want to make a contribution to improving care for others and that for some participants the process of research interviews may have positive effects.[30] Emanuel et al.[31]

argue that research interviews with terminally ill patients may be beneficial and the earlier work of Davis et al.[32] suggests that such interviews do not cause distress. The presence of an anonymous other who has promised both confidentiality and anonymity allows interviewees the opportunity to tell their own story in their own way without fear of judgment and without having to take responsibility for the emotional response of the interviewer, in this way mirroring a psychotherapeutic exchange. Even very structured interviews or interventions provide a potentially important opportunity for participants to talk in this way and may provide some psychological benefit. To our knowledge there is no published evidence to suggest that reasons for participation in and distress caused by participation in research studies is markedly different for people at the end of life than for those engaged in the research process in other areas.

Patient experiences are essential contributions to the development of patient-centred care and this is no less so in end-of-life or palliative care. If patients' views are not taken into account, care would (continue to) be provided in a rather paternalistic way with other people dictating the spectrum and mode of care delivery.[33] The views of the 'expert' patient are essential and if we do not incorporate the views of dying people we may be acting unethically and any research would lack scientific rigour.

Asking dying people to take part in research is not intrinsically unethical. It is perhaps the issue of informed consent that poses the greatest problems and it is the responsibility of the research worker to ensure that potential participants understand what is meant by informed consent and that such consent is continually sought.[34] This can be a particular challenge in studies in end-of-life and palliative care because of high levels of cognitive impairment and reduced capacity as death approaches may affect a potential subject's ability to fully understand the proposed study.[35] Cognitive impairment has been highlighted as a problem in HF. And patients with such problems need to be identified to fulfil the requirements of truly informed consent.[36]

By being clear about what participation will mean for participants, by giving them ample opportunity to refuse participation, by ensuring that participants understand that any such decision will not affect their current or future care, and by being imaginative and flexible in research designs we are acting in an ethical way. Working within a universal ethical framework, one that values and promotes beneficence, non-maleficence, respect, and justice as suggested by Beauchamp and Childress[37] may provide a firm basis for ethical decision-making.[38] If these criteria are met it is possible to allow dying patients the opportunity to potentially improve the care or experiences of others with similar conditions, something many people value, as evidenced by the growing popular literature on personal experiences of living with and dying from cancer.

Methodological challenges in conducting research at the end of life

Sampling and recruitment

Following changes in legislation in the UK with the introduction of the Data Protection Act (1998), researchers are no longer able to directly approach potential participants in research studies. Rather, research workers must rely on those holding patient details to make initial approaches to appropriate individuals. Such reliance on others to make first contact with the research cohort has a number of effects that may potentially bias results. Firstly health-care staff may exhibit selection bias and favour only those individuals they feel are appropriate for a particular study. They may be especially concerned about placing additional burdens on patients, and those caring for them, who are receiving supportive or palliative care, thereby reducing the number and clinical spectrum of potential participants through a process often referred to as 'gate keeping'.[39–41] Secondly, when research workers are reliant on health-care staff to introduce a study they are unable to control the manner in which it is described or how details of participation are explained. While participants are usually given written information about a study, these overtures may be crucial to the decision on whether to participate. Thirdly, reliance on others to approach potential study members may also result in patients being referred to the study inappropriately, which is potentially embarrassing for both patients and research staff. Finally, approaches made to a potential research sample by a third party introduces logistical risks in establishing and maintaining contact that may adversely affect data acquisition

Retention and attrition

In end-of-life care research it is not only longitudinal studies that experience difficulties in retaining patients. Patients recruited to studies are by definition suffering from an incurable illness which not only increases the likelihood that participants will die but also that they will experience a significant deterioration in their health rendering them unable to participate in research studies as planned. There are a number of strategies that can be employed to try to reduce rates of attrition and increase retention: once a patient is recruited to a study researchers should undertake the research intervention as quickly as possible, reminders about repeat interventions should be sent to participants who may already be busy with hospital or doctors' appointments, efforts should be made to keep track of participants whose care setting may change and research workers need to be vigilant in maintaining contact with recruited patients. It is important to be realistic about sample size, research design, and the time required for fieldwork.

Research methods in end-of-life care

The retrospective method

The retrospective or post-bereavement method has been used in all the major population-based surveys concerning care of the dying in the UK.[42,43] This method relies on the identification of individuals who have registered a death relevant to the proposed study and then gathering information from this person (the informant) on the nature of the death they registered. The key advantage of the retrospective method is that it allows the identification of a complete cohort of deaths from a specific cause or within a specific population. As already discussed, prognostication is difficult even in cancer and it is difficult to identify patients who are likely to die over a specified time period.

Also effectively gathering information from people in the last hours or days of life is often impossible as they are likely to be very ill and unable to participate in interviews or complete standard scales or questionnaires. However, bereaved relatives or other informants are potential sources of important information about end-of-life issues. While such proxy accounts cannot be the same as those that would have been provided by patients themselves, work by McPherson and Addington-Hall[44] indicates that the accounts of bereaved relative are more reliable than previously thought, with respondents' replies often being based on tangible evidence, such as the provision of pain control, the quality of care provided by nursing staff, and the patient's overall presentation rather than being a reflection of their own distress or bereavement.

The first study of care of the dying in the UK, Life Before Death[45] used fieldworkers to identify appropriate participants from within given communities by calling at selected addresses until a suitable respondent was found. However the Regional Study of Care for the Dying (RSCD) drew its sample from death certificates, and by doing so could sample deaths from a number of different causes and different geographical location.[43] More recently the questionnaire used in the RSCD has been redeveloped in light of developments in psychometrics and questionnaire design. The resultant version has been successfully used as a postal questionnaire in a number of studies.[46–48] The Views of Informal Cares Evaluation of Services (VOICES) questionnaire can be used by individual service providers to audit and assess the quality of the care they provide as they would have access to the names and contact details of potential sample members and this may result in higher response rates.

Retrospective case reviews such as that conducted by Thorns et al.[10] have the key advantage that a complete cohort of deaths can be included in an analysis.[49] However, such case reviews are by their nature service specific and are reliant on the quality of nursing or medical notes. The advent of computer-generated records and treatment pro formas may enhance the quality of this information in the future.

Observational studies

Observational studies have played an important part in end-of-life care research and in developing our understanding of the experience of dying, particularly within institutional settings. The seminal work of Glaser and Strauss, *Awareness of Dying*,[50] was a result of observational work at hospitals in the United States and Mills et al.'s early study of dying in a hospital in the West of Scotland[51] did much to highlight the lack of care provided to dying patients. Observational studies are reliant on a research worker being present within a care setting, gathering information from a number of different sources that may include direct observation of events such as ward rounds or multidisciplinary team meetings, formal and informal interviews with key players, and some analysis of medical notes.[52] Such researchers may assume a purely observational role or act as participant observers.[53] All types of observational studies are time-consuming and can place considerable burdens on the research worker and, initially at least, may increase feelings of anxiety among those being observed. Such studies come with their own ethical challenges.[54] If the observation is being undertaken within a care setting, consent needs to be gained from all those working or being cared for in that clinical area;[55] Dilemmas may arise if observers witness unprofessional or potentially criminal conduct. Researchers with clinical experience may be drawn or cajoled to contribute to patient care, thereby undermining the validity of the observational study.[54]

Interviews and focus groups

To date interview-based studies of patients' experiences of their diagnosis, living with and dying from an incurable condition, have been central to our growing understanding of the needs of these patients and those caring for them. They have also been important in demonstrating the value of palliative care. Interviews have been used not only to describe patients' experiences,[11,56,57] but also in the evaluation of services. Interviews with health-care professionals concerning the care they provide to dying patients or those with life-limiting conditions are also common research strategies. While face-to-face interviews are excellent in providing detailed pictures of a phenomenon, they are often expensive in terms of research workers' time, both in terms of travelling and data collection. Although they may be cost-effective, to date few studies have used telephone interviews, perhaps due to the belief that they are inappropriate. Our own research experience suggests that at least some bereaved relatives have actively asked to be interviewed over the telephone. While data gathered in this way were not as detailed as in face-to-face interviews and the interviews themselves stretched the research interviewers' powers of concentration and their emotional fortitude, it did allow people to participate in the study on their own terms.

Focus groups have also been used in end-of-life research, including studies with older people,[58,59] those from minority communities,[60] and bereaved carers. Focus groups are good ways of facilitating discussions about concrete phenomena such as GP-based care for patients with HF[61] or beliefs about and desires for end-of-life care among older people.[62] Focus groups may not provide as much detail as individual interviews but may facilitate the development of consensus among participants, often crucial to the understanding of an area of research .

We have shown that many of the major research methods and designs have been used in studies concerned with end-of-life, palliative, or supportive care. No one method has been shown to be more successful than any other in this area. As in all research it is the choice and use of the most appropriate method or methods that is most important. Ideally, all research concerning end-of-life care would be a programme of research that involved a number of questions and a natural progression from patients' experiences, development and testing of novel or new to the area treatments or interventions, and then audit or assessment of changes in clinical care. However, such comprehensive research programmes are rare and all too often end-of-life research is conducted on an *ad hoc* or one-off basis often in response to funding opportunities from governmental or national medical research councils or interested charities, all of whom have their own priorities for research and may favour some research methods over others. As such, studies should seek to account for this and try to engender original research results rather than merely replicating the earlier work of others.

Challenges in palliative care research in heart failure

Sampling and recruitment

One of the biggest barriers to research in chronic HF may be locating a sample. While many people with chronic HF will be known to cardiologists others will remain under the care of their GP or, depending on their age, be cared for by geriatricians or care of the elderly consultants. Some patients may be admitted to cardiology wards, others will be cared for on care of the elderly or general medical wards. If a representative sample is required a strategy must be devised to ensure that all patients who are eligible for inclusion are incorporated in the potential sample. The use of information technology in both acute and community-based care may facilitate case finding. However, to date, such studies are still heavily reliant on third-party recruitment, be that an acute or community-based service provider, local charity, or governmental organization such as the Office of National Statistics. As suggested earlier, steps need to be taken to address or take account of any inherent bias introduced by the method of recruitment.

Prognostication

As already noted prognosis is difficult to determine in HF; although it is known to have a high mortality rate it is difficult to predict when an individual patient is likely to die. In New York heart Association (NYHA) functional Class II, symptoms are mild and annual mortality is reported to between 5–15%, with 50–80% of individuals dying suddenly.[63] In NYHA functional Class IV annual mortality is 30–70%, but only 5–30% of deaths are sudden.[64] The relatively high risk of sudden death and high overall mortality rate make it difficult to determine when a patient is likely to die and this may have a real impact on defining populations for research concerning palliative or end-of-life care for this group. The illness trajectory in HF is typically that of organ failure with periods of acute decompensations in heart and lung function followed by periods of relative stability, albeit with progressively declining function. While the NYHA system of classification does provide some indication of a patient's condition, our own experience indicates that patients move between these groups, and as such this system presents problems in setting study inclusion criteria.

Patient knowledge of chronic heart failure

Research interviewers working with people toward the end of life often conduct interviews in which they are uncertain about interviewees' knowledge of their disease or its prognosis.[29] This is true for patients with HF who have been shown not to know or recognize the implications of their diagnosis.[6] While some patients may know they have a problem with their heart, the words 'heart failure' may be meaningless or frightening to them. This can also be true of bereaved relatives who may not know the diagnosis or who may only have been told or remember being told a diagnosis relatively late in their loved one's illness or indeed they may have learned of it for the first time from a death certificate. Alongside a lack of knowledge of their diagnosis many people with HF may not appreciate their prognosis and may be unaware that they have an incurable condition, believing instead that their medication will keep them well even if it will not cure them.

To address these two issues researchers have tended to ask people to talk 'about their heart problems' or 'health problems'. This allows patients to self-define their illness and to raise issues about prognosis or death and dying should they so wish. Methods that overcome or account for these issues need to be included or developed by those researching end-of-life in HF. It may be possible to check patients' records for documentation or preferably clarify with individual patient's health-care staff their perception of a patient's knowledge of the nature of their condition.

Co-morbidity

The older age of the majority of people with HF will often mean that their heart problem is only one among many health problems for which they receive medical care, drug treatment, or other therapeutic interventions.[65] As a consequence they may experience difficulties in attributing symptoms and side-effects to one particular condition or treatment,[54] or in assessing quality of care of individual care providers as they may not recognize which health-care team is responsible for each element of care. It might be argued that these factors may affect research outcomes and the ability of patients to provide meaningful information to research staff, and again efforts need to be made to either minimize or take account of these. Research into the effectiveness of palliative care interventions in general, but in HF in particular, may be affected by these problems. Research that aims to evaluate the effectiveness of supportive or palliative interventions, especially those provided in patients' homes, may be providing one intervention or service among many and patients may not be able to attribute increased feelings of well-being or symptom reduction to any one intervention. Palliative interventions that aim to improve coordination of service or secure additional services, such as physiotherapy, complementary therapies, or night sitting may not be immediately associated with the palliative care provider and as community nurse specialists rarely wear uniforms, it may not be obvious where they are employed.

Cognitive impairment and depression

Both cognitive impairment and depression are common among people with HF[16,17,36] and both probably affect an individual's ability to take part in research interviews or complete research-based questionnaires. With regard to cognitive deficit, there are a number of existing scales such as the Mini Mental State Examination[66,67] that can be used within the research setting to assess cognitive functioning. However, their use may introduce new problems with regard to the use of data gathered from people with impaired cognition, who by inference may not have understood the consent process for taking part in a study, and some people may question the validity or reliability of findings that include data provided by such individuals. Depression may affect an individual's ability to take part in research and may colour patients' narratives or rankings in interviews or questionnaires. A number of measures have been used in research settings to assess levels of depression, the Geriatric Depression Scale[68] and the Hospital Anxiety and

Depression Scale[69] can both be used detect clinical depression, and have been used successfully with patients with HF.

Breathlessness and weakness

Breathlessness and weakness or fatigue are common symptoms of chronic HF that may affect an individual's ability to participate in research activities, especially as their HF worsens during or following acute exacerbations. Weakness and fatigue press home the imperative that research-based interventions are short and can be undertaken at a time convenient to patients even if this requires repeated visits from research workers. There may be some value in questionnaire-based research in prioritizing the order of questions, ensuring that the most 'important' measures are completed at the beginning of the schedule. Alternatively, interviewers may start at random places within the questionnaire or different patients may be selected to complete different scales if questionnaires are lengthy. However, the best research strategy may be to limit the number of questions included and aim to get complete or near complete data from all participants. It has often being more useful and productive to use complete data from fewer measures but from a complete patient sample.

Excessive breathlessness impacts on peoples' ability to talk but can also affect the quality of their speech which in turn affects their participation in research interviews. Giving respondents plenty of time to answer questions, time to rest between questions, and the opportunity to complete an interview over two sessions may minimize these effects. If interviews are to be audio tape recorded it may be best to position the microphone close to the interviewee rather than attach it to their clothes as many manufacturers recommend, because noise associated with breathlessness can drown out the spoken word and render tapes useless.

Research workers

Until recently the support needs of research workers and particularly research interviewers were largely ignored. However, it is now recognized that any research, but especially that which focuses on the end of life, can be stressful and that adequate supervision for these workers is essential. As in many other conditions, in HF interviewers may have little first-hand experience of people with this particular condition, and may be particularly distressed by breathlessness, extreme fatigue, and depression associated with this group of patients. Interviewers, especially those without an appropriate clinical background, may find it difficult to assess what is within the 'normal' range and when someone may need extra or emergency medical or nursing care. Interviewing someone who may be at home, often alone, but who seems to be in significant distress is not uncommon, and having a clear plan of action in such instances is essential. Health-care professionals who are working as research workers or interviewers may be more competent to make patient assessments and may have more ready access to services, but they and their fellow research workers must consider their responsibility to respondents to whom they have promised confidentiality and anonymity and who may not wish to access additional help.

Conclusion

While there are many challenges to conducting appropriate, robust research with people with an incurable condition and who are towards the end of their lives, the research literature amply illustrates that it is indeed possible to complete the type of studies that have the potential to impact on both the quality of life and the quality of care for these patients. Dame Cicely Saunders' early research work on pain control improved the care of people with cancer immeasurably in the 1960s and has led to a body of evidence which continues to influence end-of-life care and treatments today. The supportive, palliative, and end-of-life care of people with chronic HF similarly needs to be improved through the provision of a sound scientific evidence base of the best treatments, interventions, service provision, and educational strategies.

End-of-life care research for people with chronic HF may be characterized by a number of challenges not often faced by those working in other areas. Patients with chronic HF may not know their diagnosis, and may be unaware of their prognosis. Additionally they may face difficulties in talking due to problems with breathing, excessive tiredness, and significant depression and may experience some degree of cognitive impairment. These factors require researchers to think imaginatively about ways of collecting valid and reliable information.

Research workers in chronic HF need to work in close alliance with health-care professionals and other care providers to ensure not only that they produce research that has the potential to improve patient care, but also to ensure access to appropriate patients and a ready source of help and advice for researchers working in the field.

When research is properly undertaken with appropriate safeguards in place for all those involved, when informed consent is routinely sought throughout the research process, and when research design is such that any findings are robust enough to contribute to improving care or quality of life there can be no ethical objections to research in this area. Indeed it might be pertinent to consider whether it would be more ethical to exclude people who are nearing the end of their life from the research process. If this were the case we would be denying dying people the opportunity to contribute to and potentially improve future care, an opportunity many have been shown to value.

References

1. Department of Health (2000). *National Service Framework for Coronary Heart Disease*. London: Department of Health.
2. Department of Health (2005). *The National Service Framework for Long-term Conditions*. London: Department of Health.
3. National Council for Palliative Care (2005). *Focus on Policy – Branching Out*. London: National Council for Palliative Care.
4. Addington-Hall JM (1997). *Reaching Out. Report of the Joint NCHSPCS and Scottish Partnership Agency Working Party on Palliative Care for Patients with Non-malignant Disease*. London: National Council for Hospice and Specialist Palliative Care Services.
5. Exley C, Field D, Jones L, Stokes T (2005). Palliative care in the community for cancer and end-stage cardiorespiratory disease: the views of patients, lay-carers and health professionals. *Palliat Med* **19**: 76–83.

6. Rogers AE, Addington-Hall JM, Aberry AJ *et al.* (2000). Knowledge and communication difficulties for patients with chronic heart failure: qualitative study. *Br Med J* **321**: 605–7.

7. Gibbs JSR (2001). Heart disease. In: *Palliative Care for Non-cancer Patients* (ed. JM Addington-Hall and IJ Higginson), pp. Oxford: Oxford University Press.

8. Murray SA, Boyd K, Kendall M, Worth A, Benton TF, Clausen H (2002). Dying of lung cancer or cardiac failure: prospective qualitative interview study of patients and their carers in the community. *Br Med J* **325**: 929–34

9. Anderson H, Ward C, Eardley A *et al.* (2001). The concerns of patients under palliative care and heart failure clinics are not being met. *Palliat Med* **15**: 279–86.

10. Thorns AR, Gibbs LME, Gibbs SJR (2001). Management of severe heart failure by specialist palliative care. *Heart* **85**: 93.

11. Horne G, Payne S (2004). Removing boundaries: palliative care for patients with heart failure. *Palliat Med* **18**: 291–6.

12. Lewis C, Stephens B (2005). Improving palliative care provision for patients with heart failure. *Br J Nurs* **14**: 563–7.

13. Stewart AL, Greenfield S, Hays RD *et al.* (1989). Functional status and well being of patients with chronic conditions. Results from a medical outcomes study. *J Am Med Assoc* **262**: 907–13.

14. Rideout E, Montemuro M (1986). Hope, morale and adaption in patients with chronic heart failure. *J Adv Nurs* **11**: 429–38.

15. Dracup K, Walden JA, Stevenson LW, Brecht ML (1992). Quality of life in patients with advanced heart failure. *J Heart Lung Transplant* **11**: 273–9.

16. Koenig HG (1998). Depression in hospitalized older patients with congestive heart failure. *Gen Hosp Psychiat* **20**: 29–43.

17. Freedland KE, Carney RM, Rich MW (1991). Depression in hospitalised older patients with congestive heart failure. *J Geriat Psychiat* **24**: 59–71

18. McCarthy M, Addington-Hall JM, Ley M (1997). Communication and choice in dying from heart disease. *J R Soc Med* **90**: 128–31.

19. Stewart S, MacIntyre K, Hole DJ, Capewell S, McMurray JJV (2001). More 'malignant' then cancer? Five year survival following readmission for heart failure. *Eur J Heart Fail* **3**: 315–22.

20. Kjekshus J (1990). Arrhythmias and mortality from congestive heart failure. *Am J Cardiol* **60**: 421–81.

21. Califf RM, Adams KF, McKenna WJ *et al.* (1997). A randomized control trial of epoprostenol therapy for severe congestive heart failure: The Flolan International Randomized Survival Trial (FIRST). *Am Heart J* **134**: 44–54.

22. Higginson IJ (2004). It would be NICE to have some evidence. *Palliat Med* **18**: 85–6.

23. Blue L, Long E, McMurray *et al.* (2001). Randomised controlled trial of specialist nurse intervention in heart failure. *Br Med J* **322**: 715–18.

24. Ellershaw J, Wilkinson S (2003). *Care of the Dying. A Pathway to Excellence*. Oxford: Oxford University Press.

25. National Council for Palliative Care (2005). *Information Exchange*.

26. Janssens R, Gordijn B (2000). Clinical trials in palliative care: an ethical evaluation. *Patient Educ Counsel* **41**: 55–62.

27. Addington-Hall JM (2002). Research sensitivities in palliative care patients. *Eur J Palliat Care* **11**: 220–4.

28. Raudonis BM (1992). Ethical considerations in qualitative research with hospice patients. *Qual Health Res* **2**: 238–49.

29. Kendall M, Harris F, Boyd K *et al.* (2007). Key challenges and ways forward in researching the 'good death': qualitative in-depth interview and focus group study. *Br Med J* **334**: 521–7.

30. Finch J. (1993). 'It's great to have somebody to talk to': ethics and politics of interviewing women. In: *Social Research: Philosophy, Politics and Practice* (ed. M Hammersley) London: Sage.

31. Emanuel EJ, Fairclough DL, Wolfe P, Emanuel LL (1997). Talking with terminally ill patients and their care givers about death, dying and bereavement: it is stressful? Is it helpful? *Palliat Med* **11**: 31–4.

32. Davis E, Hall, S, Bannon M, Hopkins A (1998). Do research interviews cause distress or interfere with management? Experience with a study of cancer patients. *J R Coll Physicians* **32**: 406–11.

33. Addington-Hall J. Introduction. In: *Palliative Research in Practice*.

34. Lawton J (2001). Gaining and maintaining informed consent: ethical concerns raised in a study of dying patients. *Qual Health Res* 11: 693–705.

35. Bruera E, Miller L, McCallon J, Macmillan K, Kefting L, Hansin J (1992). Cognitive failure (CF) in patients with terminal cancer: a prospective study. *J Pain Sympt Manage* 7: 192–5.

36. Califf RM, Adams KF, McKenna WJ *et al.* (1997). A randomized control trial of epoprostenol therapy for severe congestive heart failure: The Flolan International Randomized Survival Trial (FIRST). *Am Heart J* **134**: 44–54.

37. Beauchamp TL, Childress JF (1994). *Principles of Biomedical Ethics*. New York: Oxford University Press.

38. Sheldon F, Sargeant A. Ethical and practical issues in qualitative research. In: *Palliative Care Research in Practice* (ed. J. Addington-Hall).

39. Riley J, Ross JR (2005). Research into end of life care. *Lancet* **365**: 735–7.

40. Cook AM, Finlay AG, Butler-Keating RJ (2002). Recruiting into palliative care trials: lessons learnt from a feasibility study. *Palliat Med* **16**: 163–5.

41. Krishnasamy M (2000). Perceptions of health care need in lung cancer. Can prospective surveys provide nationally representative data? *Palliat Med* **14**: 410–18.

42. Seale CF, Cartwright A (1994). *The Year Before Death*. Aldershot: Avebury.

43. Addington-Hall JM, McCarthy M (1995). Regional study of care for the dying: methods and sample characteristics. *Palliat Med* **9**: 27–35.

44. McPherson C, Addington-Hall JM (2004). Evaluating palliative care: bereaved family members' evaluations of patients' pain, anxiety and depression. *J Pain Sympt Manage* 28, 104–14.

45. Cartwright A, Hockey L, Anderson JL (1974). *Life After Death*. London: Kegan Paul.

46. Addington-Hall JM, Walker L, Jones C, Karlsen S, McCarthy M (1998). A randomised controlled trial of postal versus interviewer administration of a questionnaire measuring satisfaction with, and use of, services received in the year before death. *J Epidemiol Commun Health* **52**: 802–7.

47. Elkington H, White P, Addington-Hall JM, Higgs R, Edmonds P (2005). The healthcare needs of chronic obstructive pulmonary disease patients in the last year of life. *Palliat Med* **19**: 487–91.

48. Rogers A, Karlsen S, Addington-Hall J (2000). 'All the services were excellent. It is when the human element comes in that things go wrong': dissatisfaction with hospital care in the last year of life. *J Adv Nurs* **31**: 768–74.

49. Formiga F, Espel E, Chivite D, Pujol R (2002). Dying from heart failure in hospital: palliative decision making analysis. *Heart* 88: 187.

50. Glaser BJ, Strauss AL (1965). *Awareness of Dying*. Chicago: Aldine.

51. Mills M, Davies HTO, Macrae WA (1994). Care of dying patients in hospital. *Br Med J* **309**: 583–6.

52. Rogers A, Addington-Hall JM (2005). Care of the dying stroke patient in the acute setting. *J Res Nurs* **10**: 153–67.

53. Kite K (1999). Participant observation, peripheral observation or apart-icipant observation? *Nurse Res* 7: 44–55.

54. Seymour J, Ingleton C (1999). Ethical issues in qualitative research at the end of life. *Int J Palliat Nurs* **5**: 65–73.

55. Merrell J, Williams A (1994). Participant observation and informed consent: relationships and tactical decision making. *Nurs Ethics* **1**: 163–72.

56. Rogers A, Addington-Hall JM, McCoy ASM *et al.* (2002). A qualitative study of chronic heart failure patients' understanding of their symptoms and drug therapy. *Eur J Heart Fail* **4**: 283–7.

57. Elkington H, White P, Addington-Hall JM, Higgs R, Pettinari C (2004). The last year of life of COPD: a qualitative study of symptoms and services. *Respir Med* **98**: 439–45.

58. Catt S, Blanchard M, Addington-Hall JM, Zis M, Blizard R, King M (2006). Older adults' attitudes to death, palliative treatment and hospice care. *Palliat Med* **19**: 402–10.

59. Catt S, Blanchard M, Addington-Hall JM, Zis M, Blizard B, King M (2006). The development of a questionnaire to assess the attitudes of older people to end-of-life issues (AEOLI). *Palliat Med* **19**: 397–401.

60. Hughes R, Saleem T, Addington-Hall J (2005). Towards a culturally acceptable end-of-life survey questionnaire: a Bengali translation of VOICES. *Int J Palliat Nurs* **11**: 116–23.

61. Hanratty B, Hibbert D, Mair F *et al.* (2002). Doctors' perceptions of palliative care for heart failure: focus group study. *Br Med J* **325**: 581–5.

62. Seymour J, Gott J, Bellamy G (2004). Planning for the end of life: views of older people about advanced care directives. *Soc Sci Med* **59**: 57–68.

63. Kjekshus J (1990). Arrhythmias and mortality from congestive heart failure. *Am J Cardiol* **65**: 421–81.

64. Lynn J, Harrell F, Cohn F *et al.* (1997). Prognosis of seriously ill hospitalized patients on the days before death: implications for patient care and public policy. *New Horizons* **5**: 56–61.

65. Taylor J, Stott DJ (2002). Chronic heart failure and cognitive impairment: co-existence of conditions or true association? Eur J Heart Fail 4: 7–9.

66. Folstein M, Folstein S, McHugh P (1975). Mini-Mental State. A practical method for grading the cognitive state of patients for the clinician. *J Psychiatr Res* **12**: 189–98.

67. Hodkinson HM (1972). Evaluation of a mental test score for assessment of mental impairment in the elderly. *Age Ageing* **1**: 233–8.

68. Yesavage JA, Brink TL, Rose TL *et al.* (1983). Development and validation of a geriatric depression screening scale: a preliminary report. *J Psychiatr Res* **17**: 37–49.

69. Zigmond AS, Snaith RP (1983). The Hospital Anxiety and Depression Scale. *Acta Psychiatr Scand* **67**: 361–70.

Chapter 27

Coping with patients' deaths

Sarah J. Goodlin and Eric J. Cassell

A 36-year-old man with a familial cardiomyopathy died suddenly in the intensive care unit while awaiting a cardiac transplant. Aggressive efforts at cardiopulmonary resuscitation were unsuccessful. His wife, 12-year-old son and 10-year-old daughter were not present and last saw him the evening prior to his death. He had not talked with them about dying as all planned on his transplantation.

An 88-year-old woman with heart failure with preserved systolic function, diabetes and atherosclerotic vascular disease underwent surgery for a colonic volvulus. She had been hospitalized three times earlier that year and both during this hospitalization and at the time of her previous discharge physicians advised the woman's adult children that death soon was likely and hospice care was appropriate given her guarded prognosis. Post-operatively she developed volume overload and then, with diuresis, progressive renal dysfunction and decreasing responsiveness, followed by death. Throughout all her daughter still hoped she would recover.

Patients' deaths are a common part of the physician's experience in heart failure (HF) care, yet physicians rarely receive support to process and cope with their deaths. Repeated patient deaths contribute to physician stress and disenchantment.[1] Doctors' responses to the death of a patient vary with the context of the death and with their relationship to the patient and their family. Nonetheless, many times death occurs in the course of a busy day and it is difficult to address the myriad of emotions, then or subsequently. Burying feelings in the day's or week's business is hurtful, and robs physicians of part of the passion of caring for patients. This chapter reflects on death of patients, the associated emotions, and approaches to processing and coping with them.

Talking with patients about dying

In physicians' work with patients to maximize health and quality of life the physician and patient must prepare for likely events in the course of HF. The subject of death should be brought up early in the care of the HF patient. If physicians talk about dying early it makes it easier for the patient and family, and the physician, to cope with death during the HF course. Physicians must become comfortable talking with patients about dying or must work with a member of the clinical team who can join them to talk with the patient. Just as oncologists began learning to talk to patients about dying three decades ago, those caring for HF patients must learn to talk about dying.

Physicians need not lecture patients about dying; rather they must learn to allow the topic of dying to come up in their interactions with patients. Because of the increased risk HF patients have for sudden death, whether to attempt resuscitation when the heart stops should be addressed at the beginning of caring for a HF patient. This conversation can be introduced as part of talking with the patient about 'what to do in an emergency', or as a routine conversation conducted with all HF patients. The conversation should end with reassurance that the physician will work with them to improve quality of life, prolong life, or to otherwise try to meet the patient's goals. The topic of dying can arise by asking patients what they know about HF, what they believe will be their course, and asking what their worries or concerns are. If the patient does not explicitly ask about dying, reflecting on concerns or the patient's belief about the next period of time opens the door for the physician to acknowledge that patients die from HF. The frame of this conversation should be to identify the fact, next tell the patient what it means for them, and end with the plan to approach the patient's care with them. ('People die from worsened HF; you are doing well now; we are going to use medications and other treatments to help you function as well as possible for as long as possible.') We suggest that it is not necessary to *tell* patients about dying, but to answer questions. It is a rare patient who has never thought he or she might die, so encouraging the question that gives you the opportunity to answer the concern is usually not difficult.

The physician's relationship with death

Death is a reality of medical care and particularly of HF care. Remarkable advances in medication and other treatments have somewhat reduced the frequency of death early after HF diagnosis. Death is nonetheless inevitable. The only reasonable approach to patients' deaths is honesty: physicians must acknowledge to themselves and with colleagues that patients die from or with HF. Honesty must extend to patients and families. While doctors cannot know who will live for years or who will die fairly soon, they must be prepared for either early or later death and so must their patients. Avoiding these conversations by saying that you do not know what is going to happen or that you cannot predict the future is not fair to patients. You may not have a crystal ball, but you have a much better idea about what will happen than the patient does.

The physician's relationships with patients

The relationship a physician builds with patients is more limited and fragmented now than in any previous period in the practice of medicine. Medicine is increasingly divided into outpatient primary care, inpatient 'hospitalist' care, specialist care, nursing home care, and hospice or palliative care. Few physicians know their patients over long periods of time, and even fewer provide their care in more than one arena. Nonetheless, the interaction between physician, patient, and their family depends on a unique relationship. This relationship demands an intimacy that comes from knowing the patient's pathophysiology and physical status, while interacting with them as persons. Physicians know patients' secrets and interpersonal dynamics to which others are not privy, and both provide medical expertise and interact with patients personally. The relationship with the family may be separate or overlap with one's relationship with the patient; however, physicians must not forget that their primary responsibility is to the patient, not the family. A physician may connect emotionally with some patients and not with others, but all relationships are based upon trust placed in physicians by the patient and/or their family.

On some level, despite the brevity or length of the relationship, the physician is given a window into the patient's experience and an opportunity to support them through their illness. When people are very sick and when the stakes of life versus death are high, physicians are intensely involved in the patient's care and the patient and family depend on the physician. Caring for patients who are dying, or who die despite efforts to postpone death, makes the doctor–patient relationship intense. It also brings enormous emotional rewards to physicians. The partnership between physicians and very ill patients and their families requires honest acknowledgement of likely events, including worsened illness and death, and a collaborative plan to approach those events when they occur.

Coping with emotions and death

Suffering is a component of the patient's experience, representing physical, psychological, and spiritual distress that occurs when a person believes that his or her intactness or integrity as a person has been threatened, injured, or disrupted.[2] Physicians also experience distress or challenge to their persons in terms of their professional role and self-image, or in non-professional personal emotions, spirituality, or even physical well-being. The death of a patient opens the door to injury to the physician's sense of adequacy and sense of self. Emotion is inherent in the very act of caring for patients and emotion is very near the surface for physicians. In medicine the emotions are more complex because of the intimacy of the doctor–patient relationship combined with impersonal medical science. It is not surprising that physicians feel emotion when a patient dies. It is surprising, but common, to see physicians hide their emotional responses to a patient's death. If not earlier then at least at the end of the day these emotions should be identified and given time. Not acknowledging one's emotional response to death carries a price. The price is often an inability to express emotion in other parts of one's life.

As the end of life, death is sad. Even when it is expected or finally arrives at the end of long period of sickness, death represents a loss to loved ones. Though families may be relieved that an ordeal has ended, the very finality of death has a great impact. It is sad that the person is no longer a part of one's life. For physicians, a patient's death often also represents a statement about their work and the care they provided, and presents an opportunity to rethink decisions or weigh outcomes of one's work. When the goal is to extend life, death is a disappointment, or worse; a failure of the physician's efforts.

As such it may provoke anger, frustration, or guilt. Almost by their nature, physicians criticize and judge their work. Even when death is anticipated, physicians second guess their actions and rethink treatments and their impact on the quality of the person's death. Ultimately, as a physician, one needs to process the death and feelings about it in order to learn and move on.

When the patient was a friend or someone the physician had true affection for, death brings personal sadness. For some, deaths recall other deaths or previous losses or failures and the grief is complex. In the absence of a personal connection, physicians witness the sadness of the patient's family and friends.

The first step in coping with these emotions is to 'name' them. Telling someone else or oneself out loud that this is sad, unfair, or disappointing makes it possible for one to respond to the emotion. Importantly, however, the response should often just be to feel the emotion. Like many life events, the finality of death does not permit negotiation or manipulation. One feels death's finality and death's sadness. Death and sadness are a part of the drama lived by physicians who care for the seriously ill. Even without a support network to help them cope with patients' deaths, simply regarding the impact of the death and their emotions is a coping mechanism for doctors. Identifying the source of one's feelings may be more complex, though it might take time and require reflection or counselling.

'Bad' and 'good' deaths

Many clinicians, having witnessed deaths that occur in various settings and ways, develop an opinion of what a 'good death' should be. Although the definition varies, a good death might be one that occurs with enough time to allow the individual and their family to prepare, to resolve issues, to say goodbye, and to accept their mortality. A stereotyped good death might occur in certain environments; usually not the hospital, not sterile – a place that is peaceful, with lovely music, soft light, and possibly even in the person's own home. In reality, such deaths are probably rare.

The deaths of some HF patients might occur as described above, though many instead are quite different. People often die as they live or according to beliefs their physician does not share. The 'beautiful music–soft light' death is not right for all. Some choose to not prepare for death. Many people die as physicians are trying to save their lives. When the patient dies in the midst of aggressive life-prolonging efforts sometimes a 'good' death is one that occurs despite having done all that medically was possible. The attempted rescue dictates that the patient be in the hospital, often in the intensive care unit. When unplanned or unanticipated, death may only be allowed after attempts at technological intervention, surgery, or cardiopulmonary resuscitation. Death may be accompanied by short or longer periods of unconsciousness, delirium, coma, or unresponsiveness. Or death may be associated with progressive multi-organ system loss with decline in critical bodily function in the presence of pain or even suffering. Such deaths can seem to rob patients and their families of a chance to say goodbye. They may seem cruel or even gruesome. Death will happen; it should come off well. Planning for the death in order to ensure that it is as smooth and humane as possible is an appropriate medical act that requires forethought.

Ultimately what matters is how the patient and their family judge the death. Regardless of the context and course to death, physicians need to acknowledge the loss it creates for the family. At best, death should occur with at least enough notice while the patient is cognitively intact to have some meaningful interaction with their family. Physicians should provide this notice. When the patient hopes not to die, the physician can say 'I also hope you survive this event. We'll do the best we can to help you live longer, but this is an opportunity to say and do what is important should you die despite our efforts.'.

In reality, the aggressive effort to postpone death cannot possibly always be successful, though its failure still sometimes shocks both physicians and the family. Some patients or families will not want to acknowledge the likelihood of dying, and for them the shock of death is greater. Coping with patients who die in the midst of efforts to save them is easier when one knows that the patient and family wished to try to prolong life. Caring for someone whose dying is characterized by long illness and progressive loss of function, independence, and the life that once was while providing yet another medical intervention is more difficult. In the multiple roles of expert, guide, or advisor, doctors can only try to do both what the patient and family prefer and what he or she thinks they can best achieve. Physicians must constantly learn how to make available the things they consider important and move constructively beyond their disappointment when they do not succeed. Physicians must accept their foibles and also accept that the needs they must try to meet are those of the patient and family.

'Closing the circle'

In *How We Die*, Sherwin Nuland wrote 'dying is for the dying and those who love them'.[3] Death ultimately is a life experience for the individual and their loved ones. Regardless of how medically involved the death, a physician's relationship with the patient, and most often with the family, ends with the patient's death. When they grieve the death, the physician's grief is different and separate from the family's grief. Acknowledging the relationship and marking its end is an important element of coping.

Finding a way to mark and acknowledge the end of the relationship is a fundamental coping strategy for physicians who regularly care for the dying. Some relationships with patients grow and develop over time, and some of these are characterized by real affection for the patient and their family on the part of the physician. Some physicians will also know a patient or their family as a friend prior to becoming their physician. The relationship that ends with death in these cases involves a greater emotional cost for physicians than a relationship characterized by brevity or distance. Bringing closure to the relationship, 'closing the circle' of the doctor–patient relationship, requires a deliberate act. At times, the physician can visit the dead, by pronouncing their death or viewing their body prior to a funeral. More often a busy life does not allow time for this and the physician must mentally say goodbye. Sometimes the act of signing the death certificate signifies the finality of the relationship. The end can be ritualized by calling or writing a note to the family. It is important to tell them good things about the patient, that their role in helping provide medical care was valued, and that the family did a good job as family or caregiver. Not surprisingly, families look for and value this acknowledgement from physicians. Family members often keep and refer repeatedly to these simple notes. A call to the family after a death allows one to solicit questions they harbor; these questions are sometimes surprising, often about an event prior to death of which the physician was unaware. A note or call to the family permits the physician to name their own emotional response; this act of telling the family that one was saddened, disappointed, or surprised by the death is a step in coping with death.

Conclusions

Caring for patients with HF who are seriously ill exposes physicians repeatedly to their patients' deaths. As a result clinicians must be honest with themselves and their patients about the reality of death. Emotions that surface at the time of death are directed by the nature of the physician's relationship with the patient and family, the goals set for their care, the context of the death, and one's prior losses. Physicians are obliged to witness the sadness at the end of a life, and mark the end of the relationship with the patient and their family. Coping with disappointment, frustration, or guilt or critically rethinking care may be inherent to the role of a physician. Death is final and very real. Acknowledging and reflecting on emotions associated with a patient's death are part of the drama and add to the passion experienced in caring for the seriously ill.

References

1. Whippen DA, Canellos GP (1991). Burnout syndrome in the practice of clinical oncology: results of a random survey of 1000 oncologists. *J Clin Oncol* **9**: 1916–20.
2. Cassell EJ (1982). The nature of suffering and the goals of medicine. *New Engl J Med* **306**: 630–45.
3. Nuland, S (1994). *How We Die: Reflections on Life's Final Chapter.* New York: Alfred A. Knopf.

Index